THE PROMISE OF ADOLESCENCE
Realizing Opportunity for All Youth

Committee on the Neurobiological and Socio-behavioral Science of
Adolescent Development and Its Applications

Richard J. Bonnie and Emily P. Backes, *Editors*

Board on Children, Youth, and Families

Division of Behavioral and Social Sciences and Education

Health and Medicine Division

A Consensus Study Report of

The National Academies of
SCIENCES · ENGINEERING · MEDICINE

THE NATIONAL ACADEMIES PRESS
Washington, DC
www.nap.edu

THE NATIONAL ACADEMIES PRESS   500 Fifth Street, NW   Washington, DC 20001

This activity was supported by contracts between the National Academy of Sciences and the Bezos Family Foundation (unnumbered), the National Public Education Support Fund (unnumbered), the Robert Wood Johnson Foundation (#75005), and the Seattle Foundation (unnumbered), which was supported by the Annie E. Casey Foundation, the Chan Zuckerberg Initiative, the Conrad N. Hilton Foundation, the Ford Foundation, and the Raikes Foundation. Any opinions, findings, conclusions, or recommendations expressed in this publication do not necessarily reflect the views of any organization or agency that provided support for the project.

International Standard Book Number-13: 978-0-309-49008-5
International Standard Book Number-10: 0-309-49008-1
Library of Congress Control Number: 2019945550
Digital Object Identifier: https://doi.org/10.17226/25388

Additional copies of this publication are available for sale from the National Academies Press, 500 Fifth Street, NW, Keck 360, Washington, DC 20001; (800) 624-6242 or (202) 334-3313; http://www.nap.edu.

Suggested citation: National Academies of Sciences, Engineering, and Medicine. (2019). *The Promise of Adolescence: Realizing Opportunity for All Youth*. Washington, DC: The National Academies Press. doi: https://doi.org/10.17226/25388.

The National Academies of
SCIENCES · ENGINEERING · MEDICINE

The **National Academy of Sciences** was established in 1863 by an Act of Congress, signed by President Lincoln, as a private, nongovernmental institution to advise the nation on issues related to science and technology. Members are elected by their peers for outstanding contributions to research. Dr. Marcia McNutt is president.

The **National Academy of Engineering** was established in 1964 under the charter of the National Academy of Sciences to bring the practices of engineering to advising the nation. Members are elected by their peers for extraordinary contributions to engineering. Dr. C. D. Mote, Jr., is president.

The **National Academy of Medicine** (formerly the Institute of Medicine) was established in 1970 under the charter of the National Academy of Sciences to advise the nation on medical and health issues. Members are elected by their peers for distinguished contributions to medicine and health. Dr. Victor J. Dzau is president.

The three Academies work together as the **National Academies of Sciences, Engineering, and Medicine** to provide independent, objective analysis and advice to the nation and conduct other activities to solve complex problems and inform public policy decisions. The National Academies also encourage education and research, recognize outstanding contributions to knowledge, and increase public understanding in matters of science, engineering, and medicine.

Learn more about the **National Academies of Sciences, Engineering, and Medicine** at www.nationalacademies.org.

The National Academies of
SCIENCES · ENGINEERING · MEDICINE

Consensus Study Reports published by the National Academies of Sciences, Engineering, and Medicine document the evidence-based consensus on the study's statement of task by an authoring committee of experts. Reports typically include findings, conclusions, and recommendations based on information gathered by the committee and the committee's deliberations. Each report has been subjected to a rigorous and independent peer-review process and it represents the position of the National Academies on the statement of task.

Proceedings published by the National Academies of Sciences, Engineering, and Medicine chronicle the presentations and discussions at a workshop, symposium, or other event convened by the National Academies. The statements and opinions contained in proceedings are those of the participants and are not endorsed by other participants, the planning committee, or the National Academies.

For information about other products and activities of the National Academies, please visit www.nationalacademies.org/about/whatwedo.

Title: Only Skin Deep

Artist: Angela Casarez (Fort Worth, TX)

Artist age: 19

Artist statement:
This collage of different facial features and anatomy illustrates the many dimensions of global health disparities that include race, ethnicity, socioeconomic status, and geography. It is critically important for both policy makers and health care providers to identify the many facets of disparities so that solutions address health security for a variety of different circumstances and lifestyles. Efforts to eliminate disparities and increase equity must be part of a broader effort to transform health care and improve the quality and breadth of care delivered to individual patients—no matter what piece of this collage they may identify with. The strongest and most evident point this piece illustrates is simply that we are all human. Yet ironically, although beneath our skin and our socioeconomic positions, we all share the same anatomy, modern medicine is not practiced with such certainty and consistency. With that, I and my piece put forth that a world in which everyone has an equal chance to be healthy, safe, and happy, is one in which health care is as undeniable as the fact that any and every human possesses a zygomaticus major to smile.

This artwork was submitted as a part of the National Academy of Medicine's Young Leaders Visualize Health Equity nationwide call for art. This call for art encouraged young people between the ages of 5 and 26 to use art to explore how the social determinants of health play a role in shaping their lives and their communities, and what it might look and feel like to one day live in a world where everyone has the same chance to be healthy, safe, and happy. More information on this project can be found at nam.edu/youngleaders.

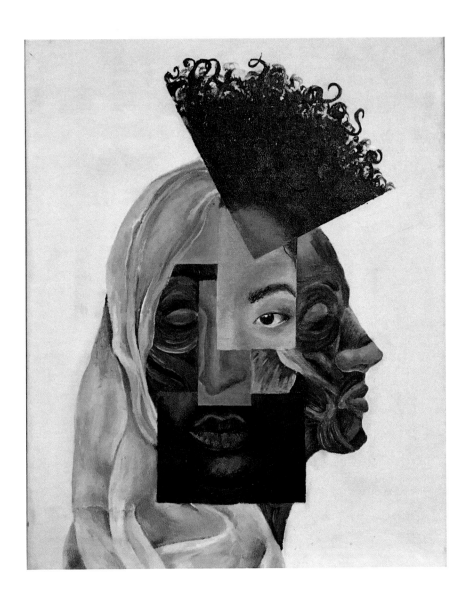

Preface

Our nation's youth hold the key to our future well-being. Investing generously in them will create a "more perfect union." That is the central message of this consensus report on the "promise of adolescence" sponsored by the Funders for Adolescent Science Translation, a consortium of foundations that came together with the aim of using science to produce more equitable and positive life outcomes for youth. This report takes its place in a sequence of National Academies of Sciences, Engineering, and Medicine reports exploring the science of child and adolescent development that began with *From Neurons to Neighborhoods*, the path-breaking Institute of Medicine study on the science of early childhood development published in 2000.

The science of adolescent development explores the neurobiological and socio-behavioral processes that underlie the unique and fascinating process of maturation. The 21st century has featured extraordinary advances in knowledge about the unique developmental processes—and challenges—of adolescence as well as the important role of this developmental period in shaping the trajectory of the life course. Our committee's assignment was to synthesize these exciting advances in the science of adolescent development and draw out their implications for the social systems charged with helping all adolescents flourish.

This committee's study is a companion to a parallel study funded by the Robert Wood Johnson Foundation exploring the neurobiological and socio-behavioral sciences' findings concerning childhood development from the prenatal period through early childhood. Together, these two reports consolidate the extraordinary advances in the science of human development in order to inform child- and youth-serving institutions and policy makers. In this respect, they also complement a 2014 Health Resources and Services Administration-funded study focused on improving the safety and well-being of young adults.

Studying adolescents provides a rich opportunity for exploring the developing mind. For one thing, the fascinating process of evolving self-awareness—indeed, a preoccupation with self—is heightened during adolescence and our individual memories of that experience tend to be especially vivid. In addition, our sense of identity—of who we are and who we want to be—is taking shape during adolescence. We all tend to remember these experiences many years later.

As the report explains, the adolescent brain undergoes a remarkable transformation between puberty and the mid-20s that underpins amazing advances in learning and creativity. The plasticity of the adolescent brain also provides the potential for resilient responses to childhood trauma and distress. Personal experience teaches us, of course, that the excitement and emotional preoccupations of adolescence can yield both opportunity and risk. As a society, we bear a collective obligation to unleash the creativity of the adolescent brain while cushioning adolescents from experiences that could endanger their future well-being.

Another central theme of this report, signified by its subtitle, is that our nation must ensure that the "promise of adolescence" is realized for *all* adolescents. As the report shows, millions of adolescents are being left behind because they have lacked equal opportunity to succeed. Disparities in developmental outcomes for disadvantaged youth are attributable to lack of adequate resources and supports in their families and in the neighborhoods where they live, as well as the effects of bias and discrimination. The committee has concluded that we have the knowledge needed to reduce these disparities and close the opportunity gap. The committee has also expressed its collective view that these remedial measures *should* be taken because it is unjust (and contrary to the nation's collective self-interest) to allow these disparities to continue. We did so because this value judgment is implicit in our charge.

On behalf of the National Academies and its Board on Children, Youth and Families, I want to thank the member foundations of Funders for Adolescent Science Translation for sponsoring this important study. I am deeply grateful to Emily Backes and the National Academies staff for their extraordinary skill and diligence, and most of all, to my fellow members of the committee. It has been a pleasure to work with such talented colleagues on this interesting and important project. I look forward to working with them, as well as our sponsors, to disseminate the committee's findings and implement its recommendations for developmentally informed youth-serving systems.

I want to close with a personal observation. The Virginia Bar Association, to which I belong, devoted the plenary session of its annual meeting in 2019 to a panel discussion lamenting the incivility of discourse in our fractious society. As we discussed what our organization can and should do about it, I observed that our current state of polarization has emerged and deepened over several decades and that remedial efforts should focus on our young people, beginning in adolescence when they are learning how people differ from one another and as they are discovering (and shaping) their own identities. As parents and teachers, our obligation is to help them develop the desire, and the skill, to listen to each other and to respect differences in their beliefs and values. We need to invest in our youngsters to repair our weakened (and imperfect) union.

Richard J. Bonnie, *Chair*
Committee on the Neurobiolgoical and
Socio-behavioral Science of Adolescent
Development and Its Applications

Acknowledgments

This report would not have been possible without the contributions of many people. First, we thank the sponsors of this study: the Funders for Adolescent Science Translation, including the Annie E. Casey Foundation, the Bezos Family Foundation, the Chan Zuckerberg Initiative, the Ford Foundation, the Conrad N. Hilton Foundation, the Raikes Foundation, the Robert Wood Johnson Foundation, and the National Public Education Support Fund.

Special thanks go to the members of the study committee, who dedicated extensive time, thought, and energy to the project. Thanks are also due to Tammy Chang (University of Michigan, Ann Arbor) who contributed her time and expertise throughout the report process, as well as Natalie Slopen (University of Maryland, College Park), who served as a liaison between our study committee and the Committee on Applying Neurobiological and Socio-behavioral Sciences from Prenatal through Early Childhood Development: A Health Equity Approach. We also extend our gratitude to Nat Kendall-Taylor, Marisa Gerstein Pineau, and Daniel Busso from the Frameworks Institute for their insights on communicating about adolescence.

In addition to its own research and deliberations, the committee received input from several outside sources, whose willingness to share their perspectives and experiences was essential to the committee's work. We thank Linda Burton (Duke University), Tammy Fields (Palm Beach County Youth Services Department), Andrew J. Fuligni (University of California, Los Angeles), Seema Gajwani (Office of the Attorney General for the District of Columbia), Roberto G. Gonzales (Harvard School of Education), Phil Hammack (University of California, Santa Cruz), Cheri Hoffman

(U.S. Department of Health and Human Services), Diane Hughes (New York University), Allyson Mackey (University of Pennsylvania), Gloria Mark (University of California, Irvine), Steve Michael (Iowa Collaboration for Youth Development), Jacqueline Nesi (Brown University), Candice Odgers (Duke University), Uma Rao (University of California, Irvine), Russell Romeo (Barnard College), Robert Sainz (Economic and Workforce Development Department, City of Los Angeles), Kaveri Subrahmanyam (California State, Los Angeles), and Roderick J. Watts (University of New York).The committee also gathered information through two commissioned analyses. We thank Monica Kirkpatrick Johnson (Washington State University) for "Contemporary Adolescents: Understanding the Demographic, Social, and Economic Changes Shaping Adolescent Life" and the University of Michigan MyVoice team for "Contemporary Adolescents: Understanding the Lived Experiences of Today's Youth."

The committee was also able to elicit input from adolescents throughout the report process. We extend our gratitude to the thoughtful young people who graciously gave their time to inform our work: Zachary Caplan, Darius Craig, Tanya Gumbs, Shyara Hill, Marcus Jarvis, Carolin Larkin, Nyla Mpofu, Jocelyn Nolasco, and Ayanna Tucker. We were truly awed by their ability to speak their truth and their impassioned commitment to bettering society. Their insights were incredibly valuable.

This Consensus Study Report was reviewed in draft form by individuals chosen for their diverse perspectives and technical expertise. The purpose of this independent review is to provide candid and critical comments that will assist the National Academies of Sciences, Engineering, and Medicine in making each published report as sound as possible and to ensure that it meets the institutional standards for quality, objectivity, evidence, and responsiveness to the study charge. The review comments and draft manuscript remain confidential to protect the integrity of the deliberative process.

We thank the following individuals for their review of this report: Sarah M. Bagley, CATALYST Clinic, Boston University School of Medicine/Boston Medical Center; Robert Wm. Blum, Department of Population, Family and Reproductive Health, Urban Health Institute, Johns Hopkins University; Catherine Bradshaw, Curry School of Education and Human Development, University of Virginia; Jeanne Brooks-Gunn, Teachers College and College of Physicians and Surgeons, Columbia University; Cleopatra Cabuz, Technology and Partnerships (retired), Honeywell Safety and Productivity Solutions; Ron E. Dahl, Institute of Human Development, University of California, Berkeley; Amy Dworksy, Chapin Hall, The University of Chicago; Adriana Galván, Department of Psychology Brain Research Institute, University of California, Los Angeles; Jonathan Guryan, Institute for Policy Research, Northwestern University; Cheri Hoffman, Division of Children and Youth Policy, Office of the Assistant Secretary for Planning and Evaluation, U.S.

Department of Health and Human Services; Velma McBride Murry, Department of Human and Organizational Development, Vanderbilt University; Anne C. Peterson, Ford School, University of Michigan; Alex R. Piquero, School of Economic, Political and Policy Sciences, The University of Texas at Dallas; Ricki Price-Baugh, Director of Academic Achievement, Council of the Great City Schools.

Although the reviewers listed above provided many constructive comments and suggestions, they were not asked to endorse the conclusions or recommendations of this report nor did they see the final draft before its release. The review of this report was overseen by Rosemary Chalk, independent consultant, Bethesda, Maryland, and Antonia M. Villarruel, School of Nursing, University of Pennsylvania. They were responsible for making certain that an independent examination of this report was carried out in accordance with the standards of the National Academies and that all review comments were carefully considered. Responsibility for the final content rests entirely with the authoring committee and the National Academies.

The committee also wishes to extend its gratitude to the staff of the National Academies of Sciences, Engineering, and Medicine, in particular to Liz Townsend and Dara Shefska, who contributed research and writing assistance to the committee's work and played an important role in editing portions of the report. Mary Ghitelman provided key administrative and logistical support and made sure that committee meetings and report production ran efficiently and smoothly. Thanks are also due to fellows Stephanie Oh, who provided valuable research assistance in the report's early stages, and Katrina Ferrara, who made important contributions during the editing process. Throughout the project, Natacha Blain, director of the Board on Children, Youth, and Families, provided helpful oversight. The committee is also grateful to Anthony Bryant and Pamella Atayi for their financial and administrative assistance on the project. From the Division of Behavioral and Social Sciences and Education Office of Reports and Communication, we thank Kirsten Sampson Snyder, Yvonne Wise, and Douglas Sprunger, who shepherded the report through the review and production process and assisted with its communication and dissemination. We also thank Marc DeFrancis for his skillful editing.

We are grateful to our colleagues and collaborators in the Health and Medicine Division (HMD) and the National Academy of Medicine's Culture of Health Program. In particular, we would like to extend our thanks to HMD's Rose Marie Martinez, Amy Geller, Yami Negussie, and Sophie Yang for their wonderful collegiality and thoughtful input throughout the endeavor. Thanks are also due to National Academy of Medicine staff Charlee Alexander, Kyra Cappelucci, Ivory Clarke, and the entire Culture of Health Program team.

Finally, the committee wishes to thank our chair, Richard Bonnie, for his time, intellectual leadership, and devotion to this study. It was an honor to work with Richard, and this report is truly better for his commitment.

Emily P. Backes, *Study Director*
Committee on the Neurobiolgoical and
Socio-behavioral Science of Adolescent
Development and Its Applications

Contents

Summary

Adolescence—beginning with the onset of puberty and ending in the mid-20s—is a critical period of development during which key areas of the brain develop and mature. These changes in brain structure, function, and connectivity mark adolescence as a period of opportunity to discover new vistas, to form relationships with peers and adults, and to explore one's developing identity. It is also a period of resilience that can ameliorate childhood setbacks and set the stage for a thriving trajectory over the life course.

Because adolescents comprise nearly one-fourth of the entire U.S. population, the nation needs policies and practices that will better leverage these developmental opportunities to harness the promise of adolescence—rather than focusing myopically on containing its risks. The National Academies of Sciences, Engineering, and Medicine were asked to convene a committee of experts to examine the neurobiological and socio-behavioral science of adolescent development and to outline how this knowledge can be applied, both to promote adolescent well-being, resilience, and development and to rectify structural barriers and inequalities in opportunity, enabling all adolescents to flourish. The challenge for a caring society is to take maximum advantage of the developmental opportunities afforded by adolescence to forge positive trajectories into adulthood for all adolescents.

ADOLESCENT DEVELOPMENT

Puberty occurs over an extended period of a young person's life during which developmental changes result in the maturation of primary and

1

secondary sex characteristics and the acquisition of reproductive maturity. Pubertal development varies greatly from one individual to the next, and the age at which an adolescent matures depends on a combination of genetic and environmental influences, including early life experiences. Socially, pubertal maturation and its accompanying physical changes also affect how adolescents perceive themselves and how they are treated by others, and in this regard early pubertal timing has been shown to have challenging social consequences. Structural changes that disrupt the systemic factors that increase risk for early puberty (e.g., resource deprivation) as well as supportive relationships can mitigate the risks associated with early puberty and foster resilient outcomes.

Neurobiologically, throughout adolescence the connections within and between brain regions become stronger and more efficient, and unused connections are pruned away. Such developmental plasticity means adolescents' brains are adaptive; they become more specialized in response to environmental demands. The timing and location of these dynamic changes are also important. The onset of puberty brings about changes in the limbic region of the brain, resulting in greater sensitivity to rewards, threats, novelty, and peers. In contrast, it takes longer for the cortical region, which is implicated in cognitive control and self-regulation, to develop.

Consequently, adolescent brains are not simply "advanced" child brains or "immature" adult brains, but have evolved to meet the needs of this stage of life. Indeed, the temporal discrepancy in the specialization of and connections between brain regions makes adolescence unique. The developmental changes heighten sensitivity to rewards, willingness to take risks, and the salience of social status, propensities that are necessary for exploring new environments and building nonfamilial relationships. Adolescents must explore and take risks to build the cognitive, social, and emotional skills necessary for productivity in adulthood.

The increased cognitive abilities gained throughout adolescence also provide the capacity for other aspects of psychosocial development, such as developing identity and capacity for self-direction. An adolescent's identity is an emerging reflection of his or her values, beliefs, and aspirations, and it can be constructed and reconstructed over time and experience. Multiple factors, including family, culture, peers, and media, shape identity development, but young people are also active agents in the process. Ultimately, how adolescents' multifaceted identities are manifested—neurobiologically, behaviorally, or otherwise—and what role identity plays in their overall well-being greatly depends on their experiences in particular social contexts.

Adolescence is also marked by a growing capacity for self-direction. Over the course of adolescence, youth gain the cognitive skills needed to reflect on complex questions about their role in the world. This enables them to question the legitimacy and fairness of everyday experiences and of social institutions. Indeed, the social systems they must navigate—schools, employment, health care, justice—are complex, and navigating them often requires independent decision making. Such skills are important not only to support the transition to adulthood but also to make adolescence itself a period that fosters a propensity to contribute to others.

In summary, although adolescence is often thought of as a time of turmoil and risk for young people, it is more accurately viewed as a developmental period rich with opportunity for youth to learn and grow. Adolescence thus forms a critical bridge between childhood and adulthood and is a window of opportunity for positive, life-shaping development.

HOW ENVIRONMENT "GETS UNDER THE SKIN": THE CONTINUOUS INTERPLAY BETWEEN BIOLOGY AND ENVIRONMENT

While the malleable brains of adolescents are adaptable to learning and innovation, they are also vulnerable to toxic exposures. The emerging science of epigenetics[1] focuses our attention on the ongoing plasticity of the brain and the reciprocal influences of the brain, body, and environment. Contrary to the common understanding that the effects of heredity are immutable and direct, contemporary studies of gene-environment interaction and epigenetics show that the way heredity is expressed in behavior depends significantly on environmental influences. The epigenetic approach also embraces a "trajectory" model of the life course: the trajectory of an individual's life may be changed, negatively or positively, at each life stage. Protective environmental factors support positive or flourishing trajectories, while adverse experiences may lead to at-risk or poor trajectories. The future condition of the brain and body will be affected by events that have changed the trajectory in the past, and interventions undertaken in the present have the potential to remediate past developmental challenges.

Adolescents' heightened sensitivity and responsiveness to environmental influences also implies "resilience," meaning adolescents have the opportunity to develop neurobiological adaptations and behaviors that leave them better equipped to handle adversities that emerge throughout the life course. Thus, investments in programs and interventions that capitalize on brain plasticity during adolescence can promote beneficial changes in developmental trajectories for youth who may have faced adverse experiences earlier in life or are facing them now and prevent future challenges and risks.

---

[1] Epigenetics studies the seamless and ongoing interaction between genes and the environment, with particular interest in cataloging the numerous environmental mechanisms comprising the nongenetic influences of gene expression.

INEQUITY AND ADOLESCENCE

The promise of adolescence can be severely curtailed by economic, social, and structural disadvantage and, in all too many cases, by racism, bias, and discrimination. These potent societal determinants shape adolescents' life-course trajectories in multiple ways, not only by reducing access to the opportunities, services, and supports enjoyed by more privileged youth but also by exposing less privileged youth to excess risks, stresses, and demands. These excess pressures "get under the skin" and adversely affect the brain and body during this critical developmental period.

Striking differences in opportunity are associated with striking differences in outcomes—in health, safety, well-being, and educational and occupational attainment—and in trajectories over the life course. Educational achievement, as measured by reading and math proficiency, high school graduation rates, and college completion, varies by race and ethnicity, socioeconomic status, and gender, with White and higher-income youth consistently experiencing better outcomes than other groups. Disparities also exist in the occurrence and impact of chronic health conditions (by socioeconomic status) and mortality (by race and ethnicity, socioeconomic status, and gender), due in part to exposure to violence. Moreover, there is consistent evidence that at all ages, LGBT youth are at higher risk of poor mental health and suicide than their heterosexual and cis-gender peers. Among adolescents, poor and Black youth are dramatically overrepresented in foster care. And in the juvenile justice system, Black youth are detained at a rate six times higher than White youth and three times higher than Latinx youth. (See Chapter 4.)

These disparities are often compounded for the youth experiencing them because they cut across the multiple systems with which they interact, and deficiencies in one area negatively affect outcomes in others. For example, poor health reduces educational attainment, while involvement in child protective services negatively affects juvenile justice outcomes. Together, these disparities grow as youth age and result in large disparities in their adult outcomes, such as poorer rates of employment and earnings, increased likelihood of criminal justice involvement, and poorer health and well-being.

However, disparities in adolescent outcomes are not immutable: they are responsive to changes in underlying conditions, and adolescents themselves show resilience and demonstrate strengths and assets that may be utilized to overcome inequities. Recent trends show that, in fact, adolescent well-being has improved over time, as illustrated by the steady decline in teen childbearing rates since 1990, which have been accompanied by significant declines in disparities by race and ethnicity.

Because a full understanding of the sources of these outcome disparities is necessary to formulate effective strategies for reducing them, we categorize the possible sources of these disparities as follows: (1) differences in family wealth and income, combined with living in neighborhoods segregated by income and race, (2) differences in institutional responses to adolescents by schools, the health system, the justice system, or the welfare system, and (3) prejudicial or discriminatory attitudes or behavior on the part of the adults or peers who interact with adolescents on a regular basis. Of course, other possible sources of outcome disparities exist, but here we point to some of the specific, quantifiable sources that have been captured empirically.

More than 9 million children and youth (ages 0 to 18) in the United States live in households with incomes below the poverty level, and rates of child poverty are highest for Black, Latinx, and American Indian and Alaska Native youth. For adolescents, growing up in poverty is associated with worse physical and mental health, as well as higher prevalence of risky behaviors and delinquency. The stagnation of wages for those in the bottom half of the income distribution over the past 50 years has reduced the resources available to lower-income families for investment in their children. Like income, wealth accumulation affects the resources families have available for investing in the next generation, especially for investments in higher education. Racial differences in wealth are three times greater than racial differences or gaps in income, with the average White household in 2010 having nearly six times the wealth of the average Black household (see Chapter 4).

In addition, because of the relatively high rates of residential segregation in the United States, adolescents from poor or minority families are much more likely than others to live in poor and segregated neighborhoods. Low-income neighborhoods, in turn, are more likely than other neighborhoods to be lacking in access to health care, youth-oriented organizations, and learning centers, and they are also more likely to be located near polluting factors, to have high levels of violence and low levels of safety, and to have low-quality housing. Moreover, poor families and minority families experience considerably more stress than others. As a result, not only are poor families less able to invest financially in their children, but also their nonfinancial investments, such as the amount and quality of their caregiving, are also affected by family disadvantage.

This disparity in family resources is often compounded by the institutions and systems with which youth interact. Segregation of schools by family income is the single most predictive factor of academic achievement gaps by race and income. The increasing income segregation of U.S. schools, compounded by rising income inequality, has most likely prevented society from achieving the full benefit of the significant, recent gains in financial parity across schools, suggesting that children from disadvantaged households likely need *more* resources (not equal resources) if society is to reduce disparities in educational outcomes. School segregation is driven largely by neighborhood segregation and, as such, the policy or institutional response to the increasing segregation of U.S. schools largely lies in housing policy, but tightness in the housing market and housing discrimination reduce the likelihood that low-income families can move to low-poverty neighborhoods. Moreover, lack of health care access and low health care quality, as well as laws and policies that drive crossover from involvement with the child welfare system into involvement in the juvenile justice system, compound disadvantage and contribute to disparities in opportunity.

A third source of disparities in adolescent outcomes derives from the explicit and implicit (or unconscious) prejudice and bias that individuals hold against groups defined by race, ethnicity, gender, LGBTQ identity, ability status, and so on. The experience of being targeted by such bias can include both singular significant interactions as well as a series of less obvious but frequent events, referred to as micro-aggressions. At a time when adolescents are especially sensitive to the attitudes and behaviors of adult members of the community, evidence suggests that educators, health professionals, child welfare system actors, and justice system actors exhibit behaviors that lead to disparate treatment of youth by race, gender, LGBTQ identity, and ability status. When aggregated in an institutional context, these biases can result in disparate outcomes for the affected groups.

An effective strategy, or set of strategies, to reduce inequities needs to address the main sources of these disparities. The committee recognizes some promising policies and programs that attempt to tackle these disparities in opportunity, including (1) policies and programs to reduce disparities in income, wealth, and neighborhood resources, such as the Supplemental Nutrition Assistance Program and the Earned Income Tax Credit; (2) trauma-informed approaches preparing adults serving youth to address differential exposure to violence and trauma among youth; and (3) emerging tools, such as predictive analytics, to erase or counteract bias in decision making by system-level actors.

With any strategy, greater coordination is needed across the multiple systems responsible for adolescents: the school system, health care system, and juvenile justice and child protection systems. Parity in public system funding is a first step, but it will not be sufficient to significantly reduce disparities. To significantly reduce or eliminate disparities, disadvantaged youth will likely require disproportionate funding.

Although progress may not be immediate, there is substantial reason for optimism. Progress has already been made in reducing disparities in adolescent outcomes, especially in the areas of education, health, and teen pregnancy. With the notable exception of the juvenile justice system, the evidence suggests that as overall adolescent health and well-being improve, disparities fall. These trends underscore the hope that with additional effort and a comprehensive approach, further reductions in outcome disparities among adolescents are indeed attainable.

USING DEVELOPMENTAL KNOWLEDGE TO ASSURE OPPORTUNITY FOR ALL YOUTH

The committee's charge requested recommendations regarding ways by which youth-serving systems—education, health, child welfare, and justice—can apply accelerating knowledge about adolescent development (and particularly knowledge from the neurobiological and socio-behavioral sciences) to their own work. Of course, investing in youth also requires investing in the adult caregivers who support them, as supportive familial, caregiver, and adult relationships play a significant role in fostering positive outcomes for adolescents. Such investments need to be multilevel and multisectoral; interventions to change parenting behavior may be futile if the systems themselves are not attuned to the pressing economic needs of parents.

The following sections briefly identify the major domains of the committee's recommendations for each of the four youth-serving systems designated in the committee's charge: education, health, child welfare, and justice. Detailed recommendations for specific actors and actions can be found in Chapters 6 through 9.

Recommendations for the Education System

Our enriched understanding of adolescence, together with major changes in the labor market, require rethinking and modernizing a public school system that was largely designed for early 20th century life. As the economy has changed over the past several decades, the skills and dispositions required to succeed in the current and future job market are increasingly interpersonal and socio-emotional. Relatedly, today's increasingly knowledge-based economy requires a mindset of learning, malleability, and expectation for growth and improvement.

When young people reach adolescence, they vary widely in their academic skills and needs and in their future career aspirations. The secondary school system of the future must meet teens "where they are" and offer differentiated and responsive academic opportunities, including individualized instruction, tutoring, tracking, and credentialing. Growing recognition of the importance of skills other than reading, writing, and arithmetic for both personal fulfillment and success in modern life requires schools to broaden their mission to incorporate the teaching of nonacademic skills such as decision making, practical knowledge, and adaptability. The growing diversity of U.S. adolescents also requires schools to better recognize adolescents' integrated needs, become more culturally sensitive, and become adept at assisting youth with issues related to identity and social competence. Moreover, recognizing the importance of caregivers in adolescents' lives, the education system will need to provide additional supports for adolescents and their families to assist them in navigating an increasingly complex education sector.

In short, secondary schools should be modernized to reflect the preparation, knowledge, and skills that youth need for the 21st century and rectify longstanding and persistent disparities in resources across the demographic backgrounds of their students. This committee's recommendations for transforming secondary education for the 21st century highlight six key areas to implement such change:

RECOMMENDATION 6-1: Rectify disparities in resources for least-advantaged schools and students.

RECOMMENDATION 6-2: Design purposeful but flexible pathways through education.

RECOMMENDATION 6-3: Teach practical knowledge and non-academic skills, such as decision making, adaptability, and socio-emotional competence.

RECOMMENDATION 6-4: Protect the overall health and well-being of each student.

RECOMMENDATION 6-5: Foster culturally sensitive learning environments.

RECOMMENDATION 6-6: Help adolescents and families navigate the education sector.

Recommendations for the Health System

Access to appropriate health care services is important to ensure adolescents' well-being both today and for a lifetime. Access is particularly important while they are developing habits that will affect their long-term health, such as diet, exercise, and substance use. Yet adolescents face a variety of barriers to accessing health care, which contributes to longstanding disparities in their use of such care that are measurable by race and ethnicity, LGBTQ status, ability status, and socioeconomic status. While limited access to health care has been most frequently associated with financial barriers, adolescents face the additional challenge that they are generally inexperienced in navigating the health care system independently, concerned that their health needs and services remain confidential, and more likely than adults to engage in risk-taking behaviors that could have both short- and long-term effects on their health.

Developmentally appropriate changes to provider practices and innovative care delivery systems can help adolescents become more engaged with their care and achieve better outcomes. To ensure the health and well-being of all adolescents, health systems should offer integrated, comprehensive health services that prepare youth for the distinct physical, cognitive, and social changes that take place during adolescence, prepare them to navigate the health system independently, and provide services that are culturally informed and attentive to the needs of all youth.

A systemic approach to prioritizing the health and well-being of adolescents is needed on a national level, including clear goals and priorities to help mobilize both the public and private sectors to improve adolescent health. The committee's recommendations draw on neurobiological and socio-behavioral research to identify more effective health policy, programs, and practices with five key aims:

RECOMMENDATION 7-1: Strengthen the financing of health care services for adolescents, including insurance coverage for uninsured or under-insured populations.

RECOMMENDATION 7-2: Improve access to comprehensive, integrated, coordinated health services for adolescents.

RECOMMENDATION 7-3: Increase access to behavioral health care and treatment services.

RECOMMENDATION 7-4: Improve the training and distribution and increase the number of adolescent health care providers.

RECOMMENDATION 7-5: Improve federal and state data collection on adolescent health and well-being, and conduct adolescent-specific health services research and disseminate the findings.

Recommendations for the Child Welfare System

The purpose of the child welfare system is to protect children at risk of abuse or neglect by their parents or guardians (or whomever the state defines as a perpetrator). Historically and up to the present day, two defining aspects of the child welfare system have been its focus on young children and its attention to preventing serious physical abuse. These foci are coupled with a funding scheme that prioritizes funding for out-of-home placement. As a result, the system is under-resourced in providing support services to *prevent* out-of-home placement and in providing support to families, particularly families with adolescents. This approach is ill-suited to helping adolescents in the child welfare system flourish, given their more advanced decision-making skills, their need for a balance of autonomy and healthy relationships, and their ability to use technology to seek solutions, relative to younger children. In addition, courts with jurisdiction over adolescents as a result of acting-out behaviors for status offenses have insufficient resources to address the underlying and presenting problems of these youth and their families.

Also of great concern are disparities within the child welfare system: poor children and children of color are disproportionately referred to the child welfare system. In general, both disproportionate need and differential treatment by community members and the child welfare system play important roles in explaining these disparities. Community reporters are more likely to report children of color to child welfare authorities, which suggests discriminatory reporting and increased surveillance for maltreatment in communities of color. A second important source of systemic disparity in treatment is that families of color are offered fewer in-home services that might prevent the placement of a child or adolescent in foster care. As a result, children of color are both more likely to be removed from a home and more likely to remain in foster placements longer without a permanent resolution.

Over the past two decades, Congress has gradually enacted statutory changes that better align the child welfare system with the developmental assets and challenges that adolescents face, including focusing attention on family reunification, prioritizing placement with relatives over strangers, and providing services for those adolescents aging out of foster care. These federal statutory changes are significant advances, but additional efforts are needed to ensure that all adolescents involved with the child welfare system have the opportunity to flourish. The committee's recommendations center on providing services and supports for adolescents that differ from those provided to their younger counterparts within the child welfare system, focusing on adolescents' need to be involved as partners in decisions affecting their housing, health and mental health, and education. The committee's six key areas of recommendation are

RECOMMENDATION 8-1: Reduce racial/ethnic disparities in child welfare system involvement.

RECOMMENDATION 8-2: Promote broad uptake by the states of federal programs that promote resilience and positive outcomes for adolescents involved in the child welfare system.

RECOMMENDATION 8-3: Provide services to adolescents and their families in the child welfare system that are developmentally informed at the individual, program, and system levels.

RECOMMENDATION 8-4: Conduct research that reflects all types and ages of adolescents in the child welfare system.

RECOMMENDATION 8-5: Foster greater collaboration between the child welfare, juvenile justice, education, and health systems.

RECOMMENDATION 8-6: Provide developmentally appropriate services for adolescents who engage in noncriminal misconduct without justice-system involvement.

Recommendations for the Justice System

Over the past 15 years, advances in the science of adolescent development have had a substantial impact on juvenile justice reform and have also focused attention on the potential value of developmentally appropriate practices for older adolescents involved in the criminal justice system. Findings regarding adolescent brain development have highlighted the diminished culpability of adolescent offenders and their potential responsiveness to preventive interventions based on evidence-based risk- and needs-assessments.

While it is clear that a developmental approach to the juvenile justice system has been widely embraced by reformers and is having a discernible impact on law and practice in many states, progress across the country is uneven, and sustained effort and attention are needed to accelerate advances and to prevent an erosion of gains. Priority areas for reform within the juvenile justice system include the need for increased family engagement and greater attention to procedural fairness, including fairness in interactions with the police, legal representation for youth, and reduced use of juvenile fines and fees. Another reform priority is reducing the unwarranted harm to juveniles' future well-being caused by justice-system involvement, including public disclosure of justice-system records, listing on sex offender registries, and solitary confinement.

Similar reform efforts recognizing the developmental needs of older adolescents and young adults are emerging within the criminal justice system, including reducing automatic transfers of juveniles to criminal courts based only on the charged offense, and creating developmentally informed correctional programs for young offenders. These efforts should be guided by the science of adolescent development and the core principles of a developmental approach.

Despite decades of attention under federal law, racial/ethnic disparities in police, prosecutorial, and judicial decision making in the juvenile justice and criminal justice systems persist, and in some contexts they are actually increasing. While the literature reflects continuing uncertainty about the relative contribution of differential offending, differential enforcement, and differential judicial processing, it is clear that the lack of progress in reducing disparities within the justice system has led to harmful outcomes for minority and other affected youth.

Previous National Academies' reports on juvenile justice outlined recommendations for needed reforms to ensure that the juvenile justice system accounts for and attends to the developmental needs of youth. This committee reaffirms those recommendations, and offers several additional recommendations in five key areas:

RECOMMENDATION 9-1: Reduce disparities based on race, ethnicity, gender, ability status, and sexual orientation or gender identity and expression among adolescents involved in the justice system.

RECOMMENDATION 9-2: Ensure that youth maintain supportive relationships while involved in the justice system and receive appropriate guidance and counsel from legal professionals and caregivers.

RECOMMENDATION 9-3: Implement policies that aim to reduce harm to justice-involved youth in accordance with knowledge from developmental science.

RECOMMENDATION 9-4: Implement developmentally appropriate and fair policies and practices for adolescents involved in the criminal justice system.

RECOMMENDATION 9-5: For those youth in the custody of the justice system, ensure that policies and practices are implemented to prioritize the health and educational needs of adolescents and avoid causing harm.

CONCLUSION

Adolescence, spanning the years from the onset of puberty to adulthood, is a formative period when changes in cognition, affect, and interpersonal behavior occur alongside the most extensive neurobiological transitions since infancy, especially with respect to pubertal and brain development. These changes make it clear that adolescent brains are not best understood as simply "advanced" child brains or "immature" adult brains. Instead they have evolved to meet the developmental needs of humans at this stage of life. Collectively, the pubertal, neurobiological, cognitive, and psychosocial changes occurring during adolescence mark this as a period of great opportunity for adolescents to flourish and thrive.

However, in the United States today many families lack adequate resources and neighborhood supports, leaving many adolescents at significant disadvantage during this critical period of development. To fail to address the sources of these disparities is to waste human capital: lower worker productivity, lost wages and employment, worse health and mental health, increased criminal justice involvement, and a drain on public support. These outcomes would reduce economic growth and exacerbate rising income inequality. Creating positive impact by improving opportunities for adolescents not only improves trajectories relevant to multiple outcomes, but also, by making use of high-impact, cost-effective interventions, it can counteract the effects of childhood stresses and deprivations and prevent negative outcomes in adulthood.

These realities also highlight a compelling scientific challenge. To understand how we can help all adolescents flourish, we need to connect two bodies of research: the deepened understanding of developmental processes needs to also encompass a richer understanding of the impact of the social environment. Achieving this will require a major commitment by our research establishment. Future research investments in adolescence should support efforts that (1) deepen our knowledge of the processes of adolescent development, (2) examine the socio-environmental contexts that offer opportunities for flourishing, and (3) understand and combat inequities that curtail the promise of adolescence for all youth.

Our society has a collective responsibility to build systems that support and promote positive adolescent development. These systems should reflect a rich understanding of the developmental needs of adolescents and a specific recognition of adolescence as a time of great opportunity to promote learning and discovery and to remediate past developmental challenges. Until society embraces this responsibility, the promise of adolescence will remain unfulfilled for millions of youth.

Part I:
Adolescence as a Period of Opportunity

1

Introduction

Although often thought of as an age span, such as the second decade of life or "the teenage years," adolescence is the distinct period of bio-developmental change in a person's life that bridges childhood and adulthood. It denotes a set of developmental transitions beginning with the onset of puberty[1] and ending during the mid-20s, characterized by maturation of the body, intensification of capacity for learning, and emergence of personal identity. From a social vantage point, the developmental tasks of adolescence include taking responsibility for oneself and forming relationships with others. This period of developmental maturation is underpinned by unique changes in brain structure and function.

All these transitions mark adolescence as a period of both opportunity and risk (see Chapter 2). Parents (or parent surrogates)[2] typically bear primary responsibility as caretakers of their children, but the whole society

---

[1] The average child in the United States experiences the onset of puberty between the age of 8 and 10 years. The onset of puberty may be defined by two biological components, adrenarche and gonadarche. Adrenarche, which refers to the maturation of the hypothalamic-pituitary-adrenal (HPA) axis typically begins in late childhood, but levels of adrenarchal hormones continue to rise throughout adolescence (Blakemore et al., 2010). Gonadarche typically begins in early adolescence, at approximately ages 9 to 11, and involves the reactivation of the hypothalamic-pituitary-gonadal (HPG) axis. See Chapter 2 for a full discussion of adolescent development and puberty.

[2] In this report, the committee uses the term "parents" to broadly encompass those adults in adolescents' lives who are their primary caretaker. For some young people, the primary caretaker is a grandparent, aunt or uncle, step-parent, or foster parent, among others.

shares the obligation to help adolescents achieve their full potential in adulthood (Casey et al., 2010; Galván, 2014; Spear, 2010).

In the past, it was thought that the brain was entirely developed before a person entered adolescence and that cognitive functions were fully mature by then. But it is now widely understood that key areas of the brain and its circuitry continue maturing from the onset of puberty and well into an individual's mid-20s (Giedd et al., 1999; Lenroot and Giedd, 2006). This demarcates adolescence as a sensitive period of neurodevelopment that is especially affected by the environment, including physical factors such as nutrition, trauma, and toxic exposures, as well as social factors such as the influence of parents and caregivers, peers, and teachers (Fuhrmann et al., 2015).

For these reasons, it is important to understand the potentially profound impact that an uneven social distribution of risks and resources can have on youth, privileging some while leaving disadvantaged populations behind (Steinberg, 2014; see also Chapter 4). The challenge for a caring society is to take maximum advantage of the developmental opportunities afforded by adolescence. The remarkable adaptability, plasticity, and heterogeneity of adolescent brains (Ismail et al., 2017) creates accompanying opportunities—and obligations—for individuals and agencies responsible for protecting and serving youth to help all adolescents flourish.

Over the past two decades, advances in neurobiology and neuroimaging have demonstrated the dramatic extent of brain maturation during adolescence. However, as a recent *Lancet* commission on adolescence has noted, this exciting advance in knowledge has not penetrated the everyday understanding of informed citizens and policy makers, including many who serve young people (Patton et al., 2016). While some youth-serving policies and programs have embraced developmentally informed changes, the wide-scale changes needed to support and bolster adolescents' development have not yet materialized.

The challenge of educating the public is compounded by a deeply ingrained tendency to view adolescence as mainly a time of vulnerability and risk—a viewpoint that may have been reinforced in recent years by oversimplified headlines about a "mismatch" in the adolescent brain between intensifying desires and emotions (akin to "stepping on the gas") and a more slowly developing capacity for self-regulation ("stepping on the brakes)." This preoccupation with risk leads to a tendency to attribute risk and vulnerability to developing young people, while overlooking society's responsibility to protect and support them in their growth. To continue the metaphor, it draws attention to "risky drivers" rather than the conditions of the roads, the presence of guardrails, and the availability of driver education. A preoccupation with risk also leads to a selective valuing of policies and practices that aim to shield adolescents from harm and relative disregard for those that create incentives for discovery and innovation.

A key theme of this report is that recent advances in neuroscientific understanding have been fundamentally misunderstood by large segments of the public. The defining characteristics of the adolescent brain are malleability and plasticity. These attributes may sometimes be worrisome but they also generate unique opportunities for learning, exploration, and growth. Our society needs policies and practices that will help us better leverage these developmental opportunities to harness the promise of adolescence—rather than focusing myopically on containing its risks.

A second important theme of the report—and a major challenge for the nation—is that the promise of adolescence is now unrealized for many of our nation's adolescents due to deeply rooted structural inequalities that underpin well-documented disparities in developmental outcomes. These structural inequalities include substantial differences in family resources, in the safety and support of neighborhoods, and the occurrence of racial/ethnic bias. (See Chapter 4.) Counteracting and erasing these disparities will require sustained, multipronged, multilevel interventions. Developmental science can tell us what to do, but only a sustained political commitment can enable us to do it.

STUDY CHARGE AND APPROACH

The National Academies of Sciences, Engineering, and Medicine appointed the Committee on the Neurobiological and Socio-behavioral Science of Adolescent Development and Its Applications ("the committee") to prepare a report examining the neurobiological and socio-behavioral science of adolescent development and outlining how this knowledge can be applied to institutions and systems (1) to promote adolescent well-being, resilience, and development and (2) to rectify structural barriers and inequalities in opportunity. (See the committee's full Statement of Task in Box 1-1.) Sixteen prominent scholars and practitioners were included on the committee, representing a broad array of disciplines including neuroscience, developmental and social psychology, economics, sociology, adolescent health and medicine, law, and education and learning. They met and deliberated over a 15-month period to reach the findings presented in this report.

The study builds on the foundation laid by the first study in the National Academy of Medicine's Culture of Health study series, *Communities in Action: Pathways to Health Equity.* The Funders for Adolescent Science Translation (FAST) provided funding for this committee's study and report. FAST members include the Annie E. Casey Foundation, the Bezos Family Foundation, the Chan Zuckerberg Initiative, the Conrad N. Hilton Foundation, the Ford Foundation, the National Public Education Support Fund, the Raikes Foundation, and the Robert Wood Johnson Foundation.

BOX 1-1
Statement of Task

An ad hoc committee will examine the neurobiological and socio-behavioral science of adolescent development, health, well-being, resilience, and agency including the science of positive youth development. The committee will also focus on how this knowledge can be applied to institutions and systems so that adolescent well-being, resilience, and development are promoted and that systems address structural barriers and inequalities in opportunity and access. The study will aim to build off the first study in the National Academy of Medicine's Culture of Health study series and outline the implications of developmental interactions with the social distribution of risks and resources identified in the first study, *Communities in Action: Pathways to Health Equity.*

As appropriate to their review, the study committee will make evidence-driven recommendations to key stakeholders serving adolescents and their families including government agencies and community institutions; federal, state, and local policy makers who guide allocation of resources; and the research community. The committee will highlight promising models, opportunities for translations, and potential policy areas to better support adolescents, and will identify three to five research gaps. The committee will also work with a communications consultant throughout the process to identify and communicate key messages.

The committee will explore

1. What are the unique neurobiological and socio-behavioral characteristics in adolescence that make this a period of unique opportunity for positive developmental trajectories? Adolescence has largely been seen as a time of heightened risk and poor decision making; however, emerging research suggests that adolescence, especially the adaptive flexibility of adolescents, is also a period of opportunity for learning and skill acquisition. How can these opportunities be maximized and harmful risks mitigated?
2. Recognizing that development begins early in life; how do early life conditions, including supports and adversity, shape adolescent development? What is the role of adolescent agency? What does science tell us about our ability, during the adolescent period, to mediate past developmental challenges?
3. As outlined in the report, *Communities in Action: Pathways to Health Equity,* areas of potential structural inequities (p. 7), include intrapersonal, interpersonal, institutional, and systemic mechanisms that guide allocation of resources along the lines of race, gender, class, sexual orientation, gender expression, and other dimensions of individual and group identity. Of these, which ones are particularly important in supporting or threatening positive adolescent development? What role does historical trauma play in health and development?
4. What does the science suggest about how systems (e.g., health, justice, education/higher education, child welfare) could be changed to improve the process and outcomes of adolescent development? How can systems recognize and support resilience, and promote adolescent agency and the development of positive youth assets to improve their services?

The central charge for the committee was to draw upon research from neurobiological and socio-behavioral science to highlight promising models, opportunities for translations, and policies to better support adolescents (see Chapters 2 through 4); identify research gaps (see Chapter 10); and develop evidence-based recommendations to key stakeholders serving adolescents and their families (see Chapters 6 through 9). Targets for these recommendations include government agencies and community institutions; federal, state, and local policy makers who guide the allocation of resources; and the research community. Taken together, these recommendations are intended to outline a vision in support of positive development for all adolescents.

Successful Development

In undertaking this task, the committee gave much thought to what successful maturation during adolescence entails or requires. How can we best ensure that all adolescents will flourish? A flourishing adolescent experiences high levels of emotional, psychological, and social well-being.[3] The psychological and philosophical literature identifies a range of possible indicators of flourishing, including happiness, satisfaction, behavioral flexibility, growth, and resilience in the aftermath of adversity (Fredrickson and Losada, 2005). Many of the current academic discussions of flourishing focus on how best to achieve it. The central challenge is to identify a core set of conditions or capabilities that need to be supported, such as bodily health, bodily integrity, and material control over one's environment (Nussbaum, 2003, 2011; Sen, 1993, 1999).[4]

The committee considered a range of capabilities that appear to be central to a flourishing adolescence and determined that the necessary conditions are good health, education, positive socialization, and the fostering of stable, supportive familial and caretaker relationships. Ultimately, the committee regards supporting and promoting flourishing during adolescence as essential for youth to transition into successful adulthood. This report therefore focuses on the youth-serving systems specifically tasked with supporting these capabilities—the health, education, child welfare, and justice systems—and discusses the role of families and neighborhoods in shaping experiences within those systems (see Chapters 6 through 9). While a number of other systems and system-level actors, ranging from religious institutions to law enforcement, also touch the lives of adolescents,

---

[3] Flourishing is a concept that originated in Aristotle's discussions of what it means to "do and live well," and it is embraced as an ideal by political philosophers and psychologists alike. See, for example, Keyes (2002, p. 210).

[4] For a useful summary, see https://plato.stanford.edu/entries/capability-approach/.

the systems outlined in the committee's charge shape many of adolescents' experiences as they develop and transition into adulthood. Each of them has a profound obligation to implement evidence-informed policies and practices to enable all adolescents to flourish.

The Age Span of Adolescence

In order to interpret the scope of its charge, the committee, inevitably, needed to define the age span of "adolescence." At the lower boundary, it is generally accepted that the onset of puberty—at approximately ages 10 to 12—signals the beginning of the developmental processes of adolescence. The more consequential question for the committee's work concerns the upper bound of adolescence. On the one hand, the unique period of brain development and heightened brain plasticity at the heart of the committee's charge continues into the mid-20s. On the other hand, the socio-emotional changes associated with adolescence (e.g., forming relationships with peers and adults and developing personal identity) occur largely during the teenage years and, in everyday life, graduation from high school and leaving the family home, mark a fairly distinct social transition to "young adulthood," typically signified by the 18th birthday (the legal "age of majority"). However, as explained in a recent National Academies report, most 18–25 year-olds experience a prolonged period of transition to *independent* adulthood, a worldwide trend that blurs the boundary between adolescence and "young adulthood," developmentally speaking.

With these considerations in mind, the committee interprets its charge to encompass youth ages 10 to 25. While there is a growing recognition that young adulthood is a critical life stage in itself, especially in educational and occupational terms, for the purposes of this report, the committee encompasses young adulthood within a broad conception of adolescence. While older adolescents (or young adults) differ greatly in their social roles and tasks from younger adolescents, it would be developmentally arbitrary in developmental terms to draw a cut-off line at age 18.

Although the committee has interpreted its charge as one including young adults (ages 18 to 25), it focuses most of its attention on the needs of adolescents ages 10 to 18), typically those living with their families and attending secondary schools. Thus, some chapters (Chapters 6, 8, and 9) clearly center on a subset of the population, typically because of legal definitions. In Chapters 6 and 9, for example, we focus on secondary schools and the juvenile justice system instead of higher education and the criminal justice system—although both chapters discuss the latter systems to a lesser degree. Because higher education (including technical education) and the criminal justice system are designed to serve individuals of all ages and to effectuate much more complex social purposes than specifically serving adolescents, the committee does not focus the majority of its recommendations on these systems. Moreover, this committee was not constituted to take on the challenges of reforming criminal justice and higher education, notwithstanding the observation that young adults ages 18 to 25 may sensibly be characterized as adolescents from a developmental point of view. (For further understanding of the need to invest in the health and well-being of young adults, see *Investing in the Health and Well-being of Young Adults* (Institute of Medicine and National Research Council, 2014).)

Even within the period of adolescence, much of the literature uses different terms for different phases or stages. In this report, the committee refers to adolescence as encompassing four periods—early adolescence (ages 10 to 12), middle adolescence (ages 13 to 15), late adolescence (ages 16 to 18), and young adulthood (ages 19 to 25). Figure 1-1 visually depicts these periods as shading into one another around these ages, recognizing that they are fluid and based, in part, on socially constructed transition points (e.g., from elementary to secondary school and so on).

The Life-Course Perspective

The well-being of adolescents is shaped by experiences during the prenatal and early childhood years. Fortunately, the prenatal and early childhood periods are already widely recognized to be sensitive times for development. Over the past several decades large-scale investments in supports for young children—such as Early Head Start, Head Start, and home visiting programs—have contributed to broader public awareness of the importance of prenatal and early childhood development in achieving positive outcomes for all young children. Of course, more can be done, as far too many young children enter adolescence bearing the scars of childhood adversity, including toxic stress, exposure to environmental toxins, child maltreatment, food insecurity, and limited access to high-quality early care and education.

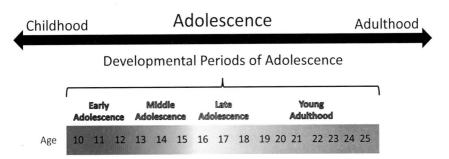

FIGURE 1-1 Developmental periods of adolescence.

A companion National Academies' study on applying the neurobiological and socio-behavioral science concerning prenatal through early childhood development was under way to address these issues during the time of this committee's investigations.[5] The resulting report discusses programs and policies designed to mitigate adverse prenatal and early childhood conditions during a child's earliest years. In accordance with our charge, this committee discusses how early life conditions, including supports and adversity, can affect adolescent development and how past developmental challenges may be mediated in adolescence (see Chapter 3). Taken together, the two reports take a life-course perspective, arguing that a strong infrastructure for young children should be extended throughout adolescence to nurture positive development for all children from birth to adulthood.

HISTORY OF ADOLESCENCE

Popular understanding of adolescence as a distinct period of neurobiological and socio-emotional development and of the duration of that period has evolved over time, shaped by social and cultural change. The first use of the word "adolescence" appears to have occurred in the 15th century, the word being derived from the Latin *adolescere*, meaning "to grow up or to grow into maturity." However, the word and the concept only gained widespread popular use at the turn of the 20th century, first in the United States and later in other Western countries. Psychologist G. Stanley Hall characterized adolescence as a "new" developmental phase resulting from social changes brought about by the industrial revolution and the introduction of public schooling occurring during the Progressive era, when reformers were advocating for compulsory education and legal restrictions on child labor (Arnett and Cravens, 2006; Hall, 1904). Yet nearly 90 years after Hall's observations, anthropologists Alice Schlegel and Herbert Barry documented evidence that the vast majority of pre-industrial societies throughout human history appear to have recognized a period that corresponds to adolescence, that is, a period when a person is no longer a child but is not yet an adult (Schlegel and Barry, 1991). More recently, anthropologists Carol Worthman and Kathy Trang have documented the biological-social mismatch that has been associated with increasingly younger ages of physical maturation accompanied by older ages of social maturation around the world, pointing to an increasingly globalized cultural construction of adolescence (Worthman and Trang, 2018).

---

[5] For more information on the Committee on Applying Neurobiological and Socio-behavioral Sciences from Prenatal through Early Childhood Development: A Health Equity Approach, see www.nationalacademies.org/earlydevelopment.

While a period of adolescence may have been recognized across time and culture, and a global understanding may now be emerging (Worthman and Trang, 2018), Hall's observations a century ago about the impact of the industrial revolution in the United States are still salient. Taking young people out of the workplace and placing them in schools erased the expectation that young teens would become "bread earners" and, instead, prolonged their dependence on their parents and families. Moreover, this change gave them an opportunity to form their own peer groups. A side effect of this change was the opportunity for adolescents to experience a period of social development and freedom without the responsibilities of adulthood.

Spurred by post-World War II economic expansion, as of mid-century a discernible youth culture had emerged in the United States, defined by distinct youth styles, behaviors, and interests. The latter half of the 20th century saw the rise of youth engagement in and creation of social and political movements, including student-led civil rights protests, anti-Vietnam War protests, and divestment and anti-apartheid initiatives, through which adolescents exerted agency and actively sought to change the contexts in which they lived.

Beginning in the late 20th century and into the early 21st century, society began to recognize the emergence of "young adulthood," sometimes thought of as an extension of adolescence. In *Investing in Young Adults* (2014), a committee of the National Academies suggested that young adulthood should be viewed as a distinct developmental period, reflecting the social and economic developments that have prolonged the transition to independent adulthood. For the purposes of this report, however, our committee encompasses young adulthood within a prolonged period of adolescence.

The 21st-century blurring of the age of adulthood reflects a larger point: that conceptions of when and how adolescence begins and ends are, in part, socially constructed and vary across time and place. Currently, we understand adolescence as beginning with the onset of puberty and ending when young people take on various socially defined tasks signifying adulthood. Due to trends toward earlier onset of puberty and changing societal dynamics around the commencement of adulthood, adolescence, which once lasted only a matter of years, is now conceived as a much longer period—lengthened at the beginning by the earlier onset of puberty and at the end by the increasingly protracted transition of young people into careers, marriages, and financial independence (Steinberg, 2014).

Ideas about the upper boundary of adolescence are also socially determined. They are connected to familial, social, legal, and cultural expectations regarding what it means to be an adult, and the point in time when youth "become adults" may be, and historically has been, defined in a variety of ways.[6] Today, included among the tasks signifying a successful transition to adulthood are completing postsecondary education, gaining financial independence, starting a career, and getting married. It is therefore of real consequence that these milestones are continually shifting. For example, Americans were delaying marriage, on average, until the age of 29 as of 2011; delaying child bearing, with the median age of first birth for females being 26.7, in 2015; and looking to their parents for continued financial support, with over half of 18–24-year-olds living with their parents in 2015.

With the onset of puberty happening earlier and earlier and marriage occurring later and later, adolescence in the United States now lasts roughly 15 years. While this lengthening has increased for all Americans, there is great variation in how the period has elongated. Puberty is most often beginning earlier among the nation's poorest children, while the transition to adulthood is increasingly delayed for more affluent adolescents, who are more likely to pursue higher education and delay marriage and parenthood (Steinberg, 2014). This pattern is extremely important, because early life experiences, including social risks and disadvantages, have been shown to lower the age of pubertal timing, whereas delayed adulthood elongates the period of novel experiences and learning. As a result, longer adolescence benefits the privileged far more than the underprivileged (Steinberg, 2014, p. 177).

CONTEMPORARY ADOLESCENTS

Today's adolescents are growing up in remarkable times. At least since the industrial revolution of the 18th and 19th centuries, each new generation has faced a progressively modernizing world with changing expectations and opportunities for young people (e.g., see Modell, 1991). This appears to be accelerating, as adolescents in the 21st century are experiencing sometimes dramatic shifts in the social, cultural, economic, and technological environments. As they navigate their adolescent years and emerge into adulthood, demographic shifts are altering community and family life in fundamental ways. For example, today's youth population in the United States is more culturally and ethnically diverse than ever before, while at the same time

---

[6]For example, legal rights associated with adulthood vary in age both across and within societies. In the United States, society imposes different legal ages for driving (ranging from ages 14 to 17 among some U.S. states, with a range of restrictions on driving and age to receive full license across states), military service (age 18, or 17 with parental consent), marriage (typically age 18, with some states allowing marriage at younger ages with parental or judicial consent), voting (typically age 18, or in recent years, 16 in some countries and U.S. localities), and drinking alcohol (age 21 in the United States. but younger in many other countries). Each of these has been in some way and in certain times a marker of adulthood.

inequalities in income and opportunity among youth continues to increase. Perhaps no societal development will have a greater impact on the lives and well-being of adolescents in the 21st century than the digital revolution. Finally, although it is still too early to predict the precise effects, the polarization and intensity of political discourse in the United States and what appears to many young people as a battle for national identity are bound to have a long-term impact on current and future cohorts of adolescents.

Demographic Trends

Adolescents currently represent nearly one-fourth of the entire U.S. population. According to the Census Bureau, there were approximately 73.5 million adolescents ages 10 to 25 in 2017, representing 22.6 percent of the U.S. population (U.S. Census Bureau, 2018b).[7] While in raw numbers the size of the adolescent population has grown recently, it is now declining slightly as a proportion of the population (U.S. Census Bureau, 2018b). Based on a projected continued decline in fertility as well as the continued aging of the population, this trend is likely to continue for several more decades (Colby and Ortman, 2014). According to U.S. Census projections, youth (10 to 24 years old) are expected to comprise about 18 percent of the population in 2040.[8] Immigration is projected to slow a little as well, although the percentage of the population that is foreign-born is expected to rise, albeit more slowly than it has been rising in recent years (Colby and Ortman, 2014).

The composition of the U.S. population overall, as well as among adolescents, has also become more racially and ethnically diverse; the U.S. population as a whole is expected to become minority majority, that is, with more than half belonging to a category other than non-Latinx White alone, by 2044 (Colby and Ortman, 2014). Because this is expected to occur more quickly among children under 18, the crossover from minority

---

[7]Although females outnumber males at older ages, males in this age range constitute a very slight majority (51%) (U.S. Census Bureau, 2018b). In the 2010 Census, 56 percent of 10–24-year-olds were non-Latinx White, 21 percent were Latinx (of any race), 14.5 percent were Black or African American, 4.6 percent were Asian, 2.6 percent reported two or more races, and less than 1 percent each were American Indian/Alaskan Native and Native Hawaiian/Pacific Islander (U.S. Census Bureau, 2018a). Just over 90 percent of adolescents are native-born; the remainder are a mix of naturalized citizens and both documented and undocumented immigrant non-citizens (U.S. Census Bureau, 2012). More than one-quarter of children in the United States had at least one foreign-born parent in 2014; 22 percent were second generation, that is, native-born but with at least one foreign-born parent (Child Trends, 2014).

[8]In 2040, it is estimated that there will be 66.1 million adolescents (10–24-year-olds) in the United States, or roughly 18 percent of the population. (See Table 3, National Population Projects Tables, U.S. Census, 2017, https://www.census.gov/data/tables/2017/demo/popproj/2017-summary-tables.html).

to majority of the population for adolescents ages 10 to 25 should occur much sooner, by 2020.

These broad trends intersect with several other key aspects of adolescents' lives that are changing due to demographic trends in the overall population: the socioeconomic status of their families, and thus their own status; how and where they live, including not only migration but also the family and institutional structures they live in; and the shifting landscape of their education as well as their employment and work experiences (adolescents' education and employment are discussed in detail in Chapter 6).

For most adolescents, socioeconomic status is linked to the status of their families. Poverty rates for families have been dropping in recent years following the Great Recession, falling from 13.2 percent in 2010 to 10.3 percent in 2017 (Fontenot et al., 2018). Poverty rates vary substantially across racial/ethnic groups, with 6.3 percent of non-Latinx White families, 7.7 percent of Asian families, 16.9 percent of Latinx families, and 19.0 percent of Black families living below the poverty line in 2017. Single-mother families have especially high rates of poverty, at almost 28 percent; one-third of Black and Latinx single-mother families were in poverty in 2017.

Youth today are also more likely to live in urban areas than in the past, a trend that has been observable for adolescents over the past 35 years. Data from the Monitoring the Future (MTF) surveys,[9] which ask adolescents where they mostly grew up, shows a decline in the percentage of those reporting that they grew up on a farm or in the country, from 24.7 percent in 1976 to 16.5 percent in 2012 (Bachman et al., 1980, 2014). More adolescents have reported over time that they were living in cities or in suburbs of medium-sized cities (fewer than 100,000 people). White adolescents are much more likely to report living or having grown up on farms or in the country than are Black adolescents, and also more likely to report living in small cities or suburbs; Black adolescents report living in medium, large, or very large cities more often.

Technology and the Digital Revolution

These demographic and social changes are happening alongside and often intertwined with an extraordinarily fast-paced changing world of technology, all in the context of shifting political and economic change. Through the Internet and social media, youth have broad access to information and ideas in ways that were never before possible, giving rise to new forms of digital community among youth, as well as new forms of social

---

[9]The Monitoring the Future surveys are funded by the National Institute on Drug Abuse. MTF is an ongoing study of the behaviors, attitudes, and values of American secondary schools students, college students, and young adults.

action and interaction. An example of the latter is the leading role youth have taken in social movements in response to gun violence. Taken together, these broad trends have global as well as local impacts and make up the broader context for the typical developmental changes that characterize the period of adolescence for all youth.

For adolescents, the technological and digital revolution have become a key context of their development, permeating nearly every aspect of their lives. In a recent survey conducted by the Pew Research Center, researchers found that approximately 76 percent of adolescents surveyed use social media, with 45 percent indicating that they are almost always online, whether by phone or computer. When these numbers are broken down by gender and race and ethnicity, they show that girls were more likely than boys (50% vs. 39%) to identify as being "almost constantly" online, as were Latinx youth when compared to Whites (54% vs. 4%) (Anderson and Jiang, 2018).

Given adolescents' near-constant interaction with digital technology, it is important to understand the ways in which this engagement may present opportunities for positive development, as well as potential risks. For example, engagement online and with digital media may help adolescents achieve a healthy level of autonomy by providing opportunities to associate with peers and cultures they might not otherwise encounter in their daily lives, opening the door to new interests (e.g., music, writing, coding, sports), which could benefit them as they move into adulthood (Boyd, 2014; Ito et al., 2008). This type of engagement can also provide a new way for youth to build social networks. LGBTQ youth, for example, are able to connect with each other and build supportive and empowering communities in ways that were unavailable to previous generations (Hammack, 2018). Further, in addition to forming new relationships, research suggests that online contact among young people's existing social networks reinforces the bonds that are made offline, making them feel more connected and supported by their peers and families (Uhls et al., 2017).[10]

Notwithstanding the many worries that have been expressed about the possible detrimental effects of social media consumption on overall adolescent well-being, strong evidence documenting such effects has not yet emerged (Orben and Przybylski, 2019). Some specific reasons for concern are generally acknowledged, however. In recent years, bullying has been

---

[10] While much of popular reporting today suggests that adolescents' use of digital and social media may be creating tension between parents and youth, research is mixed about the impact of technology on family relationships. While some research has found that technology may create a barrier and limit communication with parents, there is also evidence that the use of social media, texting, and other communication technologies may offer new ways for parents and children to relate and communicate (Lee, 2009; Schwartz et al., 2014; Subrahmanyam and Greenfield, 2008).

increasingly moving from the schoolyard to the Internet. While previous generations could usually find refuge once at home, the public nature of cyberbullying makes it difficult for youth to escape, which in turn can increase the risk of mental health issues such as depression and anxiety (National Academies of Sciences, Engineering, and Medicine, 2016). According to a recent study on adolescent well-being and social media, an adolescent's ability to cope with bullying plays a significant role in social media's overall impact on well-being (Schwartz et al., 2014; Subrahmanyam and Greenfield, 2008; Weinstein, 2018).

Adolescents are also at risk of negative consequences when sharing information online. Whereas in previous generations, such actions were often easily forgotten in time, for today's youth online personal histories become part of that person's digital footprint, which often remains connected to their name long after an initial posting (Madden et al., 2007). Laws such as the Privacy Rights for California Minors in the Digital World help by giving adolescents under age 18 the right to remove posted material, but not all states provide such protection (Costello et al., 2016). The federal Children's Online Privacy Protection Act (COPPA) of 1998 also provides some protection, but only for youth under age 13.

The rapidly changing nature of communications technology and the influx of digital media will continue to shape young people's development, and this context for development presents both opportunities and potential risks, making understanding the role of technology in adolescents' lives a critical area of future research; see Chapter 10. Moreover, technology presents another context with the potential to increase inequities as not all youth have access to the benefits of digital technologies, such as youth from low-income or rural households who may be unable to access high-speed Internet at home (Anderson and Perrin, 2018).

Civic Engagement

Another potentially significant trend among 21st-century adolescents in the United States is a burst of civic engagement, somewhat reminiscent of the period of dissent during the Vietnam conflict and the Civil Rights Movement in the 1960s and 1970s. Youth today are engaging in multiple forms of "participatory politics" to amplify their voices on issues of public concern, and increasingly they are doing so through digital media (Cohen, et al., 2012). Indeed, young people are exercising agency and capitalizing on technology as a new forum for political engagement (Finlay et al., 2010; Smith, 2013). In a recent Pew Research Center survey, two-thirds of all 18–24-year-olds reported participating in some sort of political activity in social networking spaces during the past 12 months (Smith, 2013). Young people have been major contributors to the Occupy movement and other attempts to raise awareness about inequality and promote policies that support greater equity. Through movements such as Black Lives Matter, which encompasses intersecting axes of racial and economic oppression, young people are at the forefront of advancing an intersectional approach to combatting systemic inequity and discrimination. Political organizing for school safety and reducing gun violence is another recent example.

Volunteering to serve others is another measurable indicator of civic engagement. Among 8th, 10th, and 12th graders in the MTF surveys, 27.1 percent, 34.4 percent, and 38.8 percent (respectively) reported volunteering at least once per month in 2015 (Child Trends, 2015). However, rates of volunteering and other forms of civic behavior tend to drop when young people enter their early twenties and are no longer enrolled in high schools or colleges (Finlay et al., 2010). Similarly, 18–24-year-olds' voting rates are consistently lower than those of older age groups, although early analyses of returns from the 2018 election show increased rates (File, 2014; Langer and Siu, 2018).

Much like the patterns observed among adults, for whom civic engagement is positively correlated with educational attainment, adolescents who plan to complete 4-year college degrees are more civically involved than those with plans for 2-year degrees or no higher education, as are those whose parents have higher levels of education (Syvertsen et al., 2011). Notably, this gap has been growing since the early 1990s (Syvertsen et al., 2011). Wray-Lake and Hart (2012) report a growing gap specifically in voting behavior by education level across cohorts, but not in other conventional political activities (such as attending meetings, donating money, working for a campaign, or wearing a button for a candidate). Females and minorities of all ages are less likely to engage in political activities (other than voting), although holding socioeconomic status and other demographic characteristics constant, Blacks have higher levels of political participation than do Whites (Fisher, 2012). Despite patterns of lower levels of political engagement among members of historically marginalized groups, in the United States there has been a recent uptick in the number of women, openly LGBTQ+ people, and (importantly for this report) young people elected to political positions (Caron, 2018; DeSilver, 2018).

In summary, the explosion of new communication technologies and the positive as well as compromising possibilities they offer, together with the shifting access to and demands for civic engagement that are now emerging, not only comprise key contexts shaping adolescents' lives today but also suggest the agency of young people. In each context, adolescents are themselves actively influencing change in their lives and communities, while at the same time shaping the experiences and environments of their development.

THE PROMISE OF ADOLESCENCE

Having reviewed the background and context for the report as well as the characteristics of 21st-century adolescents and the world they inhabit, we return now to the committee's basic assignment and the core themes of the report.

Adolescence is a developmental stage in which heightened neuro-sensitivity and normative changes in neural and hormonal development intersect with changes in young people's social, technological, and cultural environments, opening a critically important gateway to adulthood. Brain development is complex and ongoing throughout childhood and adolescence, with different parts of the brain experiencing major changes at different times. The nature of these changes—in brain structures, functions, and connectivity—and the developmental plasticity unique to this period of life—present remarkable opportunities for learning and growth as well as amelioration of the harmful effects of childhood exposures.

While humans retain a baseline level of neuroplasticity required for experience-based learning throughout their lives, adolescent brain circuitry is exceedingly adaptable and "experience-dependent," which means that adolescents are specially primed to learn from their particular circumstances and environments during this period (Fuhrmann et al., 2015). (See Chapter 2 for a full discussion of the developing adolescent brain.) In addition to being a period of profound cognitive transformation, adolescence is also a time of numerous biological, psychosocial, and emotional changes (see Chapter 2). The changes in the body, the brain, and behavior occurring during adolescence are interrelated and interact with one another and with the environment to shape the adolescents' pathways to adulthood.

Because pubertal, neurological, cognitive, and psychosocial changes are occurring, adolescence is a critical period of opportunity to shape developmental trajectories. With this growth and learning, each new experience is an opportunity for the adolescent to discover new interests, develop new skills, and otherwise flourish. This heightened sensitivity and responsiveness to environmental influences also suggests that adolescence is a period during which interventions—at both the individual and societal levels—may be used to redirect and remediate maladaptation in brain structure and behavior from earlier developmental periods, that is, to achieve resilience (see Chapter 3). Adolescence therefore holds great promise to realize positive trajectories for all youth.

THE POLITICAL CHALLENGE

Here, then, lies the political challenge. How does a caring society take advantage of this critical developmental opportunity in a world characterized by substantial—and worsening—disparities in resources, safety, social supports, and other necessary conditions of well-being for children and adolescents? Widening income and wealth inequality in the United States has placed individuals and families that are at the lower end of the socio-economic distribution at a historically great distance from those at the top end of the distribution (Chetty et al., 2017; Piketty and Saez, 2014). Economic inequality poses unique challenges to young people across the socioeconomic distribution and is also strongly associated with other measures of inequality.

It is well documented that economic inequality strongly influences the opportunities available to adolescents from lower socioeconomic backgrounds. Greater inequality often accompanies more severe residential segregation, such that young people from families with lower incomes and less wealth, and often families from nondominant racial groups, live in communities that are increasingly isolated and separated from economic and educational opportunities (Ananat, 2011; Oliver and Shapiro, 2006; Owens, 2016; Quillian, 2014; Reardon and Bischoff, 2011). In addition to this unequal and reduced access to resources, inequality contributes to the way young people perceive themselves, their place in the world, and the possibilities for their futures.

It is now understood that these inequalities shape individuals' developmental trajectories by "getting under the skin." For example, adolescents living in poverty often experience heightened levels of stress, which can lead not only to short-term changes in observable behavior but also to long-lasting changes in brain structure and function and in connectivity within the brain (see Chapter 3). While some of these changes may help an adolescent adapt to their particular social and physical environment, they may also make it more difficult to function in another environment should conditions change. In this way, key experiences interact with fundamental neurobiological processes to shape developmental trajectories.

The salience of environmental influences in shaping development during adolescence, together with the critical developmental importance of adolescence, make a powerful case for remedial action. The nation should ensure that all adolescents have a genuine opportunity to flourish, not only as an expression of a collective sense of justice but also as an investment in the nation's future.

STUDY METHODS

To understand the science of adolescent development and its applications, the committee reviewed the existing research literature in disciplines such as neuroscience, developmental and social psychology, adolescent health and medicine, and education and learning. To understand the roles, structures, policies, practices, and effects of social systems, we also reviewed pertinent research in social and behavioral sciences, law, and public policy. The committee held four in-person meetings and conducted additional deliberations by teleconference and electronic communications during the course of the study. The first and second in-person meetings were information-gathering meetings during which the committee heard from a variety of stakeholders, including the study's sponsors, youth, researchers and scholars, and policy makers from the federal, state, and local levels. The third and fourth meetings were closed to the public to enable the committee to deliberate and to formulate its conclusions and recommendations.

Recognizing that the lived experience of young people represents an important form of evidence itself, the committee sought to hear the voices of young people in a variety of ways. First, the committee invited six adolescents from a range of backgrounds to speak at a public session in June 2017. These young people described their experiences in the foster care and juvenile justice systems as well as the health and education systems, commented on the impact on their lives of ever-changing access to technology and social media, and reflected on their hopes for the future. Second, the committee commissioned an analysis from the University of Michigan's My Voice program to understand adolescents' own perceptions of this period of life as well as their perspectives on inequality in their communities.[11] Finally, the committee invited the Maryland Youth Advisory Council to assemble a "youth reflection panel" to comment on possible committee recommendations. In the course of all of these activities, the committee heard from youth about their priorities for the future and the greatest challenges they currently face. The insights the committee garnered from these activities are included throughout the report in text boxes highlighting "Youth Perspectives" as well as in Appendix B.

ORGANIZATION OF THE REPORT

The committee's report is organized into two parts and 10 chapters. Part I conveys the scientific findings that serve as a foundation for the report. Following this introduction, Chapter 2 summarizes the scientific literature on adolescent development, including biological, neurological, and socio-behavioral changes that show why we characterize adolescence as a period of opportunity. Chapter 3 describes the emerging science of epigenetics and the ways in which the brain, body, and environment interact to shape life-course trajectories. Chapter 4 concludes Part I by summarizing the evidence bearing on the extent to which different groups of ado-

---

[11] MyVoice is a text-message based survey of 1,480 young people (ages 14 to 24) across the United States. The program's methodology is described in DeJonckheere et al. (2017).

lescents are—and are not—achieving important developmental outcomes and highlights variations in achievement among different subpopulations of youth, posing the fundamental challenge we were asked to address— how can deploying knowledge of adolescent development help us rectify these disparities?

Part II begins with Chapter 5, which introduces the concept of using developmental knowledge to assure opportunity for all youth. Chapters 6, 7, 8, and 9 then focus on four key youth-serving systems—education, health, child welfare, and justice—in order to answer the question that lies at the heart of our charge: How can these systems be changed to help all adolescents flourish? Each of these chapters also discusses the ways in which families, neighborhoods, and communities can most successfully interact with each system to improve the process and outcomes of adolescent development.[12] Finally, Part II concludes with Chapter 10, in which the committee outlines several priorities for research on adolescent development.

---

[12] Appendix A explains the committee's approach to assessing the evidence. Appendix B summarizes the committee's activities to hear from adolescents themselves and to learn from their lived experiences. Appendix C provides biographical sketches of the committee's members and staff.

2

Adolescent Development

Adolescence is a period of significant development that begins with the onset of puberty[1] and ends in the mid-20s. Consider how different a person is at the age of 12 from the person he or she is at age 24. The trajectory between those two ages involves a profound amount of change in all domains of development—biological, cognitive, psychosocial, and emotional. Personal relationships and settings also change during this period, as peers and romantic partners become more central and as the adolescent moves into and then beyond secondary school or gains employment.

Importantly, although the developmental plasticity that characterizes the period makes adolescents malleable, malleability is not synonymous with passivity. Indeed, adolescents are increasingly active agents in their own developmental process. Yet, as they explore, experiment, and learn, they still require scaffolding and support, including environments that bolster opportunities to thrive. A toxic environment makes healthy adolescent development challenging. Ultimately, the transformations in body, brain, and behavior that occur during adolescence interact with each other and with the environment to shape pathways to adulthood.

Each stage of life depends on what has come before it, and young people certainly do not enter adolescence with a "blank slate." Rather, adolescent development is partly a consequence of earlier life experiences. However, these early life experiences are not determinative, and the adaptive plasticity of adolescence marks it as a window of opportunity for change

---

[1] The average child in the United States experiences the onset of puberty between the age of 8 and 10 years.

37

through which mechanisms of resilience, recovery, and development are possible. (Chapter 3 discusses this life-course perspective on development in detail.) This chapter explores three key domains of adolescent development: puberty, neurobiological development, and psychosocial development. Within each domain, we highlight processes that reflect the capacity for adaptive plasticity during adolescence and beyond, marking adolescence as a period of unique opportunity for positive developmental trajectories.

PUBERTY

Puberty, a normative developmental transition that all youth experience, is shaped by both social and biological processes. Although often misconstrued as an abrupt, discrete event, puberty is actually a gradual process occurring between childhood and adolescence and one that takes many years to complete (Dorn and Biro, 2011). Biologically, puberty involves a series of complex alterations at both the neural and endocrine levels over an extended period that result in changes in body shape (morphology), including the maturation of primary and secondary sex characteristics during late childhood and early adolescence and, ultimately, the acquisition of reproductive maturity (Dorn and Biro, 2011; Natsuaki et al., 2014).

Two biological components of puberty, *adrenarche* and *gonadarche*, are relevant in understanding the link between puberty and adolescent well-being. Adrenarche, which typically begins between ages 6 and 9, refers to the maturation of the hypothalamic-pituitary-adrenal (HPA) axis, during which the levels of adrenal androgens (e.g., dehydroepiandrosterone and its sulfate) begin to increase. While adrenarche begins in late childhood, levels of adrenarchal hormones continue to rise throughout adolescence, peaking in the early 20's (Blakemore et al., 2010). Adrenal androgens contribute to the growth of pubic and axillary hair. Gonadarche typically begins in early adolescence, at approximately ages 9 to 11, and involves the reactivation of the hypothalamic-pituitary-gonadal (HPG) axis (for a review, see Sisk and Foster, 2004).[2] The rise of gonadal steroid hormones to adult levels occurs as a result of HPG reactivation and is primarily responsible for breast and genital development in girls.

---

[2]HPG hormones can bind within cell nuclei and change the transcription and expression of genes to regulate further hormone production, brain function, and behavior (Melmed et al., 2012; Sisk and Foster, 2004). The process begins in the brain when a gonadotropin-releasing hormone (GnRH) is secreted from the hypothalamus. The activation of GnRH is not unique to the pubertal transition; GnRH is also active during pre- and perinatal periods of development but undergoes a quiescent period during the first year of postnatal life until it reawakens during the pubertal transition. GnRH stimulates the pituitary gland to secrete luteinizing hormone (LH) and follicle-stimulating hormones (FSH), which then stimulate the ovary and testes to secrete estradiol and testosterone.

The consequence of these complex changes in HPA and HPG axes at the neuroendocrine level is a coordinated series of visible, signature changes in body parts. These include a growth spurt, changes in skin (e.g., acne) and in body odor, the accumulation of body fat (in girls), the appearance of breast budding (in girls) and enlargement of testes and increased penis size (in boys), the growth of pubic and axillary hair, the growth of facial hair (in boys), and the arrival of the first period (i.e., menarche, in girls). Key pubertal events are highlighted in Figure 2-1; however, as discussed next, there is a great deal of variation in the timing and tempo of these events.

It is useful to distinguish three distinct yet interrelated ways to conceptualize individual differences in pubertal maturation. *Pubertal status* refers to how far along adolescents are in the continuum of pubertal maturation at any given moment. For instance, if an 11-year-old girl has just experienced menarche, she is considered to have advanced pubertal status because menarche is the last event that occurs in the process of the female pubertal transition. Pubertal status is inherently confounded with age, because older adolescents are more likely to have attained advanced pubertal status.

Pubertal timing, on the other hand, refers to how mature an adolescent is when compared to his or her same-sex peers who are of the same age. In other words, pubertal timing always includes a reference group of one's peers. For example, a girl who experiences menarche at age 10 may be an earlier maturer in the United States, because her menarcheal timing is earlier than the national average age for menarche nationwide, which was found to be 12.4 years in a cohort of girls born between 1980 and 1984 (McDowell et al., 2007). Only 10 percent of girls in the United States

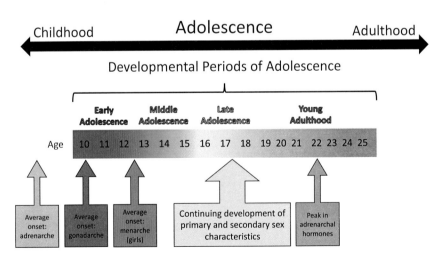

FIGURE 2-1 Key pubertal events across adolescence.

are estimated to have experienced menarche before 11.11 years of age (Chumlea et al., 2003), suggesting that the girl in this example would be considered to have early pubertal timing. Unlike pubertal status, pubertal timing is not confounded by age because, by definition, pubertal timing is inherently standardized within same-sex, same-age peers typically residing in the same country.

Pubertal tempo is a within-the-individual metric that refers to how quickly a person completes these sets of pubertal changes. For example, some boys may experience a deepening of their voice and the development of facial, axillary, and pubic hair all within a matter of months, whereas other boys may have a gap of several years between voice-deepening and the development of facial hair. Pubertal tempo has gained more attention recently with the rise of sophisticated longitudinal methodology and the resulting availability of longitudinal data on pubertal maturation (e.g., Ge et al., 2003; Marceau et al., 2011; Mendle et al., 2010).

Regardless of the metric used, most of the research on adolescent pubertal development has focused on girls. We know comparatively little about the processes, correlates, and outcomes of pubertal maturation in boys, except for the well-replicated findings that girls typically begin and complete puberty before boys. Evidence is now emerging that the relationship between puberty and structural brain development in the amygdala and hippocampus region may differ by sex (Satterthwaite et al., 2014; Vijayakumar et al., 2018). These sex differences in associations between brain development and puberty are relevant for understanding psychiatric disorders characterized by both hippocampal dysfunction and prominent gender disparities during adolescence.

It is also important to consider the pubertal development of transgender and gender-nonconforming youth. Transgender and gender-nonconforming individuals usually identify as a gender other than the one they were assigned at birth (Sylvia Rivera Law Project, 2012). Individuals who are gender-nonconforming may identify as transgender, genderqueer, gender-fluid, gender-expansive, or nonbinary. Puberty is a time that can be enormously stressful, and the fear of developing—or the actual development of—secondary sexual characteristics that do not match a child's gender identity can be intense and even destabilizing (de Vries et al., 2011). Some transgender and gender-nonconforming youth might take medications that block puberty. Although puberty blockers have the potential to ease the process of transitioning, the long-term health effects of these drugs are not yet known (Boskey, 2014; Kreukels and Cohen-Kettenis, 2011).

The Role of Early Experiences on Pubertal Timing and Tempo

As noted earlier, the timing and rate of pubertal development vary greatly. The age at which someone matures is due to a combination of genetic and environmental influences (e.g., Mustanski et al., 2004). Early life experiences, including social risks and disadvantages, have been shown to accelerate pubertal tempo and lower the age of pubertal timing (Marshall and Tanner, 1969). Specifically, accelerated pubertal tempo and early pubertal timing have been associated with stressors, including childhood sexual abuse and physical abuse, obesity, prematurity, light exposure, father absence, and exposure to endocrine disruptors (such as chemicals in plastics, pesticides, hair-care products, and many meat and dairy items) (see e.g., Steinberg, 2014, pp. 54–55). This section reviews the literature on associations between these early experiences and normative variations in pubertal timing and tempo. We close this section with a brief discussion of these associations as a marker of adaptive plasticity.

Maltreatment

One of the most widely studied early experiences related to pubertal development is child maltreatment, and in particular, sexual abuse. A series of studies shows that the age of menarche tends to be lower for girls who experienced child sexual abuse as compared to girls who have not experienced this (Bergevin et al., 2003; Natsuaki et al., 2011; Romans et al., 2003; Turner et al., 1999; Wise et al., 2009). Trickett and Putnam (1993) suggested that the trauma of child sexual abuse introduces physiological as well as psychological consequences for children, including accelerated maturation by premature activation of the HPA and HPG axes. In addition, some studies have observed a relationship between childhood physical abuse and early maturation, though less robustly and less consistently than for sexual abuse (Bergevin et al., 2003; Wise et al., 2009), and these studies do not always control for the possibility of concurrent sexual abuse (e.g., Romans et al., 2003).

In one of the few studies to examine pubertal development longitudinally in adolescents with maltreatment histories, Mendle and colleagues (2011) followed a sample of 100 girls in foster care at four points in time over 2 years, beginning in the spring of their final year of elementary school. The previously established association between sexual abuse and earlier onset of maturation and earlier age at menarche was replicated, and in addition, physical abuse was found to be related to a more rapid tempo of pubertal development. A recent longitudinal study of 84 sexually abused girls and matched-comparison girls replicated the association between sexual abuse and earlier pubertal onset (including breast development and pubic hair; Noll et al., 2017). Further, using this same sample, childhood sexual abuse predicted earlier pubertal development which, in turn, was associated with higher levels of internalizing symptoms such as depression and anxiety concurrently and 2 years later (Mendle et al., 2014). A third study with this sample found that earlier-maturing girls were more anxious in the pre- and peri-menarche periods than their later-maturing peers; however, their anxiety declined after menarche, suggesting a time-limited effect on mental health and the potential for recovery upon completion of pubertal maturation, as girls enter later adolescence (Natsuaki et al., 2011).

The association between sexual abuse and earlier pubertal development was recently replicated using a large population-based sample of adolescents, the National Longitudinal Study of Adolescent Health[3] ($N = 6,273$ girls). In that study, child sexual abuse predicted earlier menarche and development of secondary sexual characteristics, whereas other types of maltreatment did not (Mendle et al., 2016). The distinctive role for early pubertal timing suggests that the heightened sexual circumstances of puberty may be especially challenging for girls whose lives have already been disrupted by adverse early experiences, yet also suggests a potential opportunity for intervention and resilience, particularly in later adolescence, once pubertal development is complete. However, the vast majority of research in this area has focused solely on girls, and we know very little about whether maltreatment is also associated with earlier pubertal timing in boys.

Other Family and Health Factors

Other family factors that may be stress-inducing yet much less extreme than maltreatment have also been associated with pubertal timing and tempo. For example, Quinlan (2003) found that the number of caretaking transitions a child experiences was associated with earlier menarche. Sung and colleagues (2016) found that exposure to greater parental harshness (but not unpredictability) during the first 5 years of life predicted earlier menarche; and a recent meta-analysis found that father absence was significantly related to earlier menarche (Webster et al., 2014), although genetic confounding may play a role in this association (Barbaro et al., 2017).

Health factors that may affect the metabolic system are also predictive of pubertal timing. For example, in girls, low birth weight (Belsky et al., 2007) and obesity/higher body mass index (BMI) (Wagner et al., 2015) have both been associated with earlier pubertal maturation. For boys, overweight (BMI $\geq$ 85th and < 95th percentile) has been associated with earlier pubertal maturation, whereas obesity (BMI $\geq$ 95th percentile) was associ-

---

[3] For more information on the National Longitudinal Study of Adolescent Health, see https://www.cpc.unc.edu/projects/addhealth.

ated with later pubertal maturation (Lee et al., 2016), suggesting a complex association between aspects of the metabolic system and puberty in boys.

Environmental Exposures

Recently, researchers have examined whether a child's exposure to chemicals is related to pubertal maturation by serving as an endocrine disruptor (see e.g., Lomniczi et al., 2013; Simonneaux et al., 2013; Steingraber, 2007). In the first longitudinal study of age of pubertal timing and exposure to persistent organic pollutants—chemicals used in flame retardants—researchers found that the age at pubertal transition was consistently older in participants who were found to have higher chemical concentrations in collected blood samples (Windham et al., 2015). The effects of neuroendocrine disruptors on girls' pubertal timing may begin during the prenatal period, as there is evidence that female reproductive development is affected by phthalate or bisphenol A exposure during specific critical periods of development in the mother's uterus (Watkins et al., 2017).

Accelerated Maturation and Adaptive Plasticity

It is clear that early experiences can factor into accelerated pubertal timing and tempo, and theorists suggest that this may be adaptive. According to Mendle and colleagues (2011, p. 8), "age at certain stressful life transitions represents a dose-response relationship with maturation, with earlier ages at these events associated with earlier development (e.g., Ellis and Garber, 2000)." Belsky et al. (1991) posited that children who are raised in harsh, stressful environments may have accelerated pubertal development to compensate for a mistrust of commitment and of investment in social relationships. According to Belsky and colleagues, early pubertal timing may serve the evolutionary biological purpose of elongating the window for reproductivity and fertility, to permit more conceptions in a lifetime. Thus, the well-documented association between adverse early life experiences and early pubertal development may itself be an adaptive response, one that reflects the plasticity in neurobiological systems during adolescence to adapt to the specific socio-cultural context.

The Social Context of Pubertal Maturation

Despite the role that stressful early life events play in accelerating pubertal timing, it is important to note that adolescence is also a period of potential for recovery. Even when an adolescent has experienced early adversity and this has precipitated earlier pubertal maturation, the social context in which that adolescent is developing can ultimately change the trajectory of their outcomes—for better or worse. For example, closer and less conflict-laden parent-child relationships can reduce associations between pubertal maturation and behavior problems, while more conflict-laden and less close relationships exacerbate them (Booth et al., 2003; Dorn et al., 2009; Fang et al., 2009). Parental knowledge of an adolescent child's whereabouts and activities also plays a role, as the influence of pubertal timing on problematic outcomes is weakened when such parental knowledge of adolescent whereabouts and activities is high, and it is amplified when knowledge is low (Marceau et al., 2015; Westling et al., 2008). During early childhood, a secure infant-mother attachment can buffer girls from the later effects of harsh environments on earlier pubertal maturation (Sung et al., 2016).

The Context of Biological Sex and Gender Norms

The biological changes of puberty take place in social and cultural contexts, and these dynamic person-context interactions have implications for adolescent development. For instance, the physical changes associated with pubertal maturation affect an adolescent's self-image as much as the way he or she is treated and responded to by others (Graber et al., 2010), and culturally grounded gender norms may make these associations more salient for girls than boys. Indeed, in the United States, although menstruation is acknowledged as a normal biological event, it is nevertheless often accompanied by feelings of shame and the need to conceal it from others, particularly males (Stubbs, 2008). As a result, the arrival of a girl's first menstrual cycle is often accompanied by embarrassment and ambivalence (Brooks-Gunn et al., 1994; Moore, 1995; Tang et al., 2003), as well as by negative feelings (Rembeck et al., 2006), including anxiety, surprise, dismay, panic, and confusion (Brooks-Gunn and Ruble, 1982; Ruble and Brooks-Gunn, 1982).

The arrival of puberty has other social consequences, such as changing dynamics and maturing relationships with parents, siblings, and peers, as well as the emergence of peer relationships with adults. Pubertal maturation is associated with a higher incidence of sexual harassment, both by peers of the same gender and across genders (McMasters et al., 2002; Petersen and Hyde, 2009; Stattin and Magnusson, 1990). Social consequences may be exacerbated among youth experiencing early pubertal timing.

The increase in pubertal hormones (e.g., estradiol, progesterone, testosterone, dehydroepiandrosterone) and the changes they drive, such as the emergence of secondary sex characteristics, is also associated with the development of substance use (Auchus and Rainey, 2004; Grumbach, 2002; Grumbach and Styne, 2003; Havelock et al., 2004; Matchock et al., 2007; Oberfield et al., 1990; Terasawa and Fernandez, 2001; Young and Altemus, 2004). At the same time, the causal direction of these findings is somewhat mixed (Castellanos-Ryan et al., 2013; Dawes et al., 1999; Marceau et al., 2015), with variation by sex. In girls, relatively early pubertal timing and faster pubertal tempo often mark an increased risk for adolescent substance use (Cance et al., 2013; Castellanos-Ryan et al., 2013; Costello et al., 2007; Lee et al., 2014). By contrast, in boys later pubertal timing and/or slower pubertal tempo mark an increased risk for substance use (Davis et al., 2015; Marceau et al., 2015; Mendle and Ferrero, 2012). This striking gender difference in associations between pubertal maturation and substance use highlights how the same biological event (pubertal maturation) can lead to very different outcomes as a function of one's biological sex.

Puberty and Stress Sensitivity

Puberty-related hormones influence the way adolescents adjust to their environment, for example by experiencing symptoms of depression and anxiety. One mechanism through which this might occur is in pubertal hormones' ability to alter sensitivity to stress, making adolescent girls particularly sensitive to exogenous stressors. Recent studies using salivary cortisol as an index of stress regulation have documented heightened stress reactivity and delayed post-stress recovery in pubescent adolescents (Gunnar, et al., 2009; Stroud et al., 2004; Walker et al., 2004). Cortisol is a steroid hormone released by the HPA axis, and disruption to this axis has been implicated in the development of symptoms of depression and anxiety (e.g., Gold and Chrousos, 2002; Guerry and Hastings, 2011; Sapolsky, 2000).

In fact, cortisol secretion is closely intertwined with age, puberty, and sex, which together appear to contribute to adolescent girls' vulnerability to external stressors (Walker et al., 2004; Young and Altemus, 2004). As will be discussed in Chapter 3, cortisol, along with neuroendocrine, autonomic, immune, and metabolic mediators, usually promotes positive adaptation in the body and the brain, such as efficient operation of the stress response system. However, when cortisol is over- or under-produced it can, along with the other mediators, produce negative effects on the body and brain, such as forming insulin resistance and remodeling the brain circuits that alter mood and behavior. At the same time, as will be shown in Chapter 3, interventions during adolescence have the potential to mediate the harmful effects of stress.

Summary

In summary, puberty is shaped by both biological and social processes. Biologically, puberty occurs over an extended period during which neuroendocrine alterations result in the maturation of primary and secondary sex characteristics and the acquisition of reproductive maturity. The timing and tempo of pubertal development varies greatly, and the age at which an adolescent matures depends upon a combination of genetic and environmental influences, including early life experiences. Socially, pubertal maturation and its accompanying physical changes affect how adolescents perceive themselves and how they are treated by others, and early pubertal timing especially has been shown to have social consequences. While we know a great deal about the biological processes of puberty, much of the research, particularly on the role of adverse early experiences, is based on studies of girls rather than boys and excludes transgender and gender-nonconforming youth. Thus, it is important to monitor whether or not conclusions drawn from the extant research are relevant for both girls and boys, and to consider how further study of puberty in boys, transgender youth, and gender-nonconforming youth may deepen our understanding of these dynamic processes.

Despite this limitation, research on associations between stress exposure and pubertal timing and tempo makes clear the importance of early experiences and highlights the role of social determinants of health. Stressful living conditions are related to earlier pubertal timing and accelerated pubertal tempo. While early puberty may be an evolutionarily adaptive response to context that reflects neurobiological plasticity, there are important consequences that suggest it may not be adaptive in terms of supporting a long-term path to health and well-being for youth living in the 21st century. Structural changes that disrupt the systemic factors that increase risk for early puberty (e.g., resource deprivation) as well as supportive relationships can mitigate the risks associated with early puberty, can foster positive outcomes, and may promote adolescents' capability for resilience.

NEUROBIOLOGICAL DEVELOPMENT

Adolescence is a particularly dynamic period of brain development, second only to infancy in the extent and significance of the neural changes that occur. The nature of these changes—in brain structures, functions, and connectivity—allows for a remarkable amount of developmental plasticity unique to this period of life, making adolescents amenable to change.[4] These normative developments are required to prepare the brain so it can respond to the demands and challenges of adolescence and adulthood, but they may also increase vulnerability for risk behavior and psychopathology (Paus et al., 2008; Rudolph et al., 2017). To understand how to take advantage of this versatile adolescent period, it is first important to recognize how and where the dynamic changes in the brain are taking place; Figure 2-2 shows structures and regions of the brain that have been the focus of adolescent developmental neuroscience.

---

[4] See Chapter 3 for a discussion of the adaptive plasticity of adolescence and the potential of interventions during adolescence to mediate deficiencies from earlier life periods.

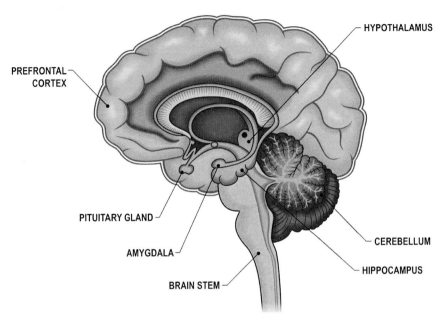

FIGURE 2-2 Brain areas important to adolescent development.
SOURCE: iStock.com/James Kopp.

In the following sections, we summarize current research on structural and functional brain changes taking place over the course of adolescence. Our summary begins with a focus on morphological changes in gray and white matter, followed by a discussion of structural changes in regions of the brain that have particular relevance for adolescent cognitive and social functioning. We then discuss current theoretical perspectives that attempt to account for the associations between neurobiological, psychological, and behavioral development in adolescence.

Notably, the field of adolescent neuroscience has grown quickly over the past several decades. Advances in technology continue to provide new insights into neurobiological development; however, there is still a lack of agreed-upon best practices, and different approaches (e.g., in equipment, in statistical modeling) can result in different findings (Vijayakumar et al., 2018). Our summary relies on the most recent evidence available and, per the committee's charge, we focus on neurobiological changes that make adolescence a period of unique opportunity for positive development. This is not intended to be an exhaustive review of the literature; moreover, studies tend to use "typically" developing adolescents, which limits our ability to comment on whether or how these processes may change for young people with developmental delays or across a broader spectrum of neurodiversity.

High Plasticity Marks the Window of Opportunity

Studies of adolescent brain development have traditionally focused on two important processes: changes in gray matter and changes in myelin. Gray matter is comprised of neural cell bodies (i.e., the location of each nerve cell's nucleus), dendrites, and all the synapses, which are the connections between neurons. Thus, increases or decreases in gray matter reflect changes in these elements, representing, for instance, the formation or disappearance of synapsis (also known as "synaptogenesis" and "synaptic pruning"). New learning and memories are stored in dynamic synaptic networks that depend equally on synapse elimination and synapse formation. That is, unused connections and cells must be pruned away as the brain matures, specializes, and tailors itself to its environment (Ismail et al., 2017).

White matter, on the other hand, is comprised of myelin. Myelin is the fatty sheath around the long projections, or axons, that neurons use to communicate with other neurons. The fatty myelin insulates the axonal "wire" so that the signal that travels down it can travel up to 100 times faster than it can on unmyelinated axons (Giedd, 2015). With myelination, neurons are also able to recover quickly from firing each signal and are thereby able to increase the frequency of information transmission (Giedd, 2015). Not only that, myelinated neurons can more efficiently integrate information from other input neurons and better coordinate their signaling, firing an outgoing signal only when information from all other incoming neurons is timed correctly (Giedd, 2015). Thus, the increase in white matter is representative of the increase in quality and speed of neuron-to-neuron communication throughout adolescence. This is comparable to upgrading from driving alone on a single-lane dirt road to driving on an eight-lane paved expressway within an organized transportation/transit authority system, since it increases not only the amount of information trafficked throughout the brain but also the brain's computational power by creating more efficient connections.

Recent advances in neuroimaging methods have greatly enhanced our understanding of adolescent brain development over the past three decades. In the mid-2000s developmental neuroscientists described differential changes in gray matter (i.e., neurons) and white matter (i.e., myelin) over the course of adolescence. Specifically, gray-matter volume was believed to follow an inverted-U shape, peaking in different regions at different ages and declining over the course of late adolescence and adulthood (Lenroot and Giedd, 2006). In contrast, cortical white matter, which reflects myelin growth, was shown to increase steadily throughout adolescence and into early adulthood, reflecting increased connectivity among brain regions (Lenroot and Giedd, 2006). The proliferation of neuroimaging studies, particularly longitudinal studies following children over the course of adolescence, has enabled researchers to examine these processes in more detail and across a larger number of participants (Vijayakumar et al., 2018).

Analyses of about 850 brain scans from four samples of participants ranging in age from 7 to 29 years (average = 15.2 years) confirm some previous trends, disconfirm others, and highlight the complexity in patterns of change over time. Researchers found that gray-matter volume was highest in childhood, decreased across early and middle adolescence, and began to stabilize in the early twenties; this pattern held even after accounting for intracranial and whole brain volume (Mills et al., 2016). Additional studies of cortical volume have also documented the highest levels occurring in childhood with decreases from late childhood throughout adolescence; the decrease appears to be due to the thinning of the cortex (Tamnes et al., 2017). Importantly, this finding contrasts with the "inverted-U shape" description of changes in gray-matter volume and disconfirms previous findings of a peak during the onset of puberty (Mills et al., 2016).

For white-matter volume, on the other hand, researchers found that across samples, increases in white-matter volume occurred from childhood through mid-adolescence and showed some stabilizing in late adolescence (Mills et al., 2016). This finding generally confirms patterns observed in other recent studies, with the exception that some researchers have found continued increases in white-matter volume into early adulthood (versus stabilizing in late adolescence; e.g., Aubert-Broche et al., 2013). Figure 2-3 shows these recent findings related to gray and white matter.

The widely held belief about a peak in cortical gray matter around puberty followed by declines throughout adolescence was based on the best available evidence at the time. New studies show steady declines in cortical volume beginning in late childhood and continuing through middle adolescence. While the decrease in volume is largely due to cortical thinning rather than changes in surface area, there appear to be complex, regionally specific associations between cortical thickness and surface area that change over the course of adolescence (Tamnes et al., 2017). Discrepant findings can be attributed to a number of factors including head motion during brain imaging procedures (more common among younger participants), different brain imaging equipment, and different approaches to statistical modeling (Tamnes et al., 2017; Vijayakumar et al., 2018). There do appear to be converging findings regarding overall directions of change; however, inconsistencies in descriptions of trajectories, peaks, and regional changes will likely continue to emerge as researchers work toward agreed-upon best practices (Vijayakumar et al., 2018). Importantly, though, as Mills and colleagues (2016, p. 279) point out, it is critical to acknowledge that "it is not possible to directly relate developmental changes in morphometric MRI measures to changes in cellular or synaptic anatomy" (also see Mills and Tamnes, 2014). In other words, patterns of change in overall gray- or

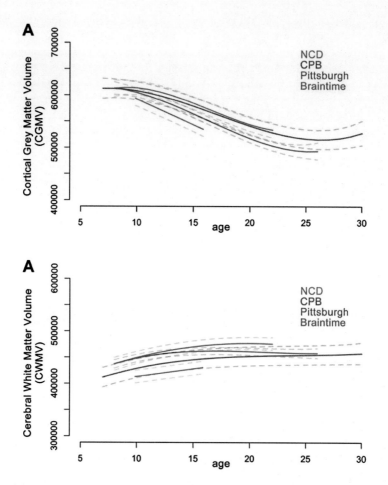

FIGURE 2-3 Cortical gray- and white-matter volume, ages 5 to 30.
NOTES: Age in years is measured along the x-axis and brain measure along the y-axis (raw values (mm³). Best fitting models are represented by the solid lines. Dashed lines represent 95-percent confidence intervals. Four longitudinal datasets from: CPB = NIH Child Psychiatry Branch (National Institute of Mental Health); NCD = Neurocognitive Development (University of Oslo); Pittsburgh = University of Pittsburgh; and Braintime = Leiden University.
SOURCE: Mills et al. (2016, pp. 277–278).

white-matter volume do not provide insight into the specific ways in which neural connections (e.g., synapses, neural networks) may change within the adolescent brain.

In fact, some neural circuitry, consisting of networks of synaptic connections, is extremely malleable during adolescence, as connections form and reform in response to a variety of novel experiences and stressors (Ismail et al., 2017; Selemon, 2013). Gray-matter reduction in the cortex is associated with white-matter organization, indicating that cortical thinning seen in adulthood may be a result of both increased connectivity of necessary circuitry and pruning of unnecessary synapses (Vandekar et al., 2015). Thus, adolescent brains can modulate the strength and quality of neuronal connections rapidly to allow for flexibility in reasoning and for leaps in cognition (Giedd, 2015).

Structural Changes in the Adolescent Brain

Two key neurodevelopmental processes are most reliably observed during adolescence. First, there is evidence of significant change and maturation in regions of the prefrontal cortex (PFC) involved in executive functioning and cognitive and impulse control capabilities (Crone and Steinbeis, 2017; Steinberg, 2005). In other words, areas of the brain that support planning and decision-making develop significantly during the second decade of life. Second, there is evidence of improved connectivity[5] within and between the cortical (i.e., outer) and subcortical (i.e., inner) regions of the brain. Moreover, in both the cortical and subcortical regions, there are age-related and hormone-related changes in neural activity and structure, such as increased volume and connectivity (Gogtay et al., 2004; Østby et al., 2009; Peper and Dahl, 2013; Wierenga et al., 2014).

Over the course of adolescence, regions of the PFC undergo protracted development and significant remodeling. Cortical circuits, especially those that inhibit behavior, continue to develop, enhancing adolescents' capacity for self-regulation (Caballero and Tseng, 2016). Compared to adults, adolescents have a significantly less mature cortical system and tend to utilize these regions less efficiently, and this impacts their top-down cognitive abilities including planning, working memory, impulsivity control, and decision-making (Casey and Caudle, 2013). Ongoing development of structures and connections within the cortical regions corresponds to more efficient balancing of inputs and outputs as adolescents interact with the world.

Changes within subcortical brain regions are also reflected in adolescent capabilities. For instance, increased volume in certain subregions of the hippocampus may predict greater capacity for memory recall and retention in adolescents (Tamnes et al., 2014). Adolescents also display heightened activity in the hippocampus, compared with adults, and differential reward processing in the striatum, which is part of the basal ganglia and plays an important role in motivation and perception of reward. This neural activ-

---

[5] "Connectivity" refers to the formation of synapses, or connections between neurons; groups of interconnected neurons form circuit-like neural networks.

ity may explain their increased sensitivity to rewards and contribute to their greater capacity for learning and habit formation, particularly when incentivized by positive outcomes (Davidow et al., 2016; Sturman and Moghaddam, 2012).

Another subcortical structure, the amygdala, undergoes significant development during puberty and gains new connections to other parts of the brain, such as the striatum and hippocampus (Scherf et al., 2013). The amygdala modulates and integrates emotional responses based on their relevance and impact in context. In conjunction with the amygdala's substantial development, adolescents show higher amygdala activity in response to threat cues[6] than do children or adults (Fuhrmann et al., 2015; Hare et al., 2008; Pattwell et al., 2012). Consequently, they are prone to impulsive action in response to potential threats[7] (Dreyfuss et al., 2014). Changes in the hippocampus and amygdala may be responsible for suppressing fear responses in certain contexts (Pattwell et al., 2011). Such fearlessness can be adaptive for adolescents as they explore new environments and make important transitions—such as entering college or starting a new job away from home. Children and adults do not tend to show the same kind of fear suppression as adolescents, suggesting that this is unique to this stage of development (Pattwell et al., 2011).

A Neurodevelopmental Perspective on Risk-Taking

In recent years, researchers have worked to reconcile contemporary neuroscience findings with decades of behavioral research on adolescents. There has been a particular emphasis on understanding "risky" behavior through the lens of developmental neuroscience. Risk-taking can be driven by a tendency for sensation-seeking, in which individuals exhibit an increased attraction toward novel and intense sensations and experiences despite their possible risks (Steinberg, 2008; Zuckerman and Kuhlman, 2000). This characteristic is heightened during adolescence and is strongly associated with reward sensitivity and drive (Cservenka et al., 2013) as well as the rise in dopamine pathways from the subcortical striatum to the PFC (Wahlstrom et al., 2010). Ironically, as executive function improves, risk-taking based on sensation-seeking also rises, likely due to these strengthened dopamine pathways from the striatum to the PFC regions (Murty et al., 2016; Wahlstrom et al., 2010). Despite these stronger sensation-seeking

---

[6]The threat cues used in the research cited here were pictures of "fearful faces," which serve as a social cue of impending danger.

[7]Impulsive action in response to potential threat was assessed using a "go/no-go" task. Simply put, this is a task in which participants are presented with two types out of three facial emotions ("happy" or "calm" or "fearful") that are randomly assigned as "go" (stimulate action = press a button) or "no-go" (inhibit action = do not press button).

tendencies, however, by mid-adolescence most youth are able to perform cognitive-control tasks at the same level as adults, signaling their capacity for executive self-control (Crone and Dahl, 2012).

Risk-taking can also be driven by impulsivity, which includes the tendency to act without thinking about consequences (impulsive action) or to choose small, immediate rewards over larger, delayed rewards (impulsive choice) (Romer et al., 2017). Impulsive action, which is based on insensitivity to risk, is a form of risk-taking that peaks during early adolescence and is inversely related to working memory ability (Romer et al., 2011). It may also be a consequence of asynchronous limbic-PFC maturation, which is described below. Notably, impulsive actions are seen most frequently in a subgroup of adolescents with pre-existing impairment in self-control and executive function (Bjork and Pardini, 2015). In contrast, impulsive choice behaviors, which are made under conditions of known risks and rewards, do not peak in adolescence. Instead, impulsive choice declines from childhood to adulthood, reflecting the trend of increasing, prefrontal-regulated executive functions throughout adolescence (van den Bos et al., 2015). Interestingly, when given the choice between two risky options with ambiguous reward guarantees, adolescents are more inclined to explore the riskier option than are adults (Levin and Hart, 2003), showing a greater tolerance for ambiguities in reward and stronger exploratory drive (Tymula et al., 2012).

Theoretical models have emerged to explain how neurobiological changes map onto normative "risk" behaviors in adolescence. While some argue that these models and accompanying metaphors may be overly simplistic (e.g., Pfeifer and Allen, 2012), the models are nevertheless utilized frequently to guide and interpret research (e.g., Steinberg et al., 2018). We briefly discuss two of them here: the "dual systems" model and the "imbalance" model.

The "dual systems" model (Shulman et al., 2016; Steinberg, 2008) represents "the product of a developmental asynchrony between an easily aroused reward system, which inclines adolescents toward sensation seeking, and still maturing self-regulatory regions, which limit the young person's ability to resist these inclinations" (Steinberg et al., 2018). The "reward system" references subcortical structures, while the "self-regulatory regions" refer to areas like the PFC. Proponents of the dual-systems model point to recent findings on sensation seeking and self-regulation from a study of more than 5,000 young people spanning ages 10 to 30 across 11 countries. A similar pattern emerged across these settings. In 7 of 11 countries there was a peak in sensation seeking in mid-to-late adolescence (around age 19) followed by a decline. Additionally, there was a steady rise in self-regulation during adolescence; self-regulation peaked in the mid-20s in four countries and continued to rise in five others. The researchers note that there were more similarities than differences across countries and suggest that the findings provide strong support for a dual-systems account of sensation seeking and self-regulation in adolescence.

A second model, the "imbalance" model, shifts the focus away from an orthogonal, dual systems account and instead emphasizes patterns of change in neural circuitry across adolescence. This fine-tuning of circuits is hypothesized to occur in a cascading fashion, beginning within subcortical regions (such as those within the limbic system), then strengthening across regions, and finally occurring within outer areas of the brain like the PFC (Casey et al., 2016). This model corresponds with observed behavioral and emotional regulation—over time, most adolescents become more goal-oriented and purposeful, and less impulsive (Casey, 2015). Proponents of the imbalance model argue that it emphasizes the "dynamic and hierarchical development of brain circuitry to explain changes in behavior throughout adolescence" (Casey et al., 2016, p. 129). Moreover, they note that research stemming from this model focuses less on studying specific regions of the brain and more on how information flows within and between neural circuits, as well as how this flow of information shifts over the course of development (e.g., "temporal changes in functional connectivity within and between brain circuits," p. 129).

Rethinking the "Mismatch" Between the Emotional and Rational Brain Systems

Regardless of whether one of these two models more accurately represents connections between adolescent neurobiological development and behavior, both perspectives converge on the same point: fundamental areas of the brain undergo asynchronous development throughout adolescence. Moreover, adolescent behavior, especially concerning increased risk-taking and still-developing self-control, has been notably attributed to asynchronous development within and between subcortical and cortical regions of the brain. The former drives emotion, and the latter acts as the control center for long-term planning, consideration of outcomes, and level-headed regulation of behavior (Galván et al., 2006; Galván, 2010; Mueller et al., 2017; Steinbeis and Crone, 2016). Thus, if connections within the limbic system develop faster than those within and between the PFC region,[8] the imbalance may favor a tendency toward heightened sensitivity to peer influence, impulsivity, risk-taking behaviors, and emotional volatility (Casey and Caudle, 2013; Giedd, 2015; Mills et al., 2014).

---

[8] While there may be asynchronous development of circuits within specific regions of the brain during adolescence, this does not mean that these regions are "fixed" by the end of adolescence; instead, people retain the ability for neural plasticity and change throughout the life course (see Chapter 3).

Indeed, adolescents are more impulsive in response to positive incentives than children or adults, although they can suppress these impulses when large rewards are at stake. Adolescents are also more sensitive than children or adults to the presence of peers and to other environmental cues, and show a heightened limbic response to threats (Casey, 2015). As the cortical regions continue to develop and activity within and across brain regions becomes more synchronized, adolescents gain the capacity to make rational, goal-directed decisions across contexts and conditions.

The idea of asynchrony or "mismatch" between the pace of subcortical development and cortical development implies that these developmental capacities are nonoptimal. Yet, even though they are associated with impulsivity and risk-taking, we should not jump to the conclusion that the gap in maturation between the emotion and control centers of the brain is without developmental benefit. As Casey (2015, p. 310) notes, "At first glance, suggesting that a propensity toward motivational or emotional cues during adolescence is adaptive may seem untenable. However, a heightened activation into action by environmental cues and decreased apparent fear of novel environments during this time may facilitate evolutionarily appropriate exploratory behavior." While an adolescent's "heart over mind" mentality may compromise judgment and facilitate unhealthy behaviors, it can also spawn creativity and exploration. Novelty seeking can be a boon to adolescents, spurring them to pursue exciting, new directions in life (Spear, 2013).

If properly monitored and cushioned by parents and the community, adolescents can learn from missteps and take advantage of what can be viewed as developmental *opportunities*. Indeed, because adolescents are more sensitive to rewards and their decision-making ability may skew more toward seeking the positive benefits of a choice and less toward avoiding potential risks, this tendency can enhance learning and drive curiosity (Davidow et al., 2016). To avoid stereotyping all adolescents as "underdeveloped" or "imbalanced," it is important to recognize the nuances in the different types of risk-taking behavior and to counterbalance a focus on negative outcomes by observing the connections between risk-taking and exploration, curiosity, and other attributes of healthy development (Romer et al., 2017).

The "mismatch" model provides one way of understanding adolescents' capacity for self-control and involvement in risky behavior. A better model of adolescent neurobiological development, some argue, is a "lifespan wisdom model," prioritizing the significance of experience on brain maturation that can only be gained through exploration (Romer et al., 2017). Indeed, growing evidence shows that adolescents have a distinctive ability for social and emotional processing that allows them to adapt readily to the capricious social contexts of adolescence, and equips them with flexibility in adjusting their motivations and prioritizing new goals (Crone and Dahl, 2012; Nigg and Nagel, 2016).

Despite differences between neurobiological models, there is agreement that distinctions between adolescent and adult behaviors necessitate policies and opportunities intended to address adolescent-specific issues. With their heightened neurocognitive capacity for change, adolescents are in a place of both great opportunity and vulnerability. Key interventions during this period may be able to ameliorate the impact of negative experiences earlier in life, providing many adolescents with a pivotal second chance to achieve their full potential and lead meaningful, healthy, and successful lives (Guyer et al., 2016; see also Chapter 3).

Cognitive Correlates of Adolescent Brain Development

Reflective of the ongoing changes in the brain described above, most teens become more efficient at processing information, learning, and reasoning over the course of adolescence (Byrnes, 2003; Kuhn, 2006, 2009). The integration of brain regions also facilitates what is called "cognitive control," the ability to think and plan rather than acting impulsively (Casey, 2015; Casey et al., 2016; Steinberg, 2014).

Changes in components of cognitive control, such as response selection/inhibition and goal selection/maintenance, along with closely associated constructs such as working memory, increase an individual's capacity for self-regulation of affect and behavior (Ochsner and Gross, 2005). Importantly, each of these aspects of cognitive control appears to have distinct developmental trajectories, and each may be most prominently associated with distinct underlying regions of the cortex (Crone and Steinbeis, 2017). For example, although the greatest developmental improvements in response inhibition and interference control may be observed prior to adolescence, improvements in flexibility, error monitoring, and working memory are more likely to occur throughout the second decade of life (Crone and Steinbeis, 2017). This suggests different developmental trajectories, whereby more basic, stimulus-driven cognitive control processes develop earlier than do more complex cognitive control processes, which rely on internal and abstract representation (Crone and Steinbeis, 2017; Dumontheil et al., 2008).

Those functions that do continue to show significant developmental change during adolescence seem to especially rely on the capacity for abstract representation, which is a capacity that has been found to undergo a distinctive increase during adolescence (Dumontheil, 2014). The capacity for abstract representation can relate to both temporal and relational processes, that is, to both long-term goals and to past or future events (temporal) and to representing higher-order relationships between representations (relational) as distinct from simple stimulus features (Dumontheil, 2014). From early through late adolescence (into adulthood), this increase in abstract thinking ability makes teens better at using evidence to draw conclusions, although they still have a tendency to generalize based on personal experience—something even adults do. Adolescents also develop greater capacity for strategic problem-solving, deductive reasoning, and information processing, due in part to their ability to reason about ideas that may be abstract or untrue; however, these skills require scaffolding and opportunities for practice (Kuhn, 2009).

Recent research on cognitive development during adolescence has focused on both cognitive and emotional (or "affective") processing, particularly to understand how these processes interact with and influence each other in the context of adolescent decision making. First, the capacity for abstract representation and for affective engagement with such representations (Davey et al., 2008) increases the capacity for self-regulation of emotions in order to achieve a goal (Ochsner and Gross, 2005). Indeed, the capacity to regulate a potent, stimulus-driven, short-term response may rely on the ability to mentally represent and affectively engage with a longer-term goal. Furthermore, such stimulus-driven, affective influences on cognitive processing, including on decision making, risk-taking, and judgment, change significantly over the course of adolescence (Hartley and Somerville, 2015; Steinberg, 2005).

Beyond individual capacities for cognitive regulation, the social and emotional context for cognitive processing matters a great deal. The presence of peers and the value of performing a task influence how motivating certain contexts may be and the extent to which cognitive processing is recruited (Johnson et al., 2009). Moreover, there is increasing evidence that some of these changes in cognitive and affective processing are linked to the onset of puberty (Crone and Dahl, 2012). Researchers have found that adolescents do better than young adults on learning and memory tasks when the reward systems of the brain are engaged (Davidow et al., 2016).

These changes in cognitive functioning may have adaptive qualities as part of normative adolescent development, even though they also make some individuals more vulnerable to psychopathology, such as depression and anxiety disorders. Notably, the flexibility of the frontal cortical network may be greater in adolescence than in adulthood (Jolles and Crone, 2012). Such flexibility may result in an improved ability to learn to navigate the increasingly complex social challenges that are part of adolescents' social worlds, and as adolescents encounter increasing opportunities for autonomy it may prove to be adaptive. In addition, the ability to shift focus in a highly motivated way could allow more learning, problem solving, and use of creativity (Kleibeuker et al., 2016). Of particular relevance, such emerging abilities may also determine the degree to which an individual can take advantage of new learning opportunities, including mental health–promoting interventions. With the right supports, this capacity for flexibility and adaptability can foster deep learning, complex problem-solving skills, and creativity (Crone and Dahl, 2012; Hauser et al., 2015; Kleibeuker et al., 2012).

Summary

The extensive neurobiological changes in adolescence enable us to reimagine this period as one of remarkable opportunity for growth. Connections within and between brain regions become stronger and more efficient, and unused connections are pruned away. Such developmental plasticity means adolescents' brains are adaptive; they become more specialized in response to environmental demands. The timing and location of the dynamic changes are also important to understand. The onset of puberty, often between ages 10 and 12, brings about changes in the limbic system region resulting in increased sensitivity to both rewards and threats, to novelty, and to peers. In contrast, it takes longer for the cortical regions, implicated in cognitive control and self-regulation, to develop (Steinberg et al., 2018).

Adolescent brains are neither simply "advanced" child brains, nor are they "immature" adult brains—they are specially tailored to meet the needs of this stage of life (Giedd, 2015). Indeed, the temporal discrepancy in the specialization of and connections between cortical and subcortical brain regions makes adolescence unique. The developmental changes heighten sensitivity to reward, willingness to take risks, and the salience of social status, propensities that are necessary for exploring new environments and building nonfamilial relationships. Adolescents must explore and take risks to build the cognitive, social, and emotional skills they will need to be productive adults. Moreover, the unique and dynamic patterns of brain development in adolescence foster flexible problem-solving and learning (Crone and Dahl, 2012). Indeed, adolescence is a seminal period for social and motivational learning (Fuligni, 2018), and this flexibility confers opportunity for adaptability and innovation.

While developmental plasticity in adolescence bears many advantages, as with all aspects of development the environment matters a great deal. The malleable brains of adolescents are not only adaptable to innovation and learning but also vulnerable to toxic experiences, such as resource deprivation, harsh, coercive or antisocial relationships, and exposure to drugs or violence. All of these can "get under the skin" as adolescents develop, or more precisely interact with the brain and body to influence development (see Chapter 3).

What is more, the majority of mental illnesses—including psychotic and substance use disorders—begin by age 24 (Casey, 2015; Giedd, 2015).

This means that we have a collective responsibility to ask, "How can we create the kinds of settings and supports needed to optimize development during this period of life?" This goes well beyond simply keeping youth out of harm's way, and instead signals an urgent need to consider how we design the systems with which adolescents engage most frequently to meet their developmental needs. Notably, scholars studying adolescent developmental neuroscience suggest the next generation of research should consider questions that shift from understanding risk to understanding thriving, and context-specific opportunities to promote it. Such questions for the field include, "How does brain development create unique opportunities for learning and problem solving?," "Is the adolescent brain more sensitive to some features of the social environment than others?," and "Are trajectories of change [in cognitive control and emotional processing] steeper or quicker during some periods than others, potentially providing key windows for input and intervention?" (Fuligni et al., 2018, p. 151).

PSYCHOSOCIAL DEVELOPMENT IN ADOLESCENCE

As described above, young people develop increased cognitive abilities throughout adolescence. These cognitive abilities provide the capacity for other aspects of psychosocial development that occur during the period. This section describes the psychosocial developmental tasks—including developing identity and a capacity for self-direction—that adolescents complete during their transition to adulthood. Understanding one's self, understanding one's place in the world, and understanding one's capacity to affect the world (i.e., agency) are all processes that begin to take shape during adolescence in tandem with the physiological, neurobiological, and cognitive changes discussed above.

The trajectory of social and emotional development in adolescence may perhaps be best characterized as a time of increasing complexity and integration. As is true of their neurobiological development during the period, adolescents' capacity for understanding and engaging with self, others, and societal institutions requires both integration and deepening. It requires adolescents to integrate multiple perspectives and experiences across contexts, and also to deepen their ability to make sense of complex and abstract phenomena.

This section begins with a summary of developmental trends in adolescent self- and identity development at a broad level, followed by a brief discussion of how these trends reflect recent findings from developmental neuroscience. From there, we discuss group-specific social identities. While there are many critical dimensions of social identity (e.g., gender, social class, religion, immigration status, disability, and others), we use race and sexuality as exemplars given the recent, monumental shifts in racial/ethnic demographics and in the social and political climate around sexual minority status in the United States. The focus on race and sexuality is not intended to minimize other dimensions of identity; indeed, identity development is a salient process for all adolescents regardless of social group memberships. Moreover, as we discuss below, developmental scientists are increasingly calling for research that examines the *intersectional* nature of identities, both at the individual level as well as in ways that reflect membership in multiple groups that have historically experienced marginalization (Santos and Toomey, 2018).

Identity

Finding an answer to the question, "Who am I?" is often viewed as a central task of adolescence. Decades ago, Erik Erikson (1968) argued that during adolescence, youth take on the challenge of developing a coherent, integrated, and stable sense of themselves, and that failing to do so may make the transition to adult roles and responsibilities more difficult. Erikson's concept of identity development assumes opportunities for exploration and choice and may or may not generalize across global contexts (Arnett, 2015; Syed, 2017). However, it has utility in the United States, where societal structures and dominant values such as independence and individuality encourage identity exploration.

Closely related to the question, "Who am I?" is the question, "*How do I see myself?*" (Harter, 2012). McAdams (2013) describes the developmental trajectory of "self" using a set of sequential metaphors: the "social actor" in childhood (because children engage in action) grows to become a "motivated agent" in adolescence (because teens are more purposeful and agent-driven, guided by values, motives, and hopes), and finally an "autobiographical author" in emerging adulthood, a time when young people work on building a coherent self-narrative. Studies of youth across the span of adolescence show that, for many young people, the sense of self and identity become more integrated, coherent, and stable over time (Harter, 2012; Klimstra et al., 2010; Meeus et al., 2010). Importantly, theory suggests and empirical evidence supports the idea that having a more "achieved" identity and integrated sense of self relates to positive well-being in adulthood and even throughout the life course (e.g., Kroger and Marcia, 2011; Meca et al., 2015; Schwartz et al., 2011).

While there is great variability across youth, there are also some distinct developmental trends in the emergence of self and identity. In early adolescence, young teens' self-definitions are increasingly differentiated relative to childhood. They see themselves in multiple ways across various social and relational contexts, for example one way when with their family and another way when with close friends in the classroom. Although a young adolescent may carry a great number of "abstractions" about his or her self, these labels tend to be fragmented and sometimes even contradictory (Harter, 2012). For instance, a 13-year-old may view herself as shy and quiet in the classroom, as loud and bubbly with close friends, and as bossy and controlling with her younger siblings. Longitudinal studies suggest that some perceptions of self (e.g., academic self-concept) decline in early adolescence as youth transition to middle school; however, there is a great deal of individual variability, variability across domains (e.g., academic vs. behavioral self-concept), and variability by gender (higher athletic self-concept among males vs. females; Cole et al., 2001; Gentile et al., 2009).

In middle adolescence, teens may still hold onto multiple and disjointed abstractions of themselves; however, their growing cognitive abilities allow for more frequent comparisons among the inconsistencies, and heightened awareness of these contradictions can create some stress (Brummelman and Thomaes, 2017; Harter, 2012). In this period, youth may also be more aware that their conflicting self-characterizations tend to occur most often across different relationship contexts. As in early adolescence, discrepancies between real and ideal selves can create stress for some youth, but as teens develop deeper meta-cognitive and self-reflection skills, they are better able to manage the discrepancies. To continue with the same hypothetical teen introduced above at age 13, at age 16 she might view being shy and quiet in the classroom and loud and bubbly with friends as parts of a more holistic, less fragmented sense of self.

Older adolescents have greater abilities to make sense of their multiple abstractions about self. They can reconcile what seem like contradictory behaviors by understanding them in context (Harter, 2012). For instance, older teens are more likely to view their different patterns of behavior across settings as reflecting a positive trait like "flexibility," or they may characterize themselves as "moody" if they vacillate between positive and negative emotions in different situations. While peers are still important in late adolescence, youth may rely on them less when making self-evaluations; they also have greater capacity for perspective-taking and attunement to others, especially in the context of supportive relationships.

Emerging adulthood provides additional opportunities for experimenting with vocational options, forming new friendships and romantic relationships, and exercising more independent decision-making (Arnett, 2015; Harter, 2012; Schwartz et al., 2005). Many young adults shift from "grand" visions of possible selves to visions that are narrower and directly related to immediate opportunities. New experiences across contexts—like attending college or transitioning into the workforce—can shape whether emerging adults develop an authentic and integrated sense of self.

With the normative development of heightened sensitivity to social information, some youth may rely heavily on peer feedback in self-evaluation;

however, parents still play an important role in supporting a positive sense of self, especially when they are attuned to youths' needs and couple their high expectations with support (Harter, 2012). Indeed, secure and supportive relationships with parents can help early and middle adolescents develop a clear sense of self (Becht et al., 2017) and can buffer youth who are socially anxious against harsh self-criticism (Peter and Gazelle, 2017).

Identity and Self: A Neurobiological Perspective

Recent advances in developmental neuroscience appear to complement decades of behavioral research on youth. For instance, the integrated-circuitry model of adolescent brain development discussed in the previous section (Casey et al., 2016), along with other models emphasizing the growing integration within and between emotionally sensitive brain regions (e.g., the limbic system) and those involved in planning and decision making (e.g., the cortical regions), correspond with the observation that adolescents develop a more coherent sense of self over time and experience. Likewise, changes observed in social and affective regions of the brain during adolescence align with behavioral tendencies toward exploration and trying new things (Crone and Dahl, 2012; Flannery et al., 2018). Although the evidence base is still growing, recent studies document how self-evaluation and relational identity processes are linked with regions of the brain like the ventromedial PFC (vmPFC) (which plays a role in the inhibition of emotional responses, in decision making, and in self-control) and the rostral/perigenual anterior cingulate cortex (which plays a role in error and conflict detection processes). In particular, activity in these regions increases from childhood through adolescence in a manner consistent with changes in identity development (Pfeifer and Berkman, 2018).

Recent theoretical models of value-based decision making suggest specific ways in which identity development and neural development are linked in adolescence (Berkman et al., 2017; Pfeifer and Berkman, 2018). An important premise is that while adolescents may be more sensitive to social stimuli such as peer norms and to rewarding outcomes such as tangible gains, their sense of self is still a critical factor influencing their behavior. In other words, while social norms and tangible gains and costs represent some of the "value inputs," their construal of self and identity are also factors in their decision making. Moreover, neural evidence, like the activation observed in the vmPFC during self- and relational identity tasks, suggests that identity and self-related processes may play a greater role in value-based decision making during adolescence than they do in childhood (Pfeifer and Berkman, 2018).

Social Identities in Adolescence

As many youth work toward building a cohesive, integrated answer to the question, "Who am I?," the answer itself is shaped by membership across multiple social identity groups: race, ethnicity, nationality, sexuality, gender, religion, political affiliation, ability status, and more. Indeed, in the context of increasingly complex cognitive abilities and social demands, youth may be more likely to contest, negotiate, elaborate upon, and internalize the meaning of membership in racial/ethnic, gender, sexual, and other social identity groups (e.g., Umaña-Taylor et al., 2014). From a developmental perspective, these tasks are paramount in a pluralistic, multiethnic and multicultural society like the United States, which, as discussed in Chapter 1, is more diverse now than in previous generations.

Ethnic-Racial Identity. Currently, our nation's population of adolescents is continuing to increase in diversity, with no single racial or ethnic group in the majority. A burgeoning area of study over the past two decades concerns ethnic-racial identity (ERI), and research in this field has found that for most youth, particularly adolescents of color, ERI exploration, centrality, and group pride are positively related to psychosocial, academic, and even health outcomes (Rivas-Drake et al., 2014). ERI is multidimensional—it includes youths' beliefs about their group and how their race or ethnicity relate to their self-definition—both of which may change over time (Umaña-Taylor et al., 2014). For immigrant youth, developing their own ERI may involve an internal negotiation between their culture of origin and that of their new host country, and most immigrant youth show a great deal of flexibility in redefining their new identity (Fuligni and Tsai, 2015). Regardless of country of origin, making sense of one's ERI is a normative developmental process that often begins in adolescence (Williams et al., 2012). Indeed, given that research has consistently found ERI to be associated with adaptive outcomes, dimensions of ERI can be understood as components of positive youth development (Williams et al., 2014).

Sexual Orientation and Gender Identity. One of the distinctive aspects of adolescence is the emergence and awareness of sexuality, and a related aspect is the emerging salience of gender roles and expression. Adolescence is also a time when identities or sense of self related to gender and sexuality are developed and solidified (Tolman, 2011), and this occurs in a period during which sexuality and gender norms are learned and regulated by peers (Galambos et al., 1990). In this developmental context, LGBTQ youth begin to understand their sexual and gender identities.

The growing societal acceptance and legal recognition of LGBTQ youth is implicated in the recent observed drop in the age at which most of these young people "come out," that is, disclose their same-sex sexual identities. Less than a generation ago, LGBTQ people in the United States typically came out as young adults in their 20s; today the average age at coming out appears to be around 14, according to several independent studies (Russell and Fish, 2017).

In the context of such changes and growing acceptance and support for LGBTQ youth developing their sexual identity, it might be expected that the longstanding health and behavior disparities between these adolescents and heterosexual and cis-gender adolescents would be lessening. Yet multiple recent studies challenge that conclusion. Things do not appear to be getting "better" for LGBTQ youth: rather than diminishing, health disparities across multiple domains appear to be stable if not widening (Russell and Fish, 2017). This pattern may be explained by several factors, including greater visibility and associated stigma and victimization for LGBTQ youth, just at the developmental period during which youth engage in more peer regulation and bullying in general, especially regarding sexuality and gender (Poteat and Russell, 2013). In fact, a meta-analysis of studies of homophobic bullying in schools showed higher levels of homophobic bullying in more recent studies (Toomey and Russell, 2016). These patterns point to the importance of policies and programs that help schools, communities, and families understand and support LGBTQ (and all) youth (see Chapter 7).

Identity Complexity. Beyond race, gender, or sexuality alone, having a strong connection to *some* dimension of social identity—which could also be cultural, religious, or national—appears to be important for psychological well-being in adolescence (Kiang et al., 2008). Recent research also suggests that young adolescents benefit from having a more complex, multi-faceted identity that goes beyond stereotypical expectations of social-group norms, especially when it comes to inclusive beliefs (Knifsend and Juvonen, 2013). For instance, a youth who identifies as a Black, 13-year-old, transgender female who plays volleyball and loves gaming is apt to have more positive attitudes toward other racial/ethnic groups than she would if she viewed racial/ethnic identity and other social identities as necessarily convergent (such as the notion that "playing volleyball and being a gamer are activities restricted to youth from specific racial/ethnic groups"; Knifsend and Juvonen, 2014).

However, context is still important, and the association between identity complexity and inclusive beliefs in early adolescence tends to be stronger for youth who have a diverse group of friends (Knifsend and Juvonen, 2014). Among college-age students there is also variation by race and ethnicity. For instance, the positive association between having a complex social identity and holding more inclusive attitudes toward others has been found most consistently among students who are members of the racial/ethnic majority; for members of racial/ethnic minority groups, convergence between racial/ethnic identity and other in-group identities is not related to attitudes toward other racial/ethnic groups (Brewer et al., 2013). Beyond outgroup attitudes, there is evidence that social identity complexity has implications for youths' own perceptions of belonging; for instance, Muslim immigrant adolescents (ages 15 to 18) with greater identity complexity reported a stronger sense of identification with their host country (Verkuyten and Martinovic, 2012).

Social Identity and Neurobiology

Cultural neuroscience provides some insight into how social identity development may manifest at the neurobiological level, although there is still much work to be done to understand the deep associations between biology and culture (Mrazek et al., 2015). In adolescence, evidence suggests, areas of the brain attuned to social information may be undergoing shifts that heighten youths' social sensitivity (Blakemore and Mills, 2014), and of course, adolescents' "social brains" develop in a cultural context. For instance, we know the amygdala responds to stimuli with heightened emotional significance; in the United States, where negative stereotypes about Blacks contribute to implicit biases and fears about them, amygdala sensitivity to Black faces has been documented in adult samples (Cunningham et al., 2004; Lieberman et al., 2005; Phelps et al., 2000).

In a study of children and adolescents (ages 4 to 16) in the United States, Telzer and colleagues (2013) found that amygdala activation in response to racial stimuli, such as images of Black faces, was greater in adolescence than during childhood. They suggest that identity processes reflecting heightened sensitivity to race, along with biological changes (e.g., those stemming from puberty) related to a "social reorientation" of the amygdala, may be among the mechanisms that explain these race-sensitive patterns of activation in adolescence (Telzer et al., 2013). Importantly, neural activation appears to vary based on the context of social experiences. Specifically, the amygdala activation observed in response to Black faces was attenuated for youth who had more friends and schoolmates of a race differing from their own (i.e., cross-race friends).

The foregoing findings converge with psychobehavioral studies that demonstrate the importance of school and friendship diversity. Attending diverse middle schools and having more cross-race friends is associated with more positive attitudes toward outsider groups, less social vulnerability, greater social and academic competence, and better mental health (Graham, 2018; Williams and Hamm, 2017). Adolescence is a period of transformation in social cognition (Blakemore and Mills, 2014; Giedd, 2015), so in

light of the findings from psychobehavioral and cultural neuroscience research on the benefits of diversity, important questions may be asked about
whether adolescence is a critical period for providing exposure to difference. For instance, should we expect the benefits of exposure to diversity to
be maximized if such exposure occurs during adolescence, or are benefits
most likely with cumulative exposure that begins well before this period?[9]

Identity Development in Context

Identity development takes place in specific socio-cultural, political, and
historical contexts. As an example, consider recent cultural and political
shifts regarding same-sex relationships in the United States: in the period
of one generation there has been dramatic social change regarding understanding and awareness of LGBTQ lives and issues. For context, consider
that less than 20 years ago, marriage between same-sex couples was just
beginning to be recognized anywhere in the world (the first country to do
so was the Netherlands in 2001); less than 20 years later, 25 countries have
legalized same-sex marriage, and recent surveys show that most young
people in the United States approve of same-sex marriages (Pew Research
Center, 2015). Moreover, the identity language and labels used among
youth who are often placed under the umbrella of LGBTQ have continued
to rapidly evolve. A growing number of LGBTQ youth say they have a
nonbinary gender identity (i.e., neither male nor female) or sexual identity
(e.g., pansexual, bisexual, queer) (Hammack, 2018). Indeed, young people
appear to be leading a movement toward challenging existing categories
and constructing new identities.

Meanwhile, in the past decade there has been a dramatic change in public awareness and understanding of transgender identities. Popular attention
to the gender changes of a number of celebrities coincided with growing
emergence and awareness of transgender children.[10] Thus, a subject that
was literally unknown by most people in the United States has within a
decade become the subject of public discussion and political debate. School
systems are grappling with gender change and accommodations for transgender students, and the typical developmental challenges of adolescence
are being navigated by a growing number of openly transgender, gender-
nonbinary, or gender-nonconforming adolescents (Wilson et al, 2017).

---

[9] For instance, rodent models suggest that empathy is shaped by social context (e.g., rats
usually assist members of their own genetic strain, but will extend their prosocial behavior to
unrelated peers if they are raised together; Bartal et al., 2011; Meyza et al., 2017).

[10] See, for example, "Beyond 'He' or 'She': The Changing Meaning of Gender and Sexuality,"
TIME Magazine, March 16, 2017.

Developmental scientists have recently called for a deeper investigation of the ways in which intersecting axes of oppression shape youth development, often referred to as "intersectionality" (Crenshaw, 1990; Santos and Toomey, 2018; Velez and Spencer, 2018). Indeed, against a backdrop of social stratification and oppression, relationships between identity, experience, and behavior may not operate the same way for all youth (Spencer, 1995). For example, the way in which knowledge is socially constructed contributes to maintaining systems and structures that control and exclude marginalized populations such as people with disabilities (Peña et al., 2016). Smart and Smart (2007) argue that society has historically viewed people with disabilities from a medical perspective, in which individuals were labeled as ill, dysfunctional, and in need of medical treatment. This approach perpetuates an ableist worldview that suggests people with disabilities should strive toward an able-bodied norm, reflecting society's perceptions that certain abilities are essential to fully function in the world (Hutcheon and Wolbring, 2012). This example highlights why an intersectional perspective is important for understanding adolescent psychosocial development in context, both for considering systemic factors that shape opportunities and for broadening the range of questions, values, samples, and experiences that have been defined and studied from a dominant-group perspective (Syed et al., 2018). Ultimately, intersectional approaches and related integrative models are needed to understand how youth development in context can lead to further marginalization for some youth (Causadias and Umaña-Taylor, 2018) or to adaptability and resilience for others (Gaylord-Harden et al., 2018; Suárez-Orozco et al., 2018).

Summary

We have long considered identity exploration as a hallmark of adolescence. An adolescent's identity is an emerging reflection of his or her values, beliefs, and aspirations, and it can be constructed and reconstructed over time and experience. Multiple factors—family, culture, peers, media—shape identity development, but young people are also active agents in the process. Movement toward stability and coherence is normative, yet there remain dynamic elements that shape the relationship between identity and behavior; teens often select activities that feel identity-congruent, and may interpret and respond to a given situation based on aspects of identity that are salient in the moment (Oyserman, 2015; Oyserman and Destin, 2010). This has implications for adolescents' experiences in important contexts such as school. Identity processes are connected to a larger set of self-development characteristics, including self-regulation, self-efficacy, and a sense of agency, all of which youth need to help develop and commit to meaningful goals. Ensuring that adolescents understand how all identities can be consistent with their current academic choices and future educational and vocational aspirations is an important consideration for the education system and is discussed further in Chapter 6.

Recent neuroscientific findings suggest that changes in social and affective regions of the brain correspond to developmental changes in identity development. Moreover, identity and self-related processes may play a greater role in decision making during adolescence than they do in childhood. Youth may also experience identity congruence, affirmation, or marginalization through their interpersonal interactions with policies, sociopolitical events, and historical factors. Ultimately, how adolescents' multifaceted identities are manifested—neurobiologically, behaviorally, and otherwise—and the role identity plays in their overall well-being depend a great deal on experiences in context. This requires us to reflect on the nature of the contexts in which adolescents are developing their identities.

Consider, for example, that a youth's likelihood of involvement in extremist organizations may be heightened as they search for meaningful in-groups, if they accept group beliefs without questioning them (i.e., identity foreclosure), and/or if they feel their personal or group identities are under threat (Dean, 2017; Schwartz et al., 2009). As Schwartz and colleagues note, "providing mainstream paths for young people, within the cultural constraints of their society, can help to alleviate the anger, frustration, and hopelessness leading many young people [towards extremism]" (Schwartz et al., 2009, p. 553). While the overwhelming majority of adolescents do not become involved in extremist groups, acknowledging this possibility underscores how the significant opportunities afforded by identity exploration in adolescence can be thwarted by conditions that increase the likelihood of marginalization.

Adolescent Capacity for Self-Direction

As adolescents ask, "Who am I?" their growing cognitive capacities also permit reflection on themselves in relation to a broader collective: "What is my role in my school? my community? my society?" As adolescents grow older, they have more opportunities to make their own choices in domains that matter for future outcomes, and their capacity to make such choices also increases; Box 2-1 describes youths' perspectives on this emerging autonomy, agency, and independence.

In the following section, we discuss developmental changes in autonomy, purpose, and agency in adolescence. One might think of these three things not only as competencies that develop within adolescents, but also as resources or opportunities they need to thrive as they transition into adult roles. Framing them as *both* capacities of the individual youth *and* as characteristics

BOX 2-1
Youth Perspectives: Sense of Agency, Purpose, and Autonomy

During adolescence, young people begin to develop autonomy, agency, and independence. When adolescent respondents age 16 to 24 were asked in a recent MyVoice poll about their perceptions of adolescence, respondents overwhelmingly spoke about this time as a period of opportunity and excitement, but with associated stressors and anxieties related to growing responsibilities and independence. (See Appendix B for a description of MyVoice and its methodology.)

"It's been exciting learning about all the things I can do with myself and preparing my life being fully independent. I can start to see my future shaping up which is cool."—21-year-old, Asian, female

"I feel that I have been able to start thinking about what I'm really passionate about and start cultivating skills that benefit those passions. It's exciting to start finding myself and see what may be the future." —17-year-old, White, female

"I have fully come to terms with what I want to do in my life and with my sexuality."—16-year-old, Black, female

"Building a stronger bond with my family and friends and learning that you have to keep pushing forward even through the hard times." —18-year-old, Hispanic, male

Many of the adolescents polled acknowledged feeling fearful about their new autonomy and independence. Lack of support, lack of knowledge of how to become an "adult," and stressors related to developing identity, relationships, increased responsibilities, and financial concerns were prominent themes.

"Stressful. You can never be quite sure what decisions to make, and if they're even the right choice." —17-year-old, White, female

"It's been rough. Becoming financially responsible was tough to learn and it took me years to finally spend and save money responsibly." —23-year-old, Hispanic, female

"Stressful because you just get thrown off the deep end." —17-year-old, Asian, male

"Very STRESSFUL. I am learning how to become an adult and it is hard, college is two years away from me and I am not ready. I am too scared to be on my own." —16-year-old, Hispanic, male

"Increasingly difficult. I have social anxiety which has made it especially hard for me to get a job and even get my driver's license. I've yet to do either thing."—19-year-old, White, male

SOURCE: Information from MyVoice, 2019.

afforded by supportive settings reminds us that developmental pathways that lead to thriving in adulthood are not forged by adolescents alone, but instead require alignment between youths' strengths and the resources available in their environments.

Striving for Autonomy While Remaining Connected

For most adolescents, establishing a level of independence and self-sufficiency is normative. This typically involves individuating from one's family. However, gaining a sense of autonomy does not mean that adolescents strive to become detached from their family. Indeed, the developmental task for most teens is about establishing a balance between autonomy and connection (McElhaney et al., 2009). While many adolescents would like more autonomy for making decisions, this varies by age and domain (Daddis, 2011; Smetana, 2011). Most youth report having enough autonomy when it comes to making moral decisions, but younger adolescents tend to desire more autonomy for personal matters (e.g., hairstyle and clothing choices) and conventional matters (e.g., cursing/swearing) than older teens. This increase in desired autonomy among younger teens maps onto findings that older teens report having more autonomy across multiple domains than their younger peers.

Not only do young adolescents have less autonomy than older youth, they also tend to overestimate how much autonomy their peers have; in other words, younger adolescents tend to think their friends are allowed to have more control over their choices and behaviors than they actually do. Adolescents who think they have low levels of autonomy over decisions also tend to believe their friends have more autonomy, whereas adolescents who feel they have enough autonomy are less influenced by perceptions of their peers (Daddis, 2011).

Autonomy and Culture

The concept of "autonomy" implies independence, which generally is accepted as a core value among cultures oriented toward individualism. In contrast, one might expect youth from cultures oriented toward collectivism and interdependence to be more inclined toward harmonious, less conflictual relationships with parents and a lower desire for individuation. However, evidence suggests that teens in many cultures, both those labeled "individualist" and those labeled "collectivist," strive to develop autonomy, and levels of parent-teen conflict are similar in immigrant and nonimmigrant families (Fuligni and Tsai, 2015; Tsai et al., 2012). Studies of youth from multiple ethnic backgrounds in the United States, including those who are U.S.-born and those from immigrant families, show that most adolescents express a desire to have control over personal choices (Phinney et al., 2005). Importantly, while youth across cultural backgrounds identify autonomy as important, there can be culturally relevant variations in how autonomy is defined. For example, some adolescents from Asian American heritage groups describe autonomy through the lens of "interdependence" (Russell et al., 2010).

Examining Autonomy and Culture "Under the Skin"

While all teens may desire autonomy from their parents and seek identities and self-definitions that go beyond their role in the family, adolescents in immigrant families in the United States may have a stronger sense of family obligation relative to youth in nonimmigrant families. Recent findings from the field of cultural neuroscience demonstrate the integration between biology and sociocultural context (Telzer et al., 2010; Fuligni and Telzer, 2013). In one study, White and Latinx older adolescents participated in laboratory-based tasks in which they were asked to allot cash rewards to themselves or to their families; during the task their patterns of brain activity were observed using functional magnetic resonance imaging (fMRI). While youth from both groups allotted cash rewards to family at the same rate, among Latinx youth the "reward centers" of the brain were more activated when they contributed to family, whereas White youth showed more brain activity in the reward centers when allotting cash to themselves. Across both groups, those who felt a stronger sense of family identification and who felt fulfilled by contributing to family had more activation in the reward centers of the brain when allotting cash to their family. Thus, the cultural meaning that youth and families make around issues of autonomy, connection, and obligation are connected to neurobiological responses in the context of family contribution.

Some studies show linkages between broad cultural orientations, such as being more individually or more collectively oriented, and patterns of neural response (Mrazek et al., 2015). Moreover, cultural neuroscientists posit that developmental growth and transitions in neural activity shape the transmission of cultural values, like preference for social hierarchy (Mrazek et al., 2015). In addition to the vmPFC and the anterior cingulate cortex regions of the brain implicated in personal identity development, researchers speculate that the temporoparietal junction may be implicated in culturally embedded identities that orient youth toward independence or interdependence (Cheon et al., 2011; Mrazek et al., 2015; Saxe et al., 2009).

Finding Meaning and Taking Action: Purpose and Agency

Purpose

Purpose has been defined as "a stable and generalized intention to accomplish something that is at once meaningful to the self and of consequence to the world beyond the self" (Damon et al., 2003, p. 121) and also as "a central, self-organizing life aim that organizes and stimulates goals, manages behaviors, and provides a sense of meaning" (McKnight and Kashdan, 2009, p. 242). Thus, one's sense of purpose can be oriented toward life aims that are self-focused or toward aims that transcend the self (Sumner et al., 2018; Yeager et al., 2012). Higher scores on measures of purpose are generally associated with more positive psychological well-being, a more consolidated identity, a deeper sense of meaning, and fewer health-compromising behaviors; a sense of purpose is also positively correlated with religiosity and spirituality (Burrow and Hill, 2011; Sumner et al., 2018). Moreover, there is evidence that purpose helps explain associations between identity commitment and positive youth adjustment (Burrow and Hill, 2011).

For all adolescents, developing a sense of purpose requires some support, particularly while their sense of orientation toward the future is still under development (Steinberg et al., 2009). For adolescents who experience marginalization—by virtue of membership in one or more groups that experience systemic oppression (García Coll et al., 1996; Causadias and Umaña-Taylor, 2018)—developing a sense of purpose may be compromised if structural discrimination makes links between present action and future outcomes unpredictable (e.g., for adolescents with an undocumented immigration status) (Gonzales, 2016; Sumner et al., 2018). Adolescents experiencing marginalization may internalize such messages as they become more aware of their own external realities; the messages may also be reinforced through family socialization practices. For example, researchers studying low-income White adolescents suggest that parents' messages of "isolation and threat, helplessness and hopelessness, and live fast, die young," which may be adaptive in the short-term and in the immediate settings where the families live, can compromise youth's sense of purpose, hope, and agency (Jones et al., 2018).

Agency to Take Action

Adolescents' growing competencies in flexible problem-solving, their awareness of and concern with others, and their openness to exploration and novelty (Crone and Dahl, 2012) make adolescence a particularly opportune time to allow for agency and leadership (Flanagan and Christens,

2011). Indeed, young people have been at the helm of social movements for centuries. For some youth, active civic engagement may be an adaptive means for coping with systemic injustice, particularly for those in histori- cally marginalized communities (Diemer and Rapa, 2016; Ginwright et al., 2006; Hope and Spencer, 2017). In a recent multi-methods study of middle and late adolescents in seven community organizations (four in the United States, two in Ireland, and one in South Africa), many of which served low-income or working class communities, researchers documented mul- tiple benefits of civic engagement. Findings suggest the context of youth organizing promoted the skills of critical thinking and analysis, social and emotional learning, and involvement in community leadership and action (Watts, 2018; Watts et al., 2011).

In relation to research on community leadership and action, recent work has examined the construct of "critical consciousness" among ado- lescents (Watts et al., 2011). Contemporary definitions of critical conscious- ness, grounded in the work of Brazilian educator Paolo Freire (1970), include the elements of critical reflection, motivation, and action (Diemer et al., 2015). These core concepts have informed the development of new mea- sures of critical consciousness for middle and late adolescents (e.g., Diemer et al., 2017; McWhirter and McWhirter, 2016; Thomas et al., 2014). Youth with higher levels of critical consciousness are more likely to recognize injustice and may feel a greater sense of agency or efficacy in responding to it (Diemer and Rapa, 2016; Shedd, 2015). Critical consciousness is also positively associated with vocational and educational attainment (Diemer et al., 2010; Luginbuhl et al., 2016; McWhirter and McWhirter, 2016).

Capacity for Self-Direction as a Developmental Opportunity

While there is general agreement about the benefits of purpose and agency in adolescence, ongoing work is needed to better understand the circumstances under which they are best fostered and the way they relate to other processes (e.g., critical consciousness) and to behavior (e.g., volun- teering, social activism). For instance, do opportunities for critical reflection contribute to an adolescent's sense of purpose? Are community service or civic action necessary for building an adolescents' belief in their own agency to create change?

Additional research might determine whether a sense of purpose that transcends the self has greater positive impact on an adolescent than one that is more self-focused. Current work in this area suggests that a self- transcendent sense of purpose better predicts academic regulation, perfor- mance, and persistence among high school students (Yeager et al., 2014); however, whether this extends beyond the school context is unclear. As research methods and methods in studies of critical consciousness continue to advance (e.g., Diemer et al., 2015), we may have a better understanding of how this particular kind of agency develops across adolescence, and for whom and under what conditions greater critical consciousness is most beneficial. Finally, an emerging body of work on adolescents' contribution mindset (i.e., giving to others; Fuligni and Telzer, 2013) and value-based decision making (Pfeifer and Berkman, 2018) may provide some insight into the neurobiological correlates underlying the cognitive and social skills needed for developing purpose.

Summary

Over the course of adolescence, youth gain the cognitive skills needed to reflect on complex questions about their aims in life and their role in the world. They can question the legitimacy and fairness of everyday experiences and of social institutions. Indeed, the social systems they must navigate—schools, employment, health care, justice—are quite complex and often require them to engage in independent decision making. Two important questions stemming from this reality are, "What experiences are needed to support adolescents' agency as they transition into adult roles?" and "What might our society look like if all adolescents felt a sense of commitment to something personally meaningful and goal-directed that extends beyond the self?" (Bronk, 2014).

Supporting opportunities for autonomy and agency and fostering a sense of purpose may help adolescents explore meaningful questions about who they are, and about their place in the world and their capacity to shape it. Continuing shifts in the social, cultural, economic, and technological contexts in which today's adolescents are developing require thoughtful consideration as to how, when, and where adolescents can find and act upon ideas and issues they find meaningful. For example, religion has traditionally been a context where youth have found purpose and meaning, and religious involvement is associated with civic engagement (Furrow et al., 2004; Pew Research Center, 2019; Sumner et al., 2018). Religion can also be protective against stressors like discrimination and against negative mental health outcomes (Hope et al., 2017). However, adolescents and young adults today are less likely to be religiously engaged than those in earlier generations (Pew Research Center, 2018). If faith-based institutions are playing a less central role in the lives of greater numbers of today's adolescents, this brings to the fore questions about the alternative settings and experiences to which youth are turning and whether these settings play a comparable role in fostering involvement and purpose.

Although there is great variation in how the skills of autonomy, purpose, and agency manifest and how they are defined and valued, adolescents should be afforded opportunities—in families, schools, or out-of-school settings—to develop them. Such skills not only are important to support the transition to adulthood, but also make adolescence itself a period that fosters a propensity to choose their own paths in life and to shape the roles they want to play in their communities (Fuligni, 2018).

CONCLUSION

Adolescence, spanning the period from the onset of puberty to adulthood, is a formative period where changes in cognition, affect, and interpersonal behavior occur alongside the most extensive biological transitions since infancy, especially with respect to pubertal and brain development. Collectively, the pubertal, neurobiological, cognitive, and psychosocial changes occurring during adolescence mark this as a period of great opportunity for adolescents to flourish and thrive.

While often thought of as a time of turmoil and risk for young people, adolescence is more accurately viewed as a developmental period rich with opportunity for youth to learn and grow. If provided with the proper supports and protection, normal processes of growth and maturation can lead youth to form healthy relationships with their peers and families, develop a sense of identity and self, and experience enriching and memorable engagements with the world. Adolescence thus forms a critical bridge between childhood and adulthood and is a critical window of opportunity for positive, life-altering development. As a positive window of opportunity, adolescence marks a period of optimism, where the assets of youth and their development may be capitalized for the betterment of society.

Important questions emerge from these findings. What are the "windows of opportunity" for promoting a positive developmental trajectory and adaptive plasticity? What are the mechanisms that shape developmental trajectories, for better or worse, during adolescence and over the life course? To begin to answer these, in the next chapter we consider the emerging science of epigenetics as it reveals the ongoing plasticity of the brain and the reciprocal influences of brain on body and vice versa.

3

How Environment
"Gets Under the Skin":
The Continuous Interplay
Between Biology and Environment

Nearly 20 years ago, the National Research Council published a landmark study on early childhood development, *From Neurons to Neighborhoods: The Science of Early Childhood Development* (National Research Council and Institute of Medicine, 2000). At a time when public discussion of child development was dominated by the question, "What is more important—nature or nurture?", the report concluded that the nature vs. nurture debate was "overly simplistic and scientifically obsolete" (p. 6). The report emphasized that there is a continuous and adaptive interaction between biology and environment from the moment of birth and through the early childhood years. Research in the years following the report has continued to demonstrate the powerful and lasting effects of in-utero, preconception, and transgenerational influences on child development (Bohacek and Mansuy, 2015; Dias and Ressler, 2014; Entringer et al., 2015).

Since the publication of *Neurons to Neighborhoods,* several scientific advances have furthered our understanding of the interaction between biology and environment. Chief among these is the emergence of the science of *epigenetics*, which synthesizes research findings from the social and biological sciences to understand the seamless and ongoing interaction between genes and the environment, with particular interest in cataloging the numerous environmental mechanisms comprising the nongenetic influences of gene expression. In this context, "environment" encompasses all exposures or influences that can affect well-being or increase or limit opportunity, such as supportive parenting and stress.

Central to the epigenetic approach is the life-course perspective, which has long been employed in both the social sciences and epidemiology to analyze demographic and social change. It starts from the position that an individual's current circumstances are at least partly a consequence of events and experiences that occurred earlier in the individual's life. The epigenetic approach embraces a "trajectory" model of the life course, which posits that the trajectory of an individual's life may be changed, negatively or positively, at each life stage (Halfon et al., 2014). The future condition of the brain and body will be affected by events that have changed the trajectory in the past and possibly by further interventions undertaken in the present.

An important feature of the trajectory model is that for much of the life course, trajectories of a person's brain circuits and body systems show *plasticity*, meaning they can be altered for better or worse. If they are positively altered, enrichment can occur with life-long benefits, and similarly, if deficits or injuries have previously occurred, the person can experience resilience and recovery through compensatory mechanisms. It is well known that early childhood comprises a period of high plasticity, when young children's brains and bodies are rapidly developing and are particularly sensitive to environmental influences. But recent scientific advances have increased our understanding of the life course such that, as described in Chapter 2, it is now clear adolescence is also a time when considerable change is possible. Adolescents exhibit heightened brain plasticity, making adolescence a sensitive period of development during which life-course trajectories can be changed for better or for worse.

Because of the interactions between the brain, the body, and the environment and the plasticity of the adolescent brain, interventions to change developmental trajectories may be particularly effective during adolescence. A healthy, or flourishing, adolescent brain is plastic and resilient and thus receptive to both individual- and societal-level influences and interventions that promote positive adaptation. By the same token, however, harmful or unhealthy influences on the brain and body can shift the trajectory for the worse.

This chapter discusses key findings from the emergent field of epigenetics that are of particular relevance to adolescence. It examines the reciprocal interactions between the brain, the body, and the environment during the adolescent period, with a focus on toxic stress and early life adversities, and reviews promising interventions for mediating and mitigating early developmental challenges in order to change trajectories.

UNDERSTANDING EPIGENETICS

Epigenetics refers to the environmental influences that shape the individual, resulting in different developmental outcomes even among individuals with the same genome (Freund et al., 2013). Advances in epigenetics have furthered our understanding of the interplay between genes and the environment, underscoring how the influences of genetics and environment on an individual's health and development are inseparable. Contrary to the traditional view that heredity is unchanging, current studies of gene-environment interaction and epigenetics show that the ways in which heredity is expressed in behavior depends on environmental influences. The emerging field of epigenetics, therefore, studies biological processes not as primary causes of social outcomes but rather as mechanisms with contingent effects that depend on social structures, relationships, and interactions (McEwen and McEwen, 2017).

An example of gene-environment interplay may be drawn from the field of mental health. Consider a pair of identical twins—who therefore share identical DNA—who carry genes predisposing them to schizophrenia or bipolar illness. The probability that one twin will develop either disease at the same time as the other twin is only in the range of 40 to 60 percent. Differential experiences and other environmental factors will influence their genes to the extent that the disorder is either prevented or precipitated. Such influences, for example, result in changes and divergence in the activity (methylation patterns) of the DNA as the identical twins grow older (Fraga et al., 2005).[1] This example illustrates how environmental conditions can alter gene expression—that is, when, how, and to what degree different genes become activated (and thus influential) or deactivated (and thus uninfluential)—in behavior and development. Thus, even though an individual's DNA does not change, the expression of the information it contains can be changed by experiences; Figure 3-1 illustrates this concept. Through these mechanistic linkages, gene-environment interactions affect lifelong behavior and brain development that are particularly consequential for developmental trajectories.

Advances in epigenetics have also helped us to understand that individuals differ in how susceptible they are to environmental influences. The expression of genes in the brain is changing continuously with each person's experiences, and each new stressor or enhancement will have different effects upon gene expression (McEwen et al., 2015b). That is, the same gene in the same person may be expressed differently through time as experiences

---

[1] DNA methylation—when methyl groups are added to the DNA molecule—can change the activity of a DNA segment without changing the sequence. The example presented above describes an epigenetic mechanism in which the environment influences the CpG methylation of DNA, but there are multiple other forms of epigenetic modification (Szyf et al., 2008). These mechanisms include histone modifications that repress or activate chromatin unfolding (Allfrey, 1970) and the actions of non-coding RNA's (Mehler, 2008), as well as transposons and retrotransposons (Griffiths and Hunter, 2014) and RNA editing (Mehler and Mattick, 2007).

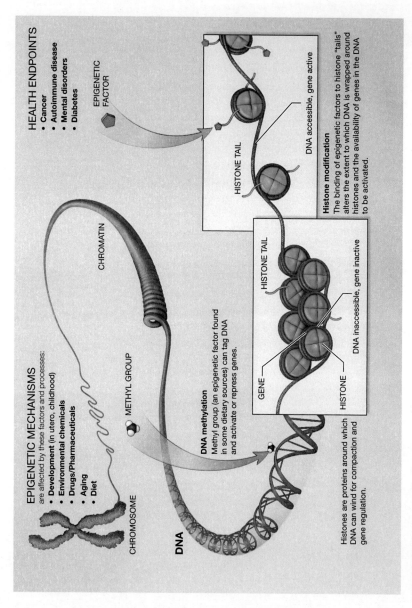

FIGURE 3-1 A scientific illustration of how epigenetic mechanisms can affect health.
SOURCE: National Institutes of Health (2018), see (https://commonfund.nih.gov/epigenomics/figure.

change. In addition, gene expression varies from person to person. Environmental adversity or support may dramatically affect some individuals, who flourish when conditions are positive but are negatively affected in poor conditions. Conversely, others appear to be less affected by environmental adversity or support, and their outcomes remain fairly consistent in both positive and negative circumstances (Boyce and Ellis, 2005; Obradovic et al., 2010). This differentiation may result because of early experiences, temperamental variability, genetic predispositions, or some combination of these factors. Taken together, however, research demonstrates that the same environmental circumstances do not affect individuals in the same way (Obradovic and Boyce, 2009).

Figure 3-2 illustrates the epigenetic life-course perspective and shows the ways in which environmental factors influence trajectories throughout the life course. It is important to recognize that these trajectories are "not straight, linear, overly determined, or immutable" (Halfon et al., 2014, p. 352). Rather, they are likely to be in a constant state of flux, determined by the various influences occurring at different times throughout the life course (Halfon et al., 2014, p. 352).

The cumulative measure of environmental factors has been referred to as the "exposome." According to Miller and Jones (2014, p. 2), "the exposome captures the essence of nurture; it is the summation and integration of external forces acting upon our genome throughout our lifespan." Environmental factors comprising the exposome include where one lives, what one eats, the quality of the air one breathes, one's social interactions and relationships, and one's lifestyle choices, among others. Related to this concept is the large literature in the field of public health on the social determinants of health, which are the upstream factors that shape behavior and influence health. These social determinants include education, employ-

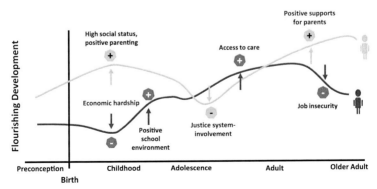

FIGURE 3-2 Epigenetic life-course perspective: Preconception to older adult.
SOURCE: Adapted from Halfon et al. (2014, p. 352).

ment, health systems and services, housing, income and wealth, the physical environment, public safety, the social environment, and transportation (National Academies of Sciences, Engineering, and Medicine, 2017).

Some factors are associated with flourishing trajectories and protect individuals from entering an at-risk trajectory. For example, having supportive relationships and having positive role models are protective factors that have been shown to be associated with lower risk for depressive symptoms and anxiety in homeless youth (Tyler et al., 2017). Supportive parenting, which may also be key to developing resilience in the face of risk factors, has been shown to mitigate some of the hormonal, metabolic, and cardiovascular changes that follow childhood adversity (Brody et al., 2017b). Additional factors associated with flourishing trajectories include positive school environments and access to quality, nutritious foods, among others.

Other factors, such as toxic stress, might consign individuals to the at-risk trajectory or move them from a flourishing trajectory to an at-risk trajectory. In addition, discrimination has been shown to affect sleep quality and duration, which has been shown to have a negative impact on psychological and physical health and academic outcomes (Asarnow et al., 2014; Barnes and Meldrum, 2015; Kuo et al., 2015; Majeno et al., 2018). Box 3-1 discusses the importance of sleep for adolescents and the ways in which environmental influences affect sleep and development. Similarly, and often related to the factors just mentioned, growing up in poverty has negative implications for the maturation of brain regions such as the hippocampus

---

BOX 3-1
Importance of Sleep for Adolescents

Sleep is a basic drive of nature (National Sleep Foundation, 2000) and plays an important role in flourishing development. Sleep helps us think more clearly, learn and retain new material, and complete tasks more efficiently (National Sleep Foundation, 2010). Adolescents often need more sleep than adults (Iglowstein et al., 2003; Huber and Born, 2014; Roffwarg et al., 1996; Jan et al., 2010; Dahl and Lewin, 2002; Telzer et al., 2015). Research suggests that during adolescence when brain maturation processes are occurring, approximately 9 hours of sleep per night is optimal in order to gain the full physical, mental, and cognitive health benefits of sleep (Eaton et al., 2010; Carskadon et al., 1980; National Sleep Foundation, 2006).

Existing research has shown that sleep problems are not uncommon among children and adolescents, with many reporting that they experience difficulty falling asleep, restless sleep, and variability in sleep patterns (Shanahan et al., 2014; Telzer et al., 2015). Sleep problems in adolescence have been associated with a number of negative outcomes, such as decreased alertness (Short et al.,

BOX 3-1 Continued

2013), higher levels of inattention (Aronen et al., 2000; Becker, 2014; Fallone et al., 2005; Paavonen et al., 2009), poor emotion regulation (Baum et al., 2014), suicidality (Lee et al., 2012; Wong and Brower, 2012), lower academic achievement (Perkinson-Gloor et al., 2013), and obesity (Mitchell et al., 2013; Suglia et al., 2014). In fact, sleep has been shown to be so influential on adolescent functioning that even one night of poor sleep can have deleterious consequences, particularly in regards to neurobehavioral performance (Louca and Short, 2014).

Studies have also identified a link between sleep disturbances and depression (Danielsson et al., 2013; Roberts and Duong, 2014; Short et al., 2013). Sleep disturbances are often comorbid with depression and anxiety in adolescents (Brunello et al., 2000; Wolfson and Carskadon, 1998), and there is evidence that these conditions have bidirectional effects that serve to mutually maintain one another (Dahl and Harvey, 2007; Harvey, 2000). At the neural level, the circuits involved in emotion regulation and those involved in sleep regulation also interact bidirectionally (Clarke and Harvey, 2013; Saper et al., 2005). Sleep issues have also been shown to increase the likelihood of recurrent depression following treatment in adolescents (Brouwer et al., 2006; Ising et al., 2007).

Research suggests a neurobiological account for the observed connection between poor sleep quality and greater risk taking and delinquent behavior in adolescence (Peach and Gaultney, 2013; Telzer et al., 2013). Telzer and colleagues (2014) found that adolescents who reported poorer sleep had less activation in the dorsolateral prefrontal cortex while performing a task that required cognitive control and greater activation in the insula during reward processing. This suggests that adolescents who do not get enough sleep may be especially oriented to rewards and are more likely to make risky decisions (Becker et al., 2015).

Despite the potential for poor sleep habits to cause long-lasting impairments during this critical stage of development (Telzer et al., 2015), there remains a significant gap in our understanding (Parthasarathy et al., 2016; Slopen et al., 2016). Issues in particular need of exploration include the impact of technology use on sleep, given adolescents' increasing use of electronic devices (see Chapter 1) and evidence showing the detrimental effects of using electronic devices before bed (Adams et al., 2013; Arora et al., 2014; Gamble et al., 2014; Hale and Guan, 2015; Hysing et al., 2015; King et al., 2013; Woods and Scott, 2016). Another important area for future research is the examination of potential racial/ethnic differences in sleep issues experienced by adolescents, as studies of adults have found that people of color are more vulnerable to sleep disturbances and negative consequences in comparison to their white counterparts (Kaufmann et al., 2016; Owens et al., 2017; Petrov and Lichstein, 2016; Roane et al., 2014). As such, future efforts need to recognize the importance of context when examining the sleep habits of youth (Jenni and O'Connor, 2005), particularly since cultural differences in sleep patterns and rituals have been demonstrated in the academic literature (Giannotti and Cortesi, 2009; Mindell et al., 2013). This is especially important since improving sleep education and addressing cultural differences in the treatment of sleep problems, especially early on in life, might serve to decrease the risk of impairments later in life.

and amygdala, which contribute to learning, memory, mood, and stress reactivity (Brody et al., 2017a). Brody and colleagues (2017a), for example, found that childhood poverty was associated with reduced volume of brain limbic regions in adulthood.

The relative contributions of risks and protective factors during childhood will therefore affect the likelihood of a flourishing trajectory, but an epigenetic life-course perspective also emphasizes that resilience and recovery are possible throughout the life course and especially during adolescence. Although one cannot *reverse* epigenetic modifications driven by environmental experiences that have occurred in previous life periods (Gray et al., 2014), recovery from earlier experiences is possible by redirecting gene expression to compensate for what has happened, through interventions such as the Strong African American Families Program, described below. That is, although each stage of life depends on what has come before, redirection, recovery, and resilience are possible, and windows of plasticity that make this possible are to be found across the entire life course. Insofar as the brain is healthy, individuals always have the capacity for resilience. Even the social and biological transitions that occur during adulthood offer opportunities for plasticity to be exploited, so that interventions may be effective beyond the early childhood and adolescent years.

RECIPROCAL INTERACTIONS BETWEEN
BRAIN, BODY, AND ENVIRONMENT

As discussed in the previous chapter, adolescence is a sensitive period of brain development, during which adolescents exhibit key developmental changes (Casey et al., 2008; Davidow et al., 2016; Steinberg, 2008). Whether these changes lead to positive or negative developmental outcomes depends on the social and physical environmental contexts of a person's development over the life course. All environments expose individuals to experiences that will produce adaptation in brain architecture and physiological processes: biological and neurological development are sensitive to social inputs and cues in the complex sociocultural environments in which adolescents live. An individual's environment, thus, influences the course of development and shapes developmental changes as either opportunities for flourishing trajectories or risk factors for poor trajectories. Given the continuous, reciprocal communication between the brain, body, and environment, each stage of development offers possibilities to change the trajectory of brain and body function, with consequences for the individual's life course from that point forward (McEwen et al., 2015b; for definitions of key terms used in this section, see Box 3-2).

While neuroscience has until recently tended to ignore the influence of the rest of the body on the brain's function, and traditional medicine

BOX 3-2
Key Terms Relevant to Brain, Body,
and Environment Interactions

Adrenal Gland
- The adrenal gland is adjacent to the kidney. The outer layer of the adrenal gland is called the **adrenal cortex**. It secretes a number of hormones—known as glucocorticoids—that are involved in stress, metabolism, and puberty.
- **Cortisol** is the main glucocorticoid hormone produced by the adrenal cortex. In addition to its role in metabolism, cortisol controls the sleep/wake cycle and is used by the body during times of stress to boost energy.

Amygdala
- The amygdala is located next to the hippocampus. It plays a key role in emotional responses, such as pleasure, fear, and anger.

Autonomic Nervous System
- The **autonomic nervous system** (ANS) regulates the body's involuntary functions, such as breathing and heart rate, blood pressure, digestion, metabolism, sexual response, and the production of body fluids (saliva, sweat, and tears). It is regulated by the hypothalamus.

Gray and White Matter
- The central nervous system is composed of two types of tissue: gray matter and white matter. **Gray matter** is pinkish-gray in color and is mainly located on the surface of the brain. **White matter** is lighter in color and is found in deeper tissues of the brain. It mainly consists of mylenated nerve fibers (axons).

Hippocampus
- The hippocampus is a region of the brain involved in emotional processing, learning, and memory formation. The hippocampal formation consists of three distinct parts: the **dentate gyrus**, the hippocampus proper, and the **subiculum**.
- The **dentate gyrus** mediates memory processing of spatially based information (Kesner, 2018).
- The **subiculum** plays a role in spatial navigation, memory processing, and control of the response to stress (O'Mara, 2005).
- The **CA3 subregion** of the hippocampus is involved in the encoding of new spatial information in short-term memory (Kesner, 2007).

HPA Axis
- The **hypothalamic-pituitary-adrenal (HPA) axis** is a hormonal system involved in the body's response to stress. It describes the interactions of the **hypothalamus** (a region of the brain involved in autonomic functions), the **pituitary gland** (a hormone-secreting gland that sits at the base of the hypothalamus), and the **adrenal gland** (see above).

Neuroendocrine Processes
- Neuroendocrine processes involve the interaction of the nervous system and the endocrine system to regulate a physiological or behavioral state.

has tended to ignore the brain, it is now understood that neural activity not only regulates the immune, metabolic, autonomic, and neuroendocrine systems but also those systems "talk to" and affect each other's activity and "talk back" to the brain, influencing its structure and function (McEwen et al., 2015b). For example, regular physical activity improves memory and mood, because activity increases neurogenesis (the formation of new neurons) in the input region (dentate gyrus) of the hippocampus, which is involved in learning and memory formation. This is mediated, in part, by the liver hormone known as insulin-like growth factor-1, entering the brain and facilitating the process (Trejo et al., 2001). In contrast, insulin resistance, which can be ameliorated by physical activity, impairs signaling mechanisms in the hippocampus, reduces neurogenesis, and contributes to depression, impaired cognitive function, and increased risk for dementia later in life (Biessels and Reagan, 2015; Grillo et al., 2015; Rasgon and McEwen, 2016).

To understand the reciprocal interactions between the brain, the body, and the environment one can consider the impact of stress on development across the life course. (In the example here we examine the effect of experiencing stress during adolescence; the pathways by which toxic stress in early childhood compromises the developing brain and body are discussed in Box 3-3.) The body and brain respond to environmental stressors through the biological stress response. Stressors range in severity from, for example, stress on the first day of school to mental or physical abuse. The type, timing, and severity of stress can have different pathophysiological outcomes (functional changes occurring with a particular disease), and stress can trigger or aggravate many diseases or pathological conditions (Yaribeygi et al., 2017).

BOX 3-3
Some Pathways by Which Toxic Stress in Early Childhood Compromises the Developing Brain and Body

The adolescent brain and body reflect events and conditions that have occurred from preconception through gestation and into childhood. The plasticity of the fetal, infant, childhood, and adolescent brain makes it particularly sensitive to the influences of systemic hormones, neural and immune feedback, and endogenous neurochemicals on its circuitry and responsiveness. Both animal and human studies reveal growing evidence that persistently elevated levels of stress-related hormones and inflammation can disrupt the brain's developing architecture in a way that makes it more difficult later for an individual to adapt to a different environment from the one in which they grew up.

BOX 3-3 Continued

For example, insulin resistance and Type 2 diabetes are two conditions made more likely by early-life toxic stress. Both are associated with cognitive impairment, a reduced volume of the hippocampus, and disrupted myelin protection in adolescents as well as in adults (Gold et al., 2007; Yau et al., 2012). Early-life toxic stress also increases both inflammatory tone, a comorbid condition in Type 2 diabetes, and body-mass index (Verstynen et al., 2012), resulting in altered myelin structure (Gianaros et al., 2013). Insulin resistance is also associated over the life course with a subtype of major depression and is a risk factor for Alzheimer's disease (Rasgon and McEwen, 2016). Yet some evidence (discussed in the last section of this chapter) shows that intervention in adolescence can redirect the brain and body to a more positive trajectory (Brody et al., 2017a, 2017b).

Glucocorticoids from the adrenal cortex play an important role, along with other mediators (Chattarji et al., 2015; McEwen et al., 2015a; McEwen and Morrison, 2013), not only in successful adaptation but also in long-lasting maladaptation. Through the process of allostatic load and overload, glucocorticoids can either prevent or contribute to permanent brain damage (e.g., from stroke, seizures, head trauma, dementia) and damage to the body (e.g., in diabetes, cardiovascular disease, and arthritis) (McEwen, 1998; McEwen and Gianaros, 2011).

Glucocorticoid receptors are abundant in the amygdala, hippocampus, and prefrontal cortex (PFC), where they help mediate exposure to stressful experiences in ways that ultimately change the size and architecture of these areas and lead to differences in learning, memory, and executive functioning (Chattarji et al., 2015; McEwen et al., 2015a; McEwen and Morrison, 2013). An example of this, during early childhood, is the effect of significant stress, such as living with a depressed mother (Lupien et al., 2011), which can trigger hypertrophic growth of the amygdala and result in a hyper-responsive or chronically activated physiologic stress response, chronic inflammation, and increased potential for fear and anxiety. This is one of the ways a child's environment and early experiences "get under the skin."

While toxic stress is associated with hypertrophy and overactivity in the amygdala and orbitofrontal cortex and in the hippocampus and medial PFC, similar levels of adversity can, conversely, lead to the *shrinkage* of neurons and neural connections (Chattarji et al., 2015; McEwen et al., 2015a; McEwen and Morrison, 2013). As a result of these structural changes, individuals may experience heightened anxiety, stemming from both hyper-activation of the amygdala and less top-down control as a result of PFC atrophy, and impaired memory and mood control as a consequence of a reduced hippocampus. These changes are actually adaptive to dangerous situations, and recovery from them is possible after danger has passed. However, recovery may require interventions. Such interventions, if they are appropriate to the developmental stage, can redirect brain plasticity in a beneficial direction, using at least some of the same mediators that, when dysregulated, may have created the problem in the first place. Without such interventions, early life adversity impairs brain development in numerous ways that create a weak foundation for later learning, behavior, and health (Teicher et al., 2016).

Specifically, the autonomic nervous system (which controls bodily functions not consciously directed, such as breathing and digestion), the hypothalamic-pituitary-adrenal (HPA) axis, and the cardiovascular, metabolic, and immune systems protect the body by reacting to internal and external stress through allostasis (the ability to achieve stability through change) (McEwen, 1998; Sterling and Eyer, 1988). Efficient allostasis involves "turning on" a physiological response when needed and turning it off efficiently when the stressor is over. Examples of this are the sudden increasing of cortisol[2] or heart rate, or releasing the neurotransmitter glutamate. In short, the brain perceives and determines what is threatening and regulates the behavioral and physiological responses to the environmental stressor.

Both adult and developing brains possess significant structural and functional plasticity in reaction to stress, including the replacement of neurons, remodeling of dendritic connections, and turnover rate of synapse activity. This plasticity may lead to three possible outcomes: positive adaptation (*good stress*), negative but remediable responses (*tolerable stress*), or long-term pathophysiological and negative behavioral responses (*toxic stress*).

Positive adaptation may occur in response to brief and mild to moderate experiences of stress. For example, this type of "good" stress might occur if an adolescent has anxiety related to the first day of a new school year or experiences moderate frustration but feels rewarded at the end of the experience. If an environment of stable and supportive relationships buffers these stressors, a young person can cope with the stressful event and the stress response systems will efficiently return to baseline status. In this context, good stress becomes a growth-promoting opportunity, allowing a young person to learn healthy, adaptive responses to adverse experiences (Shonkoff and Garner, 2012).

Remedial adaptation occurs in response to tolerable stress. This occurs when an individual is exposed to non-normative experiences that present greater adversity or threat than positive stress events do, such as a serious illness or injury or a parent's contentious divorce. These stressful events can result in tolerable stress when "protective adult relationships facilitate the child's adaptive coping and sense of control, reducing the physiologic stress response and promoting a return to baseline status" (Shonkoff and Garner, 2012, p. e236).

Toxic stress, the most dangerous form of stress, occurs when the heightened stress response persists even after the danger or stressor passes, that is,

---

[2] Cortisol is often referred to as the "stress hormone." It is a steroid hormone that is released in response to stressors. Cortisol, thus, is part of the body's "fight-or-flight" response and gives the body energy to fuel muscles during threatening conditions.

when the responses are either not turned on when needed or are not turned off appropriately. In particular, toxic stress occurs when an individual is unable to cope effectively with the stress, either due to a lack of support or less healthy brain architecture due to adverse early life experiences (McEwen and McEwen, 2017). Toxic stress contributes to long-term changes in the body and brain, referred to as "allostatic load" or "overload."[3] The maladaptation resulting from toxic stress disrupts brain circuitry and other organ and metabolic systems as well during sensitive developmental periods, which may result in damage to the regulation of these systems. That damage in turn is a precursor of later impairments in learning and behavior and can become the roots of chronic, stress-related physical and mental illness such as chronic anxiety and depression (McEwen et al., 2015b; Shonkoff and Garner, 2012).

As an example, abuse and neglect are likely to produce toxic stress in adolescents. This can lead to both short-term changes in observable behavior and less outwardly visible yet long-lasting changes in brain structure and function, including connectivity within the brain (Teicher et al., 2016). These changes may include reduced brain volume and disruption of protective myelin growth (Hair et al., 2015; Hanson et al., 2013, 2015). Exposure to toxic stress and high levels of cortisol also inhibit neurogenesis in the hippocampus, which is thought to play a role in the encoding of memory and in antidepressant functions (Cameron and Gould, 1996). The neurobiological pathways and effects of childhood and adolescent abuse and trauma are discussed in greater detail in Box 3-4.

In the absence of preventative interventions to promote positive, adaptive neuroplasticity and health-promoting behavior and physiology, stress-induced changes in the brain are likely to increase a person's vulnerability to toxic stress and resulting allostatic overload (Eckenrode et al., 2017; Shonkoff et al., 2009).

Moreover, toxic stress hampers the hippocampus's ability to promote contextual learning, which makes it difficult for a person to discriminate between dangerous situations and safe ones.[4] While some of these changes may help the individual adapt to the particular social and physical environment in which he or she currently lives, they may make it more difficult to function in a different environment in the future (Del Giudice, et al., 2011). For instance, in a safe environment a normal prefrontal cortex (PFC)

---

[3]The concepts of allostatic load and overload help us understand the cumulative and potentially damaging, as well as protective, effects of stressors on the brain and body (McEwen, 1998; see also, McEwen and Gianaros, 2011; McEwen and Stellar, 1993; McEwen and Wingfield, 2003; McEwen et al., 2015b). A related concept is that of "allostatic state," which represents a chronic deviation of the set point for an allostatic system such as heart rate or blood pressure.

[4]This reaction is common in post-traumatic stress disorder (PTSD), for example.

BOX 3-4
Neurobiological Pathways and Effects of Trauma

Childhood abuse and trauma—especially child physical abuse and neglect and child sexual abuse (CSA)—can have lasting effects into adolescence and adulthood. Although exposure to physical abuse and sexual abuse typically occurs in childhood (with the median age at onset of child sexual abuse being 7.5 years of age (Tricket et al., 2011), adolescence is a particularly vulnerable age for exposure to potentially traumatic events such as interpersonal violence, including dating violence, rape and sexual assault, and exposure to community violence. It is also a developmental period in which the impact of childhood physical and sexual abuse often begins to be behaviorally expressed.

Trauma affects brain development in a way that can have long-term consequences for individuals, including negatively affecting a person's ability to cope with stress and leading to an increased risk of cardiovascular disease, hypertension, asthma, diabetes, and activated inflammatory response, among other consequences. In the child and adolescent, trauma causes the amygdala to become hyperactive and increased in size, with weaker inhibitory input from the prefrontal cortex (PFC) and a smaller hippocampus (Herringa, 2017); autonomic and cortisol secretion becomes abnormal. Along with the hippocampus and PFC, the amygdala plays a key role in fear, anxiety, and depression as well as control of the sympathetic and cortisol response to stressors.

Adolescents may react to trauma exposure by struggling with their identity, with eating disorders, or by engaging in suicidality, hyper-sexuality, substance abuse, delinquency, or truancy. Some may report an urge to self-mutilate, an effort to relieve intense stress-induced dysphoria (Schwarz and Perry, 1994). Furthermore, trauma during childhood and adolescence can lead to future disorders—including PTSD, anxiety, depression, anger, and aggression (Finkelhor et al., 2007), substance abuse (Putnam, 2003; Simpson and Miller, 2002), and other psychopathology, as well as social and educational impairments and cardiovascular and metabolic problems (Copeland et al., 2007; van der Kolk et al., 2005). Early trauma can also lead to disruption of normal development, self-destructive behavior, and delinquency in adolescence, and vulnerability to being revictimized (Fergusson et al., 1997; McLaughlin et al., 2013).

The particular childhood trauma of CSA is noteworthy for its long-term consequences, including during adolescence. One highly consequential impact of such abuse is that victims are more vulnerable for revictimization than non-CSA youth, which further confounds their risk for yet more negative consequences (Fergusson et al., 1997). CSA victims are more likely to experience dating violence in their early romantic relationships. This vulnerability has lifelong consequences. Among females, CSA victims are up to five times more at risk of being sexually revictimized in adulthood than women who were not sexually abused in childhood (Classen et al., 2005).

regulates impulses and moods (through downstream control of the amygdala and nucleus accumbens) and facilitates decision making and proactive planning (McEwen and Morrison, 2013). In a dangerous environment, the orbitofrontal part of the PFC promotes vigilance for possible threat and danger. For children experiencing early adversity, the PFC develops in such a way that the child is continuously prepared for threat and danger, but this also makes the child, as they age, less able to control mood and impulse and less able to take part in thoughtful decision making and proactive planning (Gee et al., 2013a, 2013b).

In summary, as the example of the varying effects of stress highlights, the brain, the body, and the environment interact with one another in continuous and reciprocal ways, so that key life experiences influence basic neurobiological growth to shape developmental trajectories that may have profound long-term consequences.

AMELIORATING EARLY LIFE ADVERSITIES IN ADOLESCENCE

As discussed above and in Chapter 2, the heightened plasticity of the adolescent brain suggests that adolescence is a particularly sensitive period in which environmental influences may affect developmental trajectories, both positively and negatively, through a multitude of reciprocal interactions. In addition, this heightened sensitivity and responsiveness to environmental influences suggests that adolescence is a period when interventions can redirect and remediate maladaptation in brain structure and behavior that may have accumulated from earlier developmental periods.[5]

While preventing early life adversities is ideal,[6] research shows that ameliorating and redirecting an unhealthy developmental trajectory remains possible during adolescence and later developmental periods. A number of programs and interventions are emerging that look to take advantage of the potential of adolescence—driven by the adaptive plasticity of the brain and the developmental changes occurring in adolescence—to influence not only behavior but also systemic physiology, ensuring that youth flourish. This is an area of particular importance for future research; see Chapter 10.

One such intervention is the Strong African American Families (SAAF) Program, a developmentally and culturally responsive intervention that

---

[5]In fact, opportunities to promote better physical, mental, and cognitive health continue throughout the life course. For example, pregnancy opens a window for better parenting and family and child health, as exemplified by the Nurse Family Partnership (Eckenrode et al., 2017). This particular program may be of particular relevance to adolescents who are young mothers.

[6]For a discussion of prenatal and early childhood interventions, see the companion study authored by the Committee on Applying Neurobiological and Socio-behavioral Sciences from Prenatal through Early Childhood Development: A Health Equity Approach: www.nationalacademies.org/earlydevelopment.

promotes positive racial identity and ways for parents to learn to support youth goals and independence (Brody et al., 2017b). The program, which engaged 667 families from nine rural counties in Georgia for 7 weeks, promotes supportive parenting and the development of self-regulatory skills by the adolescents (Brody et al., 2017a, 2017b). In a randomized control trial, adolescents (ages 11 to 13) from families that received the intervention showed positive short- and long-term psychological, physiological, and neurobiological improvements, including reduced low-grade inflammation (a condition associated with many chronic diseases; see Minihane et al., 2015) (Miller et al., 2014) and reduced incidence of pre-diabetes, a condition that presumably had been elevated during adolescence due to adverse childhood experiences (Brody et al., 2017b; Yau et al., 2012). Increased locus of control (an individual's sense that they determine their experiences, rather than external forces such as luck or fate) is a likely mediator of the beneficial effects of interventions such as this (Culpin et al., 2015).

The SAAF Program demonstrated remarkable protective effects on the brain in addition to its beneficial effects on metabolic control (Brody et al., 2017a). Using magnetic resonance imaging, assessments were conducted a decade after the intervention (at age 25) to examine young adults' whole hippocampal region as well as amygdala volume. Both the control population and the participants in the SAAF Program were largely from backgrounds of low socioeconomic status, with 46.3 percent living below poverty thresholds, a situation that normally forecasts diminishment in the volume of the left dentate gyrus, the CA3 hippocampal subfields, and the left amygdala. The assessment found this diminishment among the young adults in the control condition but not among those who had participated in the SAAF Program. In addition, the SAAF Program was shown to reduce insulin resistance, another example of the ways in which brain-body interactions influence systemic disorders (Brody et al., 2017b).

In addition to family-based interventions such as the SAAF Program, stress-reduction interventions targeted directly at adolescents hold promise for undoing, or mitigating, the impact of early life stress on brain development. Mindfulness meditation has been associated with changes in brain regions associated with stress and attention (Tang et al., 2015). The DeStress for Success intervention teaches adolescents to cope with stress as they transition from elementary to middle school. Adolescents participating in the program are guided through a series of brief workshops that explain what stress is, how the body reacts to it, and problem-focused methods for coping (Lupien et al., 2013). This program has been found to lead to reductions in glucocorticoid levels and reductions in depressive symptoms in adolescents with high levels of anger (Lupien et al., 2013). Although the program has not yet been assessed for neurobiological impacts, they are likely given the changes observed in stress hormones and mental health.

Of course, research on neuroplasticity in adolescence need not only focus on ameliorating negative early life experience. There are other programs applicable across the life course that are focused on promoting emotional well-being through mindfulness and empathy-sensitizing work, programs that promote physical activity and social integration to counteract loneliness and improve sleep, and programs that promote healthier diets and mindfulness (Cacioppo et al., 2011; Erickson et al., 2011, Tasali et al., 2008; Valk et al., 2017).

Enrichment programs involving reading and mathematics instruction and music education also have established benefits. For example, reading instruction is associated with changes in cortical thickness (Romeo, 2017; Romeo et al., 2018) and structural connectivity (Huber et al., 2018; Keller and Just, 2009), especially in children from low socioeconomic status backgrounds. Math instruction is associated with structural and functional changes in math networks (Iuculano et al., 2015; Wang et al., 2017; Weng et al., 2017) and music classes have been linked to changes in neural signatures of language processing in children from high poverty neighborhoods (Kraus et al., 2014a, 2014b, 2014c). Practice with divergent thinking (e.g., coming up with alternative uses for household objects) improves creativity and leads to changes in prefrontal function (Kleibeuker et al., 2017).

CONCLUSION

Our developing understanding of epigenetics and the ways in which environmental influences shape individuals and the genome have underscored how the influences of genetics and environment on an individual's health and development are inseparable. Neurobiological processes can best be understood not as the cause of societal outcomes, but rather as mechanisms through which social structures, relationships, and interactions, together with other environmental influences, effect changes in the individual person. In this way, environment can be said to "get under the skin."

Because of the heightened plasticity of the adolescent brain and the interplay between genes and the environment, adolescence is a particularly sensitive period in which environmental influences may positively or negatively shape developmental trajectories through reciprocal interactions between the brain, the body, and the environment. This heightened sensitivity and responsiveness to environmental influences implies that adolescence is ripe with the promise of discovery and intensive learning that have a lasting imprint on the life course. Heightened neural plasticity also suggests that adolescence is a period during which well-designed interventions may be used to redirect and remediate maladaptation in brain structure and behavior from earlier developmental periods.

Thus, investments in programs and interventions that capitalize on the promise of brain plasticity during adolescence are needed to promote beneficial changes in developmental trajectories for youth who may have faced adverse experiences earlier in life or are facing them now. The challenge is to promote adaptation and change the trajectory of brain development and function so that the youth can adapt in a healthy way even when conditions change—for example from a dangerous environment to a safer one. The desired effect is to promote compensatory change in the adolescent to accommodate a more productive lifestyle in a changing environment.

Moreover, because environments and experiences interact with fundamental neurobiological developments, and because pubertal, neurobiological, cognitive, and psychosocial changes are occurring, adolescence represents a critical period of opportunity for the shaping of developmental trajectories. Adolescents are growing and learning within their environments, and each experience is an opportunity for adolescents to flourish and thrive. It is sometimes popularly said that a deviant adolescent is "incorrigible." However, what we know about the science of adolescent development strongly supports the supposition that *all adolescents have the capacity to change*. No child is without the potential to succeed. From a developmental perspective, adolescence is a time of promise, resilience, hope, and opportunity for all youth.

But few adolescents can flourish without the support of caring adults, especially if the circumstances of their childhoods yielded adversity or curtailed opportunity. The focus in this chapter has been on the developmental determinants of life-course trajectories as understood through epigenetic research. However, the harsh reality is that for many youth, opportunity is severely curtailed by economic and social disadvantage. These potent societal determinants of adolescents' life-course trajectories are discussed in the next chapter.

4

Inequity and Adolescence

Like every other society, the United States has a profound interest in promoting the well-being and successful development of all adolescents in our country. In so doing, our leaders, as well as teachers, families, and other caregivers, are naturally interested in how well our adolescents are developing as compared with adolescents in other countries or, perhaps as compared with previous generations of young people in our own country. However, this committee's charge is much more urgent and direct: its central focus is inequity among our nation's adolescents. Why are so many adolescents in the United States being left behind in relation to their own U.S. peers? What can we do about it, and what should we do to assure equal opportunity to flourish and succeed? This chapter documents disparities in adolescent well-being and performance, explores the sources of inequity, and lays the foundation for decisive social action.

For many youth in our country, the promise of adolescence is severely curtailed by economic, social, and structural disadvantage and, in all too many cases, by racism, bias, and discrimination. These potent societal determinants shape adolescents' life trajectories in multiple ways. They not only reduce access to the opportunities, services, and supports enjoyed by more privileged youth, but they also expose less privileged youth to risks, stresses, and demands that "get under the skin," adversely affecting the body and the brain during critical developmental periods. The unfortunate truth is that these striking differences in opportunity are associated with striking differences in outcomes—in health, safety, well-being, and educational and occupational attainment—and in trajectories over the life course. To the extent that these disadvantageous conditions have already impeded healthy development during childhood, failure to address the resulting deficiencies during adolescence represents a missed opportunity for remediation.

This chapter discusses the critical influences that either promote or hinder opportunity for adolescents at the individual, community, and population levels. These factors include differences in family income and wealth, differences in neighborhood resources, and racism, bias, and discrimination. The aim of this chapter is to identify disparities among adolescents in achievement, well-being, and other pertinent outcomes that stem from unwarranted and remediable differences in opportunity to succeed or in the ways particular groups of adolescents are treated by adults with authority over them, and to identify possible remediable responses. This analysis requires two tasks: We first summarize adolescent *outcomes* for which adequate data are available and identify disparities in these outcomes by race, ethnicity, gender, income, and, where possible, nativity, and sexual orientation.[1] These disparities are neither inevitable nor irremediable. The next section therefore identifies the major sources of these disparities, because a full understanding of the sources of the disparities is necessary to formulate effective strategies for reducing them.

Many factors might contribute to disparities in adolescent outcomes and they can be characterized in many different ways. Based on extensive bodies of well-accepted research as well as the framework set forth in *Communities in Action* (National Academies of Sciences, Engineering, and Medicine, 2017), we categorize the possible sources of outcome disparities as follows: (1) differences in family wealth and income, combined with living in neighborhoods segregated by income and race; (2) differences in institutional responses to adolescents by schools, the health system, the justice system, or the welfare system; and (3) prejudicial or discriminatory attitudes or behavior on the part of adults or peers who interact with adolescents on a regular basis. Of course, other possible sources of outcome disparities exist, such as immeasurable factors related to historical legacies of systemic discrimination and inequality as well as a range of other understudied factors. Here, we point to some specific, quantifiable sources that have been captured empirically by a large body of research.

Disparities among groups of adolescents in these domains not only affect developmental trajectories during adolescence but also are predictive of significant disparities in adult economic and social outcomes. Thus, to fail to address the sources of these disparities during adolescence is to con-

---

[1] Of course, as discussed in Chapter 10, there are a number of limitations to these data, including a paucity of markers of positive growth and an inability to characterize the outcomes of populations that are small in size or difficult to characterize (e.g., Native Americans and LGBTQ youth). These limitations also curtail our ability to fully capture "intersectional" inequalities, that is, those inequalities that arise from membership in multiple disadvantaged groups.

tinue to allow less than optimal development of our nation's human capital and the economic and social costs that entails, which include reduced worker productivity, lost wages and employment, worse health and mental health, and increased criminal justice involvement. These outcomes reduce overall economic growth and exacerbate rising inequality. To allow avoidable disparities to persist without making reasonable efforts to remediate them is also unjust.

We conclude the chapter by discussing some promising policies, programs, and practices that combat some of the sources of these disparities, promoting equity for all adolescents. While the challenge is large, progress can be made. Indeed, a review of trends in the extent of these disparities, underscores the point that the disparities are not immutable but are responsive to changes in underlying conditions and institutional processes. An important question, of course, is whether our society is willing to make the necessary long-term commitment to change the conditions that underpin these stark disparities.

DISPARITIES IN ADOLESCENT OUTCOMES

Recently, increasing attention has been paid to understanding adolescent outcomes and, more specifically, addressing disparities in adolescent outcomes. The recent interest in reducing adolescent disparities has resulted from a combination of deepening societal concern over inequality in the United States and recognition that the antecedents of adult inequality can be traced to disparities in adolescent development.

When considering how best to support and promote successful adolescent development, it is useful to have an eye toward three different questions. The first question is whether and to what extent adolescents as a group, or at a specific age (or grade), can achieve specific levels of performance or well-being at their given levels of physical, social, cognitive, and behavioral development at that age or grade level. (We have been referring to this question simply as measuring outcomes.) The second question is the extent to which members of different social groups achieve those levels of performance or well-being, thereby focusing attention on differences (disparities) in outcomes among groups that are not expected to differ in levels of development or capacity. The third question relates to the distribution of opportunity, that is, the extent to which members of differing social groups have the same chances of achieving desirable developmental outcomes. This section addresses the first two questions and the next section, which explores the underlying causes of disparities in outcomes, addresses equality of opportunity.

The first question of interest concerns the achievement of given levels of proficiency or development, as well as the rate of growth in proficiency and development. For example, in the early years of adolescence, it may be desirable for individuals to have achieved a certain level of competence in mathematics and reading, but we would also hope to see substantial continued growth in those skills over the course of the adolescent years. Indeed, the entire path to adulthood could be mapped by identifying desirable levels of development that we would hope for individuals to have achieved by given points in the life course, regardless of socioeconomic or racial/ethnic or other background factors.

The second important question relates to the distribution of developmental outcomes across different groups of adolescents. There are indeed significant differences in adolescent outcomes when measured by income, socioeconomic status, race, ethnicity, gender, nativity, and sexual identity, especially when taking account of the intersections among disadvantaged groups. The extent to which adolescents from these different social groups and backgrounds experience disparate outcomes is commonly treated as a presumptive measure of equality (or inequality) of outcome, or *equality* for short, based on the underlying supposition that disparities in outcomes based on group characteristics are *prima facie* unacceptable.

After this section describes inequalities in adolescent outcomes, the next section will describe their sources or origins. These sources derive largely from the socioeconomic status of the parents and the ways in which existing systems, institutions, and individuals interact with disadvantaged families, and thus they are not necessarily related to the underlying ability or human capital potential of the youth themselves. Consequently, for disadvantaged youth they reflect a daunting inequality of opportunity.

Current Disparities in Specific Outcomes

Table 4-1 presents measures of disparities in adolescent outcomes in the areas of education, justice, health, and child welfare across race and gender as well as ethnicity, income, nativity, gender identity, and sexual orientation where available. The table presents average shares (e.g., 0.11 or 11% of adolescents) or rates (number per 1,000 or 100,000) for the various outcome measures broken down by adolescent characteristic (race, gender, etc.) whenever available. In the following, we discuss the disparities in outcomes within each domain in turn.

Of course, our ability to characterize disparities is limited by the data available, concerning not only which outcomes have been measured but also the subgroups for which the outcomes have been separately measured. (A fuller discussion of data limitations is included in Chapter 10.) Moreover, it is more challenging to collect information on adolescent outcomes broken down by family income or sexuality, because information on the latter two categories are often not known or not solicited from

TABLE 4-1 Measures of Equality of Adolescent Outcomes in the Areas of Education, Justice, Health, and Child Welfare, by Race, Ethnicity, Income, Nativity, Gender Identity, and Sexual Orientation

Indicator	All	Black	White	Latinx	Male	Female	Poor	Non-Poor	Non-Native	LGBTQ youth
Math and Reading Test Scores										
Grade 4 math, share proficient[a]	0.40	0.19	0.51	0.26	0.42	0.38	0.25	0.57	0.14	-
Grade 8 math, share proficient[a]	0.34	0.13	0.44	0.2	0.35	0.33	0.18	0.48	0.06	-
Grade 12 math, share proficient[b]	0.25	0.07	0.32	0.12	0.26	0.23	0.11	0.32	0.06	-
Grade 4 reading, share proficient[a]	0.37	0.2	0.47	0.23	0.34	0.39	0.22	0.52	0.09	-
Grade 8 reading, share proficient[a]	0.36	0.18	0.45	0.23	0.31	0.41	0.21	0.48	0.05	-
Grade 12 reading, share proficient[a]	0.37	0.17	0.46	0.25	0.33	0.42	0.23	0.45	0.04	-
HS dropout (16–24-year-olds without a HS credential and not enrolled in school)[c]	0.061	0.062	0.052	0.086	0.071	0.051	0.097	0.051	-	-
HS completion (graduation within 4 years of starting 9th grade)[c]	0.84	0.76	0.88	0.79						
College completion (share of 25–34-year-olds with a B.A. or higher)	0.34	0.21	0.40	0.16	0.30	0.38	-	-	0.11*	-
School discipline (out-of-school suspensions)[d]	0.05	0.15	0.04	0.06	-	-	-	-	-	-
Juvenile Justice										
Arrest rate per 100[e]	2.5	5.4	2.4		3.5	1.5	-	-	-	-
Detention rate per 100,000[f]	-	153	25	50	-	-	-	-	-	-

continued

TABLE 4-1 Continued

Indicator	All	Black	White	Latinx	Male	Female	Poor	Non-Poor	Non-Native	LGBTQ youth
Health										
Mortality (ages 10–24, per 100,000)										
Mortality overall[g]	60.3	84.7	56	57.9	85.9	33.3				
Mortality from unintentional injury[g]	27.1	20.9	29.7	25.7	39.2	14.4				
Mortality from homicide[g]	9	32.8	2.5	12.2	15.2	2.6				
Mortality from suicide[g]	7.1	4.9	8.1	5.3	11.4	2.6				
Obesity[b]	0.148	0.182	0.125	0.182	0.175	0.121	0.189	0.1604	-	0.205
Behavioral Health										
Alcohol use[b]	0.604	0.513	0.617	0.647	0.581	0.626	-	-	-	0.722
Marijuana use[b]	0.356	0.428	0.32	0.424	0.352	0.359	-	-	-	0.504
Prescription pain medicine with a prescription use[b]	0.14	0.123	0.135	0.151	0.134	0.144	-	-	-	0.243
Depression[g]	0.128	0.091	0.138	0.127	0.064	0.194	-	-	-	-
Tobacco use[b]										
Cigarette use[b]	0.289	0.211	0.31	0.297	0.307	0.273	-	-	-	0.418
Frequent cigarette use[b]	0.026	0.011	0.036	0.017	0.027	0.026	-	-	-	0.054
Vape use[b]	0.422	0.362	0.418	0.487	0.449	0.397	-	-	-	0.505
Reproductive/Sexual Health										
Adolescent pregnancy[i]	0.0223	0.0318	0.016	0.0349	-					-
HIV[b]	0.093	0.152	0.089	0.081	0.079	0.105				0.14

Child Protective Services (CPS) ages 10+

In foster care (per 1000)[j]	9.4	19.8	9.3	7.9	9.5	9.2	18.5	3.6	–	–	–
In group home[i]	0.4	1	0.4	0.4	0.5	0.4	0.9	0.2	–	–	–
Aging out of foster care[i]	0.2	0.6	0.2	0.2	0.2	0.2	0.5	0.08	–	–	–
Child abuse and neglect[k]	0.0091	0.0139	0.0081	0.008	0.0087	0.0095	–	–			

NOTES: *Refers to non-native Latinx youth (related to 0.20 for native-born Latinx youth). For non-native Asian youth, this number is 0.66. See https://nces.ed.gov/programs/digest/d16/tables/dt16_104.60.asp.

SOURCES:

[a] National Center for Education Statistics (2017).

[b] National Center for Education Statistics (2015).

[c] Institute of Education Sciences, National Center for Education Statistics (2016).

[d] Institute of Education Sciences, National Center for Education Statistics (2015).

[e] U.S. Department of Justice, Office of Juvenile Justice and Delinquency Prevention (2016).

[f] U.S. Department of Justice, Office of Juvenile Justice and Delinquency Prevention (2015).

[g] U.S. Department of Health and Human Services, Centers for Disease Control and Prevention, National Center for Health Statistics (2016).

[h] U.S. Department of Health and Human Services, Centers for Disease Control and Prevention, National Center for Health Statistics (2017).

[i] U.S. Department of Health and Human Services, Centers for Disease Control and Prevention, Division of Reproductive Health (2015).

[j] U.S. Department of Health and Human Services, Administration for Children and Families, The Adoption and Foster Care Analysis and Reporting System; and U.S. Census Bureau, *American FactFinder* (2016).

[k] U.S. Department of Health and Human Services, Administration for Children and Families, Children's Bureau (2016).

adolescents, in contrast to gender, race, and ethnicity, which are more readily observed.

Disparities in Educational Achievement and School Discipline

Reading and math test scores as measured in the National Assessment of Educational Progress (NAEP), also known as The Nation's Report Card, are presented in Table 4-1a. Administered by the National Center for Education Statistics within the U.S. Department of Education, NAEP is the largest continuing assessment of the academic performance of U.S. students. It is administered to a nationally representative sample of students in both public and private schools, and it measures performance in math, reading, science, and several other subjects (National Center for Education Statistics, 2018). Overall, as of 2017, the NAEP results show that 40 percent of fourth graders are proficient in math and 37 percent are proficient in reading. If we break this down by race and ethnicity, 19 percent (and 20%) of Black students are proficient in math (and in reading), compared with 51 percent (47%) of White students and 26 percent (23%) of Latinx students. While fourth-grade boys are more likely than girls to be proficient in math (42% vs. 38%), for reading the reverse is true (34% vs. 39%).

Some of the greatest disparities are between poor and nonpoor students, as identified by free-lunch status.[2] These disparities emerge early: among fourth-grade students qualified for free lunch, 25 percent are proficient in math, compared with 57 percent of paid-lunch students. The disparities are similar for reading. As children age, gaps in proficiency in reading remain about the same between poor and non-poor students. Likewise, disparities by race and ethnicity largely stay the same, with reading proficiency among Black students remaining 25 percent lower than White students from Grades 4–12. For math, by contrast, over time the proficiency scores fall for all groups and, in addition, disparities by race and ethnicity appear to widen. Only in one area do disparities appear to narrow as adolescents age: females tend to improve their performance relative to males in both math and reading.

The disparities in NAEP test scores correspond to disparities seen in high school graduation rates, with graduation defined as completing school within 4 years of starting ninth grade. The highest rates of graduation (91%) are observed among Asian/Pacific Islander adolescents, followed by

---

[2]The percentage of students receiving free or reduced price lunch is often used as a proxy measure for the percentage of students living in poverty. While the percentage of students receiving free or reduced price lunch can provide some information about relative poverty, it should not be confused with the actual percentage of students in poverty enrolled in school (Snyder and Musu-Gillette, 2015).

TABLE 4-1A Measures of Equality of Adolescent Outcomes in the Area of Education, by Race, Ethnicity, Income, Nativity, Gender Identity, and Sexual Orientation

Indicator	All	Black	White	Latinx	Male	Female	Poor	Non-Poor	Non-Native	LGBTQ youth
Grade 4 math, share proficient[a]	0.40	0.19	0.51	0.26	0.42	0.38	0.25	0.57	0.14	-
Grade 8 math, share proficient[a]	0.34	0.13	0.44	0.2	0.35	0.33	0.18	0.48	0.06	-
Grade 12 math, share proficient[b]	0.25	0.07	0.32	0.12	0.26	0.23	0.11	0.32	0.06	-
Grade 4 reading, share proficient[a]	0.37	0.2	0.47	0.23	0.34	0.39	0.22	0.52	0.09	-
Grade 8 reading, share proficient[a]	0.36	0.18	0.45	0.23	0.31	0.41	0.21	0.48	0.05	-
Grade 12 reading, share proficient[a]	0.37	0.17	0.46	0.25	0.33	0.42	0.23	0.45	0.04	-
HS dropout (16–24-year-olds without a HS credential and not enrolled in school)[c]	0.061	0.062	0.052	0.086	0.071	0.051	0.097	0.051	-	-
HS completion (graduation within 4 years of starting 9th grade)[c]	0.84	0.76	0.88	0.79						
College completion (share of 25–34-year-olds with a B.A. or higher)	0.34	0.21	0.40	0.16	0.30	0.38	-	-	0.11*	-
School discipline (out of school suspensions)[d]	0.05	0.15	0.04	0.06	-	-	-	-	-	-

SOURCES:
[a]National Center for Education Statistics (2017).
[b]National Center for Education Statistics (2015).
[c]Institute of Education Sciences, National Center for Education Statistics (2016).
[d]Institute of Education Sciences, National Center for Education Statistics (2015).

88 percent for Whites, 79 percent for Latinx, and 76 percent for Blacks (National Center for Education Statistics, 2017). However, when we examine a different measure, namely the high school drop-out rate (defined as the share of 16–24-year-olds lacking a high school credential and not enrolled in school), the disparities are much smaller: only 6.2 percent of Black youth are considered drop-outs, compared with 5.2 percent of White youth, and 8.6 percent of Latinx youth. This is consistent with Black and Latinx youth taking longer to obtain their high school credential, either through delayed graduation from high school or by obtaining a GED. Importantly, female achievement outpaces male achievement by this measure as well: females (5.1%) have lower rates of high school drop-out than males (7.1%).

Racial and ethnic disparities in college completion (defined as the share of 25–34-year-olds with a B.A. degree or higher) are greater than the disparities in high school completion or rates of drop-out. Among 25–34-year-olds, 40 percent of Whites have a B.A. or higher, compared with 21 percent of Blacks and 16 percent of Latinx. The gender disparity in college completion is also greater than the gender disparity in high school drop-out rates: 38 percent of females have a B.A. or higher, compared with 30 percent for males.

As of the first quarter of 2018, the median earnings for college graduates is $1,310 per week, compared with $726 per week for high school graduates.[3] Among college graduates, median earnings are $1,550 for White male workers and $1,139 for Black males. For high school graduates, White males earn $861 relative to $604 for Black males. Thus, the growth in disparities as youth age, culminating in large differences by race, ethnicity, and gender in college completion, will likely result in continuing large disparities in adult earnings as well.

Measures of school discipline reveal significant disparities by race. For example, in 2013, 15 percent of Black students received an out-of-school suspension, compared with 4 percent of White students and 6 percent of Latinx students. Moreover, a disproportionate number of Native American, LGBTQ, and disabled youth are suspended or expelled from school as a result of discretionary disciplinary practices (Poteat et al., 2016; American Bar Association, 2018). Much of the existing research on the "school-to-prison pipeline" suggests that the disparities in school discipline by race and ethnicity are responsible in part for the disparities seen in juvenile justice involvement, including the fact that Black youth are more than twice as likely as Whites to be arrested as juveniles (5.4% compared to 2.1%). (See

---

[3] Median earnings calculated over all full-time workers ages 25 or older. This represents a significant premium in income, but because of the rising cost of college and the increasing debt of college graduates, there is more variability in terms of the college premium in wealth. (See https://fredblog.stlouisfed.org/2018/07/is-college-still-worth-it/.)

also Chapter 9, Box 9-2, "Relationship between School Disciplinary Policies and the Juvenile Justice System.")

Researchers have outlined multiple ways in which school suspension or expulsion can lead to an increase in juvenile arrest and detention. First, with the presence of school resource officers, any disciplinary infraction increases the probability of interacting with the police force (Owens, 2017). Second, suspension reduces time spent in school and increases the probability of arrest during the days of suspension (Mowen and Brent, 2016). Third, suspension and expulsion reduce attachment to school, and this in turn reduces the probability of high school graduation, which increases the probability of future criminal activity (Lochner and Moretti, 2004).

Disparities in Juvenile Justice

Table 4-1b shows measures of equality of adolescent outcomes in the area of justice. At every successive stage of the criminal/juvenile justice process, racial and (to a lesser extent) ethnic disparities increase (Rovner, 2016). There are multiple points at which decisions made by adult actors in the justice system can affect the outcomes for youth: during the decision to prosecute, during the bail-setting decision, during plea-bargaining decisions, and at sentencing. This is readily apparent in detention rates: Black youth are detained at a rate six times higher than White youth and three times higher than Latinx youth. Evidence suggests that such disparities in juvenile detention will cause significant disparities in adult outcomes including educational attainment and future incarceration (Aizer and Doyle, 2015).

In a system that is formally committed to equal and fair treatment, these comparisons suggest a serious need to study and scrutinize the sources of these growing disparities in the juvenile justice system by race and ethnicity.

Disparities in Health Outcomes and Health Behaviors

Table 4-1c shows measures of equality of adolescent outcomes in the area of health. Research examining the income gradient in child health shows that there is a positive relationship between family income and children's self-reported health and that this becomes more pronounced as children age (Case et al., 2002).[4] This age effect is not explained by insurance, health at birth, or genetics. Rather, poor children develop more chronic conditions as they age, relative to their better-off counterparts. Moreover, poor health in adolescence harms educational attainment, because sicker children miss more days of school and ultimately attain fewer years of schooling. As such, youth in low-income families enter adulthood

---

[4]The authors use self- or parent-reported health as their measure.

106

TABLE 4-1B Measures of Equality of Adolescent Outcomes in the Area of Justice, by Race, Ethnicity, Income, Nativity, Gender Identity, and Sexual Orientation

Indicator	All	Black	White	Latinx	Male	Female	Poor	Non-Poor	Non-Native	LGBTQ youth
Arrest Rate per 100[e]	2.5	5.4	2.4		3.5	1.5	-	-	-	-
Detention Rate per 100,000[f]	-	153	25	50	-	-	-	-	-	-

SOURCES:
[e]U.S. Department of Justice, Office of Juvenile Justice and Delinquency Prevention (2016).
[f]U.S. Department of Justice, Office of Juvenile Justice and Delinquency Prevention (2015).

TABLE 4-1C Measures of Equality of Adolescent Outcomes in the Area of Health, by Race, Ethnicity, Income, Nativity, Gender Identity, and Sexual Orientation

Indicator	All	Black	White	Latinx	Male	Female	Poor	Non-Poor	Non-Native	LGBTQ youth
Mortality (ages 10–24, per 100,000)										
Mortality Overall[g]	60.3	84.7	56	57.9	85.9	33.3				
Mortality from Unintentional Injury[g]	27.1	20.9	29.7	25.7	39.2	14.4				
Mortality from Homicide[g]	9	32.8	2.5	12.2	15.2	2.6				
Mortality from Suicide[g]	7.1	4.9	8.1	5.3	11.4	2.6				
Obesity[b]	0.148	0.182	0.125	0.182	0.175	0.121	0.189	0.1604	-	0.205
Alcohol Use[b]	0.604	0.513	0.617	0.647	0.581	0.626	-	-	-	0.722
Marijuana Use[b]	0.356	0.428	0.32	0.424	0.352	0.359	-	-	-	0.504
Prescription Pain Medicine with a Prescription Use[b]	0.14	0.123	0.135	0.151	0.134	0.144	-	-	-	0.243
Depression[g]	0.128	0.091	0.138	0.127	0.064	0.194	-	-	-	-
Tobacco Use[b]										
Cigarette Use[b]	0.289	0.211	0.31	0.297	0.307	0.273	-	-	-	0.418
Frequent Cigarette Use[b]	0.026	0.011	0.036	0.017	0.027	0.026	-	-	-	0.054
Vape Use[b]	0.422	0.362	0.418	0.487	0.449	0.397	-	-	-	0.505
Adolescent Pregnancy[i]	0.0223	0.0318	0.016	0.0349	-		-	-	-	-
HIV[b]	0.093	0.152	0.089	0.081	0.079	0.105	-	-	-	0.14

SOURCES:

[g]U.S. Department of Health and Human Services, Centers for Disease Control and Prevention, National Center for Health Statistics (2016).
[b]U.S. Department of Health and Human Services, Centers for Disease Control and Prevention, National Center for Health Statistics (2017).
[i]U.S. Department of Health and Human Services, Centers for Disease Control and Prevention, Division of Reproductive Health (2015).

not only poorer but also with fewer years of schooling and in worse health, and all three of these conditions predict worse outcomes in adulthood.

In addition to enduring disparities in the incidence and impact of chronic conditions, disadvantaged youth (particularly as defined by race and ethnicity) had higher rates of mortality, largely due to greater rates of violence, in 2016 (Cunningham et al., 2018). While Whites and Latinx youth ages 10 to 24 have similar rates of mortality (roughly 57 per 100,000), their Black peers have mortality rates roughly 50 percent higher (85 per 100,000) (Table 4-1c). These disparities in mortality rates by race are mainly driven by disparities in homicide rates, which are 33 per 100,000 for Blacks compared with 2.5 for Whites and 12.2 for Latinx. The only category for which White adolescents have higher rates of mortality than Black or Latinx adolescents is suicide: 8.1 per 100,000 for Whites, compared with 4.9 for Blacks and 5.3 for Latinx (Mulye et al., 2009).

There are also significant disparities in adolescent mortality by gender, with a rate of 86.6 deaths (per 100,000) for males and 33.3 for females. These disparities by gender are observable across all causes: unintentional injuries, motor vehicle accidents, homicide, and suicide. Interestingly, although rates of suicide are much higher for males, major depressive episodes are more prevalent among females (19% for females versus 6% for males in 2016).

It should be noted that while studies have documented recent increases in adult mortality in the United States among the poor, resulting in increasing disparities in mortality by income (Case and Deaton, 2015), the same is not true for child and adolescent mortality. For children and adolescents, mortality has not only continued to decline, on average, but also disparities by income have narrowed (Currie and Schwandt, 2016).

Use of alcohol and tobacco do not differ considerably by gender, but they do differ by race and ethnicity. Black adolescents generally have the lowest rates of alcohol consumption and cigarette smoking as compared to White and Latinx youth, though Black and Latinx youth have slightly higher rates of marijuana use than do White youth. LGBTQ youth have much higher rates of alcohol, marijuana, and tobacco use than the general population of adolescents (Dai, 2017; Fish and Baams, 2018; Centers for Disease Control and Prevention, 2016).

With respect to reproductive or sexual health, Black and Latinx adolescents have higher rates of teen pregnancy (roughly 3 per 100, compared with 1.5 per 100 for White non-Latinx teens). These rates, however, are currently lower than at any point in recent history, a point to which we will return later. Rates of HIV infection show similar patterns and appear to be highest for LGBTQ teens. Box 4-1 further details the health of sexual and gender minorities, proposed reasons for disparities in outcomes, and issues in measuring outcomes for this population.

Disparities in Child Protective Involvement and Outcomes

Among adolescents (age 10+), youth experiencing poverty are dramatically overrepresented in foster care (18.5 per 1,000 vs. 3.6 per 1,000 among the non-poor). They are also much more likely to be in a group home setting and more likely to age out of foster care (see Table 4-1d). Black adolescents also have higher rates of foster care and group-home placement than other youth and are more likely to age out of foster care. Similarly, American Indian and Alaska Native children are disproportionately represented in the child welfare system: while they comprise only 0.9 percent of the total child population, they comprise 1.3 percent of the children identified by Child Protective Services (CPS) as victims and 2.4 percent of the children in foster care (Children's Bureau, 2016).

Moreover, a recent analysis of nationally representative data finds that LGBT youth are overrepresented in the child welfare system generally and in foster care and other out-of-home placements specifically (Fish et al., 2019). Children in foster care do worse along a host of outcomes: they are more likely to become teen mothers and to become involved in the juvenile justice system, and as adults they are less likely to be employed. This is particularly true for adolescents, and there is evidence that this relationship is indeed causal and does not simply reflect underlying differences in the characteristics of children in and out of foster care (Doyle, 2007).

BOX 4-1
Health of Sexual and Gender Minorities

Despite trends that suggest growing social awareness and acceptance of LGBTQ youth, vexing health disparities persist for sexual- and gender-minority adolescents. There is consistent evidence that at all ages, LGBT[a] people are at higher risk for poor mental health, and multiple studies demonstrate that higher rates of compromised mental health are present among LGBT youth than among their heterosexual and cis-gender peers (Eskin et al., 2005; Fergusson et al., 2005; Fish and Pasley, 2015; Fleming et al., 2007; Marshal et al., 2011; Needham, 2012; Ueno, 2010). These higher rates of mental health issues are a fundamental predictor of a host of behavioral health disparities evident among LGBT youth, including substance use, abuse, and dependence (Marshal et al., 2008).

continued

BOX 4-1 Continued

Recent evidence suggests that sexual-minority disparities in key indicators of health have widened in recent decades. LGBT adolescents and young adults have significantly worse health outcomes than heterosexual and cis-gender youth, including higher rates of mental health problems and suicide. For example, while the consumption of alcohol has declined for all youth, high-risk alcohol behavior has increased for sexual-minority girls (Fish et al., 2017). Thus, despite a cultural shift that would suggest that things are "getting better" for sexual- and gender-minority youth, such an assertion seems premature, at least with respect to health behavior (Russell and Fish, 2016).

Reasons for these continuing and even widening health disparities for LGBT youth may be traced to the experience of stigma, discrimination, "minority stress,"[b] harassment, and other forms of victimization, which occur in families, schools, and communities (Meyer, 1995, 2003; Saewyc, 2011). Thus, experiences of rejection by families or parents due to coming out and experiences of victimization or bullying in school due to one's LGBT identity (Russell et al., 2012) are both critical predictors of compromised health for LGBT adolescents. Further, in the peer context, the declining age of coming out has coincided with more peer aggression and bullying, since younger ages of coming out now coincide with the developmental period of early adolescence, which is characterized by heightened self- and peer-regulation, especially regarding norms of gender and sexuality (Mulvey and Killen, 2015; Pasco, 2011). In fact, a recent meta-analysis documented more frequent homophobic bullying in schools in recent decades compared to earlier ones (Toomey and Russell, 2016).

Despite concerns regarding mental health problems and compromised health behaviors among LGBT youth, there is a growing body of evidence that documents family-, school-, and community-level factors and actions that are associated with positive adjustment and reduced vulnerability for LGBT youth. However, important gaps in this understanding persist due to lack of available data. The inclusion of sexual attraction, behavior, and identity measures in population-based studies (e.g., the National Longitudinal Study of Adolescent to Adult Health and the Centers for Disease Control and Prevention's Youth Risk Behavior Surveillance System) were important first steps for improving knowledge of the prevalence of LGB health disparities and the mechanisms that contribute to these inequalities for both youth and adults. However, a critical need remains for the development and inclusion of measures to identify transgender people. Lack of identification in national, population-based surveys thwarts a more complete understanding of health among transgender youth.

---

[a]In the text that follows, we use the term LGBT or LGB to reflect the current evidence being reported. In some instances, lack of available data preclude reporting of outcomes for all LGBTQ youth.

[b]Minority stress refers to the high levels of stress experienced by members of stigmatized minority groups, the most common cause of which is interpersonal discrimination and prejudice.

TABLE 4-1D Measures of Equality of Adolescent Outcomes in the Area of Child Welfare, by Race, Ethnicity, Income, Nativity, Gender Identity, and Sexual Orientation

Indicator	All	Black	White	Latinx	Male	Female	Poor	Non-Poor	Non-Native	LGBTQ youth
In Foster Care (per 1000)[j]	9.4	19.8	9.3	7.9	9.5	9.2	18.5	3.6	-	-
In Group Home[j]	0.4	1	0.4	0.4	0.5	0.4	0.9	0.2	-	-
Aging Out of Foster Care[j]	0.2	0.6	0.2	0.2	0.2	0.2	0.5	0.08	-	-
Child Abuse and Neglect[k]	0.0091	0.0139	0.0081	0.008	0.0087	0.0095	-	-	-	-

NOTE: Child Protective Services ages 10+.
SOURCES:
[j] U.S. Department of Health and Human Services, Administration for Children and Families, The Adoption and Foster Care Analysis and Reporting System; and U.S. Census Bureau, *American FactFinder* (2016).
[k] U.S. Department of Health and Human Services, Administration for Children and Families, Children's Bureau (2016).

Trends in Disparities in Adolescent Outcomes

Both Table 4-1 and the preceding discussion present a static picture of adolescent health and well-being, masking important trends over time in these measures. In fact, most measures of adolescent well-being have improved over time, and along with these general overall improvements disparities have also narrowed.

Teen childbearing is one important example. This has continued to decline steadily since 1990, accompanied by significant declines in disparities by race and ethnicity as childbearing fell disproportionately faster among Black and Latinx teens than among White teens (see Figure 4-1). Among females ages 15 to 19, the birth rate for Black teens fell by more than two-thirds from 1990 to 2016, declining from 116 to 32 per 1,000. A large but slightly smaller decline occurred among Latinx teens over the same period. The smallest decline was observed among White teenagers, whose birth rates fell from 43 to 14 per 1,000, which still represents a significant decrease (Martin et al., 2018). There is no consensus regarding the reasons for the decline, but there is some evidence that increasing use of contraception has played an important role (Boonstra, 2014).

For educational outcomes, such as test scores, high school drop-out, and college completion, the overall trend has also been one of improvement, but important differences show up in the way disparities have evolved over time across these measures. Reardon (2011) has compiled data on test scores for reading comprehension for cohorts born in the years 1943 through 2001. He calculates the average difference in standardized test scores, both by race and by income, and shows how those differences have

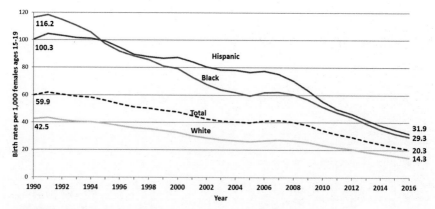

FIGURE 4-1 Trends in teen childbearing by race and ethnicity, 1990 to 2016.
SOURCE: Martin et al. (2018).

evolved over time (Figure 4-2).[5] The Black-White gap in NAEP test scores has narrowed slowly but steadily over time, declining from a difference of 1.5 standard deviations for the 1940 birth cohort to roughly 0.50 of a standard deviation by the 2001 birth cohort. The dashed line in Figure 4-2 illustrates this decline. Possible explanations include desegregation of U.S. schools and increased resource allocation to schools that predominantly serve Black students. In contrast, the "90/10 income gap" shown in the figure (defined as the difference in standardized test scores between students at the 90th percentile of family income and students at the 10th percentile) has actually increased over the decades, rising from 0.60 of a standard deviation for the 1940 birth cohort to 1.1 standard deviations by the 2001 birth cohort. This is illustrated by the solid line in Figure 4-2.

The gap in high school drop-out rates among 16–24-year-olds also narrowed from 1967 to 2016 across all racial/ethnic groups, and more so for Black and Latinx youth, significantly reducing disparities in high school dropout rates (Figure 4-3). College enrollment rates, defined as the share of 18–24-year-olds enrolled in college, increased from 32 percent to 40 percent from 1990 to 2005, but since 2005 it has remained relatively flat both overall and for most groups (Figure 4-4). The one group that has continued to enroll in college at ever higher rates over the period 2005 to 2015 is Latinx youth, whose enrollment rates increased from 25 to 37 percent during this most recent period (Musu-Gillette et al., 2017).

Perhaps some of the most dramatic improvements over time have been those seen in the juvenile justice sector. Since their peak in 1994, juvenile arrest rates have fallen dramatically overall and for all subgroups defined by race and ethnicity (Figure 4-5). Juvenile detention, while also declining over time, has done so at a slower pace and with less of a decline in disparities. For Black youth, arrest rates from 1997 to 2015 fell 64 percent, and for Whites they fell 55 percent. However, over this same period, residential placement[6] fell 55 percent for Blacks and 62 percent for White youth (Figure 4-5). Similar trends have been observed for adults.

Adolescent well-being has worsened in one important domain: suicide rates. After declining from 1995 to 2007, adolescent suicide rates have since increased steadily, particularly for males (Centers for Disease Control and Prevention, 2017). Disparities in suicide rates have largely remained

---

[5]To obtain standardized average differences, the researcher will take a test score, subtract the average score from it, and then divide this difference by the standard deviation of the test score distribution. This is also referred to as a Z-score. The mean of all standardized test scores will always be zero and the standard deviation will always be one. Standardization in this way allows for comparison across different distributions.

[6]Residential facilities include detention centers, shelters, reception/diagnostic centers, group homes, boot camps, ranch/wilderness camps, residential treatment centers, and long-term secure facilities.

114

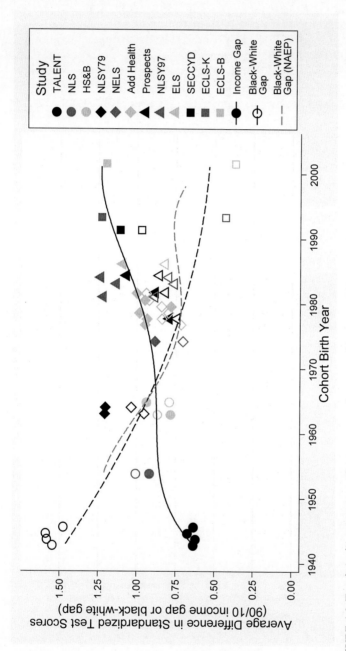

FIGURE 4-2 Trends in disparities in reading test scores by race and income, 1943 to 2001.

NOTES: Talent = Project Talent National Longitudinal Study; NLS = National Longitudinal Surveys; HS&B = High School and Beyond Longitudinal Study; NLSY79 = National Longitudinal Survey of Youth 1979; NELS = National Educational Longitudinal Study; Add Health = National Longitudinal Study of Adolescent to Adult Health; NLSY97 = National Longitudinal Survey of Youth 1997; ELS = Education Longitudinal Study; SECCYD = Study of Early Child Care and Youth Development; ECLS-K = Kindergarten Class of 1998–1999; ECLS-B = Early Childhood Longitudinal Study Birth Cohort; NAEP = National Assessment of Educational Progress.

SOURCE: Reardon (2011). Republished with permission of Russell Sage Foundation. Permission conveyed through Copyright Clearance Center, Inc.

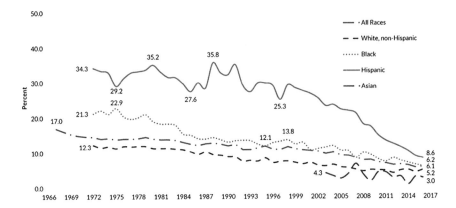

FIGURE 4-3 High school status drop-out rates among youth ages 16 to 24, by race and Hispanic origin, selected years, 1967 to 2016.

NOTES: The *status drop-out rate* measures the percentage of young adults ages 16 to 24 who were not enrolled in school and had not received a high school diploma or obtained a GED. This measure excludes people who are in the military or incarcerated but includes immigrants who never attended U.S. schools. Due to changes in race categories, estimates from 2003 are not strictly comparable to estimates from 2002 and before. After 2001, the Black race category includes some Latinx.

SOURCE: Child Trends Databank (2018).

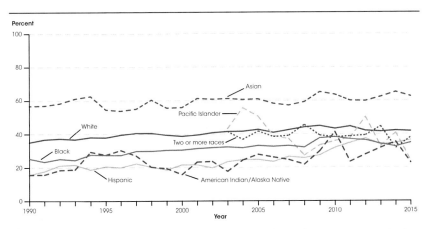

FIGURE 4-4 Total college enrollment rates of 18–24-year-olds in degree-granting institutions, by race and ethnicity, 1990 to 2015.

SOURCE: Musu-Gillette et al. (2017).

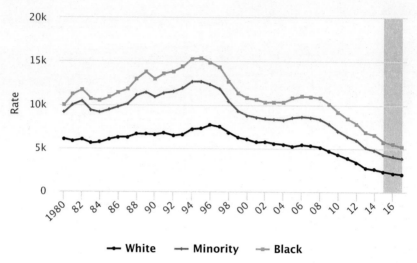

FIGURE 4-5 Trends in juvenile arrest rates, by race and ethnicity, 1980 to 2016.
NOTES: Rates are arrests of persons per 100,000 persons ages 10-17 in the resident popula-
tion. Persons of Latinx ethnicity may be of any race, i.e., White, Black, American Indian, or
Asian. Arrests of Latinx youth are not reported separately. The Office of Juvenile Justice and
Delinquency Prevention defines minority populations as American Indian and Alaska Native,
Asian, Black or African American, Hispanic or Latino, and Native Hawaiian or other Pacific
Islanders.
SOURCE: Office of Juvenile Justice and Delinquency Prevention (2018).

unchanged, with the highest rates seen among males and Whites. Research
to understand this recent rise in suicide is currently under way. Thus, the
evidence clearly shows that observed levels and disparities in adolescent
outcomes are not immutable, but are responsive to changes in underlying
conditions.

SOURCES OF DISPARITIES: INEQUALITY OF OPPORTUNITY

While what we are calling "outcome" measures refer to the extent
to which members of different groups differ with respect to a particular
developmentally significant status, equality of opportunity assesses to what
extent members of those groups had equal chances to achieve that status or
outcome. As Arneson (2015, p. 1) writes, "when equality of opportunity
prevails, the assignment of individuals to places in the social hierarchy is

determined by some form of competitive process, and all members of society are eligible to compete on equal terms."[7]

In this section, we review the main sources of differential opportunity and treatment that affect adolescent health, well-being, and performance: (1) those related to the resources of families and communities where many adolescents live; (2) institutional or systematic sources of inequities in the systems with which adolescents interact; and (3) personal biases of the adults responsible for making decisions about individual adolescents.

Differences in Family Income, Wealth, and Neighborhood Resources

Although child poverty rates have decreased since the 1960s, more than 9 million children and youth in the United States live in households with incomes below the poverty level (NASEM, 2019).[8] Rates of child poverty are highest for Black, Latinx, and American Indian and Alaska Native youth (NASEM, 2019). For adolescents, growing up in poverty is associated with worse physical and mental health, as well as increased risky behaviors, delinquency, and criminal behavior (NASEM, 2019). Together, these effects of poverty can set youth on less positive developmental trajectories, and youth of color experience the greatest gap in opportunity.

Indeed, one of the most significant features of the U.S. economy over the past 50 years has been the increasing inequality of income and wealth. Parental income and wealth are both highly predictive of child outcomes, because a key input in adolescent development consists of family resources, defined generally as financial inputs, time spent, and the quality of family interactions (Cunha and Heckman, 2007). And because of strong sorting based on income and race in the United States—often driven by systemic and institutional policies—family resources also determine the neighborhood resources available for youth.

There is a strong neurobiological link between family resources and youth outcomes. Recent advances in neuroscience show that family resources during early childhood affect the development of specific neural systems, and when those resources are limited the regions of the brain responsible for language processing and executive function are negatively affected, ultimately manifesting in worse adolescent mental health and

---

[7]Political philosophers further distinguish between *formal* equality of opportunity and *substantive* equality of opportunity. The former is assured when the formal rules regulating access to goods or outcomes are the same for members of all groups, while the latter is assured only when, in fact, individuals of equal "native talent" have equal chances of access to those goods or outcomes. Substantive equality of opportunity is often referred to as *equity* or "fair equality of opportunity" (see Arneson, 2015, for a detailed discussion).

[8]Although poverty rates are not typically reported specifically for the 10–25-year-old population, child (18 and under) poverty rates are routinely reported.

lower IQ (see Hackman et al. (2010) for a review of the evidence). More-over, growing evidence suggests that these patterns of neurobiological devel-opment are not entirely or even largely genetic, but rather are a function of prenatal and postnatal environments and investment which, again, are directly affected by family income (Hackman et al., 2010).

This last conclusion is based on a growing body of natural experiments as well as animal-based lab experiments. As an example of the former, a 2003 study in which families' incomes were (arguably) randomly affected by the opening of a casino on an American Indian reservation documented the following pattern: Even though an increase in family income was not a function of underlying family characteristics, it still resulted in a significant improvement in the mental health of children in affected families, result-ing in fewer conduct and oppositional defiant disorders (Costella et al., 2003). Animal experiments serve to support the biological mechanism and plausibility of a causal relationship between family income and offspring neurobiological outcomes.

Moreover, we know that exposure to high levels of stress negatively affects a child's developing brain, and poor families and minority families experience considerably more stress than others (Blair and Raver, 2016). A growing body of research on the impact of family stress on brain develop-ment and child health and well-being has indicated that parenting behavior serves as an important mechanism behind this effect (Blair and Raver, 2012; Feldman, 2015; McLoyd, 1998; Repetti et al., 2002). Parents who are stressed are less sensitive to children's needs and are less warm, and this ex-acerbates the negative effects of stress on a child's developing brain. A likely source of these differences in parenting behavior by socioeconomic status is the fact that (often single) mothers of poor families, as well as parents of families living in high-poverty neighborhoods, have less social support and less well-developed coping mechanisms than other parents have, and this can negatively affect the quality of their interactions with their children (Klebanov et al., 1994). As a result, not only are poor families less able to invest financially in their children, but also their nonfinancial investments, such as the amount and quality of their caregiving, are harmed by family disadvantage (Guryan et al., 2008).

Intersectional inequality is also of concern, and below we discuss exist-ing disparities by race and ethnicity in family income and wealth.

Family Income

From the end of World War II to the mid-1970s, the U.S. economy grew significantly, and incomes for those at the top and bottom of the income distribution grew at roughly the same rates, consistent with a growing prosperity that was broadly shared. However, beginning in the mid-1970s, growth slowed and income gaps grew wider. Households in the middle and bottom of the income distribution saw reduced growth and stagnation, respectively. In contrast, those in the top of the income distribution continued to see their incomes rise at a fast rate.

Scholars have attributed these changes to multiple factors: technological advances and globalization, with production and labor moving more freely across borders, a decline in union membership and rise in temporary and contingent labor, a shift from manufacturing jobs to those in the service and knowledge sectors, and higher returns to cognitive, technical, and managerial skills (Corcoran and Matsudaira, 2009; Danzinger and Ratner, 2010; Golden and Katz, 2008). Taxation policy and the eroding real value of the minimum wage have also contributed to the rising inequality witnessed since the mid-1970s (Danzinger and Ratner, 2010; Fontenot et al., 2018; Morris and Western, 1999).

These changes in the income distribution have significant implications for adolescent development and especially for disparities in their development. Rising income inequality combined with the stagnation of wages for those in the bottom half of the income distribution reduces the relative resources available to lower-income families for investment in their children. Data from the American Community Survey for 2016 show that Black and Latinx adolescents live in households characterized by significantly lower average incomes than their White counterparts: Whites ($85,000), Blacks ($38,000), Latinx ($43,000), and multiple-race households ($57,000).[9] Not only do the last three categories of families have fewer resources than White families for investment in their children, but also they suffer greater relative disadvantage.[10]

Family Wealth

Inequality in wealth accumulation has also increased steadily since 1979, and it exceeds inequality in income (Charles and Hurst, 2003; Saez and Zucman, 2014). For example, racial differences in wealth are three times greater than racial differences or gaps in income, with Whites in 2010 having on average nearly six times the wealth of Blacks (McKernan et al., 2013). One factor contributing to inequality in wealth accumulation is his-

---

[9] See https://datacenter.kidscount.org/data/tables/8782-median-family-income-among-households-with-children-by-race-and-ethnicity#detailed/1/any/false/870,573,869,36,133,35,16/4038,4040,4039,2638,2597,4758,1353/17618.

[10] The extent to which relative income matters is an area of active debate, with some research findings suggesting that proximity to more affluent peers negatively affects child outcomes (via competitive disadvantage or "negative self-evaluations" among the less well-off), while other research finds that proximity to youth of higher socioeconomic status improves outcomes for disadvantaged youth (Chetty et al., 2016; Odgers, 2015).

torical discrimination in housing and banking policies, which has reduced opportunities for wealth accumulation among Black and Latinx families in particular. More recently, the Great Recession reduced the wealth of many Americans, but disproportionately affected the wealth of Black and Latinx families, whose wealth fell by 31 and 40 percent, respectively, compared with an 11 percent loss for White families (McKernan et al., 2013). Like income, wealth accumulation affects the resources families have available for investing in the next generation, especially for investing in their higher education.

In addition, because of the relatively high rates of residential segregation in the United States, adolescents from poor or minority families are much more likely to live in poor and minority neighborhoods. The degree of residential segregation is measured by researchers using a "dissimilarity index," a measure of the evenness with which two groups are distributed across multiple geographic areas that make up a larger area. Neighborhoods with large levels of segregation will have numbers that are high on the index, which ranges from 0.0 (lowest level of segregation) to 1.0 (highest level of segregation). Current measures of dissimilarity for Black and Latinx households are 0.67 and 0.52, respectively. These dissimilarity index scores are both higher (indicating greater segregation) than those calculated for the foreign-born (0.44) and for the poor (0.37) (Boustan, 2013).

Between 1960 and 2000, Black-White residential segregation fell by a third. But importantly, that decline reflected falling segregation between neighborhoods within a jurisdiction. Over the same period, segregation actually rose between cities and suburbs and across different suburban areas. Segregation also rose for Latinx families (Frey, 2010). This high degree of segregation has meant that in 2010, Blacks were four times more likely to live in a high-poverty neighborhood (defined as greater than 40% poor) than other Americans. High levels of racial/ethnic residential segregation even affect the neighborhood characteristics of higher-income Black and Latinx families: On average, Black families with earnings of $75,000 live in higher-poverty neighborhoods than White families with earnings of just $40,000 (Logan, 2011).

Neighborhood Resources

Why does neighborhood matter so much? Neighborhoods matter because of their physical and social characteristics and the normative environment they produce. Recent work shows that neighborhoods are highly predictive of whether the offspring of poor parents escape poverty as adults (Chetty et al., 2018). Moving to a neighborhood with a higher likelihood of upward mobility is associated with improved outcomes for children when those moves occur before adolescence.[11] In this section, we describe the literature as it relates to multiple characteristics of a neighborhood including housing quality, exposure to violence, environmental supports, expectations, and social capital.

Housing Quality. First and foremost, the quality of housing in low-income neighborhoods is significantly lower, characterized by high levels of mold and lead, moisture, dust mites, and rodents. Such conditions have been linked with poor physical and mental health among the children and adolescents residing there (Coley et al., 2013; NASEM, 2019). Asthma, in particular, is likely to be exacerbated by poor housing conditions and is the chronic disease that causes the greatest number of school absences, which in turn are a contributing factor to diminished achievement, school drop-out, lower college completion, and greater welfare use and criminal justice involvement (Kreger et al., 2011).[12] Furthermore, absences can also lead directly to the loss of school revenues, since funding is tied to student attendance (Kreger et al., 2010).

Exposure to Violence. High-poverty neighborhoods are also characterized by high levels of violence and low levels of safety (Peterson and Krivo, 2010; Sampson, 2012; U.S. Department of Housing and Urban Development, 2016). Nationally, the past 20 years have witnessed significant declines in crime, including violent crime. While those declines have been greatest in the most violent and most disadvantaged neighborhoods, crime still remains concentrated in those cities characterized by the highest levels of disadvantage (Friedson and Sharkey, 2015).

Exposure to community violence—either witnessing violence or being a victim—during childhood or adolescence can trigger an adverse stress response, which has in turn been shown to be highly negatively correlated with future adult health, including increased risk of cardiovascular disease, hypertension, asthma, and diabetes (Anda et al., 2006; Fowler et al., 2009; Herringa, 2017; Lee et al., 2017; Wathen and MacMillan, 2013). Exposure to violence and trauma is associated with several mental health challenges for adolescence, including depression and anxiety. Studies of middle- and high-school aged youth in the United States and Canada have documented relationships between exposure to community violence and higher rates of

---

[11] The adult lifetime income for a child from a low-income family (defined as below the 25th percentile of the income distribution) who lives in a census tract at the 25th percentile of upward mobility is about $200,000 lower than that of a child from a similar family living in a tract at the 75th percentile of upward mobility.

[12] For most students, asthma is a controllable disease if proper diagnosis and care are administered. The schooling of Black and Latinx students appears to be disproportionally affected by asthma (Kopel et al., 2014).

depressive and anxiety symptoms (Dube et al., 2018; Heinze et al., 2018; Heleniak et al., 2017). For example, a study of urban U.S. high school students found a strong positive association between exposure to violence during adolescence and subsequent self-reported depressive and anxiety symptoms (Heinze et al., 2018). Plainly, researchers found that exposure to violence was a significant predictor of depression levels (Heinze et al., 2018). Moreover, the effects of community violence exposure can follow adolescents into adulthood: using data from the National Longitudinal Study of Adolescent to Adult Health, researchers found that exposure to violence in adolescence was predictive of depressive symptoms in adulthood (Chen et al., 2017).

Emerging research indicates that exposure to violence in early adolescence is related to changes in brain structure and function in mid-adolescence, independent of age and gender (Saxbe et al., 2018). Much of this research focuses on the relationship between community violence and sleep, which (as discussed in Chapter 3) is critical for brain development in adolescence. Heissel and colleagues (2018), for example, found that the experience of local, prior-day violence disrupted sleep and increased next-day cortisol awakening response. In addition, Heleniak and colleagues (2018) found that exposure to community violence was associated with internalizing symptoms, negative affect during peer evaluation, emotional reactivity, and infrequent problem solving. The authors found that indirect effects of community violence on internalizing problems implicate emotion dysregulation as one mechanism linking community violence exposure to adolescents' internalizing symptoms.

Importantly, low-income adolescents, as well as Black and Latinx adolescents generally, are more likely to witness violence in their neighborhoods due to residential segregation and concentrated disadvantage, resulting in "compounded community trauma" and negatively affecting behavioral health (Alegria et al., 2010). Emerging literature also explores the role of historical trauma in shaping outcomes; see Box 4-2. Such adverse childhood experiences are important factors to consider when addressing the mental health of adolescents who come from communities dealing with violence.

Environmental Supports. Low-income neighborhoods are also more likely to be lacking in access to health care, youth-oriented organizations, and learning centers, and are more likely to be located near polluting factors (Boardman and Saint Onge, 2005). Together, these environmental factors harm adolescent development through reduced access to many of the services and opportunities that provide young people with supportive, healthy environments to learn, grow, and thrive (see Box 4-3 for adolescents' perspectives on neighborhood resources). Moreover, high-poverty neighborhoods often lack employment opportunities, including job training

BOX 4-2
Historical Trauma

Historical trauma refers to trauma(s) inflicted upon a group of people who share an ethnic, national, or religious identity (Evans-Campbell, 2008). Historical trauma includes both "the legacy of numerous traumatic events a community experiences over generations and . . . the psychological and social responses to such events" among later generations (Evans-Campbell, 2008, p. 320). This kind of trauma can reach across generations, "such that contemporary members of the affected group may experience trauma-related symptoms without having been present for the past traumatizing events" (Mohatt et al., 2014, p. 2). The term originated in the study of Jewish Holocaust survivors and their children and has been applied to American Indians and Alaska Natives (AIAN) (Brave Heart and DeBruyn, 1998), Japanese American internment camp survivors, and many other communities that share a history of victimization, oppression, and collective trauma exposure (Mohatt et al., 2014). Historical trauma can also be conceptualized as a form of structural racism that shapes the opportunities, risks, and health outcomes of contemporary affected populations (National Academies of Sciences, Engineering, and Medicine, 2017).

For communities affected by historical trauma, the experiences of previous generations can reverberate into the present day in both positive and negative ways. Historical trauma is thought to impact affected groups on three levels: individual, familial, and communal (Evans-Campbell, 2008). At the individual level, descriptive studies have found higher rates of post-traumatic stress symptoms (Karenian et al., 2011; Kellermann, 2001), injection drug use (Lemstra et al., 2012), and current depressive symptoms (Bombay et al., 2011) among some offspring of trauma survivors than their non-survivor peers. At the family level, the loss of traditional parenting knowledge (e.g., due to forced separation of children from parents), impaired family communication, and stress around parenting in some survivor families have been suggested as legacies of historical trauma (Campbell and Evans-Campbell, 2011; Evans-Campbell, 2008; Kellerman, 2001). Finally, some scholars have posited that high rates of alcoholism and poor physical health seen in the AIAN population could be communal-level impacts of historical trauma (Duran et al., 1998; Evans-Campbell, 2008).

However, historical trauma can also be "the nexus of . . . communitywide transformation and resilience" (Mohatt et al., 2014). Resilient responses to historical trauma have been documented among American Indians, Holocaust survivors, and the descendants of Armenian genocide survivors (Barel et al., 2010; Denham, 2008; Fast and Collin-Vézina, 2010; Karenian et al., 2011). For example, in a cross-sectional study of Native Hawaiian adolescents and young adults in community college, Pokhrel and Herzog (2014) identified a direct, negative relationship between historical trauma and self-reported substance use, perhaps due to greater identification with their culture.

BOX 4-3
Youth Perspectives: Neighborhood Inequality

Ayanna Tucker, an intern with the American Public Health Association, shared personal and professional experiences to demonstrate how resources can differ depending on resident income levels.

"I had kind of a unique experience of growing up in a predominantly White, affluent suburb . . . but I mostly went to inner-city schools through their magnet program . . . but my sister went to our neighborhood school her entire life . . . and she was only two grades below me so we were in middle school at the same time, we were in high school around the same time. And where I had one textbook in a classroom and it was beat up, she had two textbooks, one that she got to leave at school and one that she got to take home for her homework and they were both brand new . . . when you think about the little lapses in resources that add up . . . they have huge implications on whether or not the student goes to college, can they do well in college. And we know education has huge implications for other things such as health. . . . In D.C . . . I teach nutrition in Ward 7 [which] has two grocery stores. Ward 8 has one grocery store for the entire ward. . . . Wards 2 and 3 here in Northwest [D.C.] have several grocery stores. . . . So for a child to grow up in Ward 7 or 8, they are not given the opportunity to have access to fresh produce. . . ."

Tanya Gumbs, a former foster youth and current member of the Young Women's Advisory Council and Girls for Gender Equity, shared her experience attending three high schools in three different neighborhoods, each of which had significantly different resources and expectations.

" . . . growing up I went to three different high schools in three different types of neighborhoods. My first high school was in Staten Island . . . my school was predominantly White students. . . . We used to laugh and make a joke about it and say there's only 12 Black students. . . . My next high school was in Newark, New Jersey, and that was predominantly all students of color . . . and at that school I felt like I was like a prisoner. . . . Walked in every morning . . . metal detectors. . . police with guns. . . . I'm coming to school every day in what's supposed to be a safe environment but I feel like I'm a criminal. . . . I have to wear a uniform, which was orange, and come in every day with the police officer who had a gun on him and metal detectors and they pat you down. You couldn't bring your own food in, they tell you when you can go outside, when you can eat. Sounds like prison to me. You couldn't go outside at a certain time, you had to wear certain shoes. . . . There were gates up. . . . I didn't feel like a student, I felt like I was a prisoner there. . . . The fact that I had to protest to get a teacher and they felt like I was doing too much at that school, I feel like that's because of the neighborhood I was in. . . . My next high school after that was in Harlem, it was at Life Sciences [Secondary

---

BOX 4-3 Continued

School] and I felt like I had more resources and more opportunity. That's how I got a part of GGE [Girls for Gender Equity] and I felt like I had ways to join programs where I can join the corporate world, they call it, and if it wasn't for going to that school in Harlem. . . . You can take the train to go to Brooklyn, the Bronx, and Manhattan. . . . I don't think I would probably be here today. . . . Neighborhood plays, like, a big part in the kind of person you're going to be when you get older. . . . I feel like if I had stayed in Newark, New Jersey, I probably wouldn't have went to college, because they never taught us anything about going to college, or resumes . . . or how to dress for interviews. . . ."

---

and apprenticeship pathways, which can negatively influence adolescent expectations about their own adulthood. Research has shown that this lack of job opportunities also contributes to the behavioral health disparities observed in minority adolescents, driven by feelings of hopelessness and depression (White and Borrell, 2011).

Expectations. In addition to this unequal and reduced access to family and community or neighborhood resources, inequality contributes to how young people perceive themselves, their place in the world, and the possibilities for their future. That is, evidence from multiple disciplines indicates that inequality can signal to young people that they are unlikely to be able to climb up the socioeconomic ladder (Browman et al., 2017, 2019). As a result, both correlational and experimental studies have demonstrated that greater inequality is linked to a reduced likelihood that adolescents will be able to pursue long-term goals and an increased likelihood of teen pregnancy and failure to complete high school (Kearney and Levine, 2016).

Social Capital. It should be noted that a context of increasing inequality not only shapes the opportunities available to adolescents from backgrounds of lower socioeconomic status but also influences the lives of those from families with middle and higher socioeconomic status. As shown in several studies, individuals in societies with greater inequality feel a weaker sense of trust, connection, community, and purpose (Elgar, 2010; Vergolini, 2011). Conversely, young people in more equal societies are more likely to express prosocial behaviors, like offering help to neighbors or strangers in need, and more likely to feel and express gratitude about various aspects of their lives (DeCelles and Norton, 2016; Piff and Robinson, 2017).

Altogether, the ways that inequality can lead to the disintegration of social connections and weaken the social integration of communities can inevitably have a negative influence on the individual well-being of people. It is not surprising, therefore, that the level of inequality that people experience is a consistent predictor of happiness in life, which matters regardless of where a person falls on the income or wealth distribution (Oishi and Kesebir, 2015; Oishi et al., 2011).

Institutional and Systemic Sources of Inequities

Differences in family income, wealth, and neighborhood resources are often compounded by the institutions and systems in which youth interact. Although adolescent interactions with formal institutions present opportunities to decrease disparities through either the direct provision of services, or effective screening, diagnosis, and referral to appropriate services, in practice institutions and systems often reinforce disparate outcomes through unequal funding and segregation based on income, race, and ethnicity. This section discusses how various educational, health, welfare, and justice institutions and policies serve to increase disparities in adolescent outcomes, beginning with the school, an institution that almost all adolescents will interact with over a prolonged period. The next section addresses additional disparities that can arise in the design and operation of social systems as they interact with groups of adolescents.

Schools: Segregation and Financing

Historically, schools in the United States were segregated by race and funded largely through local property taxes. As a result, there were huge disparities in both the family resources of the students attending school as well as the public resources devoted to the administration of each school. The courts have been responsible for substantial changes to both. As a result of the landmark 1954 *Brown v. Board of Education* Supreme Court decision, U.S. schools desegregated (racially) between 1968 (the first year of adequate data) and 1980, with the greatest changes occurring in the South (Boozer et al., 1992). However, while within-school-district segregation fell, between-district segregation rose because of greater residential segregation by race and income across districts as a result of White flight, gentrification, and housing patterns and practices.

Since 1980, with the end of much court-ordered desegregation, there has been no further reduction in race-based school segregation. Segregation in practice (though not by law) stemming from economic or family-income differences has been rising since 1970, and Black and Latinx students are disproportionately served by high-minority, high-poverty schools (Owens et al., 2016). While most of the existing work on school segregation has focused on race and income, a 2016 Government Accountability Office report documented that Latinx youth comprise the largest group attending high-poverty schools, defined as 75 percent free lunch eligible (U.S. Government Accountability Office, 2016).[13]

However, while schools have become increasingly disparate in terms of the share of students from low-income families and racial/ethnic minorities, school financing has converged considerably over time (Lafortune et al., 2017). In 1990, low-income districts (defined as those in the bottom quantile of mean household income in the district) collected 20 percent less in school funding, but by 2001 these districts received funding equal to those in the top quantile. This parity was achieved by overall increases in funding for all schools, with disproportionately greater increases in low-income districts, stemming from reforms to state education funding formulas implemented in response to court orders. The increase in parity with respect to school financing corresponds to increasing parity with respect to teacher training and wages, which no longer vary significantly based on the racial or ethnic composition of the student body (U.S. Department of Education, Office of Civil Rights, 2015). This is not to imply that there are no differences in school resources for students based on income, race, and ethnicity. Black and Latinx students, for example, still have less access to advanced coursework such as calculus and physics as well as advanced placement courses in high school. The effects of such disparities on student achievement often carry on long after secondary school as this lack of early access fails to help prepare students for college and the workforce (U.S. Department of Education, Office of Civil Rights, 2015).

The increase in parity with respect to school financing has resulted in significant gains in test scores for students in low-income districts across the United States (they rose by 0.1 standard deviation, or one-fifth of the baseline gap between high- and low-income districts, over a 10-year period) (Lafortune et al., 2017). The fact that parity in funding did not result in an even greater parity in test scores suggests that increasing disparities in the family resources of students attending schools has continued to exert significant influence. Children from disadvantaged families enter kindergarten with lower rates of preliteracy and school readiness. One reason is that they are less likely to attend preschool, and if they have attended preschool it is likely one of lower quality (Magnuson and Waldfogel, 2005; Magnuson et al., 2004). In order to compensate for this starting-from-behind position,

---

[13]U.S. Government Accountability Office (2016) documented that the number of schools in which more than 75 percent of children were free lunch-eligible and more than 75 percent were Black or Latinx grew from 9 percent in 2001 to 16 percent in 2014.

children from disadvantaged households likely need *more* resources, and not simply equal resources, if society is to help reduce disparities in educational outcomes.

Moreover, in addition to fewer family resources being a source of disadvantage for some families when it comes to school readiness, there is also evidence that the collective resources of the families whose children attend a given school also matters. Segregation of schools by family income is the single most predictive factor of academic achievement gaps by race and income (Reardon, 2015). The increasing income segregation of American schools, along with rising income inequality, has most likely prevented society from achieving the full benefit of the significant gains in financial parity across schools in terms of improved outcomes and decreased disparities in test scores.

Housing: Segregation and Financing

School segregation is driven largely by neighborhood segregation and, as such, the policy or institutional response to the increasing segregation of American schools largely lies in housing policy. The Fair Housing Act of 1968 requires that all municipalities follow policies to "affirmatively further fair housing," but to date this has not been pursued with vigor. There is a severe shortage of affordable homes generally in the United States today. The federal housing voucher program, which subsidizes the rent of low- and middle-income families, in theory, allows families to move to more integrated neighborhoods, but it currently funds only 5.3 million individuals in 2.2 million households. Moreover, tightness in the housing market and housing discrimination serve to reduce the likelihood that low-income families can move to low-poverty neighborhoods, even with a housing voucher (Chetty et al., 2016; Katz et al., 2001).

The federal government has dramatically reduced its direct role in the construction of low-income housing, in part because public housing projects served to exacerbate the segregation of low-income families in high-poverty areas. Instead, the government has increasingly relied on making low-income housing tax credits available to developers to increase their construction of housing for low-income populations. However, evidence suggests that these construction projects have not resulted in meaningful integration. Rather, this program is more likely to provide higher-quality housing in poor neighborhoods than to build affordable housing in low-poverty neighborhoods (Cummings and DiPasquale, 1999).

Health Care: Access and Quality

Unlike education, health care is not freely available to all adolescents, and some of the disparities in their health arise from disparate access to health care for certain groups. Recent policy efforts, including the Affordable Care Act (ACA), have reduced one important source of disparities in medical care: access to health insurance. In assessing the impact of the ACA on health care access, a recent analysis of the national Medical Expenditure Panel Survey found significant increases in full-year public insurance coverage among adolescents, namely that their coverage rate of 23 percent before the ACA rose to 30 percent afterwards. There were also significant decreases among adolescents in partial coverage (dropping from 14 to 11%) and full-year uninsured status (from 9 to 5%) (Adams et al., 2017). This increase in insurance coverage was accompanied by an increase in the proportion of adolescents receiving a preventive care visit, which rose from 41 to 48 percent, with minority and low-income groups experiencing the greatest increases.[14]

Although the ACA brought about significant improvements in overall health insurance coverage and declines in disparities in coverage, severe inequities in access to and quality of care remain. Roughly 15 to 20 million children—the majority of whom are Black, Latinx, and low-income adolescents[15]—reside in medically underserved areas, thereby limiting their access to comprehensive and coordinated health care. "Medical homes" is defined as "an approach to providing comprehensive primary care that facilitates partnerships between patients, clinicians, medical staff, and fami-

---

[14] Measuring the change between pre- and post-ACA, non-White Latinx adolescents saw an increase from 33 to 43 percent. There was also a significant increase among Black adolescents from 37 to 46 percent in the proportion who had received a preventive visit. The largest increase in preventive care visits was seen among the lowest-income group (<100% of the federal poverty level or FPL), which rose from 33 to 43 percent, followed by adolescents with household incomes between 100 and 200 percent of FPL, which rose from 34 to 43 percent. The highest-income group only saw a 3 percent increase pre-to-post-ACA (51 to 54%, respectively) in the proportion reporting accessing preventive health visits.

[15] Based upon the National Survey of Children's Health, 2016 data, 48 percent of adolescents (ages 12 to 17) *without special health care needs* have a medical home; this includes 36 percent of Latinx adolescents, 40 percent of Black adolescents, and 60 percent of White adolescents. Income level also impacts whether *any child* (ages 0 to 17) without special health care needs will have a medical home. For these children, among those below poverty (using the FPL), 36 percent have a medical home; among those between 100 and 199 percent of FPL, 41 percent do; among those between 200 and 399 percent of FPL, 53 percent do; and among those above 400 percent of FPL, 63 percent do (National Adolescent and Young Health Information Center, University of San Francisco, 2016).

lies" by the American Academy of Pediatrics.[16] Related to this, young people in rural areas have less access to primary health care and mental health care than their urban peers (Sanders et al., 2017).

"Crossover Youth": Dual Involvement in Child Welfare and Justice System

The experiences of youth in the child welfare system are closely related to their experiences in the juvenile justice system, as the same adolescents are disproportionately represented in both systems (Smith et al., 2005).[17] Adolescents in the child welfare system often face (or have faced) challenges within the home that may increase the likelihood that they will engage in behaviors such as truancy or running away from home. Although non-criminal, these behaviors, known as "status offenses,"[18] are often the primary mechanism by which youth in the child welfare system "crossover" into the juvenile justice system. Adolescents that engage in status offenses often have higher rates of mental health and substance abuse disorders, and abuse and neglect during childhood have also been found to be highly predictive of committing status offenses (Herz and Ryan, 2008a).[19] Moreover, when youth in the child welfare system become involved in the juvenile justice system, they are more likely to be treated harshly, such as being sentenced to detention instead of probation.[20] Some have argued that the disproportionate share of minority adolescents in CPS is one of the main drivers of the disproportionate share of minority adolescents in juvenile detention. Child welfare involvement is an especially important avenue or pathway to the juvenile justice system for female adolescents (Ryan et al., 2007). (For further discussion of the status offense system, see Chapter 8.)

---

[16] The goal of the medical home approach to providing care is to "produce higher quality care and improved cost efficiency." See *Engaging Patients and Families: What Is Medical Home?* from the American Academy of Pediatrics, available at https://www.aap.org/en-us/professional-resources/practice-transformation/managing-patients/Pages/what-is-medical-home.aspx.

[17] Based on statistics collected from individual studies of local areas, it is estimated that 30 percent of children in the child welfare system have future involvement in juvenile justice system as well.

[18] Status offenses are defined as offenses considered crimes if committed by persons under the age of 18.

[19] Herz and Ryan (2008a) found that 80 percent and 61 percent of dual system-involved youth had substance abuse and mental health disorders in a study of Arizona youth. LGBTQ youth, who are more likely to face bullying and harassment in school, are also more likely to run away from home and be truant (Gay, Lesbian, and Straight Education Network, 2017).

[20] Again, there are no national statistics, only local studies. In Los Angeles County, for example, the probability of probation rather than placement or corrections was only 58 percent for CPS involved youth as compared to 73 percent for non-CPS involved youth (Herz and Ryan, 2008b; Ryan et al., 2007).

"Crossover youth"—youth involved in *both* CPS and juvenile justice—have the most significant needs and, therefore, require greater services, but they often experience service disruptions when they transition to the juvenile justice system (Pumariega et al., 1999). For female crossover youth in particular, who are at greater risk of pregnancy, there are few gender-specific programs to address their needs. The degree of service disruption is a function of the type of arrangements made between the two systems, which is determined by state statute. States that give the agencies concurrent jurisdictions afford the greatest amount of coordination for crossover youth, who thereby remain eligible for services provided by both systems. In contrast, in states with separate jurisdictions there is much less coordination, and adolescents lose eligibility for services when they become involved in the juvenile justice system.

Because of their greater underlying risk, their disparate treatment in the juvenile justice systems, and the disruptions in service provision they experience, crossover youth (who are disproportionately Black), have worse outcomes than other youth in both the short and the long term. They are more likely to be arrested as adults, less likely to be employed, and more likely to receive public assistance in adulthood (Culhane et al., 2011). Chapter 8, which addresses adolescents in the child welfare system, explores how the system's processes affect adolescent outcomes in greater detail.

Racism, Bias, and Discrimination

A third source of disparities in adolescent outcomes derives from the explicit and implicit (or unconscious) biases that individuals hold against groups defined by race, ethnicity, gender, LGBTQ identity, ability status, and other categories. These biases can be expressed in both singular significant interactions as well as in a series of less obvious but frequent events, referred to as micro-aggressions.[21] When aggregated in an institutional context, these biases can result in disparate outcomes for the affected groups.

Adolescents are especially sensitive to the attitudes and behaviors of adult members of the community, on whom they rely for information and encouragement with respect to care-seeking behavior, effort exerted in school, and so on. Community attitudes and behaviors can influence both the probability of mental health disorders as well as the probability of treatment. With regard to the former, the experience of bias and discrimination can harm the behavioral health of adolescents, with affected adolescents demonstrating greater depressive and anxiety symptoms (Chithambo et

---

[21] A microaggression is defined as "brief and commonplace daily verbal, behavioral, or environmental indignities, whether intentional or unintentional, that communicate hostile, derogatory, or negative . . . slights and insults" (Sue et al., 2007, p. 1).

al., 2014; Davis et al., 2016; Park et al., 2017) and outward expressions of anger (Umaña-Taylor, 2016). These effects can be long-lasting. Assari and colleagues (2017) found that Black adolescent males who perceived discrimination during adolescence suffered greater negative effects on anxiety and depression in adulthood than Black females, which may suggest one potential source for the relatively worse outcomes of adolescent Black males relative to females in terms of their educational, health, and justice-system outcomes. Bias among peers and families might also affect adolescent outcomes and explain disparities; Box 4-4 discusses the impact of family or peer acceptance and support of LGBTQ adolescents.

Researchers have also hypothesized that exposure to discrimination results in worse physical health, moderated by higher levels of stress as measured by elevated cortisol.[22] Consistent with this, Russell and colleagues (2012) found that adolescents experiencing bias-based harassment are at greater risk for compromised health outcomes in adulthood than those experiencing non-bias-based harassment (Russell et al., 2012).

In the following, we discuss the evidence regarding the bias behaviors of adults who regularly interact with adolescents and how they may help explain disparities in adolescent outcomes. By "those who regularly interact with adolescents" we mean teachers, health professionals, case workers, police officers, and other official participants in the juvenile justice system (including lawyers, judges, and corrections officers).

Educators

In the domain of education, teachers often have different expectations and standards for their students based on students' race, ethnicity, gender, and sexuality, which show up when it comes to evaluating student achievement and behavior. When a teacher has lower expectations of an adolescent's achievement based on the adolescent's group identity, this has a harmful influence on actual achievement (Jussim and Harber, 2005).

Recent research finds that Black teachers have expectations of their Black students that are 30 to 40 percent higher than the expectations that White teachers have of the same students (Gershenson et al., 2016). The same research shows evidence of intersectional inequality: these differences are larger for Black male students than for Black female students (Gershenson et al., 2016). These findings are consistent with research, finding that, for elementary-school-age Black children, having a Black teacher in third through fifth grades increased the probability of graduation from high school (Gershenson et al., 2017). These findings underscore the consid-

---

[22] See Richman and Jonassaint (2008) for evidence linking experimental exposure to discrimination and cortisol.

BOX 4-4
Impact of Family or Peer
Acceptance and Support for LGBTQ Adolescents

LGBTQ adolescents often face additional obstacles when parents and families are not accepting or supportive of their sexual identity. LGBTQ youth often report lower levels of parental closeness and elevated rates of parental abuse and homelessness (Katz-Wise et al., 2016). LGBTQ youth who report higher rates of family acceptance have greater self-esteem, social support, and better general health status than those who report lower rates of family acceptance. Family acceptance also protects against depression, substance abuse, and suicidal ideation and behaviors (Ryan et al., 2010).

Researchers have hypothesized that the common lack of acceptance of LGBTQ adolescents by their families explains why LGBTQ adolescents are overrepresented in the juvenile justice system: LGBTQ adolescents who represent 5 to 7 percent of the overall adolescent population represent 13 to 15 percent of those currently in the juvenile justice system (Hunt and Moodie-Mills, 2012; Majd et al., 2009). Researchers have also linked their higher rates of detention to the higher occurrence of out-of-home placements and homelessness among these youths (Irvine, 2010), as well as to lack of family support, which may be cited by judges as a rationale for residential placement (Majd et al., 2009).

erable cost associated with the continuing shortage of Black teachers in U.S. schools (Madkins, 2011). (For further discussion, see "Creating Culturally Sensitive Learning Environments" in Chapter 7).[23]

Disparate treatment of students when it comes to disciplinary actions, such as suspension or expulsion, is well documented (see, e.g., Gordon, 2018). Most of the previous work has focused on racial/ethnic differences, finding that Black and Latinx high school students, for example, are only slightly more likely than White or Asian students to be "sent to the principal's office" for disciplinary infractions but are two to four times more likely to be suspended or expelled (Wallace et al., 2008). They find that the differences by race and ethnicity cannot be explained by differences in income. More recently, researchers have examined the disparate treatment of LGBTQ students as well as students with disabilities (see, e.g., Skiba et al., 2016).

Interestingly, the reasons why White and minority students are reported for discipline differs significantly, with minority students being referred more often for more subjective reasons, such as "disrespect" and "perceived

---

[23] Eighty-two percent of teachers are White, compared with 8 percent who are Black. Among students, only 47 percent are White and 17 percent are Black. See https://nces.ed.gov/surveys/sass/tables/sass1112_2013314_t1s_001.asp.

threat," and White students referred more often for more objectively identi-fiable reasons, such smoking or vandalism (Skiba et al., 2002). The higher rates of suspension for Black and Latinx students for subjective infractions is consistent with differences in teacher and school personnel treatment of students based on race and ethnicity. Experimental evidence confirms racial bias in disciplinary decisions. Okonofua and Eberhardt (2015) found that when presented with identical descriptions of student behavior, teachers viewed two minimal infractions as more troubling and deserving of harsher punishment when committed by a Black student than by a White student. Mendez (2003) found that unequal treatment based on race, ethnicity, gen-der, sexuality, or disability status results in disparate outcomes for children, as out-of-school suspensions are highly predictive of future involvement with the criminal justice system and reduced educational achievement.[24] Recent initiatives have sought to reduce the suspensions and expulsions of youth of color from schools, but to date these initiatives have been small in scope.[25] (See also Chapter 9, Box 9-2, "Relationship Between School Disciplinary Policies and the Juvenile Justice System.")

Health Care Professionals

Health care professionals have also been found to treat adolescents from different social and racial/ethnic groups differently (Valenzuela and Smith, 2015). Provider attitudes have been identified as an important determinant of the quality of care provided to adolescents (Alegria et al., 2011).[26] In a clinical setting, even the most well-intentioned providers can contribute to racial/ethnic disparities in adolescent health care because of unconscious stereotyping (Burgess et al., 2004). One study that examined the way alcohol and other drug use was screened for in the primary care setting revealed that adolescents from minority groups were less likely to be screened than their non-Latinx White counterparts (Meredith et al., 2018). Since many of these adolescents are not being asked about alcohol and other drug use by their doctors, their harmful behaviors could be going unnoticed, perpetuating the consequences associated with substance abuse.

---

[24] Moreover, there is little evidence that school disciplinary actions result in reductions in the "misbehavior" they are intended to modify (Mendez, 2003).

[25] For example, the California Endowment has supported special projects in Oakland Schools geared to the retention of Black males in particular—rather than losing them. See https://philanthropynewsdigest.org/news/california-endowment-commits-50-million-to-keep-boys-and-young-men-of-color-in-school.

[26] Nevertheless, matching adolescents with providers of the same ethnicity or race has not been consistently shown to reduce disparities in the quality of care received.

Child Welfare System Actors

There are multiple reasons why Black and Latinx children are much more likely to be referred to CPS. Disproportionate need (typically stemming from poverty) and differential treatment by both community members and the child welfare system play important roles in explaining the disparities. Research on the sources of these disparities has been summarized elsewhere (Alliance for Racial Equity in Child Welfare, 2011). In general, both observational and experimental research has found that community reporters (e.g., teachers and doctors) are more likely to report children of color to CPS than other children. The experimental results suggest a role for personal bias, but the observational results are consistent with a more systematic source, such as increased maltreatment surveillance in communities of color (Chaffin and Bard, 2006).

Not only are children of color more likely to be referred to CPS, but also, conditional on observable characteristics, they are more likely to be removed for reasons not related to underlying risk. Two Texas-based studies documented that although Black families tended to be assessed as lower risk than White families, they were more likely to have substantiated cases and their children removed (Dettlaff et al., 2011; Rivaux et al., 2008). Additional research has found that Black caseworkers on average assessed all families (regardless of race) as higher risk than did White caseworkers. The fact that Black families are more likely to be assigned to Black caseworkers may explain some of the higher rates of substantiated maltreatment observed for Black families (Font et al., 2012).

A second important source of systemic disparity in treatment is the offering of fewer in-home services to families of color that might prevent the placement of a child or adolescent in foster care (Fluke et al., 2011). A Michigan-based study found that contracted agencies were not providing services in Black communities although they were required to do so (Center for the Study of Social Policy, 2009). As a result, children of color were both more likely to be removed from a home and more likely to remain in their foster placement longer without permanent resolution.

Justice System Actors

The area in which disparate treatment of adolescents has received the most public attention is the criminal and juvenile justice systems. As of 2013, Black adolescents were four times more likely to be committed to residential placements as White adolescents, Native Americans were three times as likely, and Latinx adolescents were 61 percent more likely (Rovner, 2016) (Figure 4-6). Although the available data are difficult to assess because of the nature of self-reports, they suggest that White and Black

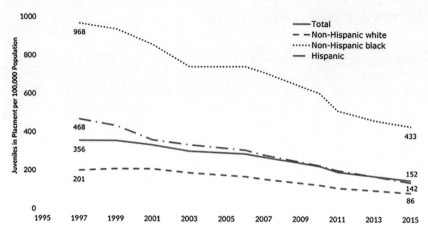

FIGURE 4-6 Trends in juvenile residential placement by race and ethnicity, 1997-2015.
NOTES: The Census of Juveniles in Residential Placement collects data on all juvenile residential custody facilities in the United States, asking for information on each youth assigned a bed in each facility on the last Wednesday in October. Residential facilities include detention centers, shelters, reception/diagnostic centers, group homes, boot camps, ranch/wilderness camps, residential treatment centers, and long-term secure facilities. Rates are calculated per 100,000 juveniles ages 10 through the upper age of each state's juvenile court jurisdiction.
SOURCE: Child Trends (2018).

high school students do not differ in the probability of either committing property crime or engaging in violent behavior (Bureau of Justice Statistics, 2000). The disparate treatment they nevertheless receive is particularly troubling given the system's stated emphasis on fairness, suggesting that much of the disparate treatment stems from interpersonal sources of bias.

The fact that there have been significant declines in juvenile arrest and detention in the United States since 1995 has not translated into declines in disparities by race and ethnicity; in fact, disparities appear to have increased over this period. These disparities seem to widen at every stage of the process, from arrest, to the decision to prosecute and remove to adult court, to sentencing and type of confinement (DeLone and DeLone, 2017; Fader et al., 2014; Sickmund et al., 2014). A possible explanation for the increase in disparate treatment over the past two decades is the decline in the rate of serious offenses for which there is less discretion in the decision making (e.g., in deciding to prosecute or how to sentence). As the number of less-serious offenses has risen as a proportion of all offenses, there may have been more discretion exercised by practitioners at every stage of the process, potentially resulting in a greater proportion of biased decisions. For further discussion of disparities in the justice system, see Chapter 9.

ACHIEVING EQUITY FOR ADOLESCENTS

While inequalities in opportunity are deeply rooted in U.S. society, progress can be achieved. Recent improvements in adolescent health and well-being, education, and justice-system involvement inspire some confidence that change is possible. In this section, we discuss promising policies and programs that attempt to tackle some of the disparities in opportunity outlined above, including (1) policies and programs aiming to reduce disparities in income, wealth, and neighborhood resources to rectify disparities in financing and policy implementation in youth-serving systems; (2) trauma-informed approaches preparing adults serving youth in youth-serving systems to address differential exposure to violence and trauma among youth; and (3) emerging tools to erase or counteract bias in decision making by system-level actors. Specific policies to combat disparities in institutions and systems are discussed in Chapters 6 through 9.

It is also important to note that existing research demonstrates the great resilience and strength of youth traditionally considered disadvantaged or at risk (Task Force Report on Resilience and Strength in African-American Children and Adolescents, n.d.). Box 4-5 summarizes the extant literature on resilience in adolescence; see also Chapter 3. Defining resilience as "a dynamic process encompassing positive adaptation within the context of significant adversity" (Luthar et al., 2000, p. 543), resilient youth have exhibited positive outcomes in a host of domains: education, health, and psychological well-being. Indeed, researchers have documented many instances of adolescents in adverse circumstances becoming very high achievers (Hoxby and Avery, 2012). It is important to keep this in mind when interpreting existing research on disparities. Identifying and promoting resilience and strength among disadvantaged and at-risk youth, while encouraging the development of further protective factors, holds promise for enhancing opportunity for all adolescents.

Reducing Disparities in Income, Wealth, and Neighborhood Resources

As described above, one of the key sources of inequality in opportunity and treatment that affects adolescents is disparities in the resources of families and communities where adolescents live. However, such disparities are not intractable; solutions to child poverty are achievable.

Existing programs, such as the Supplemental Nutrition Assistance Program (SNAP) and the Earned Income Tax Credit (EITC), have been found to reduce child poverty and improve child and adult outcomes (NASEM, 2019). SNAP, and its predecessor, the Food Stamp Program, have been shown to improve child health in both the short- and the long-term. For example, Hoynes and colleagues (2016) found that participation in SNAP

BOX 4-5
Resilience in Adolescence

Despite growing up in adverse circumstances, some children are able to thrive or "adapt well" to the stressors of their environment. A growing body of research has examined factors and mechanisms that have a protective effect against negative outcomes associated with living in disadvantaged communities, where resources are scarce and negative social and affective experiences are common (Chiang et al., 2015; Conger et al., 2010). These *resiliency characteristics* are conceptualized as intrapersonal psychological traits such as perseverance, self-reliance, and emotional stamina (Edwards et al., 2014; Wagnild and Young, 1993; Wingo et al., 2014) and can be understood as a process or the adaptive capacity of multiple systems in a person's life (Masten, 2011; Southwick et al., 2014; Tlapek et al., 2017).

Over the past decade, studies identified the neurobiological factors of risk and resilience. For example, recent studies have considered the relationship between neural development and physiological response to chronic stress: Teenagers living in high-crime neighborhoods who have stronger and more efficient central executive networks (brain areas governing the regulation of emotion) are also the ones who show lower biological indicators of stress and better cardiovascular health (Pinker, 2018; Miller et al., 2018).

Parents play an important role in supporting the resiliency of their children. Parenting that includes high levels of warmth, sensitivity, and emotional support can help to mitigate both the psychosocial disadvantages (Brody et al., 2012b; Rutter, 2005) and hormonal, metabolic, and cardiovascular changes that are associated with exposure to poverty (Brody et al., 2014, 2017b). Furthermore, children and adolescents who have a strong attachment to their family and strong family cohesion have lower levels of mental health problems, such as anxiety and depressive symptoms and obsessive-compulsive disorder (Bond et al., 2005; Dray et al., 2017; Hjemdal et al., 2007, 2011). Support from natural mentors (nonparental adults) is also a key form of social connectedness and can mitigate risk in cases where parents are not central figures, as may be the case for homeless youth (Dang et al., 2014; Thompson et al., 2016).

Building upon this knowledge of preventative factors, preventative parent and family-centered interventions have been shown to have stress-buffering capacities for a range of psychosocial outcomes such as self-control, drug use, and conduct problems (Brody et al., 2012a). A randomized control trial using the Strong African American Families (SAAF) Program showed that these effects even have long-term consequences for patterns of brain development (see Chapter 3). School-based universal interventions targeted at adolescents themselves also show great promise in supporting mental health and resilience (Brunwasser et al., 2009; Seligman et al., 2009; Weisz et al., 2005). To help young people thrive in the face of adversity, interventions can be developed to further capitalize on the unique characteristics of the population of interest and the protective factors associated with healthy outcomes for that particular group (Zolkoski and Bullock, 2012).

in childhood is related to reduced incidence of metabolic syndrome in adulthood. For adolescents, who need adequate energy and nutrient intake to support their physical growth, SNAP benefits can play a particularly important role in their healthy development.

Yet families with teenagers face higher rates of food insecurity than families with younger children (Nord, 2009). This may be partly due to the fact that SNAP benefit allocations are based on the assumption that all children in a household are 12 years old or younger (Ziliak, 2016), thereby failing to take into account the increased dietary needs of adolescents. However, a recent National Academies report, *A Roadmap to Reducing Child Poverty* ("Reducing Child Poverty report") found that expanding SNAP benefits, accounting for the needs of adolescents, and increasing benefits during the summer months could decrease child poverty rates by as much as 2.3 percent, depending on how large the expansion is (NASEM, 2019).[27]

Similarly, the EITC—a refundable tax credit for low- and moderate-income workers—has been shown to improve the longer-term health and human capital of children and youth in families who receive it. Several studies have found a consistent positive impact of larger EITC payments on children's and adolescents' education outcomes (NASEM, 2019). For example, Maxfield (2013) found that larger EITC payments increase the odds of youth in low-income families graduating from high school and completing 1 or more years of college by age 19. Similarly, Manoli and Turner (2014) found that more generous EITC payments lead to a greater number of youth in low-income families attending college. Further expanding the EITC could decrease child poverty rates by up to 2.1 percent, lifting 1.5 million children and youth out of poverty, according to the Reducing Child Poverty report (NASEM, 2019).

In addition to expanding existing programs, implementing innovative new programs could cut child poverty rates further and improve the material circumstances of adolescents living in poverty (NASEM, 2019). For example, implementing a child allowance program—which would provide a monthly cash payment to families for each child under 18 in the household—has the potential to reduce child poverty in the United States by as much as 40 percent (NASEM, 2019). Child allowance programs are already in effect in 17 other nations, including Australia, Canada, Ireland, and the United Kingdom (NASEM, 2019). In addition to benefiting adolescents under 18 and their families, a child allowance program would also support adolescents who are parents.

---

[27] The report presents data from a microsimulation model called TRIM3. For more on this proposal and the study methodology, visit nap.edu/reducingchildpoverty.

In summary, the child poverty rate in the United States can be reduced substantially through the expansion of existing programs and the implementation of new ones. Living in poverty significantly curtails economic opportunity for adolescents and youth of color who are disproportionately disadvantaged by growing up in poverty. By reducing child poverty, society can make a timely long-term investment to overcome the inequities faced by adolescents from low-income families and unleash new opportunities.

Addressing Differential Exposure to Violence and Trauma

Research from across disciplines has highlighted the potential impact of trauma on all aspects of an adolescent's development and functioning and recognized that in many different settings it is essential that those who encounter adolescents routinely understand how trauma may be manifested in the particular context of the encounters. This viewpoint is becoming increasingly developed under the umbrella of *trauma-informed youth services*. To be trauma-informed means to know the history of past and current abuse in the life of the person one is serving, no matter what the service setting. Because trauma's impact is manifested during adolescence in ways that cut across all aspects of their development and behavior, the major initial challenge in becoming trauma-informed is how to recognize and identify trauma victims across the many varied settings that serve young people and places they congregate. The second challenge is how to engage these young people in services that can help them.

In calling for a trauma-informed service system, Harris and Fallot (2001) write:

> Systems serve survivors of childhood trauma without treating them for the consequences of that trauma; more significant, systems serve individuals without even being aware of the trauma that occurred. This lack of awareness can result in failures to make appropriate referrals for trauma services. It can also result in inadvertent re-traumatization when a service system's usual operating procedures trigger a reemergence or an exacerbation of trauma symptoms (p. 3).

Further, Harris and Fallot (2001) identify the following requirements for services to be truly trauma-informed:

1. administrative commitment to change, including allocating resources to ensure this;
2. universal screening;
3. trauma-specific training and education;

4. ensuring that hiring practices are designed to recruit expertise in trauma; and

5. ensuring that policies and procedures are sensitive to the issues faced by trauma victims.

So, for example, in schools teachers and school support staff need to be informed about how, in the school setting, adolescent victims are frequently misidentified as presenting with attention deficit disorder, oppositional-defiant disorder, or conduct disorder. Such a diagnosis may prevent consideration of effective interventions for curtailing or remediating the effects of trauma (Perry, 2006).

McInerney and McKlindon (2014) note that some states, such as Massachusetts and Washington, are implementing trauma-informed approaches in schools. These states have adopted models, such as the Sanctuary Model,[28] which engage educational leaders and staff to develop a culture where educators model and students develop safety, emotional management, self-control, and conflict resolution skills. They note that for schools, being trauma-informed requires being informed about and responsive to trauma, and providing a safe and stable environment for both students and staff, acknowledging trauma and its triggers, and avoiding stigmatizing and punishing students. One of the goals is to prevent re-traumatization (McInerney and McKlindon, 2014). Another example of trauma-specific interventions designed for use in schools is the Cognitive Behavioral Intervention for Trauma in Schools, an evidence-based intervention that can be delivered in group settings or individually and that includes psychoeducation for parents and training for teachers.

In systems that work with adolescent populations that are disproportionately affected by trauma—child welfare and juvenile justice—there is an emerging literature on the implementation of trauma-informed approaches. For example, Ford and Blaustein (2013) describe trauma-informed approaches developed for juvenile justice systems and present guidelines for one model: Trauma Affect Regulation: Guide for Education and Therapy (TARGET). TARGET is an educational and therapeutic intervention for adolescents and adults that can be implemented as individual or group therapy and focuses on trauma-related dysregulation, reframing symptoms as adaptive responses.

Hodgdon and colleagues (2013) describe the application of an evidenced-based, trauma-informed treatment framework known as Attachment, Regulation and Competency (ARC), used with youth involved in the justice system (Hodgdon et al., 2013). Initial data demonstrated a significant reduction in post-traumatic stress disorder symptoms and externalizing

---

[28] See http://www.sanctuaryweb.com/schools.php.

and internalizing behaviors, outcomes that are supportive of its clinical utility as a practice in residential contexts.

In addition, Riebschleger and colleagues (2015) have called for bringing a trauma-informed lens to the child welfare system. Noting that foster care youth commonly experience complex trauma as a result of family-of-origin maltreatment and separations from their families, youth involved in the study identified strategies for supporting children in foster care and reducing trauma before, during, and after foster care placement. They noted that foster parents need more training and support for dealing with traumatized youth, and asked for greater efforts to help them remain connected with their families, especially siblings.

Using Predictive Analytics to Reduce Bias in Decision Making

As discussed above, racism, bias, and discrimination contribute to differences in opportunity for youth, particularly when system-level actors exhibit such behaviors in their decision making. Although it is possible for data to have biases—as much data derive from systems and individuals that internalize societal biases and discrimination—predictive analytics (the use of historical data to predict the likelihood of future events) have the *potential* to greatly improve outcomes for youth. So long as algorithms are thoughtfully designed to avoid duplicating common human preferences and biases, such as those favoring a particular race, ethnicity, gender, or other group, and are deployed with datasets that are equally clean of bias, then algorithms, unlike human beings, do not have any intrinsic preferences to favor any particular race, ethnicity, gender, or other groups and are better able to make accurate predictions at the group level, which can lead to gains in societal outcomes that benefit disadvantaged groups. Thus, the committee views predictive analytics as promising for two reasons: (1) Algorithms use the same data that individuals use to make predictions and decisions. While individuals in the course of their decision making may add their own biases on top of those biases inherent in the data, algorithms can be structured so as to not add additional bias in their decision-making process. (2) Because algorithms can be more transparent in their operations, it is easier to detect whether any bias in the data are leading to biased decisions, and then make corrections. When individuals use data to predict and decide, given the opacity of the human condition, it is difficult to determine how data is influencing decision making, and therefore, similar course corrections to reverse bias are much more difficult to implement.

Although predictive analytics were first used as early as the late 1990s, the predictive models they built were not very accurate, mostly because of the paucity of data available to model risk. Since then, state and local governments have embarked on efforts to consolidate and integrate their data systems, and this has generated a much richer source of data upon which to build predictive tools.

Adolescent-serving systems across the United States have begun developing and refining predictive analytic techniques. The child welfare system, for example, uses predictive analytic techniques in an effort to improve decision making regarding initial investigations and placement decisions for youth in its care. Predictive analytic techniques, such as algorithms, may also be used to prioritize which adolescents will receive an educational or social science intervention when the need for the program outweighs the resources available to supply the program, to predict which social workers or teachers are likely to be the most productive and effective in their jobs, or to inform justice system-placement decisions based on risk of reoffending.

To specifically illustrate the use of predictive analytics, we detail perhaps the most prominent use of predictive analytics in child welfare and consider potential future uses in that system. Alleghany County, Pennsylvania, adopted a sophisticated screening tool based on data integrated from multiple agencies to predict risk of future maltreatment at the time of initial referral. The tool uses 100 risk factors related to the child, family, and incident to predict future risk of maltreatment. Importantly, the tool is not used in isolation, but rather, it is used in conjunction with clinical judgment to augment standardized screening decisions. When a case is referred, the tool is applied, generating a risk score from 1 to 20. Then, following a clinical assessment, only the cases deemed highest risk are investigated further (Vaithianathan et al., 2017). Studies have shown that predictive analytic tools such as those used in Alleghany County can help protect children who otherwise would not have been identified as being at high risk, and can also reduce the number of "false positives," thereby protecting families wrongly targeted and reducing the over-representation of ethnic and racial minority children in the system.

Although to date, predictive analytic tools have primarily been used to help inform initial investigations and subsequent placement decisions during childhood, there is potential for historical data and predictive analytic tools to be incorporated as one source of data in determining optimal services and treatments for adolescents in the child welfare system as well as in other systems. For example, in tandem with caseworker and adolescent judgement, machine-learning techniques could be refined to identify clusters of risk and protective factors that would increase the likelihood that a specific service or intervention might benefit a particular adolescent. Similar tools could be used to help guide decisions related to the timing of when an adolescent may be ready to successfully exit the child welfare system. There may also be a role for the use of predictive analytics in identifying youth in need of mental health services. Machine-learning analytic approaches, for example, might be applied to youth's social media activity to provide effective and timely services to high-risk youth to prevent events such as adolescent suicide and related self-harm behavior.

Use of predictive analytic techniques by adolescent-serving systems has the potential to lead to positive outcomes for youth, reduce discrimination as compared to human decision making, and remediate some of the disparate impacts produced by past reliance on biased data (Kleinberg et al., forthcoming). Kleinberg and colleagues (2018), for example, studied decisions made by New York judges in determining which defendants would be detained and then compared those decisions to decisions made by computational prediction to determine whether the judges might have made better decisions using an algorithm. They discovered when they reduced the number of Blacks and Latinx jailed by 40.8 percent and 44.6 percent, respectively, they were able to achieve the same crime rate, which suggests that it is possible for an algorithm to reduce racial/ethnic inequalities (Kleinberg et al., 2018).

However, machine-learning approaches are only as effective as the data and the human designers they draw upon, and algorithms must be transparent and auditable, use fair and nondiscriminatory choice of data, and undertake reasonable algorithmic objectives in order to realize these potential benefits (Kleinberg et al., forthcoming). These new tools have great potential for improving the lives of adolescents and their families and reducing disparities in U.S. society, but, like all technologies, they can be used well or poorly. To ensure that they realize their potential for positive social impact, regulatory systems and oversight are needed.

CONCLUSION

Certain categories of youth, often defined by race, ethnicity, income, gender, or sexuality, enter adolescence already at a disadvantage in terms of their school achievement, health, and family stability. Although the neurobiological evidence suggests that adolescence presents an opportunity for significant remediation, the data suggest that, if anything, developmental disparities increase as youth age.

Disparities in adolescent outcomes by income, race and ethnicity, and gender will continue to translate into inequality in future adult outcomes, including, but not limited to, employment, criminal justice involvement, and health, unless significant steps are taken to reduce them. Addressing disparities in adolescent outcomes will require multipronged and multilevel interventions, as the differences in opportunity are both complex and interwoven. An effective strategy, or set of strategies, must address the main sources of these disparities: rising inequality in family income and wealth accumulation; neighborhood segregation by income and race that has direct and indirect effects on youth and their families; and personal biases that subvert the very systems that are supposed to ensure the equal treatment of all youth.

Moreover, greater coordination is needed across the multiple systems responsible for adolescents: the school system, health care system, and juvenile justice and child protection systems have traditionally operated independently. We now know, however, that many of the obstacles to healthy youth development cut across multiple systems and that systemic deficiencies in one arena negatively impact outcomes in other arenas. Examples include the way poor health reduces educational attainment and the way involvement in CPS negatively affects juvenile justice outcomes.

Parity in public system funding is a first step, but will not be sufficient to significantly reduce disparities. While increasing parity in funding in the educational sector did reduce disparities, it did not eliminate them. Rather, the research suggests that the lack of parity in family and neighborhood resources remains an important predictor of the continued disparities in adolescent educational outcomes, despite improvements in system funding. To significantly reduce or eliminate disparities, disadvantaged youth will likely require disproportionate funding. Moreover, any solutions are likely to require a significant amount of time to be effective. It will likely take years, for example, to counter patterns of neighborhood segregation that were produced over many years of policies and practices aimed at reducing Blacks' access to certain neighborhoods.

Although progress may not be immediate, there is substantial reason for optimism—progress has already been made in reducing disparities in adolescent outcomes, especially in the areas of education, health, and teen pregnancy. With one notable exception in the juvenile justice system, the evidence suggests that as overall adolescent health and well-being improve, disparities fall. These trends underscore the hope that with additional effort and a comprehensive approach, further reductions in outcome disparities among adolescents are indeed attainable. Finally, while the focus of this chapter has been to provide a context for understanding various disparities in adolescent outcomes, existing research also highlights the importance of identifying and promoting resilience and strength among those traditionally considered disadvantaged or at-risk (Task Force Report on Resilience and Strength in African-American Children and Adolescents, n.d.). Appreciating existing levels of resilience among at-risk youth, while encouraging the development of further protective factors, holds considerable promise as the nation works toward enhancing positive outcomes for all adolescents. However, promoting resilience and strength should not be considered a sufficient response alone; ending the disparities in adolescent development will also require sustained and effective system change.

Part II:
Using Developmental Knowledge to Assure Opportunity for All Youth

5

Introduction

As adolescents mature, their lives project more and more into the social world, and they interact with social systems and organizations, including schools, law enforcement, businesses, and social services and health systems. The importance to their development of the ecosystem of institutions within which adolescents grow has been widely recognized since it was first highlighted in Bronfenbrenner's (1974, 1977, 1979) "ecological" theory of child development. A flourishing adolescence depends on all the institutions that surround youth, contributing to their learning and socioemotional development as well as protecting their safety. The social ecosystems within which today's youth are maturing reflect sweeping social changes, many of which were touched on in the preceding chapters.

The committee's charge directs us to help child-serving systems apply the accelerating knowledge about adolescent development to their own work. The following chapters will carry out that charge. Our prefatory comments here will address three important topics. The first is the increasing complexity of the tasks that all these systems face in a rapidly changing world. The second is the pivotal importance of supporting parents and families in helping their adolescents flourish, a topic of personal as well as scientific interest to us all. Finally, we conclude by discussing faith-based institutions as an example of the many community-based organizations that can be utilized to support youth—beyond the four systems specifically named in the committee's charge.

GROWING SYSTEM COMPLEXITY

The path to adulthood in contemporary society entails navigating a highly complex ecosystem of specialized social institutions. A successful college application, for example, might require an adolescent to navigate government systems (e.g., a FAFSA application as well as state financial aid forms), private company systems (e.g., the SAT, administered by the College Board), the education system (e.g., college applications, facilitating school-college communication), and the private consumer education market (e.g., private SAT tutoring). An institutional ecosystem such as this, made up of a large number of differentiated and specialized institutions, poses distinct challenges, particularly for socioeconomically disadvantaged youth. While socioeconomically advantaged families have the resources to "knit together" this patchwork of institutional demands, choices, and costs, disadvantaged youth may have less success in integrating them without guidance (Jackson, 2019). So, for example, even if an adolescent from a socioeconomically disadvantaged family can navigate the education system and the SAT, she may make mistakes in navigating the financial aid systems required to fund her college education.

In many ways, these increasingly complex challenges have altered what it means to be an adolescent today. Systems and organizations that were created for prior generations to guide and support adolescents—especially their schools—in many ways have not kept pace with the changing contexts and needs of today's adolescents.

Part II of this report, comprising Chapters 6 through 9, stresses that to meet the developmental needs of today's adolescents, the nation needs systems and strategies that are different from those designed for prior generations. Adolescents need all sectors in society—including government, schools, and other community institutions—as well as their families to share responsibility for identifying new settings and pathways that create possibilities for adolescents to flourish and thrive.

These four chapters discuss the four adolescent-serving systems named in the committee's charge: education, health, child welfare, and justice. Although we discuss the systems separately, the committee notes that to best serve adolescents these systems cannot continue to operate in siloes. Collaboration and coordination across systems are needed. Several approaches at the federal, state, and local levels have been implemented to break these siloes down, with varying levels of success. For example, states across the country have created "Children's Cabinets," which create a formal setting for interaction and collaboration across adolescent-serving sectors at the state level.[1] Other states and localities have begun to develop global budgets, which break down silos in funding and allow for greater collaboration across systems. Given the committee's charge, we do not detail the efficacy of these efforts but, rather, focus on specific opportunities for cross-system collaboration. These opportunities are noted throughout the subsequent chapters.

It is also important to note that the committee's recommendations for systems change in the following chapters are not the only ways for society to support and promote positive adolescent development and ensure that all adolescents have the opportunity to flourish. As discussed in Chapter 4, one of the vexing problems facing adolescents and their families today is growing inequality in income and wealth and the compounding impacts of growing up poor in this country. Thus, one might envision a set of policies and programs that combat economic inequality through provisions in the tax code or the implementation of a universal basic income, which may in turn reduce rates of child and adolescent poverty and lead to better outcomes for youth. While such proposed policies merit serious consideration and Chapter 4 discusses some of them, the committee does not make specific recommendations along these lines, as they are outside the scope of this report.[2]

Key to any consideration of systems change are the availability of funds and the prudent allocation of resources to evidence-based programs. Many of the health, social, and educational supports needed by adolescents require long-term investment rather than brief episodic or categorical responses. While successful models of interventions that promote positive outcomes for youth have been demonstrated in the field, institutions and policy makers often failed to take advantage of these models by disseminating them and scaling up their implementation. Emerging research in the neurobiological and socio-behavioral sciences provides a renewed opportunity to further enhance and improve existing services, programs, and policies by ascertaining what works, for whom, and under what circumstances. The political challenge, as mentioned in Chapter 1, is to take the necessary steps to assure a long-term commitment grounded in heightened awareness of the importance of investing in young people during this critical developmental period, an investment that will affect the life-course trajectory of future generations of adults.

---

[1] Children's Cabinets are typically made up of the heads of all government agencies with child- and youth-serving programs. They meet regularly to coordinate services, develop a common set of outcomes, and collaboratively decide upon and implement plans to foster the well-being of young people (Forum for Youth Investment, 2018).

[2] For further consideration of policies and programs to reduce childhood poverty, see National Academies of Sciences, Engineering, and Medicine (2019).

PARENTS AND CAREGIVERS

When adults prepare to become parents for the first time, they are often bombarded with advice. And while the advice may be subject to debate—formula or breast milk? co-sleeping or crib?—resources on how to best raise an infant or young child are readily available. Moreover, everyone understands that the stakes at this time in a child's life are quite high. Indeed, amidst widespread agreement about the critical nature of the first few years of life, investments in supports for parenting and early childhood education continue to garner support.

But the reality is that parents and other adult caregivers are no less important for adolescents than they are for young children: both young children and adolescents need secure attachment from parents as a foundation for healthy development and strong relationships. In fact, during this critical period of development, parents are essential for ensuring that adolescents flourish and thrive. While the *role* of parents certainly changes compared to early in life—adolescents are very different from young children—their *significance* does not. The process also remains much the same: the relationship between parents and adolescents continues to be "transactional," meaning the parents and adolescents respond to one another in a reciprocal fashion, and both of them continue to change through this process (Sameroff and Fiese, 2000). Indeed, sometimes an adolescent's behavior can have more of an effect on how parents behave than parents' behavior has on their adolescent children (Lansford et al., 2018). Despite this reality, parents of adolescents are often left to navigate the changing terrain on their own or are told to expect nothing but challenge and conflict.

A few current trends are especially salient for current parents of adolescents. First, earlier onset of puberty and later transitions to adult roles have lengthened the adolescent period, which may mean protracted parental involvement and a need for flexibility as youths' needs change (Steinberg, 2014). Second, today's adolescents are digital natives,[3] which creates new kinds of opportunities for parental monitoring and communication (Ball et al., 2013; Hussong et al., 2018). Third, the U.S. population is more racially and ethnically diverse than in previous generations, and family structures (e.g., blended families, grandparents as caregivers) are more diverse as well (Pearce et al., 2018). Last, amidst the trend of widening economic inequality, some parents are raising adolescents under great financial strain, postponing their own expectations while continuing to support their young adult offspring (Hussong and Jones, 2018; Mullainathan and Datta, 2011).

---

[3] "Digital natives" is a term first coined in 2001 by Marc Prensky (Kennedy et al., 2008). "Digital natives" are individuals who were born roughly after 1980 (Guo et al., 2008).

Diversity in personal values, cultural norms, relationship dynamics, and access to resources means the relationship between adolescents and their primary adult caregivers can look quite different across families, neighborhoods, and geographic locales. Family socialization practices, wherein adult caregivers transmit their values and norms and model behaviors, always occur in context and are impacted by social position and resource availability. For example, when parents experience marginalization as a function of their race and ethnicity, socioeconomic status, or stigmatized family structure, this often necessitates that they practice particular kinds of socialization with the intention of preparing or buffering the youth in their households against discrimination as well as to instill a sense of group and self-pride (Jones et al., 2018; McBride Murry and Lippold, 2018; Stein et al., 2018).

While there is no prescription for being the "perfect parent" to an adolescent, decades of research suggest a few practices that are consistently associated with positive youth outcomes across contexts (Lansford et al., 2018; Steinberg, 2014). The first recommended parental practice is being supportive. While the details of what support and "warmth" look like is informed by cultural norms and family contexts, adolescents need to feel valued, loved, and safe, just as they did in early childhood. Being attuned to young people's emotional needs and knowing what is going on in their lives has important benefits for development throughout adolescence (Steinberg, 2014).

A second vitally important parental practice is being firm. This involves setting boundaries and expectations around appropriate behavior, and consistently communicating these expectations to adolescents. Being firm *while* also showing support is particularly important. In practice, supporting adolescents during this period of time necessitates flexibility, since the needs of a 13-year-old can be quite different from those of a 19-year-old. The goal is to provide just enough support so a young person can learn how to address challenges and make decisions on her or his own (Steinberg, 2014).

Being both firm and supportive likely sounds easy enough; however, the reality is that parents and other primary caregivers are living in the same context of inequality as adolescents. The spaces and places where families live impact opportunities, and parents are no more immune to toxic environments than are adolescents. In addition to its direct impact on adolescents, stress impacts parenting, and in the context of limited economic resources and financial stress, parents' emotional, psychological, and temporal resources are often taxed (Mullainathan and Datta, 2012).

Beyond the immediate family context, there are important ways in which parents and families intersect with institutions and systems (e.g., education, health), and those intersections can directly or indirectly shape trajectories of adolescent development. Maximizing the opportunity of adolescence in the context of inequities goes beyond direct support to adolescents themselves. While it is outside the scope of this report to detail all the intersections between families and other systems, a few cross-cutting issues are worth highlighting:

- As noted in the following systems chapters, parents' engagement with youth, through parenting practices and other forms of socialization, is an important lever for minimizing negative system contact (e.g., preventing justice-system involvement) and maximizing optimal system engagement (e.g., promoting positive school and health outcomes). Thus, resources to support meaningful parent-adolescent relationships are needed, but as noted earlier, such resources are often targeted exclusively toward parents of young children.

- Interventions aimed at parents and other adult caregivers can benefit youth. For instance, parent training and family-based/multi-system interventions are among the most effective at preventing or reducing child maltreatment (see Chapter 8). In the education sector, sending messages to parents about their child's school absences has been found to improve student attendance (Rogers and Feller, 2018). It may be that contemporary approaches aimed at "nudging" people toward behavioral changes (e.g., text message reminders to complete financial aid forms; Castleman, 2015) could be leveraged to benefit parents, which in turn would benefit youth.

- While parents can be important partners for optimizing adolescent outcomes, there are also ways in which parental involvement in systems can exacerbate challenges. The education, health, child welfare, and juvenile justice systems are complex and difficult to navigate. Resources to help parents understand these systems are often lacking, and when under duress parents may make uninformed, rushed decisions or defer to those in positions of authority to determine the fate of their adolescent child. Parents and adolescents from historically marginalized racial/ethnic or low-socioeconomic groups are most likely to be effectively disenfranchised in this process.

- Structural barriers can tax families, especially those most in need of support, making decision making more complex and stressful. Improving access to resources accessibility—for example, by minimizing technical jargon, complicated enrollment processes, and extraneous restrictions and maximizing geographic and temporal availability and "one-stop" access—may increase the cognitive and emotional bandwidth parents need to support adolescents more effectively, as will enacting policy changes that lower structural barriers for families, such as establishing flexible workplace and family-leave policies (Daminger et al., 2015).

Ultimately, the immediate family setting remains one of the most important and influential contexts for adolescent development. Parental support and involvement play a critical role across all four sectors—education, health, justice, and welfare—by maximizing their adolescent child's optimal outcomes, mitigating any negative outcomes, and (or) preventing the child's involvement in the child welfare or justice system. As starkly illustrated in Chapter 4, "family resources"—which refers not only to income and wealth but also to time, protection, and emotional support—represents one of the most important determinants of adolescent outcomes. Although parenting is not something easily measured, in all the ways this report has illuminated concerning neurobiological and behavioral development it too "gets under the skin" in an adolescent's development.

As Chapter 4 discusses, parents differ widely in all the domains of resources that they can bring to bear in rearing their children, including their own time and energy. The least advantaged parents need resources through social assistance to effectively support adolescents during this period of opportunity, so investing in youth also requires investing in the adult caregivers who support them. Such investments must be multilevel and multisectoral; interventions to change parenting behavior may be futile if systems themselves are not attuned to parents' most pressing needs.

FAITH-BASED INSTITUTIONS

Many community-based organizations interact with and support youth and families. One important type of community-based organization is faith-based institutions. Religious faith, and its attendant institutions, can play an important role for adolescents and their families. In the United States, faith is common among young people (ages 18 to 29): 73 percent are at least fairly certain that they believe in God, and 64 percent attend religious services at least a few times a year. Among young adults ages 18 to 29 in the United States, 36 percent identify as Protestant, 36 percent as unaffiliated with any religion, 20 percent as Catholic, and 2 percent as Jewish, Mormon, Muslim, or some other faith, respectively (Pew Research Center, 2014).

The extant literature on adolescent religiosity and spirituality and mental and emotional health shows a largely positive effect of religion in young people's lives. In a systematic review of studies on religiosity and spirituality and related adolescent mental health outcomes published between 1998 and 2004, 18 of the 20 studies examined showed a positive relationship (Wong et al., 2006). More recently, a study of Latter Day Saints students at Brigham Young University found that greater religiosity predicted lower levels of depression and anxiety (Sanders et al., 2015), while in another study religious social support was found to mediate the effect of discrimination on psychiatric disorders among Black adolescents (Hope et al., 2017). In a small qualitative study of Black youth ages 12 to 20 in East Oakland, California, young people reported using faith, prayer, and religious practices to cope with stressors in their environments and family lives (Dill, 2017). For some of the youth in this last study, their faith directly informed their drive to serve their communities (Dill, 2017). However, religious engagement may not be protective for all adolescents: among lesbian, gay, and bisexual youth, religiosity has been associated with greater rates of internalized homophobia (Shilo and Savaya, 2012) and suicide behavior (Gibbs and Goldbach, 2015).

In addition to the religious services they offer, houses of worship serve as hubs of both religious and secular community life. Churches, synagogues, mosques, and other religious institutions offer educational, spiritual, and civic resources to their communities (Nguyen et al., 2013), including, importantly, an opportunity to engage. As discussed in Chapter 2, the neurobiological and socio-emotional changes that occur during adolescence prime youth to become active participants in community life. As such, offering opportunities for positive youth engagement is essential for supporting the development of adolescents, as well as the health of their communities. Community and faith-based organizations can play an important role in providing opportunities for youth to engage.

In addition to engagement, faith-based organizations may support adolescent development through identity formation. In this key task of adolescent development, young people work to establish a coherent identity independent of their families. Many faiths include rituals to mark a child's transition into adolescence, and with it, a greater role within the spiritual or religious community. For example, some Jewish youth have a bat mitzvah (for girls) or bar mitzvah (for boys) at age 12 or 13, which cements their status as full participants in Jewish religious life. In preparation for the ceremony, youth are taught and mentored by clergy and lay leaders in the congregation to take on the responsibility of Jewish adulthood (National Research Council and Institute of Medicine, 2002).[4] In Navajo culture, the kinaalda ceremony celebrates the coming-of-age of young women in a ritual that lasts 2 to 4 days. Kinaalda engages family members and community elders in support of an adolescent girl's growth and development, instilling pride in Navajo culture, identity, and community (National Research Council and Institute of Medicine, 2002).

---

[4] In some congregations, the bar/bat mitzvah includes a service project that engages youth in the broader community.

ENVISIONING DEVELOPMENTALLY INFORMED
YOUTH-SERVING SYSTEMS

These introductory comments emphasize the growing complexity of youth-serving systems and the need for greater collaboration across systems to better support youth. Key to fostering better youth outcomes and coordination across systems is supporting parents, caregivers, and families in navigating these increasingly complex institutions. While the education, health, child welfare, and justice systems are the focus of the committee's charge, community-based institutions, including faith-based organizations, play a very important role, particularly in neighborhoods where they provide a safe haven from stress of violence. Promoting a flourishing adolescence will require the engagement of all society's sectors.

In the following chapters, the committee outlines recommendations for reforming the education, health, child welfare, and justice systems. Taken together, these recommendations constitute a blueprint for developmentally informed systems change. Although each set of recommendations is targeted to a particular system, the blueprints reflect several cross-cutting themes—informed by the neurobiological and socio-behavioral science of adolescent development (discussed in Chapters 2 and 3) and an understanding of the troubling and increasing disparities in opportunity outlined in Chapter 4.

Adolescence is a sensitive period for discovery and learning, providing opportunities for life-long impact. The adolescent brain has evolved to meet the needs of this critical stage of life. Human developmental processes are now conceptualized as continuous, rather than occurring in discrete stages as was originally thought. A sequence of sensitive periods of brain maturation proceed from conception through adulthood. In adolescence, these developmental changes heighten reward sensitivity, a willingness to take risks, and the salience of social status, necessary propensities for exploring new environments and building non-familial relationships. By exploring and taking risks, adolescents build cognitive, social, and emotional skills necessary for productive contributions in adulthood.

Learning how to make decisions and to take responsibility for shaping one's own life are key developmental tasks of adolescence. Adolescents are active participants in their own development. Their developing competencies in flexible problem solving, their awareness of and concern with others, and their openness to exploration and novelty make this a particularly opportune time to support agency and leadership and promote engagement. While parents and other responsible adults must respect the developing agency of adolescents, they must also provide guidance to guard against impulsive or ill-considered decisions.

Forming personal identity is a key task of adolescence. The increasing diversity of U.S. adolescents and the nation as a whole requires youth-

serving systems to be culturally sensitive and to be attuned to the integrated needs of each adolescent. Young people become increasingly aware of and attuned to their social status during adolescence, and institutions, policies, and practices may reinforce status hierarchies and stereotypes about members of groups that are nondominant or stigmatized in society. Moreover, adolescents have distinct physiological, socio-emotional, and cognitive needs that must be recognized and addressed as they mature.

Supportive familial, caregiver, and adult relationships play a significant role in fostering positive outcomes for adolescents. Adult caregivers are no less important for adolescents than they are for young children. Adolescents need secure attachment from adults as a foundation for healthy development and strong relationships.

Adolescence provides an opportunity for recovery and repair. Because of the malleability and plasticity of the adolescent brain, maladaptation in behavior and brain structure stemming from stressful and harmful exposures during earlier developmental periods may be remediated during adolescence. Redirection, recovery, and resilience are possible. Insofar as the brain is healthy, individuals have the capacity for resilience.

Disparities in family and neighborhood resources and supports, biased and discriminatory interactions with important social systems, and resulting inequalities in opportunity and access severely curtail the promise of adolescence for many youth. Potent structural inequalities and other societal determinants shape adolescents' life trajectories, reducing access to the opportunities, services, and supports as well as exposing youth to risks, stresses, and demands that "get under the skin," adversely affecting the body and brain during this critical developmental period. These striking differences in opportunity are associated with differences in outcomes—in health, safety, well-being, and educational and occupational attainment—and in trajectories over the life course.

6

Education

Public education has long been claimed as a hallmark of democracy in the United States, a core element of the country's self-image. It ensures informed self-government, and it has helped nurture a unified national identity across several generations of diverse immigrants. In the form in which it is known today, public education first emerged in the late 19th century, driven by industrialization and urbanization. At that time, most people in the United States lived in rural areas, and about two-thirds of all workers were employed in farming. Given the conception of adolescence at the time, and the fact that average life expectancy then was only about 37 years, a common assumption was that adolescents should take on work responsibilities as quickly as possible (Kett, 2003).

As secondary schools were established across the country during the post-Civil War period, they were often designed to educate youth for routinized jobs in factories in the new industrial age and, implicitly, to socialize conformity in increasingly diverse and complex urban centers. Many of the key features of these early high schools remain with us today. Yet much has changed over the past 150 years, and the needs of American society today bear little resemblance to those that were served by secondary education in the early industrial age.

Life expectancy has more than doubled since that time, to about 79 years, so the period over which the benefits of human capital developed during adolescence can accrue has increased substantially. And changes in society have made formal schooling increasingly important for labor market success (Goldin and Katz, 2010).[1] The share of U.S. workers employed in manufacturing today is just 11 percent, while the share employed in agriculture is under 1 percent. Fully three of every five workers in America are now in what one might think of as knowledge-based "white collar" jobs.[2] At the same time, the United States is losing its competitive advantage in education. In a survey of nearly 10,000 Harvard Business School alumni judging the United States' competitiveness in global markets, the K–12 education system was deemed a weakness and to be deteriorating (Porter and Rivkin, 2012). The economic strength that America enjoys—for now—is attributed instead to our nation's universities, innovation, entrepreneurship, and capital markets, which are relied upon to help overcome our current deficiencies in K–12 education.

Changes in the labor market have also increased the returns to "non-academic" skills (Deming, 2017; Goldin and Katz, 2010). Some schools have taken a more expansive view of skill development. But most secondary schools remain large, highly structured bureaucracies where youth follow rules, with few opportunities to create, solve problems, and practice decision making, despite the fact that these skills are becoming increasingly important for economic success and these opportunities are the very things youth need to fully develop (Eccles et al., 1993).

Moreover, the country itself has changed. The United States has become increasingly diverse with respect to race and ethnicity, as Whites will soon make up less than half of the population under age 18. Gender roles have changed as well. Women have increased their participation in schools, the labor market, and other key social institutions. In 1890, fewer than 20 percent of all women were working in the formal labor market in the United States. Today, the figure is closer to 60 percent, gradually approaching the figure for men.[3]

The nation today also confronts persistent disparities in how adolescents perform in school. Differences in high school graduation rates between youth of color and White youth remain large, with a Black-White gap of 12 percentage points and a gap between Latinx and White youth equal to 9 percentage points in the 2015-2016 school year (National Center for Education Statistics, 2018). Similar disparities are found in achievement test scores. By age 13, the Black-White gap in the National Assessment of Educational Progress (NAEP) equals 0.62 standard deviations in reading and 0.80 standard deviations in math. The difference in achievement test

---

[1] While the returns to a college degree for men declined around the time of World War II, since 1950 we have seen a large rise in the difference in earnings between those with a degree versus those without one. Similarly, the returns to a high school diploma for men declined in the period leading up to 1950, but have increased steadily since (Goldin and Katz, 2010).

[2] Finance, insurance and real estate; government; education and health; and information.

[3] See https://ourworldindata.org/female-labor-force-participation-key-facts.

scores between rich and poor (the 90th versus 10th percentiles of the income distribution) is also large and has increased substantially since 1940 (Reardon, 2011). As shown in Chapter 4, these disparities in educational outcomes are linked to demonstrable disparities in educational opportunity stemming from differences in family resources (income and wealth) as well as the stability, stress, and safety of neighborhoods where students grow up.

The system of public education that emerged in the last half of the 19th and early 20th centuries was also driven by prescientific suppositions about adolescent development. During the late 20th and early 21st centuries we have learned an enormous amount about adolescence that bears on the aims and design of formal education. Research from psychology and other social sciences has taught us that development does not end at puberty with the emergence of abstract thinking skills as a final stage, as was once thought. Rather, youth have a great capacity for growth and change, retaining substantial neurobiological and developmental plasticity into their early to mid-20s (Hohnen and Murphy, 2016; Steinberg, 2014; see also Chapters 2 and 3). Moreover, research from neuroscience helps us understand how this plasticity relates to the architecture of the brain itself, creating new opportunities throughout the teen years and into the early 20s for youth to continue and sharpen their development.

These major changes in our understanding of adolescence itself, together with major changes in society and its needs, require rethinking and modernizing a public school system that was largely designed for 19th century life. We now understand that when young people reach adolescence, they vary widely in their academic skills and needs and in their future career aspirations. There are also dynamic and unique neurobiological changes taking place in tandem with cognitive, social, and behavioral development (see Chapter 2), all of which factor into educational experiences. The secondary school system of the future must do a much better job of meeting teens where they are and personalizing instruction, much as the field of health care, for instance, is increasingly shifting toward "personalized medicine." The growing recognition of the importance of skills other than reading, writing, and arithmetic for both personal fulfillment and success in modern-day life will require schools to broaden their mission.

The growing diversity of U.S. adolescents will also require schools to become more culturally competent, to have a focus on understanding differences in background and identify and assist youth with issues related to identity and social competence. Rather than become more integrated, evidence suggests that schools are becoming increasingly segregated along racial, ethnic, and socioeconomic lines (Hill and Torres, 2010; Hill, 2011). Modern society is unfortunately characterized by substantial inequalities in income, wealth, and neighborhood opportunity, which have translated into inequalities in educational opportunities (see Chapter 4). Given the growing importance of education over the past 200 years, addressing almost any form of social or economic inequality in the United States will be difficult without also addressing these educational inequalities. This includes supplementing the different resources the families of adolescents can bring to bear, including help navigating the education sector.

In the remainder of this chapter, we first highlight changes within society that are relevant for the education sector. We then discuss what social science and neuroscience have discovered about adolescence, before turning to key changes that these trends will require of the education sector in the United States, broadly defined.

SOCIETAL CHANGES

While the current system of secondary education was largely designed to meet 19th century educational needs, rapid changes in American life in the 20th and 21st centuries have affected both the contexts in which young people grow up and the skills and competencies they need to garner from the education system in order to become productive adult members of society. This section discusses these societal changes—changes in the labor market returns to education, in the growing importance of nonacademic skills, and in out-of-school learning environments—and their relevance for the education sector. Potential responses to these developments are discussed in the following section.

Changes in Labor Market Returns to Education

Adolescents today are increasingly transitioning into a labor market where technological innovation and automation are providing higher returns to education and skills, particularly for those holding a college degree (Goldin and Katz, 2010). Although the economic returns to a college degree have increased for the past three decades, the real wages of individuals in the middle of the income distribution have stagnated, at least when measured before tax and transfers (Autor et al., 2006, 2008; Cass, 2018).[4] In fact, as the top of the income distribution has pulled farther away from the middle, the before-tax wages of those with mid-range qualifications have closely tracked the before-tax wages of high school dropouts and high school graduates (Acemoglu and Autor, 2012).

---

[4]The available data suggest that there has been more growth in the middle and bottom of the income distribution with respect to income measured after taxes and transfers compared to pre-tax income (Congressional Budget Office, 2018). We focus here on trends in pre-tax income, since that seems most relevant for understanding how different types of occupations and skills are being valued in the labor market and how those valuations change over time.

The fact that the labor market returns on schooling have increased so substantially in recent decades tells us that the supply of skills we are developing among young people is not keeping up with the demand for skills in today's society (Goldin and Katz, 2010). Moreover, we may not be developing the right *mix* of skills. More than half of U.S. employers have expressed difficulty in finding and hiring people with appropriate skills, while the proportion of U.S. college graduates working in jobs that are below their skill set has increased (Porter and Rivkin, 2012). It is currently unclear whether this mismatch is due to student preferences for and values placed in aspects of jobs beyond the wages they pay, or due to misinformation about the labor market demand for different occupations. In either case, improved understanding about how academic work links to postsecondary goals and plans gives meaning and motivation to schoolwork and is associated with higher levels of academic engagement (Hill and Wang, 2015; Hill et al., 2018).

This also raises the question of whether the curricular focus and the set of skills our education system seeks to develop have become too narrow. The "college-for-all" movement has resulted in a diminished emphasis on vocational education as a purpose-driven pathway through high school that prepares youth for the workforce (Cass, 2018). However, currently only 36 percent of adults between the ages of 25 and 44 in the United States have a 4-year college degree (U.S. Census Bureau, 2017). Thus, a single high school diploma, and the curriculum that goes with it, may not provide the kind of credential that most students need to navigate the job market, which particularly disadvantages low-income students and students who are not planning to attend college. Put differently, the types of skills that the economy increasingly requires are not limited to those skills associated with college attendance; yet high school graduates are not generally well-equipped to enter the labor market.

A randomized controlled trial of Career Academies by Kemple (2008) suggests that there may be higher returns to career-oriented or vocational education than the usual college-for-all track, at least for some students. These secondary schools "combine academic and technical curricula around a career theme, and establish partnerships with local employers to provide work-based learning opportunities" (Kemple, 2008, p. iii). Relative to other high schools, Career Academies did not increase graduation rates, but they did increase annual earnings by 11 percent overall and by 17 percent for men. One challenge is to ensure that these types of vocational options are available to those students who believe they would benefit from them without closing the door to college for those who decide that is the right path for them by, for instance, not making available academic courses that are required for college attendance.

Future technological changes, and in particular the expected increase in the use of automation and artificial intelligence, are predicted to create further challenges for all workers, but perhaps particularly for lower-skilled workers (Acemoglu and Autor, 2012; Acemoglu and Restrepo, 2018a, 2018b; Agrawal et al., 2018). Increasing automation is likely to allow for substantial increases in productivity, to the benefit of the whole society, but the displacement effects of automation may produce negative consequences for many lower-skilled workers.

One question is whether potential changes in the labor market over time should lead schools to focus more on developing skills that are generally useful across all occupations (what Becker [1964] called "general human capital") or instead try to forecast what occupation-specific skills ("specific human capital") will be most helpful in the future and develop those skills. This choice partly depends on the degree to which the education system can adequately forecast the skills and disposition that match the needs of the job market, and how those requirements might vary both over time and across local micro-economies of cities and communities across the nation (Brighouse et al., 2018; Porter and Rivkin, 2012). Because most current mid-skill jobs include at least some tasks that could not easily be automated (Acemoglu and Autor, 2012), understanding and forecasting which jobs are likely to be the first to be either fully or partially automated is essential if the goal is to develop "specific" human capital. Among other things, it will be important to forecast how the increasing focus on "human augmented artificial intelligence" might change the labor market returns to different skills over time, and to identify the occupations in which humans will have comparative advantage so that we can train youth for those roles.

Growing Importance of Non-Academic Skills

For most of human history (200,000 years or so), the "economy" of human life consisted of hunting and gathering.[5] About 13,000 years ago humans shifted to farming and agriculture, which greatly improved the ability of populations to feed themselves but still required most people to spend most of their time engaged in food production. About 250 years ago, the industrial revolution fundamentally changed society in this regard, greatly improving the efficiency of agriculture and freeing up workers for entirely new types of jobs that would have been previously unimaginable. By the middle of the 20th century, in the United States, the share of workers in agriculture had declined to 8 percent, and about one-quarter of all workers were engaged in manufacturing (Thompson, 2012). The invention of computers and the early Internet about 50 years ago dramatically transformed the economy yet again. With this wide-frame view of history, the picture

---

[5] See http://www.foodsystemprimer.org/food-production/history-of-agriculture/index.html.

that emerges is not only one of an ever-changing world, but also one in which the *rate of change* itself seems to be increasing.

If the world is changing at an increasing rate, then a potentially important goal for modern-day education systems is to help adolescents prepare to deal with uncertainty and change and see how the skills learned in one occupational context can transfer and then be applied to another. Such transferable skills and dispositions are both skill based and socio-emotional.

As the economy has changed over the past several decades, the skills and dispositions required to succeed in the job market have become increasingly interpersonal and socio-emotional (Deming, 2017; Goldin and Katz, 2010; West, 2014). These dispositions include having a strong sense of identity and purpose, along with strong interpersonal skills. Indeed, youth with higher levels of self-control also have more frequent job search preparations and stronger intentions to search for jobs and, later, they have greater intrinsic and extrinsic career success (Baay et al., 2014; Converse et al., 2012).

Related to the growing need for nonacademic (or psychosocial) skills, demographic changes in society—namely the increasing racial/ethnic diversity of the U.S. population described in Chapter 1—will also make it ever more important to be able to interact with people from different backgrounds and life experiences. The socio-demographic changes in American society also change the way the education sector itself must operate. Schools must now become more culturally competent, and they must deal with the large and growing inequality in socioeconomic advantage (or disadvantage) in American society (see Chapter 4).

Changes in the Out-of-School Learning Environment

Public and private schools have long played the primary role in educating youth, with the support of parents, but agencies and programs outside of school are playing a growing role in supporting education, including providing tutorials and online learning opportunities. These and other out-of-school learning contexts remind us that the education sector continues to be broader than just schools.

While the most obvious element of the education sector is public K–12 and postsecondary schools, the sector also includes private schools, ancillary services, and agencies that provide tutoring programs, alternative education, credit recovery programs, and professional development for teachers that serve adolescents. Further, and also relevant to adolescents, the education sector includes private and public organizations designed to mentor youth and assist in making the postsecondary school transition, including apprenticeships, vocational training, internships, after-school programs, and job training, along with programs designed to help youth prepare for college applications and standardized tests. Often missed among these educational agencies designed for adolescents is the role of the military in training youth, as well as the roles of on-the-job training and gap-year programming and experiences.

Finally, while not unique to adolescence, the increased role and presence of online learning, a platform that might be more readily accessible to millennial and later generations, provides youth with many more options to gain access to information and knowledge than are available through their home and community educational institutions. Helping youth navigate these myriad online educational opportunities is increasingly important in light of evidence from Escueta and colleagues (2017) suggesting that different computer learning platforms may differ considerably in their effectiveness.

These out-of-school learning contexts are often developed to make up for differential access across socioeconomic status, such as access to enriching experiences in the summer or weekends, in order to increase equity and reduce demographic achievement gaps. However, they are also utilized by wealthier parents to ensure a competitive advantage and to cultivate their children's interests and talents (Lareau and Weininger, 2003). For instance, it is common for schools serving wealthier districts to help their students navigate the college admissions process. These schools provide coaching in how to request recommendation letters, how to choose the appropriate balance of "reach" and "safety" schools when applying for college, how to write college applications, when to take the SAT, and so on.

Schools serving poorer districts may play a similar coordinating role, but they face challenges that schools in wealthier districts do not. Most importantly, adolescents from disadvantaged backgrounds may lack access to some of the family- or community-based resources to meet basic needs (e.g., food, health care, safety) that might be required if the adolescent is to develop to full potential. Clearly, if the basic needs of an adolescent simply cannot be met by their institutional ecosystem, the school's coordinator role will be of limited value (Jackson, 2019). This is another key aspect of the education sector where significant inequities have emerged.

IMPROVED UNDERSTANDING OF ADOLESCENCE

In addition to these broad societal changes, the education system will need to be responsive to developments in neuroscience and social science that have improved our understanding of adolescence. Education, and learning more generally, can capitalize on our new understanding of the significant neurobiological development that occurs during adolescence (Hohnen and Murphy, 2016). This section reviews the scientific literature related to cognitive development and learning and identity development in adolescence that is particularly relevant for the education sector.

Cognitive Development and Learning

Neural development, including the strengthening (myelinization) and pruning of synaptic connections, increases the efficiency of cognitive processes, reducing the cognitive load of basic thinking processes and enabling youth to think and plan more abstractly, to think metacognitively about themselves and others (i.e., to "think about thinking"), and to draw connections between emotional arousal and experiences (Goldman-Rakic, 1995; Hohnen and Murphy, 2016; Petanjek et al., 2011; Rakic et al., 1994; see also Chapter 2). These emerging cognitive capacities enable youth to see themselves in the world and to understand how they might simultaneously achieve their own goals and contribute to the common good of society (Damon et al., 2003). Because of their emerging cognitive capacities, adolescents begin to take ownership of and responsibility for their schoolwork and their long-term goals (Jodl et al., 2001; Seiffge-Krenke et al., 2010), to integrate their goals into their identities (Oyserman et al., 2006; Savitz-Romerj and Bouffard, 2012), and to launch successfully into their adult life.

Neurobiological development requires practice and experiences that elicit critical, analytical, and creative thinking for those skills to develop, in a process known as experience-expectant plasticity (Greenough et al., 1987; Hohnen and Murphy, 2016; Nowakowski, 2006). This experience and practice, which contribute to the building of neural connections, synaptic pruning, and improved cognitive efficiencies, is characteristic of adolescence (Petanjek et al., 2011). Only by practicing planning and decision making can youth develop the skills and dispositions necessary to successfully navigate postsecondary school transitions and prepare for college and careers.

Current school systems are not well-aligned with this changed understanding. For example, scientific advances have demonstrated that adolescence is a time when optimal development is stimulated through exploration, making and learning from mistakes, and trying on identities (Hohnen and Murphy, 2016; Steinberg, 2014). Requirements for stringent adherence to rule-following and conformity in secondary schools may be at odds with such self-discovery. Investigation into the elements of rule-following and conformity that are currently required of students is needed to generate policies and practices to better align the structure of secondary schools with the developmental needs of adolescents. In addition, the ways in which families engage youth and become involved in their education is different during adolescence, as compared to the elementary school years (Hill and Tyson, 2009; Hill et al., 2018). Yet, these developmentally appropriate responsive changes in families' practices are not easily supported by schools.

Current knowledge about how youth learn and what contexts support their developmental needs enables us to *create* the kinds of learning environments that capitalize on the neural plasticity of adolescence, which in turn makes it possible to recover from earlier developmental setbacks in childhood as well as to embrace the socio-emotional and hormonal fluctuations of adolescence and help youth prepare to take on the responsibilities of adulthood (Hohnen and Murphy, 2016; Rakic et al., 1994; Steinberg, 2014; see also Chapter 3). Enrichment programs involving reading and mathematics instruction and music education, for example, have established benefits for brain development, such as changes in cortical thickness and structural connectivity (Huber et al., 2018; Iuculano et al., 2015; Keller and Just, 2009; Kraus et al., 2014a, 2014b, 2014c; Romeo, 2017; Romeo et al., 2018).

Another measured instructional practice is the encouragement of divergent thinking, such as asking students to come up with alternative uses for household objects; this practice improves creativity and leads to changes in prefrontal function (Kleibeuker et al., 2017). Given the brain's high plasticity during adolescence, it is very likely that novel educational experiences shape adolescent brain development for the better. However, neither schools nor the broader education sector has kept pace with this accumulating knowledge of the ways cognitive and social factors during adolescence can be guided to improve educational opportunities for all.

We have also learned that high schools, in particular, struggle with the heterogeneity in students' academic levels and needs. Cascio and Staiger (2012) show that variance in student achievement grows wider as youth progress in school. The end result, by middle or high school, is great variability in academic levels and needs, which are particularly pronounced in urban school districts. For example, in the 2017 NAEP, 38 percent of eighth graders in Chicago were below basic level in math, 27 percent were at basic level, 27 percent were proficient, and 8 percent were advanced. Keeley (2011) found that although many of the most economically and socially vulnerable adolescents in Chicago—those in contact with the criminal justice system—had academic skills at grade level, on average these youth were 2 years behind grade level in reading, with some up to 7 years behind, and they were 4 years behind grade level in math, with some up to 10 years below grade level.

Identity Development

Adolescence is also a period when young people develop a more elaborate sense of their identities, including who they are, the groups they belong to, and their possible futures. As described in Chapter 2, the meaning young people attach to their membership in social groups, also known as social identity, can support a range of positive outcomes, especially for racial-ethnic minorities (French et al., 2006; Yip et al., 2006). Educational institutions can encourage this type of identity development by providing experiences that promote identity exploration and affirmation through exposure to knowledge and role models (Umaña-Taylor et al., 2018).

Identity is a broad concept, one that incorporates aspects of how young people make sense of their life stories thus far and how they imagine the possibilities for their futures (Destin and Oyserman, 2010; McLean and Breen, 2009). Similarly, developing sense of purpose simultaneously gives and reflects meaning for oneself and benefits society (Damon et al., 2003). It grows out of identity development and leads youth in finding their place in society. Both identity and sense of purpose develop in the context of exploration and affirmation. Identity development involves a combination of exploration and commitment over time and unfolds from dynamic interactions between the self and one's social contexts, such as school, family, and peers (Koepke and Denissen, 2012; McLean and Mansfield, 2012). Broadly speaking, adolescents select into contexts that either match their understanding of their identity or reflect identities they wish to cultivate. Reciprocally, feedback from these contexts encourages, discourages, and shapes students' understanding of themselves. Identity is "rooted in emotion, emerging in relationships, developing as dynamic, self-organizing system" (Bosma and Kunnen, 2001, p. 5).

Identity processes are related to a larger set of self-development characteristics, including self-regulation and "agentic capacities"—the ability of individuals, as independent agents, to shape their own lives—that youth need to help develop and commit to meaningful goals. Youth need to develop a sense of efficacy, which includes confidence in their ability to effect change in their world. In addition, they need self-motivation, internal locus of control, and emotional stability (Hoover-Dempsey et al., 2009; Schwartz et al., 2005). These characteristics enable and equip youth to persevere toward their goals and remain true to them in the face of challenges in an individualistic culture. The development of both identity and self-regulation are facilitated by the neurobiological development that occurs during adolescence. As the human brain develops within the experience-expectant framework discussed above (Greenough et al., 1987), the experiences that result in identity development lead to the neural connections and myelination that solidify youths' sense of self and the emotional reactions associated with their experiences.

The linkages between one's social identity and future goals are captured by theories related to "possible selves of future identities" (Oyserman, 2015; Oyserman and Destin, 2010) and sense of purpose (Damon et al., 2003). Educational and career goals and aspirations, the type of goals often promoted in schools both implicitly and explicitly, reflect what youth can *do* rather than who they *are*. But adolescents quintessentially pursue more fundamental questions of "Who am I?" and "Why am I here?" In contrast to career and educational goals, it is this growing sense of purpose, and the accompanying exploration of possible selves, that reflect who youth are and why they are here. These are admittedly more philosophical preoccupations than career goals, but for that same reason they are more meaningful to youth, and having them to hold onto is a preoccupying developmental task in an otherwise volatile social world. Understanding their emerging goals and talents broadens youths' possible career paths and facilitates their ability to adapt to fluctuating economic realities and see where they have transferrable skills.

Adolescence is also an important time in which young people begin to understand how they fit into the larger society and develop the interpersonal skills that undergird their emerging sense of civic life and community. Adolescents ascertain which groups they belong to, what those groups mean to them, and how others in society perceive their group membership. They use this knowledge to help guide their behaviors as they engage with the wider world and cultivate a sense of belonging and security (Ellemers et al., 2002). These social identities include interpersonal relationships, connections to clubs and organizations, categorization within demographic groups, and even a sense of local, national, and global citizenship.

Social identities matter not only for individuals' own lives but also in shaping society as a whole. Importantly, a sense of efficacy for civic engagement, or a sense that one can make positive changes in society, is useful for promoting democratic ideals (Brighouse et al., 2018). Adolescence is therefore an important opportunity to develop all of these inclinations and skills—academic, socio-emotional, civic, and dispositional (Brighouse et al., 2018).

Our current understanding of adolescence raises questions about whether the education system needs to do a better job developing the academic, socio-emotional, and civic commitments and skills that prepare youth to find a meaningful and productive role in society and in our political and economic structures. There are signs that the education sector may need to focus on a broader set of outcomes or "educational goods" than it currently does (Brighouse et al., 2018). By the end of adolescence, youth should ideally have developed not only a means of economic productivity but also autonomy, democratic competence, healthy personal relationships, the ability and propensity to treat others as equals, and personal fulfillment (Brighouse et al., 2018). The traditional emphasis on grades and test scores, and even on graduation rates, which dates back decades or centuries, may no longer be sufficient and, potentially, may be shortchanging both youth and society.

Summary

In summary, the education system has the potential to capitalize on new understandings of the significant neurobiological and psychosocial development occurring during adolescence. Emerging cognitive capacities allow youth to develop goals and identities; build critical, analytical, and creative thinking skills; and take responsibility for their own education. However, today's school systems are not aligned with these new understandings, and many schools struggle to meet the increasingly divergent academic levels and needs of adolescents.

CREATING THE EDUCATION SECTOR OF THE FUTURE

Both to meet the needs of a changing society and to realize the promise of adolescent development, changes to the education sector are needed. This section discusses the evidence for reforming the education sector to better meet the needs of adolescents and society and to assure that all adolescents have the opportunity to flourish and thrive. We first discuss the need for differentiated and responsive academic opportunities—helping teachers learn to individualize instruction and using tutoring, technology, tracking, and credentialing. Then we discuss the development of nonacademic skills such as decision making, practical knowledge, and adaptability. Next, the section examines how schools can better recognize adolescents' integrated needs and create culturally sensitive learning environments. Finally, we conclude by exploring the supports adolescents and their families need to navigate an increasingly complex education sector.

Differentiated and Responsive Academic Opportunities

One of the most challenging aspects of teaching in general is dealing with academic variability across students. Social science study of education has shown that the variability of young people's academic levels—and hence in their needs—increases as they progress through school (Cascio and Staiger, 2012). This variation in students' academic skills or levels within a school creates challenges for successful instruction, given the risk of mismatch between the academic level at which regular classroom teaching is directed and the academic level of any given student. By the time students enter adolescence, the provision of a "one-size-fits-all" education has become increasingly problematic. As an alternative to "one-size-fits-all" approaches, "personalized medicine" may provide a useful comparison for education during adolescence.

Previous research suggests that adolescents' social environments may not be aligned with their developmental needs, something known as "stage-environment fit" (see Hunt, 1975; Eccles et al., 1993). Research also suggests a similar mismatch may occur for youth's academic needs. Engel and colleagues (2013), for example, find a mismatch in math instruction among young children in the opposite direction of what we see during adolescence—namely, that many kindergarten classrooms teach math content that is too easy. The problem becomes even more severe in high school, given the growing variation in what youth know, coupled with increased inflexibility in curricular options, inflexibility in the ability to move between academic and vocational offerings, and difficulty in making up work when students fall behind.

While the optimal approach for better individualized instruction in the United States remains somewhat unclear, candidate strategies worth exploring further include efforts to help teachers learn to better individualize instruction; opportunities for tutoring; the creation of technologies and staffing that will facilitate more intensive instruction in adequate doses, levels, and topics; efforts aimed at helping students acquire appropriate grade-level skills and knowledge and catch up on missed work or topics not mastered; and opportunities for specialization in topics of interest. We review each of these strategies in turn.

Helping Teachers Learn to Individualize Instruction

Cook and colleagues (2015) analyzed data from the School and Staffing Survey (SASS) that suggests that fully 41 percent of new elementary school teachers and 44 percent of new secondary school teachers said they were unprepared or only somewhat prepared to differentiate instruction. By way of comparison, the proportions of teachers feeling unprepared or only somewhat prepared to teach their subject matter were just 21 percent and 14 percent for new elementary and secondary school teachers, respectively. Is there some way to help teachers learn how to do this better?

While a majority of American public school teachers receive some form of professional development each year, most of this development is neither very intensive (less than 8 hours per year) nor very effective. For example, Jacob and Lefgren (2004) studied teacher professional development as part of an accountability reform in Chicago, which provided additional training to all teachers in schools with test scores below a specified cutoff. The existence of the cutoff created the opportunity for an unusually rigorous regression discontinuity study, which suggests that the relatively modest in-service training that was provided had no statistically significant impact on student learning outcomes. This finding is consistent with the generally pessimistic assessment of most existing teacher professional development efforts by the U.S. Department of Education's What Works Clearinghouse.

On the other hand, there is some suggestive evidence that more intensive professional development could improve teacher effectiveness. For
example, Allen and colleagues (2011) conducted a year-long teacher coaching intervention called My Teaching Partner. Secondary school teachers
videotaped themselves delivering a lesson and submitted the videotapes
to trained teaching consultants, who viewed the videos and then provided
20- to 30-minute coaching sessions roughly twice a month covering what
worked well and what could be improved. The randomized controlled trial
found increases in student learning of 0.22 standard deviations. While the
cost per teacher of this intervention initially seems high (about $3,700),
perhaps a more useful metric is to compare the cost per student from a gain
of this magnitude to other candidate interventions. By that standard this
intervention is remarkably cost effective.

Under the right conditions, principals can also coach teachers to help
them improve their instruction. For example, working in the Houston
public schools, Fryer (2017) studied the effect of providing principals with
300 hours of training over 2 years to teach them how to help teachers
improve instruction, carried out in a mix of elementary, middle, and high
schools. This included training principals on lesson planning and use of
data-driven instruction, and having them observe classroom lessons and
carry out one-on-one coaching with teachers (in-person analogs in some
ways to the online coaching sessions in My Teaching Partner). The intervention improved student test scores in reading and math by between 0.10
and 0.19 standard deviations. While the cost per principal is not trivial, the
cost per student for these student-level learning gains is on the order of $10.
There would seem to be enormous value in learning more about how to
optimally carry out professional development strategies that help teachers
better individualize instruction, among other key teaching tasks, and how
this compares to other candidate strategies.

Tutoring

Another way to deal with this heterogeneity in student academic needs
is through tutoring. For example, Bloom (1984) summarizes a series of
randomized controlled trials (RCTs) with K-through-8 students, in which
they are taught new subjects (such as cartography and probability), which
found that when students were assigned to 1:1 or small-group (3:1) tutoring, test scores increased by fully 2 standard deviations when compared
with regular classroom instruction alone. Tutoring also generated large increases in time-on-task, improved student attitudes and interest, increased
the amount of feedback and correction between student and instructor
(a key characteristic of effective teaching), and ensured that all students
received this attention—including those students who were struggling in

school (Bloom, 1984). While teachers in regular classrooms tend to focus their attention on students performing at the top third of the achievement distribution, tutoring allows for specialized instruction—focusing on the particular academic needs of each student or a small group of students. In this way, the mismatch between what is taught and what the students need is alleviated.

The challenge for education policy has been that such intensive small-group instruction is very costly, so in practice students lack access to appropriate, high-quality targeted tutoring, especially if their parents cannot afford to procure it for their children. Whereas many public school systems use federal funding from the Title I program (intended to provide resources to help low-income students) to support tutoring programs, most of those programs involve hiring former teachers at salaries that are close to what full-time teachers currently make, resulting in a high hourly cost. The result is that students who are far from grade level and in need of extra help and remediation often get only a very modest amount of tutoring help per week, not nearly enough to bring them up to grade level. As a consequence, they continue to sit in classrooms hearing instruction that is mismatched with what they need.

The "two sigma problem," as articulated by Bloom (1984), is to identify lower-cost instructional alternatives that are as effective as tutoring. One possible approach is to rethink who is required to deliver small-group instruction; that is, whether we can reduce the labor costs associated with this instructional model by hiring nontraditional instructors who are less costly than traditional teachers. There are encouraging signs of promise for this approach from several RCTs carried out in the Chicago Public Schools (Cook et al., 2015). An RCT with 2,700 male high school students from disadvantaged communities showed that 1 year of tutoring, at a cost of between $2,500 and $3,800 per participant, increased math achievement test scores by 0.19 to 0.31 standard deviations, increased math grades by 0.5 standard deviations, and reduced course failures in math by one-half, in addition to reducing failures in non-math courses. Fryer (2014) found similarly large impacts from this type of tutoring, which relies on instructors who have fewer credentials than regular public school teachers (and hence lower salaries), in the Houston Public Schools.

The approach remains somewhat expensive although if implemented as part of a public school system's regular operations it might not need to provide tutoring to every student every year, since the goal is primarily to help students who have fallen behind so they can re-engage with grade-level classroom instruction. Other challenges beyond cost remain. It may require incorporating tutoring into the school day itself, which raises a number of logistical challenges relative to after-school tutoring.[6] How to measure and monitor the quality of these tutoring sessions is not yet well understood. And, relatedly, whether tutoring can be delivered on a large scale remains an open question, although this is a generic challenge for most social policies or programs (Banerjee et al., 2017; Davis et al., 2017).

Technology

In principle, some of the challenges of tutoring associated with cost and scale could be addressed by making greater use of technology, though how to achieve that in practice is not yet fully understood. In a developing country context, Banerjee and colleagues (2007) studied the effects of giving elementary school children in India access to 2 hours per week on a computer to play math games that emphasized basic math competencies and were tailored to their level of math skill. The result was gains in math test scores at the end of the academic year on the order of 0.35 to 0.47 standard deviation, although 1 year later these effects had faded to 0.10 standard deviations. Similarly, Muralidharan and colleagues (2019) studied the effects of a technology-assisted after-school instruction program for middle school students in India and found after 4.5 months that there were gains of 0.37 standard deviation in math and 0.23 standard deviation in language (the equivalent of reading/English scores in the United States).

In the United States and other developed countries, Escueta and colleagues (2017) identified 29 RCTs of computer-assisted learning programs, which help tailor the level of instruction to student needs. Two-thirds of these RCTs found beneficial effects on learning, particularly in mathematics, with effect sizes on the order of 0.2 to 0.6 standard deviation. These programs can personalize instruction for each student working on the computer, while also generating data that helps teachers understand where students are and what skills or concepts they are struggling with. In addition to helping personalize instruction, both computer-assisted learning and tutoring have the potential to improve time-on-task by reducing the

---

[6] Fryer and Howard-Noveck (forthcoming) find no detectable overall effects of after-school reading tutoring on middle school students in New York City. Whether the contrast between these results and the math tutoring results in Chicago, which involved in-school tutoring, is due to the difference between in-school and after-school tutoring or instead due to a focus on reading vs. math tutoring remains somewhat unclear, although some other work in Chicago has found sizable gains in reading scores from reading tutoring (albeit in school and with younger elementary school–age children).

chances that disruptive behavior by other students in the class impede the instruction.[7]

The advantages of technology are several. Not only is it easier to scale up an automated instructional program than human instruction, but also technology-based systems are increasingly able to adapt to user input, making them more dynamic and responsive to students' learning. Further, because the skills that make people good instructors may be in short supply, as programs increase in size the average quality of instructors is likely to decline unless programs raise wages and hence program costs (Davis et al., 2017). Finally, because today's adolescents are "digital natives," computer-assisted learning may be a natural adjustment for many.

However, research on implementing such automated systems is sorely lacking, and given the centrality of social experiences to students during this period of life it is important to investigate the advantages and disadvantages of placing students in potentially isolating computer-assisted learning environments. Teachers and technology might best be viewed as complements, not substitutes. For example, teachers may be able to help keep students motivated to continue with computer-assisted instruction by connecting the content to the specific interests of each student, or by helping ensure students' needs are well-matched to the specific computer program's design.

Tracking

In principle, an alternative approach is to reduce the heterogeneity in academic levels and needs within a regular classroom setting by sorting youth together based on how they are performing academically—that is, tracking.[8] Some of the strongest empirical evidence about the effects of this practice come from developing countries. For example, a large-scale RCT in Kenya found benefits (Duflo et al., 2011), with learning outcomes higher in "tracked" schools for students in *both* the top *and* bottom halves of the achievement distribution. The study suggests the benefits of reducing academic mismatch through better-targeted instruction are potentially large enough to outweigh adverse peer effects from having lower-achieving classmates, at least for initially low-performing students.

These encouraging findings for internal tracking in the Kenyan context do not necessarily mean this is the right approach in the U.S. context. One

---

[7]Research in the United States finds that simply providing students with access to computers will increase computer use, but seems to have mixed impacts on learning outcomes (Escueta et al., 2017). The results tend to be more promising for postsecondary students than for secondary or elementary school students.

[8]On the stratification of educational systems, see Kerckhoff (1995).

concern with tracking is the potential for tracked students to get stuck in lower academic levels without a means to catch up and take on more challenging work. Moreover, a recent study of mathematics tracking shows that in the United States, high school students in the highest level math courses had a significantly higher math self-concept compared to students in lower level math courses. This pattern held when tracking occurred on a course-by-course basis (versus tracking between schools, which is less common in the United States). The authors concluded that "when students are grouped only for certain courses, they observe the grouping process on an everyday basis and are thus constantly reminded of the relative status of their track" (Chmielewski et al., 2013, p. 948). Tracking may have the adverse effect of widening the gap among students. A student who would want to move to a higher track may find that the students in the higher track have already moved to an even greater command of the content area and vocabulary needed to perform in that area than the struggling student has had an opportunity to access. This is especially concerning in the U.S. context where we find a greater proportion of traditionally underserved students in lower tracks. Another concern is that if teachers prefer to work with higher-achieving students, all else equal, grouping students by academic level (tracking) may expose struggling students to relatively less effective teachers. It could also limit the possibilities for social network equity, since tracking can segregate students in ways that deprive them of social capital and other relational resources (Gamoran and Mare, 1989). Ultimately, whether tracking generates *net* benefits in the United States remains unclear.

Credentialing

At the very least, the U.S. education sector needs to recognize that college may not be the right fit for all students and needs to find other ways to help students succeed in the labor market—including by providing them with the necessary credentials to succeed. When high schools were initially formed in the late 19th century and postsecondary plans were more circumscribed, a high school diploma signaled to employers that its holder was ready for a job in the surrounding community, largely factory jobs or apprenticeships. However, today, the kinds of skills needed to navigate the job market have broadened markedly, the pathways from high school to jobs that pay a living wage are more heterogeneous, and a greater number of individuals are using high school to prepare for college. A single high school diploma, and the curriculum that goes with it, does not provide the kind of credential that most students need to navigate the job market, which particularly disadvantages low-income students and students who are not planning to attend college.

As noted above, secondary schools today tend to deemphasize vocational education as a purpose-driven pathway through high school meant to prepare youth for direct entry into the workforce (Cass, 2018). Given that only 36 percent of adults between the ages of 25 and 44 in the United States today have a 4-year college degree (U.S. Census Bureau, 2017), it is essential that meaningful high school–based vocational training, which leads to the certification of occupation-specific skills and licensing, be developed to open the door to jobs that would otherwise be inaccessible. Obtaining certification through credentials and licensing offers adolescents opportunities to access valuable and secure labor market positions. Further, credentials and licensure, which ensure skills and knowledge, have been shown to reduce racial inequities in pay for Blacks (Blair and Chung, 2018).

There have been calls for national workforce credentialing systems, many of which emphasize the role of community colleges, to address the growing need for mid-skilled employees (ACT, 2011). Consistent with Porter and Rivkin (2012), who argued that the connections between skills and the economy is local, the Abell Foundation conducted a study of the mid-level job market and high school graduates in Baltimore, Maryland. To understand how to connect high school graduates to mid-skilled jobs that do not require a college degree, the Abell Foundation identified the "best prospect" jobs for youth and matched them with training and certification programs at Baltimore community colleges (Hopkins, 2015). These "best prospect" jobs are mid-skilled occupations that pay a living wage, have future mobility, and require little postsecondary training—often even less than an associates' degree. They found that although there are continuing education and certification programs aligned with the "best prospect" jobs, most high school graduates were unaware of them. Although the data are limited, there was a consistent positive impact on earnings 2 years post-credentialing, especially for those in health care jobs (Hopkins, 2015). Similar to what Porter and Rivkin (2012) found, there are more "best prospect" jobs than qualified employees in Baltimore. Credentialing and the curricula that undergird credentials would ensure that youth today (and in the future) do not emerge from secondary education with a diffuse and unhelpful "one-size-fits-none" high school diploma, ill-prepared to succeed in a changing job market.

While the best way to differentiate educational opportunities for adolescents still remains unclear, there is undoubtedly real value in achieving this goal where possible. Taken together, additional research to better understand how to differentiate these opportunities and more policy attention to ensuring that differential and responsive educational opportunities for all adolescents are implemented could yield high returns.

Decision-Making and Psychosocial Skills

Deepened understanding of adolescence also underlines the importance of various non-academic skills—such as decision-making and psychosocial skills—that extend beyond schools' traditional focus on reading, writing, and arithmetic. Changes in the economy and other parts of society have further served to increase the importance of such skills. Youth themselves have reported their desire for schools to teach a wider range of skills, as illustrated in Box 6-1. The education sector of the future will need to accommodate these changes. In this section, we discuss ways the education sector can better support the development of decision-making skills, practical knowledge, adaptability, and psychosocial skills for adolescents.

Decision-Making Skills

To take advantage of the choices and opportunities available to them, adolescents must have ample opportunities to practice sound decision making (Eccles, 2007; Steinberg et al., 2009). The ability to make sound decisions is enhanced by the neurobiological development that occurs during adolescence, resulting in increased "processing speed" and reaction times. Further, cognitive automaticity—the ability to carry out cognitive processes quickly and without effort or intention—which results from myelization and synaptic pruning (see Chapter 2), decreases the cognitive load of everyday decision making, freeing cognitive capacity that can be devoted to more complex thinking (Petanjek et al., 2011; Rakic et al., 1994). This means that as youth mature they are better able to see abstract connections among ideas, and engage in thinking and other cognitive activities with more flexibility and feedback utilization (Vera-Estay et al., 2015).

To make good decisions about schoolwork, as well as in other areas, youth need to practice their emerging abstract reasoning and good decision-making skills and to learn from their mistakes (Byrnes et al., 1999; Fan et al., 2012; Halpern-Felsher and Cauffman, 2001; Steinberg, 2005).

Youth are capable of exercising good decision-making skills, but research also shows that some contexts facilitate mature decision making better than others. Sound decision making can easily be disrupted during adolescence by emotional arousal (Casey et al., 2001; see also Chapter 2). Youth make good decisions when those decisions are not emotionally charged, when they have had prior practice making similar decisions, when the people they admire make similar decisions, and when an immediate "reward" is not offset by a consequence well into the future (Steinberg, 2005).

BOX 6-1
Youth Perspectives: Beyond Reading, Writing, and Arithmetic

In a recent MyVoice survey, adolescents were asked what resources programs, policies, or systems might have helped them during their transition into
college or career after high school. Many reported their wish for more structured
classes in schools on how to perform practical tasks such as applying for college
and filing their taxes. Overall, youth reported wanting more guidance, more knowledge, and more social support from family and friends during this transition. (See
Appendix B for a description of MyVoice and its methodology.)

> More guidance on how to set long-term goals, how to deal with challenges
> such as meeting others as adults, learning about taxes, etc. A primer on
> adult life would be much appreciated.—23-year-old, White, undefined gender

> If schools taught you how to apply for jobs, 401k, taught about human rights,
> and how to vote, how to be an adult able to think for myself.—17-year-old,
> Latinx, male

> Clear, straightforward guidance!!! I don't know anything about going to
> college!!! It's very scary!!!!!—16-year-old, White, female

> If there were actual adulting classes in school. School doesn't prepare us for
> the real world, just for school. I don't know how to cook, I hardly know about
> finances, and I have no idea how health care works. I don't wanna have to
> learn this stuff the hard way, but I'm going to. Nothing has really prepared
> me at all.—17-year-old, White, undefined gender

> [L]ess stressors from school and more emotional intelligence education.
> —17-year-old, Asian, male

> Learning #howtoadult—17-year-old, White, male

> Better help from my parents and my school, more clarity on what I want to
> do in life, confidence in the economy and the political state of this country.
> —15-year-old, Black, female

SOURCE: Information from MyVoice, 2018.

Practical Knowledge

In addition to these dispositions and skill sets related to decision making, youth need practical knowledge about how to function in a complex
social world. With the traditional emphasis on grades and test scores,
an additional area of competence that has lagged is the type of practical

knowledge that will help adolescents to establish independent adult lives and flourish. Social science research has helped us understand that there are important inequities in youths' exposure to such knowledge outside of the school setting. Lower income youth, for example, are significantly less likely to have basic savings accounts than their more advantaged peers (Friedline et al., 2011). Whereas financial literacy is a primary focus of policies and programs directed at the developing world (Clark et al., 2018), they have diminished in focus in the United States.

For most purposes, adolescents reach "legal" adulthood at the age of 18, and genuine independence in adulthood requires youth to be financially literate. They need the skills to "read, analyze, manage and communicate about personal financial conditions that affect material wellbeing" (Vitt et al., 2000, p. 2). Youth need to be able to understand how to develop and live by a budget, enter contracts for housing leases and mortgages, understand how to negotiate health, auto, and housing insurance, make financial plans, and otherwise engage in economic life (Johnson and Sherraden, 2007; Nussbaum and Sen, 1993; Nussbaum, 2011). Poor financial decisions during this critical transition period can result in high levels of debt and derail youths' ability to meet their basic needs as they continue to mature (Lyons, 2004; Norvilitis et al., 2003). Despite the need to develop these skills to successfully transition into adulthood, schools and other agencies have decreased their emphasis on financial literacy and competency (Johnson and Sherraden, 2007). This is especially concerning considering that adolescence is a time when marketers, retailers, and credit card companies are increasingly targeting youth, enticed by their more than $211 billion in spending power (FONA, 2014).

Many successful programs for improving practical knowledge and financial skills build on "asset theory" (Beverly et al., 2008; Karimli et al., 2015), which is focused more on developing assets rather than income because of the sustaining power of assets in times of income volatility. For adolescents, secondary school experiences that provide "experiential" learning opportunities have been found to yield the most gains in knowledge, intent, and practice (Amagir et al., 2018). Amagir and colleagues (2018) did not find differences in program effectiveness among programs teaching financial literacy as stand-alone offerings and those programs that were integrated into existing curricula in secondary schools. For young adults, participating in financial education programs in college led to increased understanding of financial concepts, the intention to engage in responsible credit card use, the use of budgeting and planning, and fewer compulsive spending decisions (Anderson and Card, 2015; Borden et al., 2008; Bowen and Jones, 2006; Maurer and Lee, 2011).

Adaptability

More than in decades past, adolescents need practice to develop skills in thinking critically and analytically. Whereas in the past, it was only important for a small proportion of our population to become life-long learners, the current and emerging economy requires workers who have developed skill sets applicable to many types of jobs and who are also prepared for continuous learning and problem solving. Throughout their working lives, these skills, dispositions, and ways of engaging the world enable youth to create opportunities and pathways into adulthood.

Relatedly, today's increasingly knowledge-based economy, which yields innovation and entrepreneurship, requires a "mindset" of learning, malleability, and expectation for growth and improvement (Blackwell et al., 2007; Dweck, 2006; Yeager and Dweck, 2012). When young people come to recognize that intelligence is malleable and continues to develop, they are more likely to respond to mistakes and failures as opportunities to learn rather than risks to avoid. These are the kinds of mindsets that succeed in a knowledge-based economy. Adolescent mindsets do not develop in isolation. Schools, teachers, and experiences that encourage opportunities for students to embrace challenges and learn from them support the development of a "growth mindset."

Psychosocial Skills

A growing understanding of the importance of psychosocial skills, especially in the labor market, highlights the value of having the education sector include them in its focus. There are numerous established approaches for supporting adolescent psychosocial skill development in secondary schools. The select strategies described next have shown some promise, although the evidence base regarding their effectiveness and scalability is still in its infancy.

Project-based Learning. One of the potential ways to support psychosocial development in secondary schools is through project-based learning (PBL). This method differs from regular classroom instruction in that instead of relying on a standard classroom lecture format, students are asked to work on a problem-based project over a sustained period of time. The potential benefits, especially in middle and high school, include leading students to see connections between the classroom and the world, increasing students' ownership of their work, and developing critical thinking skills (Friedlaender and Darling-Hammond, 2007). This is related to the core idea first proposed many years ago by, among others, John Dewey: "Learning by doing." The potential advantages of PBL relative to standard classroom instruction are in developing additional skills related to creativity, organization, and group collaboration that may be particularly relevant for how the modern economy works and—ideally—to engage students in projects they find interesting (Blumenfeld et al., 1991). This may also help address concerns about the motivation levels of high school students in the United States (National Research Council, 2003).

The effectiveness of PBL remains unclear. Existing studies of PBL implementations tend to focus on comparing student test scores in a district before versus after PBL practices are adopted (Marx et al., 2004; Rivet and Krajcik, 2004). Learning more about the effectiveness of this and other strategies to improve psychosocial skills is an important priority for research.

PBL is not currently widespread in American schools, perhaps because it asks a great deal of teachers that differs from what they learned to do in university or on the job.[9] Presumably, most teachers already have some lesson plans in place, and given the relatively limited diffusion of PBL most teachers were likely taught in a regular classroom setting themselves. Learning how to plan projects and manage students during this process will require additional work and perhaps training and assistance as well, as will learning how to assess the work product and skills of individual students if they work in groups. More research is needed on the effectiveness of PBL and possibilities for implementation and scalability.

Provision of Feedback. Development of psychosocial skills can also be infused into regular classroom settings, for example by changing how classroom teachers provide feedback to students. Because adolescents tend to be vigilant to feedback, educators have the occasion to harness everyday mistakes as learning opportunities. When mistakes occur in class, on assignments, or during exams, adolescents often draw cues from authority figures on how to respond. If they are not given a chance to reexamine their work or perhaps even a second chance to resubmit their work, it signals that mistakes are evaluative rather than formative (Smeding et al., 2013; Yeager et al., 2013). In other words, without feedback assessments appear to be provided only to sort high-ability from low-ability students, which conveys to students that they are unlikely to be able to learn and improve. On the other hand, when adolescents are provided feedback on mistakes along with assurance that educators recognize their potential and expect improvement, they experience greater motivation to exert effort and embrace challenges.

---

[9] See https://www.edsurge.com/news/2016-08-01-why-do-so-many-schools-want-to-implement-project-based-learning-but-so-few-actually-do.

Promoting Belief in Malleability. Other experimental demonstrations with high school and college students also show it is possible to promote the idea that ability is malleable rather than fixed; students with whom this has been done show better academic outcomes than those in control groups, especially if they all had low levels of previous academic performance (Paunesku et al., 2015; Yeager et al., 2016a, 2016b). The experimental demonstrations reviewed suggest that educational institutions and experiences can be designed, tailored, and facilitated within local contexts to genuinely engage students in ways that encourage learning-growth mindsets.

For example, in a study of ninth graders across 10 high schools in the United States, Yeager and colleagues (2016a) found that a mindset intervention using design thinking improved core course grades for previously low-achieving students and increased the learning-oriented attitudes and beliefs of both low and high performers. As discussed above, mindset interventions are designed to change how students interpret and approach challenges and increase their resilience by exposing and affecting their central beliefs about education and school. Growth mindset interventions seek to explain to students that intelligence can grow with hard work, reframing their struggle with learning as an opportunity to grow rather than a lack of ability. The two-session mindset program used by Yeager and colleagues (2016a) was created through an iterative, user-centered design process.

Promoting Development of Future Identities. Developing their own possible selves and future identities helps young people ascribe meaning to difficult tasks such as schoolwork. As a result, those who have the opportunity to explore and develop the possibilities and pathways for their futures tend to demonstrate more effective self-regulation than those who do not. Experimental studies demonstrate programs that effectively help students to develop motivating future identities with positive consequences for academic trajectories, whether facilitated by trained professionals, by teachers, or even by near-peers (Destin et al., 2018; Horowitz et al., 2018; Oyserman et al., 2006).

Mindfulness and Related Practices. Current evidence suggests favorable academic and psychological outcomes in secondary schools implementing mindfulness practices (Raes et al., 2014; Zenner et al., 2014). Informed by current findings in neuroscience, recommendations for secondary schools include training teens in executive functioning skills (e.g., working memory tasks), providing opportunities for mindfulness activities such as meditation, and deepening self-regulation skills through sequenced, active, focused, and explicit (SAFE) socio-emotional learning programs (Steinberg, 2014). Teacher preparation programs can also serve a critical role in exposing future educators to relevant studies of adolescent brain development so that they are equipped to understand the efficacy of these practices in their classrooms. Furthermore, the same practices may be appropriate and beneficial for learning in certain university classrooms.

Cultivating Meta-Cognition. Finally, meta-cognition itself is a critically important skill for helping youth recognize when their automatic responses, which may be adaptive in most settings, are maladaptive and therefore should be "slowed down" so they can devote more mental energy to conscious reasoning. Several RCTs in Chicago show that it is possible to improve high school graduation rates and reduce rates of violence involvement through such programs (Heller et al., 2017). Similar findings have been found for young men in developing-country contexts (see, e.g., Blattman et al., 2017). Since programs with this focus rely on providers with skills that may be in short supply, it can be a challenge to deliver them effectively at scale. But assuming this problem can be solved, such interventions could be widely scaled, because they require a limited number of contact hours—typically between 10 and 30 total.

Advocates of socio-emotional learning programs suggest, although they are critical, socio-emotional learning programs are often overlooked in secondary schools (AEI/Brookings Working Group on Poverty and Opportunity, 2015; Belfield et al., 2015; Cervone and Cushman, 2015; DePaoli et al., 2017). Given their documented impact on the risk of violence involvement, and the fact that injuries (including from violence) are the leading cause of death to adolescents, incorporating this type of instruction into the health curriculum offered by high schools may yield positive results.

Strengthening Students' Health and Well-being

Adolescents have distinct physiological, socio-emotional, and cognitive tendencies and needs that must be recognized and addressed as they mature. This section discusses five ways in which schools can recognize these needs: through the assessment of school start times; the provision of physical activity and nutrition programs and activities; the adoption of trauma-informed practices and delivery of mental health services; the creation of safe and supportive school environments; and attention to wraparound services.

School Start Times

Natural neurological changes in circadian rhythms during adolescence due to hormonal fluctuations cause a misalignment between natural wake times and school schedules (Kirby et al., 2011; Wright et al., 2012; see also Chapter 3). The neurobiological changes lead to wakefulness later in the day and later in the evening, resulting in an accumulation of "sleep debt" and less optimal cognitive functioning during school, especially in the morning hours. Multiple studies document an association between sleep loss and negative academic capacity and performance (Dewald et al., 2010; Shochat et al., 2014). Advanced cognitive capacities for planning and decision making, for which adolescence is a period of rapid growth, may also be impaired by sleep loss (Beebe, 2011; Owens, 2014).

The American Academy of Pediatrics (2014) issued a policy statement in 2014 calling for later school start times as an effective solution for addressing poor sleep hygiene among adolescents. Specifically, it recommended that secondary schools start at 8:30 a.m. or later. While starting the school day later in the morning will not address all the factors contributing to insufficient sleep during adolescence, several studies show that teens get more sleep when school starts later (Owens et al., 2010; Wahlstrom et al., 2014). Moreover, later school start times seem to be associated with improvements in academic achievement (Carrell et al., 2011) and in behavior and mental health, including decreases in teen driving accidents, fewer depressive symptoms, and increased motivation (Danner and Phillips, 2008; Owens et al., 2010; Wahlstrom et al., 2014). Positive outcomes for youth pay off at the societal level: a macroeconomic modeling study found that delaying school start times resulted in significant economic gains at the national level over a relatively short period of time (Hafner et al., 2017).

School districts that have attempted to change the start times have encountered concerns about the impact of doing so on after-school activities (e.g., athletics, employment, caring for younger siblings), student access to public resources (e.g., public library), teacher schedules (e.g., less time with their own families), and the family schedules of students themselves.[10] For school districts, the potential impact on transportation costs is often the primary argument for maintaining current, early start times.[11] Given the importance of sleep for adolescents, there would be great value in more research to understand ways to mitigate the costs of later start times, and school district–wide policy changes in school start times provide a naturalistic experimental opportunity to examine associations between adolescent sleep, health, and educational metrics such as absenteeism, grade point average (GPA), and behavioral reports. At the very least, school systems should fully consider the benefits of sleep for adolescents in their planning.

---

[10] See http://www.sleepfoundation.org.

[11] However, a recent analysis suggests that delaying secondary school start times could actually be cost-effective in the long-run, particularly considering factors such as improved student academic performance and reduced rates of teen car crashes (Hafner et al., 2017).

Physical Activity and Nutrition in Schools

Adolescents gain much of their adult height and weight during puberty, and the speed and intensity of growth during this period increases an adolescent's need for energy, protein, and certain micronutrients (Institute of Medicine, 2007). When those needs are not met, adolescents experience slower growth rates, later sexual maturation, lower bone mass, and low body reserves of micronutrients, which can have lifelong health implications (Story et al., 2002). Similarly, adolescence is a critical period for bone mass development, making adequate intake of calcium crucial (Heaney et al., 2000). Between the ages of 9 and 17, adolescents gain about 45 percent of the adult skeleton (Institute of Medicine, 2007; Weaver and Heaney, 2006), and by age 20, they have gained 90 percent of their lifetime bone mass (Santos et al., 2017).

Not only has research shown that physical activity has a host of positive physical and mental health benefits for adolescents, such as reducing symptoms of depression and anxiety and improving mood (Institute of Medicine, 2013), but research has also shown a positive association between physical activity and academic achievement for adolescents (Esteban-Cornejo et al., 2015; Institute of Medicine, 2013; Kristjánsson et al., 2010; Rasberry et al., 2011). Physical activity in youth has also been associated with positive psychosocial traits, including self-efficacy, self-concept and self-worth, social behaviors, and goal-orientation (Institute of Medicine, 2013).

These critical nutritional and physical needs during adolescence call for special environmental supports to encourage healthy physical development. The school day presents numerous opportunities to improve the nutrition and physical activity levels of adolescents. Several federal initiatives aim to improve the nutrition and, to a lesser extent, the physical activity of U.S. adolescents. Most notably, the Healthy, Hunger-Free Kids Act of 2010 (HHFKA) directed the U.S. Department of Agriculture (USDA) to update the nutrition standards for the federal government's core childhood nutrition programs: The National School Lunch Program (NSLP), the School Breakfast Program, and the Special Supplemental Nutrition Program for Women, Infants, and Children (WIC), among others. The National School Lunch Program serves 30 million children every school day, many of whom are low-income (U.S. Department of Agriculture, Food and Nutrition Service, 2017). The updated nutrition standards for this program, implemented in 2010 and revised in 2019, require school cafeterias to serve meals that align with the Dietary Guidelines for Americans and regulate the sale of unhealthy foods throughout the school. The goal is to increase the consumption of healthy foods and create a healthy food environment for students. A study of students at 12 middle schools in a low-income, urban school districts found that students consumed more fruit and ate more of their vegetables and entrees after changes to the National School Lunch Program were implemented in their cafeterias (Schwartz et al., 2015).

The Community Preventive Services Task Force (2016) found that meal and snack interventions are effective at increasing fruit and vegetable consumption and reducing or maintaining the rate of obesity and overweight among students (Community Preventive Services Task Force, 2016). These interventions include school meal policies, programs that provide fresh fruits and vegetables to students during lunches and snacks, healthy food marketing initiatives, and nutrition education opportunities that empower students to make healthier choices. In addition, the task force found that combining these interventions into multicomponent interventions was also effective at reducing or maintaining the rate of obesity and overweight in schools.

Federal- and state-level policies also affect adolescents' access to and engagement with physical activity, most clearly through regulations on schools. The majority of states mandate some amount of physical education for students in middle and high schools (80% and 86%, respectively), although the quality and quantity of physical education provided typically fails to meet recommended standards for daily physical activity: only 27 percent of adolescents in the United States met the Centers for Disease Control and Prevention's recommendation of 60 minutes or more of physical activity per day every day of the week in 2016[12] (Carlson et al., 2013; Subcommittee of the President's Council on Fitness, Sports and Nutrition, 2012).

The Physical Activity Guidelines for Americans Midcourse Report Subcommittee of the President's Council on Fitness, Sports, and Nutrition found evidence that multicomponent physical activity interventions in schools can increase physical activity during school hours. These multicomponent interventions, which have been shown to increase physical activity during school hours, typically combine enhanced physical education with other strategies such as health education, classroom physical activity, social marketing initiatives, active transportation to school, and physical environment improvements, among others. These interventions are effective at increasing physical activity during the school day, and when combined with community- and family-based interventions they show strong evidence of increasing physical activity for adolescents outside of school (Subcommittee of the President's Council on Fitness, Sports and Nutrition, 2012).

---

[12] See https://www.cdc.gov/healthyschools/physicalactivity/facts.htm.

Trauma-Informed Practices and Mental Health Services

A third example of how recognizing the wholeness of adolescents may change the way schools operate is the recognition that many students, particularly from economically disadvantaged communities, come to school after having experienced significant distress and trauma outside of school, whether due to natural disasters, neighborhood violence, or other adversity. These experiences can affect not only students' health but also their academic achievement. For example, students (including adolescents) who have had a homicide occur within their neighborhood in the recent past exhibit test scores that are one-half to two-thirds of a standard deviation lower than the scores of other teens (Sharkey, 2010). Even youth from advantaged homes and backgrounds come to school with significant unmet mental health needs (Luthar et al., 2013). Among a nationally representative sample of adolescents, fully 40 percent experienced a mental illness over a 12-month period (Kessler et al., 2012). While the mental health services received by youth are most likely to be delivered in the school setting, overall only 45 percent of students with psychiatric disorders receive mental health care (Costello et al., 2014).

The unmet mental health needs of U.S. adolescents pose a key challenge to their ability to succeed in school, something that should be as significant a concern to the education sector as it is to the health sector. There are limits to the role schools can play in resolving this issue, of course, and providing mental health services in the school setting is just one way to help students. Although schools themselves cannot do it all, they can create opportunities for identification and treatment by providing mental health services (Green et al., 2013), although the quality and magnitude of services matters (Paschall and Bersamin, 2018). (See also the discussion of "School-based Health Centers" in Chapter 7). Finally, unmet mental health needs among U.S. adolescents pose a key challenge to their ability to succeed in school, something that should be of as great a concern to the education sector as it is to the health sector.

Safe and Supportive School Environments

Not all youth feel safe and supported while at school. For example, as discussed in the following chapter, weight-based victimization is widespread in schools, and can lead to poorer emotional health outcomes for students of all weight statuses (Buchianneri et al., 2013; Calzo et al., 2012; Puhl et al., 2011; Pont et al., 2017).[13] In addition, lesbian, gay, bisexual,

---

[13] While their bodies are changing, adolescents are becoming more sensitive to the thoughts and perceptions of others (Steinberg, 2014) and attempting to establish a sense of self (Chapter 2). This greater tendency toward social comparison may exacerbate body dissatisfaction and body image issues (Steinberg, 2017; Markey, 2010; Neumark-Sztainer et al., 2006).

transgender, queer, and questioning (LGBTQ) students report high rates of discriminatory bullying based on their sexual orientation and their gender identity. A number of negative health behaviors and outcomes for LGBTQ youth have been linked to such negative experiences at school (Russell et al., 2011).

During the past decade, a body of research has identified a number of policies, programs, and practices that help to create a safe and supportive school climate for LGBTQ students and indeed for all students. These include inclusive, enumerated policies; professional development on LGBTQ issues for educators and other professionals in the school setting; LGBTQ-related resources; and the presence of Genders and Sexualities Alliance clubs (GSAs, or Gay-Straight Alliances) in schools (see, e.g., Russell et al., 2010; Walker and Shinn, 2002). Policies that specifically identify sexual orientation and gender identity or gender expression as protected statuses in schools are associated with positive school experiences and health for all youth, including LGBTQ youth (Russell et al., 2010; Hatzenbuehler, 2011). Professional development for educators and other school personnel related to LGBTQ issues can equip them with skills to support all students (Hatzenbuehler, 2011; Kosciw et al., 2016). In addition, there are multiple personal and academic benefits when sexual orientation and gender identity are incorporated into the school curriculum (Black et al., 2012; Snapp et al., 2015). Relatedly, the presence of GSA clubs has been linked with individual student well-being, as well as with positive overall school climate (Ioverno et al., 2016; Poteat et al., 2015; Walls et al., 2009).

Wraparound Services

Addressing the integrated needs of adolescents is critical, especially for youth from socioeconomically disadvantaged backgrounds. While adolescents raised in households toward the top of the socioeconomic hierarchy are likely to have access to high-quality schools, safe and supportive communities, and well-functioning social systems, it is clear that adolescents from socioeconomically disadvantaged backgrounds face special challenges in accessing a well-functioning institutional ecosystem (Jackson, 2019). To this end, schools may come to provide services more commonly provided by other social institutions. These services might include free meals, laundry services, or health care. One of the best-known examples of schools operating in this "wraparound" mode is the Harlem Children's Zone, at the heart of which is a set of well-funded charter schools that aim to create a "pipeline of support" through the provision of food and health care (Harlem Children's Zone 2009, 2010; Tough,

2009).[14] It is still too early to provide a full assessment of the effects of this pipeline approach, although Harlem Children's Zone has shown positive results, particularly with respect to test scores (Hanson 2013; Page and Stone, 2010). Dobbie and Fryer (2011, 2013), for example, examine the effects of the Harlem Children's Zone on student outcomes and find that there are sizable impacts not only on test scores in the short term, but also on longer-term outcomes such as increased college attendance and reduced teen fertility (for females) and incarceration (for males).

Creating Culturally Sensitive Learning Environments

Adolescence is also a period when young people become increasingly aware of and attuned to their social status (Yeager et al., 2018). Educational institutions can consider this by critically evaluating the extent to which these practices reinforce status hierarchies and stereotypes about members of groups that are nondominant or stigmatized in society. Although the school curriculum is often based on a majority-White cultural point of view, the U.S. school population is increasingly diverse ethnically, racially, and economically. Further, while today's school population is racially diverse, teachers remain overwhelmingly White and female. These patterns highlight the potential for cultural mismatch and marginalization of youth of color at school as well as diminished opportunities for their full exploration and affirmation of identity. Disciplinary practices, staff, and curriculum are key contexts where this issue of culturally sensitive learning environments comes into relief.

Disciplinary Practices

Pressing boundaries, taking risks, and seeking autonomy and independence are hallmark features of adolescence (Steinberg, 2005), yet they often lead to misbehavior and rule violations at schools, especially when coupled with adolescents' general sensitivity to cues of respect or disrespect (Hohnen and Murphy, 2016). These tendencies can have serious consequences if they lead to formal remediation or disciplinary processes. For this reason, it is wise to frame remediation and disciplinary processes in a way that conveys greater respect for adolescents and more effectively encourages and supports academic and behavioral improvement (Okonofua et al., 2016). For example, sending a formal suspension letter to a student emphasizing the positive goals of the suspension is more likely to lead to

---

[14]For a similar example of a wraparound approach, see Communities in Schools at https://www.communitiesinschools.org/ (Figlio, 2015).

a successful return to school than sending a purely disciplinary message (Brady et al., 2017; Brady et al., 2018).

A starkly punitive disciplinary orientation is problematic for all youth, but it is all the more harmful when it is administered with an unequal hand. Unfortunately, youth of color, LGBTQ youth, and youth with disabilities are more likely to experience harsh and punitive discipline, even for similar infractions, than other students (Fabelo et al., 2011; Losen and Gillespie, 2012). Having disciplinary policies in schools that are developmentally appropriate may be particularly important given evidence that students of color are disciplined more often and receive more punitive discipline than White students, as noted in Chapter 4. Black students are also more likely than White students to be suspended from school and receive in-school detentions that exclude them from the classroom (Fabelo et al., 2011; Losen and Gillespie, 2012). However, there is no evidence that Black youth, LGBTQ youth, or youth with disabilities violate rules more often or behave worse than other students (Losen and Skiba, 2010; Skiba et al., 2015). The disparities are greatest for infractions that require subjective judgment, such as insubordination, defiance, and disruption (Fabelo et al., 2011; also see Chapter 4 and Box 9-2).

Conflict Prevention and Intervention

In the pluralistic communities our nation sometimes idealizes, diversity is a source of strength and enrichment. However, it is sometimes a source of tension and conflict as well. As a result, contemporary secondary schools are well-advised to undertake systematic efforts to prevent and resolve conflicts among their students (Gregory et al., 2014; Gregory et al., 2017). Conditions that foster conflict prevention include supportive student-educator relationships, academic rigor, culturally responsive teaching, bias-free and respectful classrooms and schools, and opportunities for learning and correcting behavior. Equity-driven principles of conflict intervention include inquiring about the cause of the conflict, problem solving, recognizing student and family voices in identifying causes and solutions, and reintegrating students after conflicts. Finally, a multitiered system of supports that match supports with student needs can contribute to both conflict prevention and intervention. These changes may be enhanced by proactive acknowledgement of racial and cultural inequalities in discipline (Carter et al., 2017; Gregory et al., 2014; Gregory et al., 2017).

Staff and Curriculum

While school populations are increasingly diverse ethnically, racially, and economically, the education workforce is largely White. Indeed, 82 percent of the U.S. education workforce is White. Similarly, only 20 percent of school principals are people of color. In contrast, 51 percent of U.S. school children are of color, and this proportion will increase in the coming decades (Child Trends, 2018).

Because adolescence is a time during which young people are honing their identities, it is important for schools to create learning environments that affirm the cultural backgrounds of all of their students. Mounting evidence suggests benefits for students when they have teachers who share their racial background (Dee, 2004; Egalite et al., 2015; Gershenson et al., 2017); this finding has even been replicated for community college students (Fairlie et al., 2014). For Black students in particular, having just one Black teacher in elementary school is positively related to high school completion and college aspirations (Gershenon et al., 2017). Having a Black teacher is also related to a reduced likelihood of exclusionary discipline such as suspension or expulsion for Black students at all grade levels (Lindsay and Hart, 2017).

The increasing divergence between the demographic backgrounds of secondary school teachers and their students makes the risks of a "hidden curriculum"—one not explicit in textbooks but embedded in the attitudes and behaviors of school staff—even more acute. The concern is that schools may remain places that are fundamentally driven by a single cultural narrative, since the cultural aspects of schooling also matter for students (Carter, 2013). Schools are important contexts for socializing youth, sending messages about appropriate behavior, who is or is not considered "smart" or "successful," and how to get along with peers and adults (Warikoo and Carter, 2009).

Some studies suggest that more culturally diverse curricula may benefit student outcomes during adolescence. A recent study by Dee and Penner (2017) found that students of various racial/ethnic backgrounds who were assigned to take an ethnic studies course in eighth grade because their GPA was below a certain threshold had increased attendance, a higher GPA, and more credits earned in ninth grade. Similarly, students who took courses in Mexican American studies had higher rates of high school graduation and higher passing rates on state standardized tests compared to students who did not participate in the courses; this was true despite course participants starting off with lower ninth- and tenth-grade GPAs than the nonparticipants (Cabrera et al., 2014). Thus, opportunities for diverse content and exposure to the perspectives of nondominant groups in the curriculum may be beneficial for all adolescents. However, more research is necessary to determine whether there may be any unanticipated effects.

Addressing Stereotypes

As students become more aware of their social identities, including their race, class, gender, and sexuality, schools have an opportunity to positively shape the meaning of those identities rather than reinforcing negative connotations (Umaña-Taylor et al., 2014). However, institutions and educators can sometimes convey, whether intentionally or unintentionally, impressions that students from racial-ethnic minority groups and students from lower-socioeconomic backgrounds have lower academic abilities. Teacher behavior may also reinforce stereotypes that girls have less potential to excel in science and math than boys do. These negative messages can impair students' actual performance and discourage them from pursuing endeavors where they might otherwise be likely to succeed (Murphy et al., 2007). On the other hand, when learning environments positively embrace students' social identities and allow them to consider how their backgrounds may help them to succeed, their sensitivity to social status can serve as a support for motivation and achievement.

Biases held against students from particular social groups can be especially consequential when held by teachers and other school personnel (Tenenbaum and Ruck, 2007). Based on a meta-analysis, teachers hold differential expectations for students based on students' racial background. On average, they have the highest expectations for Asian students and hold the lowest expectations for Black and Latinx students (Tenenbaum and Ruck, 2007). Teachers judge Black and Latinx students to be putting less effort into their studies, compared to White students, even though the students themselves report similar effort (Kozlowski, 2015). Further, teachers have more positive interactions with and make more positive referrals for Whites and Asians, compared to Black and Latinx youth (Tenenbaum and Ruck, 2007). When shown ambiguous facial expressions, teachers interpreted them as expressing anger and made more hostile attributions about those expressions when they were expressed by Black youth than when they were expressed by White youth (Halberstadt et al., 2018).

Biases and stereotypes are accentuated in contexts where an outgroup is easily identified, where there is little or no opportunity for individual interactions, and where there is mixed or confirming evidence regarding a negative stereotype, such as when there are demographic gaps in achievement or tracking that marginalizes an ethnic group (Banaji and Greenwald, 2013; Tajfel and Bruner, 1981). Large secondary schools make it more difficult for teachers to connect with students individually and avoid relying on pre-existing biases and stereotypes. Based on a review of evidence on school size, researchers recommend that secondary schools limit enrollments to between 600 and 1,000 students; the lower end of this range is recommended in particular for schools serving a large proportion of students from communities with limited economic resources (Leithwood and Jantzi, 2009). However, contrary to what students need, 30 percent of high schools have 1,000 or more students (U.S. Department of Education, 2017).

An RCT of small high schools in New York City carried out by the Manpower Demonstration Research Corporation, which exploited randomized admission lotteries to follow students, found that attendance at the small schools increased high school graduation rates by 9.4 percentage points overall (Unterman, 2014). The effects in this study were even larger for Black males, equal to a 12.2 percentage point improvement in graduation rates. The data thereby suggest that small schools may be particularly helpful for adolescents who suffer from stereotypes in larger school settings. Small high schools were also found to increase postsecondary enrollment rates by 8 percentage points[15] although some of the evidence regarding student outcomes in small schools is mixed (Barrow et al., 2015; Wyse et al., 2008).

Helping Adolescents and Families Navigate the Education Sector

The educational needs of youth and the education sector itself have become increasingly varied and complex. As a result, youth need more support in navigating their educational opportunities and linking their education to meaningful and sustaining postsecondary opportunities. Families are, in principle, an important resource for help in navigating these options and complexities. Youth rely on their parents and caregivers to select schools through school-choice assignment systems, to advocate for the right programs and courses in high school, and to help them find resources and programs outside of school (DeLuca and Rosenblatt, 2010; Hill et al., 2017; Kimelberg, 2014). Moreover, while youth are internalizing their own values and developing a sense of purpose around education and future goals, families can support them by communicating parental expectations for achievement and the value or utility of education, linking school work to future success, fostering their aspirations, and helping them make preparations and plans for the future (Hill and Tyson, 2009; Hill et al., 2018). These strategies help youth see how education fits into their larger goals and helps direct and motivate their educational pursuits.

Because effective parental involvement in education is different during adolescence than during elementary school (Hill and Tyson, 2009; Hill et al., 2018), many parents may require some adjustment period to under-

---

[15] Observational studies, which are less reliable because they may confound the causal effects of small schools on outcomes with those of unobserved student, family, teacher, or school-level factors that are correlated with school size, yield more mixed results (Crosnoe et al., 2004; Eccles and Roeser, 2011; Gottfredson and DiPietro, 2010; Klein and Cornell, 2010).

stand this new terrain, particularly for their oldest children. With little real guidance, there is a risk of making uninformed decisions with long-term impacts as families struggle to figure things out, especially for parents who did not attend college. In addition, the adolescent drive for autonomy and independence, which is a natural part of development, can make parents feel marginalized, even when youth state that they want their parents involved to help them navigate schooling, link education to their future, and successfully make postsecondary plans (Hill et al., 2018).

Correlational evidence suggests that promoting parental engagement in the education of their adolescent child may have a protective effect against declines in achievement and engagement as children progress through middle and high school (Hill et al., 2004; Hill and Tyson, 2009; Ratelle et al., 2004). Indeed, parental involvement in education is more strongly correlated to academic outcomes in middle and high school than in elementary school and has longer-term implications for school success (Kim and Hill, 2015). Given the reluctance of many adolescents to share information with their parents, studies have found evidence that providing parents with more (and more frequent) information about how their child is doing in school can improve academic outcomes (Bergman, forthcoming; Rogers and Feller, 2018).

Parent engagement may be particularly challenging for families from economically disadvantaged circumstances. Adolescents develop in the context of an institutional ecosystem that encompasses schools, the family, the community, and systems that provide social services. Adolescents are likely to develop their educational capacities to the fullest extent only when all of the institutions within their ecosystem are operating well (see, e.g., Bronfenbrenner, 1974, 1979). However, there are inequities in adolescents' access to advocates and in their families' varying ability to help them navigate the education sector and plan for their future. Moreover, there is some evidence that when adolescents from lower socioeconomic backgrounds reach high levels of academic achievement and progress to selective colleges and universities, they may experience a sense of conflict between their past and current status (Hermann and Varnum, 2018), or uncertainty about their changing socioeconomic identity (Destin et al., 2017). Further, these students often experience surprising levels of marginalization and ostracization that systematically work against their sense of belonging and ability to achieve success. These include experiencing homelessness and hunger during college breaks when their dormatories and cafeterias close, and needing to work in positions that serve the rest of the student body (e.g., in the cafeteria) that ultimately confirms stereotypes that they do not belong and are "workers," rather than scholars (Jack, 2018). These experiences make it more difficult for low-income students to succeed academically and build social capital that will aid in their upward mobility. This body of research suggests that when educational institutions include activities and opportunities that allow students to integrate their dynamic and multifaceted socioeconomic identities, students are likely to have stronger well-being and to more effectively pursue their academic goals.

RECOMMENDATIONS

The organization and focus of U.S. public secondary schools might have made perfect sense for the 19th century industrializing nation for which they were originally designed. But our improved understanding of adolescent development, together with transformative societal changes, have created a mismatch between what adolescents need and what secondary schools are currently designed to deliver. The launching of Sputnik in 1957 catalyzed the space race between the United States and the Soviet Union and inspired a major investment in and resolve to improve our public education system.

Striking individual events such as the Sputnik launch, capable of catalyzing transformative changes in domestic policy, are few and far between, but today a similar catalyst may be the competition between the United States and China for global economic and technological leadership. We have to prepare ourselves by enlisting the talents of generations of Americans born in the 21st century. This can only be done by rethinking adolescent education.

To this end, the committee puts forth recommendations for modernizing the nation's secondary schools. Taken together, these recommendations constitute a blueprint for achieving a developmentally appropriate education sector that reflects the preparation, knowledge, and skills that youth need for the 21st century and that rectifies longstanding and persistent disparities in resources across demographic backgrounds. This blueprint should be considered in tandem with companion proposals for strengthening community colleges and innovations in technical education as alternatives to traditional 4-year colleges. One pertinent example can be found in the 2014 National Academies report, *Investing in the Health and Wellbeing of Young Adults* (Institute of Medicine and National Research Council, 2015, Chapter 4, pp. 123–170).

This committee's recommendations for transforming secondary education for the 21st century highlight general principles as well as specific actions that policy makers, educators, and administrators can take to implement such change; see Box 6-2. In the following, we focus on the six recommendations of the blueprint, discussing each in turn.

BOX 6-2
Blueprint for a Developmentally Informed
Secondary Education System for Adolescents

Recommendation 6-1: Rectify disparities in resources for least-advantaged schools and students.
   A. All states should take steps to eliminate resource disparities across districts and schools by exploring methods or formulas for financing education to augment or replace municipal tax bases.
   B. In coordination with states and localities, the federal government should develop "NextStep," a program targeting underprivileged adolescents to promote both their academic and non-academic development.

Recommendation 6-2: Design purposeful but flexible pathways through education.
   A. Recognizing the enormous heterogeneity in the academic levels and needs of adolescents, school districts should be funded to improve their capacity to adapt to individual students' needs, including pace of learning and need to make up work.
   B. School districts should facilitate diverse pathways and postsecondary plans for adolescents, including for those students interested in career-oriented or vocational education and training as well as those who are college-bound, and ensure that students have the skills and access to coursework necessary for the option to switch between the two as their interests may evolve.
   C. School districts should design flexible schedules for course offerings during the academic year and the summer to enable youth to easily make up classes, recover lost credits, and advance in their course work, especially for youth who are over-age and under-credited. In addition, school personnel should help youth and families create specific plans to recover lost credits, to advance in their course work, and to pursue postsecondary job and career opportunities.
   D. Schools should provide flexible and diverse opportunities for students to develop interests, talents, and dispositions to foster their general well-being and facilitate their civic engagement.
   E. States and localities should provide funding to allow schools to hire sufficient career, vocational, and college counselors who are knowledgeable about the local job markets in order to prepare youth for 21st century jobs and identify internships and apprenticeships to facilitate the training youth need to transition to the job market.
   F. Local businesses and school districts should create robust relationships and specific programmatic linkages to ensure that school curricula enable youth to learn the skills and information needed to prepare them for meaningful jobs and careers in the local economy.
   G. Local businesses, local colleges, and school districts should create specific internships and apprenticeship training programs to prepare youth for, and provide credentials for, meaningful jobs and careers.

BOX 6-2 Continued

Recommendation 6-3: Teach practical knowledge and non-academic skills, such as decision making, adaptability, and socio-emotional competence.
   A. Schools should create significant opportunities for youth to develop nonacademic skills, including project-based learning, socio-emotional learning, and practices encouraging reflection on intellectual growth and personal identity.
   B. Schools should teach adolescents specifically about brain development so that they understand its connections to their own health and well-being.
   C. Schools should provide opportunities to youth both within classrooms and within the larger school context to regularly make impactful decisions in order to develop both decision-making skills and efficacy for civic engagement.
   D. The U.S. Department of Education should create guidelines for, and school districts should create, curricula to ensure mastery of practical life skills for youth upon graduation, either through specific courses or integration into existing courses. Practical knowledge includes finance management, budgeting, and banking; obtaining and managing insurance (e.g., health, auto); housing (e.g.,renting, leasing, mortgages, contracts); and transportation (e.g., drivers licenses, identification and processes for using public transportation such as trains, buses, and air travel).
   E. To foster civic engagement and decision making and to empower youth to effect change in their communities, school districts and local governments should provide youth with opportunities to participate in research designed to improve the agencies that are directed to serve them (e.g., by designing and identifying appropriate research questions, analyzing appropriate data, and drawing recommendations and conclusions).

Recommendation 6-4: Protect the overall health and well-being of each student.
   A. Given the importance of sleep for adolescents, researchers and policy makers should prioritize identifying ways to mitigate the potential challenges of later school start times and fully consider the benefits of sleep for adolescents. School staff should consider the value of sleep as they plan the school day and design homework and assignments.
   B. School districts should enact policies and practices that promote supportive school climates and ensure safety for all students.
   C. States and localities should provide funding for, and direct schools to provide, increased access to mental health services for students.
   D. School districts, in coordination with their local communities, should ensure that adolescents have the time and opportunity to engage in sufficient health-promoting physical activity each day and that healthy food options are available.

continued

BOX 6-2 Continued

Recommendation 6-5: Foster culturally sensitive learning environments.
A. State and federal agencies, school districts, and schools should require that teachers, counselors, administrators, and staff engage in regular training on implicit bias and cultural sensitivity, generally and as they relate to specific populations within the school.
B. Schools should recruit and retain a diverse workforce to mirror the diversity of their student bodies.
C. College and university schools of education and other teacher training programs should require coursework that assures mastery of adolescent development and culturally inclusive pedagogy and implicit bias in their training of teachers.
D. School districts and schools should implement curricula that are culturally inclusive and affirm the value of the diverse ethnic and cultural backgrounds represented among students, both in content and learning styles.
E. Schools and school districts should create curricular opportunities for culturally relevant content and exposure to perspectives of nondominant groups.
F. Schools and districts should establish and utilize disciplinary policies and practices that are developmentally appropriate and ensure that disciplinary measures are applied equitably and fairly. School leaders should assess and monitor their disciplinary practices to assure that they are free of biases by race, gender, socioeconomic status, or ability status.
G. School districts and schools should implement equity-driven principles of conflict intervention.

Recommendation 6-6: Help adolescents and families navigate the education sector.
A. Schools should support adolescents and families by serving as a coordinator of institutional services, such as providing assistance in identifying internships, apprenticeships, mentoring, and training for career and vocational transitions, along with navigating the college admissions process.
B. School districts should assist families in navigating the education sector to identify opportunities and resources to meet the specific educational needs of their adolescents.

RECOMMENDATION 6-1: Rectify disparities in resources for least-advantaged schools and students.

The committee acknowledges that implementing its proposals will require additional resources, as well as the thoughtful deployment of existing resources to where they are needed most. A demand for additional resources is likely to be particularly challenging for the least-well-resourced communities, given the ongoing reliance of our nation's K–12 system on local financing (namely, local property taxes). Funding schools at the municipality level leads to large inequalities in educational opportunities, and disparities in school funding across states only exacerbate the problem (see Jackson et al., 2016). All states should take steps to eliminate resource disparities across districts and schools by exploring methods or formulas for financing education to augment or replace municipal tax bases.

While state-level financing reforms are a necessary first step, additional efforts are needed. Although many states have addressed these inequalities in recent years, often prodded by constitutional litigation, the country is far from eliminating resource disparities across schools. Moreover, as demonstrated in Chapter 4, even when states have closed the gap in public resources, disparities in family resources and in neighborhood supports have continued to produce disparities in educational outcomes. Unfortunately, it appears that the increasing income segregation of school districts across the country, along with rising income inequality, has prevented society from realizing the full benefit of the significant gains in financial parity among school districts as measured by improving educational outcomes and decreasing disparities in test scores. Thus, the committee envisions a major commitment to eliminate disparities in educational spending for the explicit purpose of creating equal opportunity for a large proportion of the adolescent population now being left behind.

This is a national problem, and it requires a national initiative. While primary responsibility for K–12 education lies with the states and localities, the federal role in education has gradually evolved to assist the states in achieving equal opportunity and support other national priorities. For example, the federal government has played a large role in education in recent years, beginning with the federal No Child Left Behind statute and including the current Common Core provisions. Moreover, jurisprudence surrounding the Fourteenth Amendment's Equal Protection Clause gives the federal government a role in education, particularly related to reducing inequality (Harris et al., 2016).

In the committee's view, worsening inequalities in secondary education now threaten the nation's economic well-being. The committee is convinced that a more aggressive federal role will be required to address and eliminate these persistent disparities. Such a federal initiative could take many forms. It would be well beyond the committee's charge or expertise to review the financing of secondary education, with its many complexities, but the committee does believe that setting the goal and inviting a national conversation on strategies for achieving it are well within our charge.

The goal should be to ensure that every adolescent has a genuine opportunity to reach his or her full potential and to take full advantage of the resources and services that a transformed system of secondary education can provide. Implementing the educational vision outlined in this chapter is a necessary step, and states and localities will need to make the case to their lawmakers to invest in the programs and services set forth in this blueprint. However, these changes will not be sufficient in themselves to enable all their students to flourish. The evidence reviewed in Chapter 4 demonstrates that special attention—and additional resources—will need to be devoted to the students who are already falling behind. This is where the need for a federal initiative is most compelling. In coordination with states and localities, the federal government should develop a program with the explicit goal of improving both the academic and the non-academic development of underprivileged adolescents. The program envisioned by the committee might be called "NextStep."

NextStep would be modeled on Head Start, the successful early childhood program.[16] Just as Head Start expanded the mission of the educational sector to break the cycle of poverty by targeting the needs of younger children and their families, NextStep would task the sector with promoting positive adolescent development through targeted instruction, services, and supports to disadvantaged and underperforming students. Federal financing for NextStep would supplement state-level efforts to equalize funding within and across districts by targeting additional funds to those students most in need. These programs would expand the mission of our educational sector to promote both the academic and the non-academic development of adolescents and would help adolescents develop a foundation of practical, noncognitive, and social skills, as well as academic skills, in preparation for a successful transition to life as a young adult.

Aside from NextStep, the strengthened federal role in financing secondary education could provide a backstop for the states by allowing countercyclical spending during economic downturns. During these times, when the labor market opportunity costs of human capital development are lower, the federal government could support older adolescents to obtain additional postsecondary schooling or job training.

---

[16]Head Start aims to "promote school readiness of children ages birth to five from low-income families by supporting their development in a comprehensive way" (Office of Head Start, 2017). According to the National Academies of Sciences, Engineering, and Medicine (2018, p. 63), "Head Start began as a program for prekindergarten-age children and was later expanded to include Early Head Start, which directs services to infants, toddlers, and pregnant women. The majority of Head Start funding is used to support prekindergarten programs for 3- and 4-year-olds, but funds are also used for family-oriented services such as home visits, health screenings, and parental support, as well as ECE funding for infants and toddlers." Bitler and colleagues (2016), for example, found positive short-term effects for children participating in Head Start programs, including cognitive gains for those children at the lowest achievement levels, and long-term effects on well-being in early adolescence.

RECOMMENDATION 6-2: Design purposeful but flexible pathways through education.

To respond to the enormous heterogeneity in the academic levels and needs of adolescents, school districts should be funded to improve their capacity to adapt to students' needs, including pace of learning and need to make up work. In addition, schools need curricula and course sequences that are responsive to students' strengths, interests, and postsecondary goals and plans. While the optimal approach for better individualizing instruction in the U.S. context remains somewhat unclear, candidate strategies worth exploring further include creating technologies and staffing that will facilitate more intensive instruction in adequate doses, levels, and topics that are aimed at helping students acquire appropriate grade-level skills and knowledge, catch up on missed work or topics not mastered, and specialize in topics of interest.

School districts should also facilitate diverse pathways and post-secondary plans for adolescents—including those students interested in career-oriented or vocational education and training as well as those who are college-bound—and ensure that all students have the skills and access to coursework necessary for the option to switch between the two as their interests may evolve over time. Students should be guided in developing postsecondary career goals and the educational pathways to reach these goals, whether they include preparation for college or targeted and strategic vocational and career training that leads to the certification of occupation-specific skills and licensing necessary to compete in the changing job market. School districts should design flexible schedules for course offerings during the academic year and the summer to enable youth to easily make up classes, recover lost credits, and advance in their course work, especially for youth who are over-age and under-credited. In addition, school personnel should help youth and families create specific plans to recover lost credits, to advance in their course work, and to pursue post-secondary job and career opportunities. In addition, schools should provide flexible and diverse opportunities for students to develop interests, talents, and dispositions to foster their more general wellbeing and facilitate their civic engagement.

In order to do so, states and localities should provide funding to allow schools to hire sufficient career, vocational, and college counselors who are knowledgeable about the local job markets in order to prepare youth for 21st century jobs and identify internships and apprenticeships to facilitate in training youth for their transition to the job market.

Local businesses and school districts should create robust relationships and specific programmatic linkages to ensure that school curricula enable youth to learn the skills and information needed to prepare them for meaningful jobs and careers in the local economy; local businesses, local colleges, and school districts should create specific internships and apprenticeship training programs to prepare youth for, and provide credentials for, meaningful jobs and careers. Given the potential for substantial change in the labor market of the future, one challenge for school systems will be to balance the development of general skills that (by definition; see Becker, 1964) are useful across all industries and occupations, versus more occupation-specific skills that would require forecasting future labor market demand in different sectors and jobs. Indeed, Porter and Rivkin (2012) described how economies and economic impact is localized, despite calls for national solutions. The type of analysis of job prospects and training needs at a local level is modeled in Baltimore by Hopkins (2015) and the Abell Foundation. As noted above, this report linked an assessment of mid-skilled job needs in Baltimore with the training and credentialing opportunities at local community college. Creating stronger linkages between high schools and community colleges with the specific and intentional goal of creating clearer and more flexible pathways from high schools to jobs is essential. Research is needed on effective collaborations between school districts and the actors in the local economy to develop theories of change and to design effective interventions and programs, to ensure that youth leave high school with skills, knowledge, and access to meaningful jobs and careers in the local economy, and that they are able to adapt to changing social conditions and be lifelong learners.

> **RECOMMENDATION 6-3: Teach** practical knowledge and non-academic skills, such as decision making, adaptability, and socio-emotional competence.

Research in education and psychology have helped the field understand the growing importance of skills beyond academics for success in the labor market and other aspects of life, and indeed research has shown that these psychosocial skills have become increasingly important over time. Schools should create significant opportunities to develop these skills, including project-based learning, socio-emotional learning, and practices encouraging reflection on intellectual growth and personal identity. Schools should teach adolescents specifically about brain development, so that they understand its connections to their own health and well-being. All hold potential for developing such skills as part of regular academic instruction, although more research is needed to understand the exact effects of these approaches and how to implement them most successfully.

Schools may also encourage the development of non-academic skills, for example, by changing the curricular focus of the school day, including explicit instruction targeting these skills. The U.S. Department of Education should create guidelines for, and school districts should create curricula to ensure, mastery of practical life skills for youth upon graduation, either through specific courses or integration into existing courses. Practical knowledge includes finance management, budgeting and banking; obtaining and managing insurance (e.g., health, auto); housing (e.g., renting, leasing, mortgages, contracts); and transportation (e.g., drivers licenses, identification and processes for using public transportation such as trains, buses, and air travel)

In addition, students should be provided with opportunities both within classrooms and within the larger school context to regularly make high-impact decisions in order to develop both decision-making skills and efficacy for civic engagement. To foster civic engagement and decision making and to empower youth to effect change in their communities, school districts and local governments should provide youth with opportunities to participate in research designed to improve the agencies that are directed to serve them (e.g., by designing and identifying appropriate research questions, analyzing appropriate data, and drawing recommendations and conclusions). These opportunities to practice decision making align with adolescents' neurological developmental needs. As the adolescent brain develops myelinated associations between experiences, emotional experiences, contexts, and decisions, practicing decisions making at a time of peak brain development will increase the likelihood that they will make good decisions in the future (Steinberg et al., 2009).

RECOMMENDATION 6-4: Protect the overall health and well-being of each student.

Given the importance of sleep for adolescents, researchers and policy makers should prioritize identifying ways to mitigate the potential challenges of later school start times and fully consider the benefits of better sleep for adolescents, and school staff should consider the value of sleep as they plan the school day and design homework and assignments. As described above, one of the most discussed recommendations for improving adolescent sleep duration and quality was made by the American Academy of Pediatrics, which recommended in 2014 that schools delay their start times to accommodate the natural sleep cycles of adolescents. Other recommendations with promising results have included raising community awareness of good sleep hygiene (Blunden and Rigney, 2015) and encouraging parents to enforce bedtime routines at earlier ages (Mindell et al., 2017; Mindell and Williamson, 2018). Evidence-based practices have demonstrated the potential of school-based sleep interventions (Cassoff et al., 2013; Kira et al., 2014; Tan et al., 2012), including those that use motivational interviewing (Bonnar et al., 2015) and mindfulness approaches (Bei et al., 2013). Still, more work is needed to determine best practices for improving sleep among adolescent populations.

School districts should enact policies and practices that promote supportive school climates and ensure safety for all students. In addition, school districts need to be funded and directed to provide access to mental health services for students. For example, districts and school leaders can create positions within school counseling departments and hire counselors trained in trauma-informed practices and mental health services or create partnerships with local agencies to provide these services. (See also discussion of "School-based Health Centers" in Chapter 7.)

School districts, in coordination with their local communities, should ensure that adolescents have the time and opportunity to gain sufficient health-promoting physical activity each day. One way to increase physical activity for adolescents is to deploy multicomponent interventions in schools, as recommended by the Subcommittee of the President's Council on Fitness, Sports and Nutrition (2012).

RECOMMENDATION 6-5: Foster culturally sensitive learning environments.

State and federal agencies and school districts and schools should require that teachers, counselors, administrators, and staff engage in regular training on implicit bias and cultural sensitivity, both generally and as they relate to specific populations within the school. Schools should recruit and retain a diverse workforce to mirror the diversity of their student bodies. Schools of Education and other teacher training programs should require coursework assuring mastery of culturally inclusive pedagogy and implicit bias in their training of teachers, as well as having requirements for basic training in adolescent development, including the neurobiological and psychosocial development of adolescents.

School districts and schools should implement curricula that are culturally inclusive and affirm the value of the diverse ethnic and cultural backgrounds represented among U.S. students, both in their content and in learning styles. Schools and school districts should create curricular opportunities for culturally relevant content and exposure to the perspectives of nondominant groups.

Schools and districts need to establish and utilize disciplinary policies and practices that are developmentally appropriate and ensure that disciplinary measures are applied equitably and fairly. School leaders need to assess and monitor their disciplinary practices to assure that they are free of biases by race, gender, socioeconomic, or ability status. In addition, school districts and schools should implement equity-driven principles of conflict intervention.

RECOMMENDATION 6-6: Help adolescents and families navigate the education sector.

Schools should support adolescents and families by serving formally and aggressively as placement coordinators for educational and vocational assistance, including identifying internships, apprenticeships, and training for career and vocational transitions and helping students navigate the education sector to identify opportunities and resources to meet their specific educational needs, including in the college admissions process. School districts should assist families in navigating the education sector to identify opportunities and resources to meet the specific educational needs of their adolescents.

Summary

To meet the challenges of the 21st century, we need an educational system that elicits and supports the development of the whole adolescent. To promote the educational system's core goal of developing adolescents academically, we need a system that elicits and supports other aspects of the adolescent as well—socially, physically, and cognitively. We need an educational system that is responsive to adolescents' neurological assets and opportunities. We need an educational sector that is flexible enough to meet students where they are, help them make up for early setbacks, and identify and hone their interests and talents in a way that leads all to productive and meaningful places in society—including college and career. We need an education sector that is responsive to and reflective of the increasing racial/ethnic diversity of the American population.

Finally, we need an education sector that is committed to the flourishing of every adolescent. The new research understandings of the nature of adolescence itself, summarized here, help show us how we might better conceive of an education sector that is more responsive to the needs of adolescents and, therefore, of society as a whole.

7

Health System

A ccess to appropriate health care services is important for adolescents, both to ensure their well-being today, as they experience the bumps and stresses of adolescent life, and to ensure their well-being for a lifetime by addressing habits that impact their long-term health, such as diet, exercise, and substance use (Brindis et al., 2002; National Research Council and Institute of Medicine, 2009; Patton et al., 2016). Yet adolescents—particularly ethnic and racial minority adolescents—face a variety of barriers to accessing health care (Alegría et al., 2016; Costello et al., 2014; Cummings et al., 2014; Lau et al., 2012). Additionally, many of the health issues adolescents confront are rooted in the social determinants of health and driven by underlying social and economic inequalities (Brindis et al., 2005; Philbin et al., 2014; Richardson et al., 2017; Tebb et al., 2018).

These barriers are troubling given our new understanding of how the brain, body, and environment interact during adolescence (see Chapters 2 and 3). The period of adolescence presents an opportunity for the health care system to support the optimal growth and development of all adolescents. In this distinct period of development, young people are strengthening the abstract reasoning and executive function skills that help them to set long-term goals and make rational decisions. At the same time, their heightened neurobiological flexibility and resilience make them more amenable to interventions that can maintain or improve their developmental trajectories. But this increased flexibility also makes adolescents more vulnerable to harmful or unhealthy influences that can set them on less positive paths. The health care system can work to support adolescents' growth and potential through programs, policies, and practices specifically aimed at young people.

This chapter sets out a vision for financing and delivering adolescent-friendly health services, an essential condition for every adolescent to flourish (Mazur et al., 2018). It then discusses some of the critical components of adolescent-friendly services: access to services, including sexual and reproductive health care and behavioral health care; confidentiality and parental consent; a workforce trained in adolescent care; the provision of care in nontraditional settings, including school-based health centers and through eHealth; and the creation of safe environments. The chapter concludes with a blueprint for achieving adolescent-friendly services and system-level policies to improve adolescent health.

THE VISION: SEAMLESS ACCESS TO ADOLESCENT-FRIENDLY HEALTH SERVICES

Adolescents are distinct from both children and adults when it comes to health care. In general, they are inexperienced in navigating the health care system independently and are especially concerned that their health needs and the services they receive remain confidential (Britto et al., 2010; Copen et al., 2016; Grilo et al., 2019). Moreover, adolescents are also more likely than adults to engage in risk-taking behaviors that could have both short- and long-term effects on their health (Patton et al., 2016). These distinct characteristics require health care delivery approaches tailored to adolescents' developmental needs. When such developmentally appropriate care is not available, youth have been shown to forego care and become disengaged with the health care system (Ford, 1999; Lehrer et al., 2007).

Developmentally appropriate changes to provider practices and innovative care delivery systems can help adolescents become more engaged with their care and achieve better outcomes. This section discusses the health-service wants and needs of adolescents and lays out the characteristics of adolescent-friendly health services. The goal of such services is to ensure the health and well-being of all adolescents, through integrated, comprehensive health services that prepare youth for the distinct physical, cognitive, and social changes that take place during adolescence, ready them to navigate the health system independently, and provide services that are culturally informed and attentive to the needs of all youth (see Box 7-1).

Characteristics of Adolescent-Friendly Health Services

To design services to meet the needs of adolescents, we must first understand what adolescents, as consumers of health services, expect and need from their primary care providers (Daley et al., 2017). A meta-analysis

---

BOX 7-1
Vision for an Adolescent-Friendly Health System

VISION: To ensure the health and well-being of all adolescents, through integrated, comprehensive health services that prepare youth for the distinct physical, cognitive, and social changes that take place during adolescence, ready them to navigate the health system independently, and provide services that are culturally informed and attentive to the needs of all youth.

---

of 12 qualitative studies found that adolescents have five overarching desires for their interactions with health care providers: (1) to be engaged in conversations, not lectures; (2) to have their privacy and confidentiality respected; (3) to be accepted; (4) to be treated with respect, competence, and professionalism; and (5) to be offered a trusted relationship with their providers (Daley et al., 2017). Moreover, adolescents place greater valence on the characteristics of the health care provider than any other group does, and they wish to feel welcomed, attended to, and understood (Ambresin et al., 2013; Blum et al., 1996; Daley et al., 2017; Ginsburg et al., 2002a; Mazur et al., 2018). Adolescents may find health services unfriendly if they are not accessible (too far away or expensive) or not accepting of them, for example if they fear being judged or fear breeches of confidentiality (World Health Organization, 2012). Understanding what adolescents themselves want out of the health care system is crucial for developing adolescent-friendly health services.

Comprehensive, integrated, and coordinated services represent a critical feature of adolescent-friendly services.

Comprehensive health care aims to take into account the entirety of a person's needs, from medical to social. The power of social determinants of health, as well as the social and cultural context that young people live in, require a blending of services beyond those traditionally encompassed in the health sector, such as education, social and economic development, and other family and community supports.

Integrated services address a patient's physical and behavioral health concerns. As adolescent health—and adolescence itself—has been reconceptualized over the past decades, and as new research in neurobiological development emerges, the necessity of integrating physical and mental health services has become increasingly apparent and important. Integration between physical and behavioral health providers becomes more pressing as the number of adolescents with mental or behavioral health issues grows (see "Behavioral Health Care" below). An integrated system aims to promote communication, collaboration, and coordination between physical health and mental health care providers, youth, and their families (National Alliance on Mental Illness, 2011). Ideally, both primary care and behavioral care are established within the same setting or co-located.

Coordinated services seek to break down silos in health care by synchronizing the delivery of care between multiple providers and specialists.[1] Coordinated care aims both to improve health outcomes by breaking down silos between disparate providers and to reduce health care costs by preventing duplication in tests and procedures (New England Journal of Medicine Catalyst, 2018). Thus, having highly coordinated services lessens the burden on adolescents to know exactly which services they need so that they show up at the "right" service door. For young people who often perceive their health care needs as interrelated (Brown et al., 2007; Gray et al., 2005; Manganello, 2008), and are new to navigating the health system on their own, integrated, coordinated and comprehensive services may be especially helpful. Moreover, coordination and continuity of services are especially important for adolescents with special health care needs, including physical health, mental health, and substance abuse treatment, but all adolescents need support in transitioning between systems of care (e.g., from pediatrics or primary care to internal medicine or obstetrics and gynecology). In addition, coordination within a system can decrease fragmentation and maximize available resources at the local, state, and federal levels.

The holistic approach to assessment and care is well-suited to addressing the health behaviors, concerns, and problems of young people, because the risks and vulnerabilities they face are multifaceted and highly interrelated. Providers need to be attuned to the whole adolescent and not just to the presenting issue, as adolescents often experience a range of health needs at the same time. For example, among U.S. high school students, of those whose last sexual intercourse was unprotected, 43.5 percent reported persistent sadness, 41.5 percent reported suicidal thoughts and plans, and 45.9 percent reported either binge drinking or drinking while driving (Fox et al., 2010c). This challenges us to think about young people's physical health, sexual and reproductive health, and emotional well-being in a highly connected and coordinated way.

Adolescent-friendly health service models seek to provide services that are comprehensive, accessible, confidential, developmentally appropriate,

---

[1] Coordinated care has four elements: (1) patients have ready access to a range of health care services and providers, (2) providers communicate effectively and execute effective care plan transitions, (3) the patient's total health needs are the focus, and (4) information is presented to patients clearly and simply to promote understanding (New England Journal of Medicine Catalyst, 2018).

and equitable (Daley et al., 2017; Diaz et al., 2004; Fox et al., 2010a; Ginsburg et al., 2002b; Mt. Sinai Adolescent Health Center, 2017; Sadler and Daley, 2002; Tylee et al., 2007; World Health Organization, 2003). These models seek to remove barriers to care and improve engagement in the health system among young people. They have been adopted in a number of health care settings; see Box 7-2. Several studies and frameworks have been developed to conceptualize youth-friendly health care services (Ambresin et al., 2013; Huppert and Adams Hillard, 2003; Mazur et al., 2018; Mount Sinai Adolescent Health Center, 2017; World Health Organization, 2012), but they all share some common characteristics. Adolescent-friendly health services are

- *accessible and convenient* (e.g., have convenient opening hours and youth-only hours; allow ease of scheduling appointments and follow-ups);
- *affordable* (without significant financial barriers, regardless of insurance coverage);
- *appropriate* (geared to their stage of development and needs);
- *equitable* (welcome to all, regardless of race and ethnicity, sexual orientation, or gender identity);
- *effective;*
- *competent;*
- *confidential;*
- *comprehensive* (addressing the full range of adolescent health concerns, including appropriate health education);
- *safe and respectful* (delivered in a fitting environment, such as a "safe space" where adolescents can raise questions without stigma or judgment); and
- *coordinated and integrated (*providing continuity with the same provider, and meeting all of the adolescent's needs).

Although the evidence on the relationship between providing youth-friendly services on health outcomes is still emerging, the existing evidence suggests that the barriers to access, use, and acceptability that young people face in the health system need to be removed (Santa Maria et al, 2017; Tylee et al., 2007).

Financing Health Care for All Adolescents

The Affordable Care Act (ACA) included several provisions designed to improve access to and the receipt of preventive health services for ado-

---

BOX 7-2
Models of Adolescent-Friendly Health Care Services

Several models of adolescent-friendly health services are in use today. For example, the *Mount Sinai Adolescent Health Center* (MSAHC), based in New York City, serves young people ages 10 to 24. The MSAHC model seeks to go beyond primary medical care to treat a wide range of adolescent health needs. MSAHC provides integrated and coordinated physical, sexual and reproductive, dental, optical, behavioral, and mental health care, along with preventive and supportive services, in a welcoming and nonjudgmental environment. The goal of MSAHC is to empower young people to maintain control of their health and become knowledgeable and engaged consumers of health care.

The services are confidential and free to young people. As part of its model, MSAHC also offers two types of specialized services. The first, enhanced services, aim to address issues or situations that can put any young person's health and well-being at risk. These services include violence intervention and prevention; care for survivors of sexual abuse and sexual assault; human trafficking education and treatment; obesity and eating disorder education and treatment; and substance abuse treatment and legal assistance. Second, population services aim to address the unique needs of special populations of youth, including LGBTQ youth, youth experiencing homelessness, youth living with HIV, immigrant and refugee youth, and young parents.

MSAHC supports its integrated model of wellness and health care at no cost to patients with a combination of public, private, and philanthropic funding. In addition to Medicaid billing, MSAHC receives funding from other federal and state medical reimbursement programs, public and private grants, fundraising events, and individual philanthropy.

In addition, several efforts have been made to define and implement best practices in adolescent-friendly health services. The MSAHC *Blueprint for Adolescent and Young Adult Healthcare* (Mount Sinai Adolescent Health Center, 2017), the National Adolescent and Young Adult Health Information Center, Advocates for Youth, the Office of Adolescent Health in the Department of Health and Human Services, and the World Health Organization describe best practices and provide resources to improve access to preventive services, train staff and workflows at

---

lescents, addressing both public and private insurance.[2] It allowed states to expand Medicaid up to 133 percent of the federal poverty level and to create a health insurance exchange (or "Marketplace") to offer financial assistance for insurance to low-income individuals and families. In addition, the ACA required that adolescents be enrolled in either Medicaid or a private health insurance program with access to an annual preventive health

---

[2]The ACA also included initiatives benefitting adolescents, including funding for school-based health centers, teen pregnancy preventive programs, and community health centers.

the clinic level, and improve state- and systems-level policies and practices to promote adolescent-centered health care. In addition, evidence-based curricula for youth-serving health professionals (the Adolescent Reproductive and Sexual Health Education Program) also exist that use free online modules and standardized case videos to train providers on best practices in the care of adolescents.

Innovative programs designed to improve health care delivery also include the Adolescent-Centered Environment Assessment Process and the Adolescent Champion Model.

The *Adolescent-Centered Environment Assessment Process* (ACE-AP) is a tool for health care practices to ensure that their clinical environments and practices are adolescent-centered. Developed and maintained by a multidisciplinary group of adolescent health professionals at the University of Michigan, the ACE-AP includes a comprehensive self-assessment followed by a facilitated improvement process that addresses 12 key areas, including access to care, adolescent appropriate environment, confidentiality, best practices and standards of care, reproductive and sexual health, behavioral health, nutritional health, cultural responsiveness, staff attitudes and respectful treatment, adolescent engagement and empowerment, parent engagement, and outreach and marketing.

The *Adolescent Champion Model* is a quality improvement program designed to help primary care sites become more adolescent-centered, also developed at the University of Michigan. The process is centered on identifying a multidisciplinary "adolescent champion" team to undergo training in adolescent-centered care. These adolescent champion teams deliver prepared trainings to other staff and providers in the clinic, facilitate youth-friendly site changes (rainbow stickers, youth-friendly signage), implement a standardized flow to screen for risky behaviors confidentially, and complete a quality-improvement assessment of confidentiality practices. Preliminary assessment of this program demonstrated sustained improvements in measures of adolescent-centeredness including improved care as reported by adolescent patients and providers, and improved provider knowledge of adolescent health issues and policies (Riley et al., 2018).

While a number of models exist, at the heart of each is a competent, considerate, and respectful provider who treats the adolescent in a holistic and developmentally appropriate way.

visit and allowed adolescents to stay on their parents' health insurance program until age 26, increasing stability during major points of life transition.

The ACA also required most private health plans to cover certain preventive services without cost to the patient. Covered preventive services for adolescents that require no copayments include annual wellness visits, evidence-based screening and counseling for mental health (i.e., depression, suicide) and substance use (i.e., alcohol, tobacco, and illicit drugs), and access to contraceptive services and methods. These preventive services were part of the 10 "Essential Health Benefits" offered in health plans through state health insurance exchanges. Preventive health care services provide a vital opportunity to help adolescents in establishing and maintaining a healthy lifestyle and an increasingly independent role in navigating the health care system, although parents often continue to play a substantial role in their enrollment in health insurance and accessing care.

While evidence suggests that the ACA has been effective at increasing coverage and receipt of services of adolescents (Adams et al., 2018), as of 2014, about 20 percent of young people ages 18 to 24 nationwide lacked health insurance coverage, and these rates vary widely across states and by race and ethnicity, LGBTQ status, homelessness, socioeconomic status, and ability status[3] (Okoro et al., 2017; Centers for Disease Control and Prevention, 2017). While health insurance coverage matters, with full-year publicly insured adolescents receiving wellness visits at higher rates, insurance in itself is not sufficient, as less than half of insured adolescents received wellness care. These findings reinforce the need for greater efforts to engage adolescents in wellness care and improve provider delivery of preventive care, particularly for underserved groups (Adams et al., 2018).

Troublingly, recent legislative efforts have rolled back some aspects of the ACA. In 2018, as part of the American Tax Cuts and Jobs Act, Congress passed legislation removing the ACA's insurance coverage mandate, effective January 2019. This potentially threatens the gains in health care access achieved under the ACA. Further, Congress reduced funding for community outreach regarding purchasing insurance on the exchanges and reduced the period of time during which families can enroll or re-enroll in health coverage (from a 3-month period to 6 weeks).

SEXUAL AND REPRODUCTIVE HEALTH CARE

As discussed in Chapter 2, developmental changes in the brain's limbic regions during adolescence contribute to novelty seeking and the intensification of emotional and social learning. As adolescents become more autonomous, shape their identity, and establish new relationships with peers and romantic partners, many start engaging in sexual behaviors. Sexual desire and behavior represent normative features of adolescent development that have the potential to foster the building of healthy relationships and enhance the happiness, psychological development, and well-being of youth. Parents, caretakers, systems—particularly the health

---

[3] For disparities by race and ethnicity, see Alexandre et al. (2009); Avila and Bramlett (2013); Brindis et al. (2005); Costello et al. (2014); and Cummings and Druss (2011). For disparities by LGBTQ status, see Russell et al. (2012). For disparities affecting youth experiencing homelessness, see Baer et al. (2003) and Edidin et al. (2012). For disparities by socioeconomic status, see English et al. (2014). For disparities by ability status, see Green et al. (2013); National Conference of State Legislatures (2011); and Vo and Park (2008).

system—and adolescents themselves can contribute to environments in which adolescent sexuality is positive and health-promoting and adverse risks can be minimized.

Recent advances in neuroimaging illuminate the neurocognitive mechanisms between response inhibition and adolescent decision making related to sexual behavior. These studies suggest the relevance of the right prefrontal cortex in response inhibition among adolescents and an association between adolescent risky sex and blood oxygen level dependent response in the inferior frontal gyrus, consistent with prior studies of executive control (Feldstein Ewing et al., 2015; Goldenberg et al., 2017; Hansen et al., 2018). According to the authors, "This emerging research, thus, begins to explain why many adolescents may be aware of the risks associated with unprotected sex and the protective efficacy of condoms, yet often do not translate this knowledge into prudent sexual decision making." Moreover, decision making related to sexual behavior is shaped by adolescents' desire for social status or intimacy and young people may choose to engage in risky behaviors in order to gain these immediate benefits (see, e.g., Rivers et al., 2008).

Engaging in sexual behavior is a normative part of adolescent development, and the health system plays a critical role in ensuring that adolescents receive the sexual and reproductive health care they need. Moreover, our growing understanding of the neurobiological basis of adolescent sexual decision making can inform the health system's approach to providing appropriate sexual and reproductive health care to adolescents and young adults. The next two sections focus on two aspects of the negative consequences of unprotected sexual experiences in adolescence: unintended pregnancy and sexually transmitted infections. That is followed by a discussion of the role the health system can play in reducing these risks.

Unintended Pregnancy

A major focus of adolescent health policy for the past decades has been, and remains, lowering the rates of unintended pregnancies and teenage births. Teen pregnancy and teen births commonly have negative consequences for adolescents. Though many teen mothers are disadvantaged before becoming parents, early parenthood is associated with lifelong high poverty, low educational achievement, and lower behavioral well-being among their children (Manlove et al., 2015). Social determinants associated with teen childbearing include low parental educational attainment and limited education and employment opportunities (Romero et al., 2016). These determinants are far more common in communities with higher proportions of racial and ethnic minorities (Romero et al., 2016).

Fortunately, teen pregnancies and birth rates have been declining since the late 1990s (Finer and Zolna, 2014), especially between 2007 and

2012. Several researchers identify improvements in contraceptive use as the proximal determinants of the significant decline in adolescent pregnancies and birth rates that occurred between 2007 and 2012 (Finer and Zolna, 2014; Lindberg et al., 2016). In 2015 teen birth rates reached a historic low—22.3 births per 1,000 adolescents ages 15 through 19 (Martin et al., 2018; Romero et al., 2017).

Despite this decline in adolescent pregnancies and birth rates, it is generally recognized that the rates are still far too high (Hall et al., 2016; Santelli, 2008; Schalet et al., 2014; Singh, 2000; Singh et al., 2001). The actual number of pregnancies for 10–14-year-olds (614,000 in 2014), a rate of 0.45 in 1,000, is considered exceptionally high, especially compared to other advanced industrial nations (Sedgh et al., 2015). Furthermore, birth rates among those ages 15 to 19 are approximately two times higher for Latinx, non-Latinx black, and American Indian and Alaska Native (AIAN) adolescents compared with non-Latinx White and Asian teens in the United States (Martin et al., 2018). In addition, disparities by geography persist: from 2007 to 2015, the teen birth rate among 15–19-year-olds declined by 50 percent in large urban counties, 44 percent in medium and small urban counties, and only 37 percent in rural counties (Hamilton et al., 2016).

Sexually Transmitted Infection (STI)

Levels of STI diagnosis in the United States are high, with an estimated 20 million new cases identified each year. Adolescents and young adults (ages 15 to 24) acquire one-half of all new STIs, including one-quarter of all new cases of HIV, while adolescents and young adult women have the highest rates of cervical human papillomavirus (HPV) (Forhan et al., 2009; Santa Maria et al., 2017; Satterwhite et al., 2013).

Human Papillomavirus

HPV is the most common sexually transmitted viral infection and the primary cause of cervical cancer as well as other anogenital and oropharyngeal cancers (Ford, 2011).[4] HPV prevalence reached 24.5 percent among females ages 14 to 19, and 44.8 percent among women ages 20 to 24 in 2007 (Dunne et al., 2007). Racial disparities exist in HPV infection rates as well as in cervical cancer and mortality rates. Thirty-five percent of non-Latinx Black women ages 18 to 25 are HPV-infected compared with 25 percent of their non-Latinx White peers (Busen et al., 2016). This is concerning since non-Latinx Black women experience higher mortality rates than any other racial or ethnic group in the United States.

---

[4]HPV in males is also associated with anogenital and oropharyngeal cancers.

Misinformation and risk factors may contribute to HPV disparities in adolescents. While a vaccine is available to protect against some of the most common strains of HPV, many young women are misinformed about HPV and do not consider themselves at risk, particularly migrant youth and non-English speakers (Ford, 2011). Despite evidence that supports use of the vaccine, rates of HPV vaccination among 13–17-year-olds remain sub-optimal but continue to rise steadily and reached 60 percent for the first time, in 2016 (Walker et al., 2017). Furthermore, the gap between vaccination rates for boys as compared to girls is beginning to close (Walker et al., 2017).

However, significant disparities in vaccination rates based on socio-economic status (SES) and geography persist. In 2016, HPV vaccine coverage varied considerably by income, with higher rates among families living below the poverty line (Walker et al., 2017). Differences between urban and non-urban youth were even more dramatic (Walker et al., 2017). These rates likely reflect differences in adolescent health care delivery, the emphasis of immunization programs on adolescent vaccination activities, and the prevalence of factors associated with lower vaccination coverage, such as contact with the medical system and provider failure to document risky health behaviors (Walker et al., 2017).

HIV and AIDS

Approximately 60,300 youth ages 13 to 24 were living with HIV in the United States at the end of 2015, with an estimated 51 percent living with undiagnosed HIV (Centers for Disease Control and Prevention, 2018a).[5] The HIV epidemic in the United States disproportionately affects vulnerable youth and minority men who have sex with men (MSM) populations (Prejean et al., 2011). The Centers for Disease Control and Prevention (CDC HIV youth index) reports that in 2016, 8,451 youth ages 13 to 24 received an HIV diagnosis, with the highest diagnosis rates among young people ages 20 to 24 (80%) and young gay and bisexual men (81%) (Centers for Disease Control and Prevention, 2018a). Furthermore, a majority (54%) of new infections among young gay and bisexual males are in Blacks while Latinos accounted for 25 percent (Centers for Disease Control and Prevention, 2018a). Normative adolescent risk-taking behaviors do not sufficiently explain the far higher rates of HIV infection among Black young MSM.

Among the youth diagnosed and living with HIV, in 2014, less than one-half received HIV medical care (41%), were retained in care (31%),

---

[5]Rates of HIV among adolescents may continue to increase in connection with the ongoing opioid epidemic, given the risk of contracting blood-borne infections through injecting drug use (Van Handle et al., 2016; Peters et al., 2016; Zibell et al., 2018).

and had a suppressed viral load (27%) (Centers for Disease Control and Prevention, 2018a).[6] To benefit from antiretroviral therapy and suppress viral load, those with HIV must successfully link to—and remain connected to—health care to prevent disease progression and HIV transmission (Eisinger et al., 2019). While adult studies suggest that approximately 75 percent of newly diagnosed adults are linked to care within 1 year (Zanoni and Mayer, 2014), studies of adolescents and young adults show a much greater range with some reporting alarmingly low rates, ranging from between 29 percent and 73 percent within the first year of diagnosis (Torian et al., 2008; Craw et al., 2008; Molitor, 2006; Olatosi, 2009). Additionally, younger patients (ages 18 to 24) are significantly less likely to be retained in care than adults (American Academy of Pediatrics, 2002). The high cost ($1,100 to $3,300 a month) for pre-exposure prophylaxis may also contribute to these disparities (Pace et al., 2013).

A combination approach to HIV prevention, which combines evidence-based behavioral, structural, and biomedical prevention strategies (Coates et al., 2008), is recognized as one of the best approaches for reducing risky behavior and decreasing contraction of HIV and other sexually transmitted infections (Marshall and Woods, 2010). Further research on the implementation of these prevention interventions in vulnerable youth is essential to identify psychosocially, developmentally, and culturally relevant behavioral interventions with on-the-ground applicability among high-risk youth.

Sexual and Reproductive Health Care Services

Despite the great need among adolescents for sexual and reproductive health care services, particularly for youth of color and LGBTQ youth, in 2015 one in four sexually experienced adolescent females and one in three adolescent males (ages 15 to 19) had not received a reproductive health service (Romero et al., 2017). In the United States, the gap between age of sexual debut and receipt of sexual and reproductive health services is much greater than in other countries (Hock-Long et al., 2003).

Adolescents may face multiple barriers to accessing quality sexual and reproductive health care services, and confidentiality is chief among them (see "Confidentiality and Parental Consent Requirements," below, for a discussion of the importance of privacy in adolescent health care). The barriers to adequate sexual and reproductive health care can be particularly high for LGBTQ adolescents, who face elevated sexual health risks and underutilize routine reproductive health care (Charlton et al., 2001). For the many who may find it difficult to share their sexual identities with

---

[6]Individuals with a sustained undetectable viral load have effectively no risk of exposing HIV-negative partners to HIV (Eisinger et al., 2019).

their health care providers, there is often a poor therapeutic alliance, lack of appropriate health-related education, and inadequate interventions to prevent STIs (Hafeez, 2017).

One way to increase access to sexual and reproductive health services for adolescents is to make such care available across a variety of settings (Santa Maria et al., 2017). Adolescents use health care services for a range of needs—sickness, sports physicals, immunizations, and emergency care—all of which provide opportunities to offer sexual and reproductive health care (Santa Maria et al., 2017). For instance, every year 15 million adolescents use emergency rooms for care. Compared to non-ER users, they are at substantially high risk for pregnancy (Chernick at al., 2015). Chernick and colleagues (2015) have suggested that sexual and reproductive health care services be provided in the emergency room.

A 2016 summit held by ETR on adolescent brain development and sexual and reproductive health produced three key messages: "(1) programs and theories that focus on teens must address developmental changes including how social, emotional, and cognitive processing influence adolescent decision making; (2) relationships are a fundamental context for adolescent sexual health; and (3) multiple support systems are essential to scaffold youth through positive growth and development"(ETR Associates, 2016, p. 1).[7] The summit recommendations include the need to adopt measures relevant to sexual health in developmental neuroscience research; the need to imbed the understanding of adolescent development and neurobiology in sexual and reproductive health program development and implementation, training and technical assistance; and the need for research and funding mechanisms to be reflective of emerging understandings.

BEHAVIORAL HEALTH CARE

Recent research has helped to identify existing behavioral health issues in adolescent populations, including the understanding of risk factors and the implications of trauma and stress on brain development, areas of genetic susceptibility, the protective factors and interventions that can help youth, and the patterns of help-seeking. The subsequent section discusses five behavioral and mental health disorders of particular concern to adolescents—suicide, depression, anxiety, substance use disorder, and disordered eating—and the ways in which the health system can better serve adolescents experiencing these conditions.

---

[7]The full summit report is available from https://www.etr.org/kirby-summit/.

Suicide

Suicide is the second leading cause of death among people ages 10 to 34 in the United States (National Institute of Mental Health, 2018). Reports of suicide risk, based on the Youth Risk Behavior Survey, state that 18 percent of high school students seriously contemplated attempting suicide in the past year and 30 percent report feeling "sad or hopeless almost every day for 2 or more weeks in a row so that they stopped doing some usual activities" during the past 12 months (Office of Adolescent Health, 2017). Studies also suggest that suicide ideation[8] intensifies between the ages of 12 and 17, with almost two-thirds of adolescents moving from ideation to planning and more than three-fourths from ideation to attempt during the first year of onset of ideation (Nock et al., 2013).

Consistent with several decades of prior research on community and regional samples, the 2015 Youth Risk Behavior Survey data also show higher risk for suicidal thoughts and behaviors among sexual minority youth. Greater than 40 percent of LGB students have seriously considered suicide, and 29 percent report suicidal behavior during the past 12 months (Kann et al., 2016). Although to date there are no nationally representative data on suicide risk among transgender youth, a recent representative study of California students showed that the prevalence of self-reported suicidal ideation was nearly two times higher for transgender students compared to the general student population (Perez-Brumer et al., 2017).

The risk for suicidal behaviors among adolescents may be partly attributed to neurobiological mechanisms. Multiple studies (Brent and Melhem, 2008; Voracek and Loibl, 2007; Ruderfer et al., 2019) suggest that suicidal behavior can be genetically inherited, and heritability (i.e., the extent to which a characteristic is determined by genetic rather than environmental factors) of suicidal behaviors ranges from 30 percent to 55 percent (Sokolowski et al., 2015).

Of course, environment and context also play a role in suicidal risk, particularly the quality of familial relationships. Adolescents with a history of suicide attempts rated their maternal and paternal attachment significantly lower than those with no history of suicide and less adaptable and cohesive (Sheftall et al., 2013). A review conducted by Pelkonen et al. (2011) revealed that mental disorders and high levels of familial distress are major risk factors for youth suicide. Unique to the adolescent developmental stage, high levels of emotional reactivity and engagement in risk-taking behaviors as adolescents strive for autonomy and rely less on parental support could manifest in suicidal behaviors (Pelkonen et al., 2011). The dual effects of autonomy-seeking behavior and turbulent family support may

---

[8]Suicide ideation includes self-reported thoughts of suicide and a preoccupation with suicide.

even intensify the risk for suicide. Furthermore, feelings of social disconnectedness could increase risk of suicidal behavior (Sheftall et al., 2013).

Many interventions have been tested to reduce suicidal risk and mental health problems among youth. The literature in this area highlights a number of promising strategies, including those incorporating mindfulness (Fung et al., 2018), family involvement (Prado et al., 2013), and motivational enhancement and cognitive behavioral therapy (Belur et al., 2014). For example, *Familias Unidas* is an evidence-based preventive intervention that focuses on parent-adolescent relationships and has been very effective in reducing Latinx adolescents' internalizing and externalizing disorders,[9] substance use, and risky sexual practices (Pantin et al., 2009; Perrino et al., 2014; Prado et al., 2013; Prado and Pantin, 2011). Further, the most effective services for addressing suicidality in adolescents seem to be those that affect multiple contexts, including family and home, and that recognize the developmental complexities of adolescence (Daniel and Goldston, 2009).

Depression

Mojtabai et al. (2016) examined the 12-month prevalence of major depressive episodes in a sample of adolescents (ages 12 to 17) and young adults (ages 18 to 25) and found a significant increase in these episodes between 2005 and 2014. During the period observed, depressive episodes rose in prevalence from 8.7 to 11.3 percent in adolescents and from 8.8 to 9.6 percent in young adults, which remained significant even after adjusting for substance use disorder and sociodemographic factors. Depression in adolescents is linked to systemic disorders such as diabetes, and it may be increasing in adolescents, especially among females.[10]

Wide disparities by gender and race and ethnicity are evident in the onset and incidence of depression as well. Breslau and colleagues (2017) found sex differences in both onset and incidence of depression in adolescents. Diagnostic differences have also been observed, with non-Latinx White adolescents more than two times as likely to report a prior diagnosis of depression compared to Latinx adolescents (Thomas et al., 2011).

---

[9] Internalizing-externalizing is a broad classification of behaviors and disorders among children and youth. Externalizing behaviors and disorders are mainly characterized by actions in the external world, such as acting out, antisocial behavior, and aggression. Processes within the self, such as depression, anxiety, and somatization, characterize internalizing behaviors and disorders.

[10] Depression has been linked to early-life adversity, which increases both metabolic dysregulation and a treatment-resistant type of depression. Early-life adversities contribute disproportionately to many health problems, both physical and mental.

A recent study found that adolescents who demonstrated stronger activation in the ventral striatum when making socially positive decisions for their families showed declines in depressive symptoms over time. This suggests that neural sensitivity to eudaimonic rewards—rewards that are intrinsically meaningful and provide a sense of social connection and belonging—predicts changes in depressive symptoms over time. For adolescents, therefore, "the striatal response to eudaimonic rewards may represent a motivational orientation toward engaging in inherently meaningful activities that may increase feelings of value, meaningfulness, and intrinsic reward" (Telzer et al., 2014, p. 6603). If this is the case, this striatal response provides additional psychological and social resources, leading to better well-being over time (Telzer et al., 2014).

Recent research also suggests that as peer relationships gain importance during adolescence, the experience of peer rejection (either firsthand or witnessed among one's social group) can have long-term consequences for development (Masten et al., 2013; Nishina et al., 2005; Prinstein and Aikins, 2004; Prinstein et al., 2005; Rigby, 2003). Youth facing higher levels of social risk may be especially sensitive to social information. This in turn means they are more likely to experience greater distress and difficulty regulating their emotions in response to negative social stimuli. It has been hypothesized that, as these vulnerable youth enter into a developmental period characterized by growing neural plasticity and more frequent exposure to social stressors, peer victimization and the fear of being negatively evaluated contribute to a type of long-term neural development that underlies emotion processing and regulation in social contexts. Alterations in the development of neural function, such as blunted functioning of the DLPFC[11] area, may lead to increased vulnerability to or worsening of depressive symptoms among adolescent youth (Lee et al., 2018). These findings suggest that improving DLPFC function in social contexts may be a valuable neural target for prevention efforts or interventions geared toward breaking the cycle of social difficulties and depressive symptoms in adolescents. According to Lee and colleagues (2018), interventions that use emotion-regulation strategies and repeated practice and training may improve emotion regulation by engaging greater recruitment of the DLPFC. Such interventions hold the potential to alter developmental trajectories toward depression among adolescents with social risk.

Anxiety

According to the National Comorbidity Survey of Adolescents in 2002–2004, 31.9 percent of adolescents met the criteria for an anxiety disorder

---

[11]The dorsolateral prefrontal cortex (DLPFC) is an area in the prefrontal cortex of the brain.

in the United States (Merikangas et al., 2010). The most frequent disorders among adolescents are separation anxiety disorder and specific and social phobias (Beesdo et al., 2009). Females were more likely than males to report an anxiety disorder. Non-Latinx Black adolescents have higher rates of anxiety disorders compared to their non-Latinx White counterparts. Additionally, the prevalence rates of anxiety disorders were higher for adolescents from households with divorced or separated parents, indicating a possible association between family composition and anxiety (Beesdo et al., 2009).

Studies have examined the neurobiological and genetic underpinnings of anxiety (Hettema et al., 2001; Norrholm and Ressler, 2014). Beyond genetic influences, other studies reveal the role that parenting and parental anxiety diagnosis may have on the onset of adolescent anxiety (Beesdo et al., 2009; Eley et al., 2015; Kendler et al., 2000; Lieb et al., 2000). A meta-analysis conducted by Siegel and Dickstein (2012) indicated that children and adolescents who have a parent diagnosed with anxiety are more likely to display symptoms of anxiety themselves. Kendler et al. (2000) found that high levels of coldness and authoritarianism in parents were modestly associated with a higher risk for nearly all anxiety disorders, thereby suggesting that parenting style might also influence the onset of anxiety disorders (Beesdo et al., 2009). However, they also found that the impact of parent protectiveness was variable, given that some anxiety disorders, such as generalized anxiety disorder, panic disorder, and phobia, were significantly associated with protectiveness, whereas other disorders, such as bulimia, substance use disorder, and alcohol dependence, were not (Beesdo et al., 2009).

As reviewed in Chapter 2, adolescence is a key developmental period of significant brain maturation and changes in neuroendocrine function (Ojeda and Terasawa, 2002). These characteristics likely contribute to enhanced neural susceptibility to the negative consequences of anxiety and stress (Eiland and Romeo, 2013), particularly because the limbic and cortical regions of the brain that continue to develop during adolescence are some of the most stress reactive areas (McEwen, 2005; Eiland and Romeo, 2013). As described above, the heightened focus on social acceptance in adolescence can promote a corresponding fear of rejection, which may contribute to social anxiety and depression (Klapwijk et al., 2013; Nelson et al., 2014; Pfeifer et al., 2013). Research suggests that social anxiety and maladaptive social responding in adolescence is linked to dysfunction of the striatum, involved in behavior and learning related to rewards (O'Doherty, 2004; Yin et al., 2009), and its connections to the medial prefrontal cortex, which updates predictions based on outcomes (Britton et al., 2013; Fitzgerald et al., 2011; Haber et al., 2006; Jarcho et al., 2015; O'Doherty, 2004; Roy et al., 2013).

A number of treatment and intervention approaches show promise for reducing anxiety and stress among adolescents. A meta-analysis examining anxiety prevention programs for adolescents concluded that universal anxiety programs, in comparison to those targeting other mental health disorders, are particularly effective. The effect size of universal anxiety prevention programs was 0.17, whereas the effect sizes for universal depression, eating disorder, and substance use prevention disorders were 0.12, 0.08, and 0.5, respectively (Fisak et al., 2011). Expanding the breadth and accessibility of anxiety prevention resources is essential since there is growing concern that many cases of anxiety are undiagnosed among adolescents (Siegel and Dickstein, 2012).

Anxiety may present itself differently during adolescence than at other time periods. Garland (2001) found that for some adolescents, physical symptoms of anxiety, such as stomach or headaches, may go unrecognized. Compounded with hormonal changes during this time, symptoms may also manifest as behavioral defiance instead of the more typical cognitive symptoms, such as worrying (Frick et al., 1999). Beesdo and colleagues (2009) call for the integration of a developmental perspective into the next revision of the Diagnostic and Statistical Manual of Mental Disorders (DSM) to consider the differences in age of onset, symptomology, and outcome to further understand how anxiety disorders manifest in childhood and adolescence. Recognizing the nuances of anxiety disorders in adolescence is critical both to better address the needs of those already diagnosed and to reduce prevalence in the future.

Substance Use Disorder and Addiction

Substance use disorder is characterized in the DSM-5 as a problematic pattern in the use of an intoxicating substance that results in significant impairment or distress (National Institute on Drug Abuse, 2018). In its most severe form, substance use disorder can be classified as addiction, which is a chronic disorder marked by compulsive behavior, continued substance use despite negative consequences, and long-lasting neurological changes (National Institute of Drug Abuse, 2018). Because the prefrontal cortex continues to mature through the adolescent period and into adulthood, its sensitivity to early-life adversity is a factor in impairing self-regulation and increasing the likelihood of addictive behavior (see Chapter 2).

Data from the CDC's 2017 Youth Risk Behavior Survey indicate that 15.5 percent of middle and high school students surveyed have tried alcohol before age 13 (Centers for Disease Control and Prevention, 2018b). The survey also found that 19.8 percent of all surveyed adolescents used marijuana at least once during the same time frame (Centers for Disease Control and Prevention, 2018b, 2018c). However, trend data obtained from the same survey suggest that student use of marijuana and alcohol use has declined since 2009, when the corresponding rates for alcohol and marijuana use within 30 days of the survey were 41.1 percent and 20.8 percent, respectively (Centers for Disease Control and Prevention, 2018b, 2018c).

While youth cigarette use has continuously declined since 2000, e-cigarette use has been rising dramatically. Among high school students e-cigarette use increased from 11.7 percent in 2017 to 20.8 percent in 2018, and among middle schoolers over the same brief period from 3.3 percent to 4.9 percent. Current use of any tobacco product for both high school and middle school students has also increased since 2015 (Food and Drug Administration, 2018). Although survey data suggest that youth are less likely to use opioids than alcohol or marijuana, recent findings from the National Survey on Drug Use and Health suggest that adolescents under the age of 26 may be more likely to use heroin and pain relievers than adults (National Institute on Drug Abuse, 2018). Overall, between 1999 and 2007, the death rate due to drug overdose among adolescents ages 15 to 19 more than doubled, rising from 1.6 per 100,000 deaths to 4.2 per 100,000. It then declined by 26 percent from 2007 to 2014 (dropping to 3.1), and then subsequently increased in 2015 (3.7). Death rates for drug overdoses among those ages 15 to 19 in 2015 were highest for opioids, specifically heroin (Curtin et al., 2017).

The environment can have a strong relation with substance misuse. For example, in the case of opioid misuse, Ford et al. (2017) found that neighborhood social disorganization (e.g., levels of crime, disinvestment, and population turnover) and social capital (the degree to which members of a community are engaged in communal life) were significantly related to opioid misuse in adolescents. Compared to adolescents living in urban areas, adolescents living in suburban and rural areas were more likely to report misuse of prescription opioids (Ford and Wright, 2017).

The relationship of youth to the health care system also appears crucial. Ensuring confidentiality has been found to be central to facilitating honest disclosure from adolescents about all sensitive subjects, including substance use and need for treatment (see the following section, "Confidentiality and Parental Consent Requirements"). In addition, health care providers may not be equipped to address substance use among adolescents. Wilson and colleagues (2018) found that pediatric physicians were not reaching adolescents using opioids. Of the pediatric residents whom completed the survey, 82 percent reported that they provided care to patients who misused opioids and another 82 percent reported caring for patients who they assessed as at risk for opioid overdose but only 42 percent had ever counseled patients on ways to prevent overdose and only 10 percent had ever prescribed the opioid reversal drug naloxone to eligible patients (Wilson et al., 2018).

An important aspect of substance use in adolescence is comorbidity with other mental health conditions such as anxiety and depression (Deas and Brown, 2006; Insel, 2014). The co-occurrence of marijuana use and anxiety is one such example, as individuals with marijuana use disorder are more than five times more likely than other people to also suffer from an anxiety disorder (Stinson et al., 2006). Marijuana is the most common illicit drug used by adolescents in the United States (Johnson et al., 2014), and many adolescents report using it to reduce anxiety (Patrick et al., 2011). Research indicates that the effects of marijuana use on brain structure and function can further contribute to issues with emotional processing, memory, and attention (Mashhoon et al., 2015; Mechoulam et al., 2007; Quickfall and Crockford, 2006; Cancilliere et al., 2018).

Body Dissatisfaction and Eating Disorders

For youth, body image is related to identity development and mental health, as well as family, peer, and romantic relationships. When youth are dissatisfied with their physical appearance, it can hamper their ability to complete the physical and socio-emotional tasks of development, as well as damage their physical and mental health.

Body dissatisfaction is common among U.S. adolescents (Neumark-Sztainer et al., 2002), seems to increase with age (Calzo et al., 2012), and can remain with adolescents into adulthood (Neumark-Sztainer et al., 2006). As discussed in Chapter 2, adolescence is a time of greater sensitivity to peer influence, social acceptance and rejection, and social stimuli. These changes seem to be due to greater activity in the brain regions that make up the "social brain"—regions that regulate our reactions to other people (Steinberg, 2014). These changes are an important part of adolescents' socio-emotional and cognitive development, but when coupled with a greater tendency toward social comparison, body changes, and stronger pressure to conform to gender roles, they may exacerbate body dissatisfaction in some adolescents (Markey, 2010; Steinberg, 2014).

Adolescents with overweight or obesity may be particularly vulnerable to body dissatisfaction because of weight stigma (the societal devaluation of people with overweight or obesity), which is widespread in the United States (Andreyeva et al., 2008; Pont et al., 2017). Weight-based harassment, including teasing, bullying, and victimization, is widespread among school-age adolescents, especially for girls (Bucchianeri et al., 2013; Puhl et al., 2011; Pont et al., 2017). However, body dissatisfaction is not limited to adolescents with overweight: adolescent boys with underweight also report high levels of body dissatisfaction (Calzo et al., 2012). Experiencing weight-based victimization at the hands of peers increases adolescents' risk of low self-esteem and poor body image, two aspects of self-concept (Pont et al., 2017; Calzo et al., 2012; Davison and Birch, 2002). In addition, weight-based bullying and teasing increases the risk of adverse mental and physical health outcomes, such as depression, anxiety, suicidality, self-harm behaviors, substance use, and disordered eating behaviors (Pont et al., 2017; Calzo et al., 2012; Neumark-Sztainer et al., 2002).

Eating disorders (anorexia nervosa, bulimia nervosa, subthreshold anorexia nervosa, subthreshold bulimia nervosa, and subthreshold binge eating disorder[12]), which are often associated with body dissatisfaction, affect adolescents of all genders, races, ages, and weight statuses. Estimates of the national prevalence of eating disorders among adolescents ages 13 to 18 range from 0.3 percent for anorexia nervosa to 2.5 percent for subthreshold binge eating disorder (Swanson et al., 2011). Swanson and colleagues (2011) found that among these five eating disorders, the median age of onset ranged from 12.3 to 12.6 years. Bulimia nervosa, binge eating disorder, and subthreshold anorexia nervosa were significantly more prevalent among girls than boys, though no significant differences emerged by gender for anorexia nervosa and subthreshold binge eating disorder. Latinx and non-Latinx Black youth had higher rates of all four eating disorders that were assessed, although the difference was only significant for bulimia nervosa and subthreshold binge eating disorder (Swanson et al., 2011); and sexual minority youth report higher rates of eating disorder symptoms (Austin et al., 2013) and disordered eating behaviors (Watson et al., 2017, Matthews-Ewald et al., 2014).

Adolescent eating disorders are often accompanied by other psychiatric disorders (Lock, 2015), with most adolescents with an eating disorder also meeting criteria for at least one other psychiatric disorder (Swanson et al., 2011). Adolescents with eating disorders are also more likely than other adolescents to have higher levels of suicide ideation (Swanson et al., 2011), and suicide accounts for about half of deaths from anorexia nervosa (Birmingham et al., 2005).

Although eating disorders are often thought to mostly affect girls and women, boys and men are also at risk (Allen et al., 2013; Mitchison et al., 2014; Limbers et al., 2018), and the prevalence of eating disorders among boys and men has increased (Campbell and Peebles, 2015; Lavendar et al., 2017). Disordered eating behaviors among adolescent males are of particu-

---

[12] Subthreshold eating disorders were those that did not meet the diagnostic criteria for anorexia nervosa (as defined by the DSM-IV), or binge eating disorder (as defined by the DSM-5). Subthreshold bulimia nervosa was not assessed. The definition of subthreshold anorexia nervosa included (1) lowest body weight less than 90 percent of the adolescent's ideal body weight; (2) intense fear of weight gain at the time of the lowest weight; and (3) no history of another threshold-level eating disorder. The definition of subthreshold bulimia eating disorder included (1) binge eating at least twice a week for several months; (2) perceived loss of control; and (3) no history of another threshold-level eating disorder or subthreshold anorexia nervosa.

lar public health concern because males experiencing them are less likely to seek and receive treatment for eating disorders due to greater shame and stigma (Lavendar et al., 2017; Limbers et al., 2018).

The precise etiology of eating disorders is unknown, but recent studies suggest that to some degree eating disorders are heritable (Bulick et al., 2019). Brain imaging studies have been used to examine potential neurobiological pathways that may contribute to the onset of anorexia, with mixed results (Kaye et al., 2013).

Behavioral Health Care Services

Despite a documented need for behavioral health care services, adolescents and young adults remain an underserved population. Data from the Medical Expenditure Panel Surveys show significant increases in the use of any outpatient mental health service among adolescents ages 12 to 17, from 9.0 percent in 1996–1998, to 11.5 percent in 2003–2005, to 14.0 percent in 2010–2012 (Olfson et al., 2015). Still, many adolescents and young adults underuse behavioral health services, despite documented need (e.g., Han et al., 2015; Hunt et al., 2015; Mojtabai et al., 2016). Only one-third of adolescents with any mental disorder report receiving treatment (Merikangas et al., 2011).[13] In a survey of 51 adolescents diagnosed with depression, the emotional toll of seeking treatment and the inability to access treatment (i.e., distance from home and longer referral delays than help-seeking delays) were the two most frequently reported barriers to access (Boyd et al., 2018; MacDonald et al., 2018). Some adolescents also expressed their desire to have greater access to behavioral health services, such as more frequent interaction with their providers or a longer duration of treatment (Boyd et al., 2018).

Additionally, the unique patterns and needs demonstrated by adolescents and young adults in their use of behavioral health services may contribute to the services' underutilization. For example, because youth in these age ranges tend to greatly value social relationships, concerns about negative social repercussions for seeking help can be a significant barrier to seeking treatment (Scott and Davis, 2006; Spence et al., 2016). Moreover, adolescents and young adults have specific provider preferences that may prevent them from obtaining appropriate outpatient care. Youth from minority racial/ethnic backgrounds have expressed concerns about receiving culturally and linguistically appropriate care from largely White providers (Lee et al., 2009). (See Box 7-3 for a discussion of "Disparities in Behavioral Health Care.") Young adults have reported that mental health providers from older generations do not adequately understand their expe-

---

[13] For adolescents with any psychiatric disorder, the rate is 45 percent (Costello et al., 2014).

riences (Draucker, 2005). In fact, when age-specific outpatient services are available, service use among young people increases (Gilmer et al., 2012).

Given their unique social, behavioral, and neurobiological characteristics, adolescents are susceptible to mental and behavioral health disorders and in need of tailored treatment approaches. In the absence of age-specific services, many adolescents and young adults rely on emergency departments, crisis services, school services, and inpatient substance use treatment facilities to obtain mental health care (e.g., Jin et al., 2003; Lin et al., 2012). Youth themselves have reported their desire for more access to behavioral health services in schools, as illustrated by Box 7-4. In addition, there is concern that the transition from childhood to adult behavioral health services for adolescents can disrupt the continuum of care, resulting in poor behavioral health outcomes (Macdonald et al., 2018).

For many adolescents, primary care physicians are the first contact for those seeking help, so it is important that these physicians be equipped to recognize the symptoms of behavioral health issues to refer patients to specialized resources (Macdonald et al., 2018). In specialized care settings, treatment strategies that are tailored for adolescents can be used. For example, for adolescents with substance use disorders, some of the leading behavioral health interventions are cognitive behavioral therapy, medication, and recovery support services. High efficacy has been noted for psychosocial services that combine individual behavioral approaches with community-based or family interventions (Chadi et al., 2018). As adolescents transition from pediatric to adult health care, health care systems can support their mental and behavioral health by smoothing the transition of services.

CONFIDENTIALITY AND PARENTAL CONSENT REQUIREMENTS

As described above, confidential care is a core principle of adolescent-friendly health services. As adolescents develop, their capacity for autonomous decision-making and abstract thinking grows (Patton et al., 2016; see also Chapter 2). Providers can enable this growth by facilitating adolescents' meaningful participation in their own health care decisions, in a confidential setting, as appropriate. Likewise, counseling on sensitive issues is particularly important for adolescent health care, as adolescence is a time when risky behaviors, mental disorders, and sexual behaviors emerge. Adolescents ages 15 to 17 express the most concerns about confidentiality, but those ages 18 to 25 also have concerns, particularly since many of these young adults remain on their parents' health insurance plans (Sedlander et al., 2015). Ensuring confidentiality and protecting patients' privacy are essential to screening for these sensitive issues. Adolescents who were counseled on confidentiality and spent time alone with their providers are more likely to discuss sensitive topics with their providers (Grilo

---

BOX 7-3
Disparities in Behavioral Health Care

Despite recent advancements and the growing advocacy surrounding behavioral health, equitable care continues to evade racial/ethnic minority, immigrant, homeless, and rural populations due to persistent disparities throughout the continuum of care (Tebb et al., 2015). Over the years, research has worked to identify disparities and disentangle the underlying mechanisms perpetuating these disparities. This work highlights the breadth of inequity in behavioral health care at multiple levels, from federal policies and regulations to patient-provider interactions, and points to the need for evidence-based care that is culturally and linguistically tailored to each patient (Alegría et al., 2010, 2011, 2016). Mental health services must become equitably accessible to reduce health disparities among adolescents.

Research has shown that ethnic and racial minorities face severe disparities in access to behavioral health care (Alegría et al., 2015). For example, compared to their White counterparts, Black youth are more likely to use the emergency room for mental health treatment, less likely to have psychopharmacology visits, significantly more likely to have been assigned two or more comorbid mental health diagnoses, and more likely to have Medicaid than private insurance (Carson et al., 2010). Additionally, research has suggested that only a small percentage of Asian youth (8.6%) seek any mental health-related services (Abe-Kim et al., 2007).

Disparities are also observed in service delivery. For example, 40 percent of Latinx children who have been diagnosed with Attention Deficit Hyperactivity Disorder (ADHD) do not receive stimulant treatment, with Latinx children from ethnically isolated neighborhoods being less likely to receive an ADHD diagnosis or stimulant medication than those from less isolated areas (Pennap et al., 2017). Even treatment models designed with the intention of better treating underserved populations perpetuate disparities in the care of youth. Park and colleagues (2014) examined patient-centered medical homes, a model of care utilizing a comprehensive, team-based strategy. They found that both Latinx and Black children with ADHD had a lower likelihood of having a medical home than non-Latinx White children. This reduced likelihood also held true for Latinx children with developmental delays and Black children with depression (Park et al., 2014).

Substance use is another area in which the quality of care differs by race and ethnicity. Both Black and Latinx youth with substance abuse in the past year reported receiving less services for their substance use disorders than their White counterparts, with Latinx adolescents reporting receiving less informal ser-

---

et al., 2019), increasing their likelihood of receiving appropriate services. Furthermore, a secondary analysis of adolescent primary care patients ages 12 to 17 revealed that disclosure of rates of substance use and substance use problems was three to four times higher when reported in anonymous interviews as compared to the rates disclosed in routine clinical screening

vices and Black adolescents reporting less of both informal and specialty services (Alegría et al., 2011).

Another important factor that leads to disparities in the behavioral health of youth is the experience of bias-based discrimination, that is, discrimination based on personal characteristics, such as race, ethnicity, or sexual orientation. Russell et al. (2012) found that youth experiencing bias-based harassment are at an even greater risk for compromised health outcomes than those experiencing non-bias-based harassment (Russell et al., 2012). More specifically, research has shown that youth who have experienced discrimination demonstrate greater depressive and anxiety symptoms (Chithambo and Cespedes-Knadle, 2014; Davis et al., 2016; Park et al., 2017) and outward expressions of anger (Park et al., 2017), with other serious potential consequences also being noted in the literature base (Umaña-Taylor, 2016). These experiences of bias can also occur in clinical settings through interactions with providers (Valenzuela and Smith, 2015), where even the most well-intentioned can contribute to racial/ethnic disparities in youth health care due to unconscious processes, such as stereotyping (Burgess et al., 2004; see also Chapter 4).

In addition, young people from rural areas have less access to mental health care than their urban peers (National Rural Health Association, 2015). Many rural counties have no practicing psychiatrists or social workers (Kaiser Family Foundation, 2018). Racial/ethnic disparities in behavioral health care access and treatment can be compounded by rurality. In response to the growing concern surrounding mental health and substance use in rural America, some studies have sought to assess the risk of mental health and substance use disorders in rural youth as compared to their urban counterparts (Kogan et al., 2006). Some of these studies examine reasons for differences in patterns of mental health by geography, and report on mediating/moderating effects of protective factors (Brody et al., 2014; Carlo et al., 2011). For example, Kogan and colleagues (2006) found reports of substance use by Black students living in rural areas to be at equal or higher rates than among their Black peers living in suburban or urban areas.

Youth experiencing homelessness are more likely than those in stable living situations to report compromised health, often linked to preventable risk behaviors (e.g., substance and polysubstance use). These behaviors often continue into adulthood. Despite the documented need for behavioral health care services, youth experiencing homelessness have trouble accessing behavioral and other health care services (Davies and Allen, 2017; Hudson et al., 2009, 2010; Kushel et al., 2007).

(Gryczynski et al., 2019). However, studies have found that providers discuss confidentiality with their adolescent patients in only 31 to 55 percent of routine visits (Lau et al., 2013; Grilo et al., 2019), and that barely a third of all adolescents with a wellness visit in the prior year spent any time alone with a clinician (Alexander et al., 2014; Irwin et al., 2009). Assur-

---

BOX 7-4
Youth Perspectives: Behavioral Health Care

Throughout its deliberative process, the committee sought the input of a diverse group of adolescents to better understand the issues facing young people today (the full methodology and results are described in Appendix B). Behavioral health came up repeatedly as an issue that youth believed deserved greater attention. In particular, youth identified a need for more and better behavioral health services in schools, including colleges and universities. As one participant noted: "We are in dire need of more mental health resources in high school and in college because adolescence doesn't stop as soon as you get to college."

Participants reported that even when behavioral health services were available in their schools, they still faced barriers to access, such as long waiting lists, limits on the amount of accessible school-based services, and stigma. For one participant, the school counselor's focus on college and career caused a roadblock to addressing a more immediate mental health concern:

When I was going through a personal time in my life where . . . I felt very alone, there were times where I had thoughts of suicide and self-harm issues. I really needed to see somebody immediately. I walk into the [school] counselor's office. I said I really need to talk to somebody. [I was told] 'we're in the midst of college applications right now. The soonest we can put you in is like two to three weeks.' . . . I think that our guidance counselors in our schools are getting psychology degrees from these amazing universities and then they are going to be doing class registration all day, not actually being able to help students who need help. I think that is a huge roadblock.

In addition, participants noted that mental and behavioral health support in schools could come from multiple sources. Teachers, school resource officers, and mentors could all play a role in supporting adolescents to cope with stress. Participants argued for better training for all school personnel in identifying and responding to behavioral health concerns, and noted that ending stigma around behavioral health issues would need to come from adults. "Adults need to be the ones to teach kids at a young age that there is nothing wrong with going and asking for help," said one participant.

---

ing confidentiality in health care settings is key, as many adolescents fail to seek the services they need or discuss sensitive issues because they fear their confidential information will become known, especially to a parent (Ford et al., 1997; Carlisle et al., 2006; Lehrer et al., 2007; Sedlander et al., 2015; Copen et al., 2016).

Despite its importance in adolescent health care, confidential care is not guaranteed for youth (Tylee et al., 2007). While adolescent health experts and youth-serving organizations have endorsed and supported the need for confidential care for youth, access to confidential care varies greatly by state and by medical condition (English et al., 2010; Society for Adolescent Health and Medicine and American Academy of Pediatrics, 2016). For example, all states currently allow minors to consent for STI diagnosis and treatment, although some states have age restrictions (with minimum ages ranging from 12 to 16), and others allow physicians to inform parents (Guttmacher Institute, 2019a). Mental health and contraceptive care are other sensitive services where policies vary depending on age or living situations (i.e., married, emancipated, or living apart from parents) (English et al., 2010; Guttmacher Institute, 2019b).

Even when a state allows minors to consent to services without parental consent, confidentiality is not necessarily guaranteed. For instance, an adolescent covered by her parent's health insurance can have a confidential visit with a health care provider, and later have this confidentiality breached when a bill, known as an explanation of benefits, is sent to their parents detailing the charges for the confidential services. Some jurisdictions, such as Erie County, New York, and Massachusetts, require that sensitive services such as contraceptive and STI care be suppressed from the explanation of benefits (Tebb et al., 2014). Others do not require that an explanation of benefits be sent when there is no balance due (the states of New York, Massachusetts, and Wisconsin) (Tebb et al., 2014).

Health care providers themselves can also be barriers to confidential services, because practices and policies regarding confidentiality and youths' rights are not well known or used by all health care providers and institutions. Parents are not always asked to leave during health care visits (McKee et al., 2011), and youth often report that their providers do not inform them about confidentiality policies (Gleeson et al., 2002). Many youth do not know what type of care is confidential and what will be shared with others, resulting in mistrust and poor communication (Gleeson et al., 2002). In addition, providers do not always ask about sensitive subjects. For example, a survey of school-based health center directors and clinicians in New York state who work with middle and high school students revealed that one of the most common perceived barriers to discussing substance use with students was their belief that students would not be truthful about their substance use (Harris et al., 2016).

While there is a tension between parental interests in shaping the development of their children and the society's interest in ensuring the reduction of risks, health care providers can play a key role in helping parents and youth navigate these issues and in ensuring that the rights of adolescent clients are protected (Fox et al., 2010b; Ringheim, 2007). Of course, adolescents at different stages of development have different needs, and health care settings will need to assess and adapt their procedures to ensure that age-appropriate care is offered.

ADOLESCENT HEALTH CARE WORKFORCE

At the core of an adolescent-friendly health system is the health care workforce, which delivers services and interacts directly with young people. As noted in Chapter 2, adolescence is a critical developmental period in which many important physical, neurobiological, and socio-behavioral changes occur, in which young people experiment with new behaviors and activities, and for some, when mental disorders begin (see preceding section, "Behavioral Health Care"). It is also a time in which lifelong health behaviors are often established, laying the foundation for future health and well-being or setting the adolescent on an unhealthy course (Patton et al., 2016). As such, adolescents need health care providers who understand the unique needs of their development. Providers caring for adolescents need the knowledge and training to discuss sensitive health topics in a respectful and effective manner, protect adolescents' rights and privacy, and prepare young people to be independent consumers of health care.

Adolescents receive care from a variety of providers, including pediatricians, internists, family medicine physicians, advance practice nurses, physician assistants, and obstetricians/gynecologists, depending on their gender, age, and health care needs. Among these providers, the level of comfort in providing adolescent health care services may vary. According to surveys of pediatric residents and residency directors, most pediatric training programs do not adequately cover sensitive adolescent health topics, such as mental and behavioral health, interpersonal violence, reproductive health, chronic illness, and community adolescent health (Davis et al., 2018; Fox et al., 2010a; Kershnar et al., 2009). This lack of training among pediatricians is particularly noticeable around sexual and reproductive health care services. Surveys of pediatric and family medicine residents have found that these residents have significantly less training and comfort in providing sexual and reproductive health services, such as conducting pelvic exams, prescribing contraception, and counseling about pregnancy termination, than their peers in obstetrics-gynecology (Davis et al., 2018; Kershnar et al., 2009). Providers may also be unprepared or uncomfortable navigating their state's minor consent laws (see the above section, "Confidentiality and Parental Consent Requirements," for a more detailed discussion) (Santa Maria et al. 2017; Fox et al., 2010a). Given that adolescents may withhold information or even delay or forego care if they fear that their confidentiality will be violated, this is particularly concerning, especially for sexual-minority teens, who face elevated sexual health risks and who underutilize routine reproductive health care (Charlton et al., 2011; see also "Confidentiality and Parental Consent Requirements," above).

Furthermore, young people frequently report that their health providers fail to ask about sensitive issues, including sex and sexuality, substance use and other risky behaviors, as well as abuse and violence and other trauma exposure, all of which are often at the core of adolescents' and young adults' experiences and concerns (Klein and Wilson, 2002; Schoen et al., 1997).[14] (Box 7-5 discusses the need for health care providers serving adolescents to be trained in and understand trauma.) Klein and Wilson (2002), analyzing data from a nationally representative sample of 6,278 adolescents, reported that while 71 percent reported at least one of eight potential health risks, 63 percent had not spoken to their doctor about any of these risks. They further reported that the highest-risk adolescents had the lowest rates of being asked about risky health behaviors. In addition, Alexander and colleagues (2014), in an observational study of 253 adolescents and 49 physicians in 11 clinics in North Carolina, reported that while 65 percent of the visits had some conversations about sexuality, the average time spent talking about sexuality was only 36 seconds.

Adolescents understand their need for providers to engage in unrestricted, honest conversations about their health (Daley et al., 2017), but providers frequently fail to have these essential conversations. Adolescents report that health care providers do not spend enough time to get to know them, and that they focus on their problems rather than on their strengths (Fox et al., 2010b). Unfortunately, most health services providers may be ill-informed about the concerns that young people have when seeking care: young people report that they are infrequently asked to give any feedback regarding the health services they receive (Fox et al., 2013).

MEETING ADOLESCENTS WHERE THEY ARE: SERVICES IN NONCLINICAL SETTINGS

Outside of clinical settings, innovative methods for delivering health services to adolescents have emerged over the past several decades. These programs seek to meet adolescents where they are, delivering services in other locations to remove barriers in access to care. One such nonclinical setting is schools. Because school-age adolescents spend much of their day at school during the academic year, schools have often been utilized as a

---

[14] Providers report that a major obstacle to asking about abuse is the concern that inquiry will lead to reactions and consequences for patients that the health care provider may not be equipped to handle (Leder et al., 1999). Physicians' failure to inquire is also, in part, due to the lack of commonly accepted measures (i.e., screening instruments) (Savell, 2005) and lack of strategies for incorporating the use of measures into their practice (i.e., how to practically implement screening measures) (Weinreb et al., 2007). DiLillo and colleagues (2006), for example, have pointed out that health care providers lack an understanding as to what mode of administering abuse screens (e.g., paper-and-pencil questionnaire, computer-assisted survey, or face-to-face structured interview) is most effective, decreases levels of discomfort, and increases willingness to disclose.

BOX 7-5
Adolescent Health Care Workforce and Trauma

For health providers, understanding the prevalence of both childhood physical abuse and childhood sexual abuse and how a trauma history may present itself is essential. Trauma histories may present not only through mental health conditions but also, for example, through high-risk behaviors, early sexual activity, and risky sexual behaviors. Likewise, understanding how these histories impact patterns of health care utilization as well as the perception of health, and then finding ways to identify abuse histories, is also a necessary challenge (Diaz and Peake, 2017). For providers of after-school youth programs, which serve huge numbers of adolescents across the country, knowledge of the ways trauma is manifested and an understanding of community and family violence are both equally important if adolescent victims are to be helped.

In these settings and many others, as the trauma-informed lens is developed and extended, research suggests that the identification of trauma is a process that occurs over time through dialogue (Reitsema and Grietens, 2016). Thus, the adolescent's disclosure is a relational process, one renegotiated by each interaction and that evolves over an extended period. Just as important to this process as the behavior and words of young people themselves are the characteristics, skills, and reactions of the provider. In health services, there needs to be a recognition that adolescents will talk if they trust the providers and staff and if these adults demonstrate interest and respectfully but actively question them about their lives (Diaz and Peake, in press).

Unfortunately, adolescents report that their health care providers frequently fail to ask about these salient issues (Alexander et al., 2014; Klein and Wilson, 2002; Schoen et al., 1997). However, at present health care providers who serve adolescents are frequently too poorly prepared to ask about the key issues adolescents face, including abuse and trauma, when they see young people, and they lack the screening tools that might be useful in this endeavor (Blum et al., 1996; Fox et al., 2010a; Schuster, 1996).

---

setting for health interventions. This includes expansion of school-based health services, in which school psychologists, social workers, and other allied health professionals are involved in primary prevention activities, as well as screening and treatment at the school or after-school site, if services are available. However, policy makers and health systems must ensure that measures to increase screening of behavioral health problems among adolescents are accompanied by knowledge of places to refer for treatment, a warm handoff to treatment providers, and, most importantly, adequate resources for treatment.

School-Based Care Delivery

School-based health centers (SBHCs) can be an effective way of reaching adolescents and providing them with preventive, reproductive, and mental health care (Allison et al., 2007; Juszczak et al., 2003; School Based Health Alliance, 2014). These services address many of the shortfalls and limitations of the school-nurse model (Gustafson, 2005), and there is evidence that access to SBHCs increase the use of primary care, reduce the use of emergency rooms, reduce hospitalizations, and expand access to and quality of care for underserved adolescents, even those without insurance, compared to traditional outpatient clinics (Soleimanpour et al., 2010). School-based health centers are also popular among adolescents, who report feeling greater comfort in using them as compared to primary care settings (Mason-Jones et al., 2012). As of 2014, there were 2,315 SBHCs that served students and communities in 49 of 50 states and the District of Columbia, serving more than 2 million students each year. More than one-half of SBHCs were located in urban areas. Furthermore, the students served were disproportionately low-income students and students of color who were uninsured or underinsured and had limited access to other sources of health care (School-Based Health Alliance, 2014).

While SBHCs play an important role for underserved adolescents and can greatly increase access for underinsured and uninsured teens and other who find care hard to find, including teens living in rural areas (Mason-Jones et al., 2012), there has been little high-quality research evaluating these health centers and their impact (Soleimanpour et al., 2010). Constraints on most SBHCs—especially regarding sexual and reproductive health care and access to contraception and HIV testing—greatly limit their ability to provide teens with the most needed services. Moreover, only a small proportion of schools throughout the country have SBHCs, and many schools do not have the resources to replicate this model.

While it may not be feasible for all schools to contain an SBHC, offering health services to adolescents in the school setting is critical to meeting young people where they are. For example, one in three adolescents who do receive treatment for mental illness do so in a school setting (Merikangas et al., 2011), and the presence and magnitude of mental health services available in schools can significantly impact suicide risk and substance abuse in adolescents (Paschall and Bersamin, 2018). Adolescents with mild to moderate mental and behavioral disorders are more likely to use school mental health services in schools that provide early identification resources (Green et al., 2013). Students at schools with mental health services had significantly lower likelihoods of suicide ideation, suicide attempts, and cigarette smoking compared to students at other public schools (Paschall and Bersamin, 2018).

These findings support the necessity to expand school-based health services through SBHCs, which provide integrated medical, sexual, and reproductive and mental health services, or through additional mental health services on site or through linkages to mental health services in communities. Integrating health services into the schools setting, whether through increased behavioral health options or SBHCs, can increase access to care through viable, youth-friendly services. However, for adolescents who do not attend school, other mechanisms for service delivery are required.

eHealth

An emerging setting through which to reach adolescents is digital. Digital delivery of health services, commonly referred to as "eHealth," has increased in recent years and may be a particularly important method for delivering services to adolescents, given their propensity for using digital and social media. These vehicles can play a constructive role in improving adolescent access to health care and making the health-seeking experience easier (Divecha et al., 2012; Guse et al., 2012), although their use among adolescents is still relatively new (Shaw et al., 2015). Currently use of digital media has largely focused on the use of social media for health education and is limited by the need for more rigorous methodological studies and by a lack of information on how adolescents use social media (Shaw et al., 2015).

Some qualitative studies, in which adolescents and parents were asked their views about the use of digital technology in health care, also suggest that digital and social media can be used to make communication with adolescents easier—and to help in their communications with their parents—perhaps resulting in improved preventive care (Coker et al., 2010; Shakibnia et al., 2018). Lin and Zhu (2012) have suggested that health care providers can take advantage of adolescents' frequent social media engagement to follow patients between office visits and to increase compliance with health recommendations made during visits, such as increased exercise and healthy diet choices, with the motivation of online peer support and social gaming. Wong and colleagues (2014) suggest that social media and Web-based strategies can be used to improve adolescent engagement in care, especially for those who might be harder to reach. They recommend increased and early collaboration with adolescents and young adults to include their perspectives along with those of health experts when developing content; with technology experts to develop applications; and with research teams to measure effectiveness with data collection tools built into social media platforms.

In response to adolescents' reliance on technology, recent behavioral health interventions have sought to engage adolescents through the internet and smartphones. In general, these freestanding behavioral health internet interventions to address depressive disorders have been found by some studies to show modest effectiveness, but they have shown much greater effectiveness when combined with simple face-to-face interventions in the primary care setting, such as brief advice or interviews with the physician.

For example, Van Voorhees and colleagues (2009) examined the feasibility and efficacy of a low-cost and accessible behavioral health intervention in the primary care setting to engage primary care physicians with their adolescent patients who exhibited depressive symptoms. After dividing the patients into two treatment groups—a "BA" group given brief advice recommendations (of 1 to 3 minutes) and an "MI" group given collaborative motivational interviews (of 10 to 15 minutes)—and combining that intervention with an Internet-based resiliency intervention, both the BA and the MI groups exhibited significant declines in depressive disorder symptoms at 6 weeks after baseline and again after 12 weeks (Van Voorhees et al., 2009). The results also suggested significant increase in adherence to the internet intervention. Other freestanding behavioral health internet intervention trials resulted in 30 to 50 percent adherence, whereas in the MI group and BA group, respectively, they reported 91 percent and 78 percent adherence (Christensen et al., 2002; Santor et al., 2007; Van Voorhees et al., 2009). These findings indicate the promise of combining primary care physicians' involvement with internet interventions to maximize adherence and decrease depressive symptomology among adolescents.

Similarly, Kennard and colleagues (2018) tested a behavioral health intervention that complemented in-person suicide prevention programming with a smartphone application designed to assist adolescents recently discharged from the hospital due to suicidal behavior. The As Safe As Possible (ASAP) intervention is a 3-hour program focused on emotional regulation and safety planning and is administered to the adolescents in their inpatient unit. It promotes the utilization of a smartphone app, which sends daily text messages to rate levels of emotional distress and provides helpful resources. Although the researchers had a small sample size and their results did not produce any significant clinical effects, the rate of suicide attempts among participants in the ASAP intervention who were also undergoing usual treatment (inpatient contact with unit therapist) was one-half the rate among patients using usual treatment alone. Accordingly, interventions that emphasize the integration of technology with face-to-face behavioral health services, such as ASAP, merit further study.

Although more research and development is still needed, digital media strategies can assist in reaching adolescents—perhaps assist providers in being more comfortable, too. They can supplement in-person behavioral health interventions, providing adolescents with health education that is reliable and accurate, helping them find and access services, preparing them for their health care visits, and eliciting their much-needed feedback on the experience of care.

RECOMMENDATIONS

A systemic approach to prioritizing the health and well-being of adolescents is needed on a national level, including clear goals and priorities established to help mobilize both the public and private sectors to improve adolescent health. Simultaneously, society needs to recognize its ambivalence about adolescents (discussed at greater length in Chapter 1) and the roles government can play in their lives. The committee's vision for an adolescent-friendly health system is presented in Box 7-1, and its recommendations to incorporate neurobiological and socio-behavioral research into the development of more effective health policy, programs, and practices aimed at improving the health and well-being of adolescents are presented in Box 7-6. Taken together, these recommendations constitute a blueprint for achieving a developmentally appropriate health system to better meet the needs of today's youth.

The committee also recognizes the need to build a cross-system, national prevention policy that focuses on adolescents. Many of the funding efforts to date have treated the health problems of adolescents in a fragmented manner, with limited recognition of their interwoven causes and effects. For example, previous efforts have focused mainly on providing information and education, sometimes resulting in adolescents receiving fragmented and disconnected messages from different stakeholders in their lives. Few previous efforts have addressed income distribution and access to resources, poor educational experiences, and limited job and other life opportunities—which affect health status during adolescence as well as impacting adult health, with consequences for the health system and the delivery of health services.

Risk prevention models need to consider the social determinants of adolescent behavior, and prevention efforts must acknowledge that risk taking is an inherent and normative aspect of adolescent development (Ostaszewski, 2015). Unfortunately, traditional health education generally fails to account for these environmental factors, and thus addresses only a small part of what influences adolescent risk taking. For example, prolonged exposure to neighborhood poverty greatly increases the risk for teenage pregnancy (Wodtke, 2013), perhaps due to lack of economic or job training opportunities and viable alternatives to early childbearing, but few sexual and reproductive health education interventions address these factors (Brindis and Moore, 2014).

BOX 7-6
Blueprint for Creating an Adolescent-Friendly Health System

Recommendation 7-1: Strengthen the financing of health care services for adolescents, including insurance coverage for uninsured or underinsured populations.
    A. Federal and state policy makers should make changes within Medicaid to increase access for adolescents, including expanding Medicaid in states that have not yet done so, increasing Medicaid reimbursement rates for pediatric health services to be on par with those for Medicare, allowing equitable reimbursement for comprehensive health services, and eliminating the 5-year eligibility restriction on the use of Medicaid for documented immigrant adolescents.
    B. Federal, state, and local agencies, in partnership with philanthropic foundations and the private sector, should ensure adequate financial support for comprehensive, high-quality, culturally informed, and integrated physical and behavioral health services for adolescents.
    C. To finance comprehensive, adolescent-friendly health services, federal and state policy makers should adapt eligibility requirements to allow blending of existing funding mechanisms across sectors at the local level.

Recommendation 7-2: Improve access to comprehensive, integrated, coordinated health services for adolescents.
    A. State and federal agencies, health systems, and health care providers should collaborate to provide comprehensive, integrated, and coordinated care for adolescents, linking physical and behavioral health providers as well as other vital support services to the health sector.
    B. With help from federal agencies and designated funding, health care providers, public and private health organizations, and community agencies should work to develop or enhance coordinated, linked, and interdisciplinary adolescent health services. This includes funding community outreach efforts to attract and retain adolescents and their families in the health care system.
    C. To better understand effective methods for delivering coordinated care, federal research agencies and other research funders should encourage and replicate pilot programs and interventions that aim to decrease fragmentation and alleviate the complicated maze of services for adolescents and their families.
    D. Health care providers and health organizations should implement policies and practices that support adolescents' emerging sense of agency and independence, such as ensuring that all adolescents receive confidential health care for sensitive services as appropriate, such as empowering youth to meaningfully participate in their health care.
    E. Health care providers, public and private health organizations, health insurers, and state governments should ensure that all adolescents receive confidential care for sensitive services. Policies and ethical guidelines

continued

BOX 7-6 Continued

should enable adolescents who are minors to give their own consent for health services and to receive those services on a confidential basis when necessary to protect their health, and states should enact stronger regulations that ensure confidential access to sensitive services.

Recommendation 7-3: Increase access to behavioral health care and treatment services.
A. Federal agencies and behavioral health education institutions should work together to grow the behavioral health workforce available to adolescents, particularly those in underserved areas by expanding Health Resources and Services Administration's Behavioral Health Workforce Education and Training Program and the National Health Service Corps' scholarship program to include mental and behavioral health providers.
B. Federal, state, and local policy makers should develop and implement behavioral health programs for prevention, screening, and treatment that better meet the needs of all adolescents, with particular attention to vulnerable groups. Adolescents should actively participate in program development and implementation.

Recommendation 7-4: Improve the training and distribution and increase the number of adolescent health care providers.
A. Regulatory bodies for health professions in which an appreciable number of providers offer care to adolescents—such as the American College of Obstetrics and Gynecology, American Academy of Family Medicine, American Academy of Pediatrics, American Academy of Physician Assistants, and state boards of nursing and social work—should include

---

RECOMMENDATION 7-1: Strengthen financing of health care services for adolescents, including insurance coverage for uninsured or underinsured populations.

The importance of health insurance coverage has been well documented, and strengthening health insurance coverage for adolescents is a cornerstone for advancing adolescent health. Adolescents need comprehensive, continuous health insurance coverage, regardless of their parents' health coverage. Federal, state, and local agencies, in partnership with philanthropic foundations and the private sector, should assure adequate financial support for comprehensive, high-quality, culturally informed, and integrated physical and behavioral health services for adolescents.

Medicaid is a key lever for increasing health insurance coverage and health care access among the nation's youth, providing health insurance

a minimum set of competencies in adolescent health care and development into their licensing, certification, and accreditation requirements, and all pediatricians and primary care providers should have a minimum level of competency in adolescent medicine.

B. Public agencies and private organizations should work together to expand the number of training sites for board-certified adolescent medicine fellowships across multiple academic training centers.

C. HRSA, medical and nursing schools, and other key stakeholders should work together to create new pathways for medical students and other health professionals to become adolescent health specialists.

Recommendation 7-5: Improve federal and state data collection on adolescent health and well-being, and conduct adolescent-specific health services research and disseminate the findings.

A. The Federal Interagency Forum on Child and Family Statistics should work with federal agencies and, when possible, states to organize and disseminate data on the health of and health services for adolescents, including developmental and behavioral health.

B. To improve the health of adolescents, data must be used to assess whether existing programs and services are working. State and local health agencies should work with community-level adolescent service providers to identify opportunities for improvement in their programs.

C. Federal health agencies and private foundations should prepare a research agenda for improving adolescent health services that includes assessing existing service models, developing new models for providing adolescent-friendly health services, piloting projects to develop and test innovative approaches for incorporating neurodevelopmental and sociobehavioral sciences in the delivery of health care to adolescents, and evaluating the effectiveness of collaborations.

coverage for 35 million children and youth ages 18 and under and for 8.5 million young people ages 19 to 26 (Kaiser Family Foundation, 2019). The following recommended adjustments within Medicaid would increase access for adolescents:

- Expand Medicaid within the states that have not yet done so.
- Increase Medicaid reimbursement rates for pediatric health services to be on par with those for Medicare.[15]

---

[15]Nationwide, primary care services provided under Medicaid are reimbursed at significantly lower rates than those provided under Medicare. When Medicaid reimbursement rates were temporarily increased to be on par with Medicare, participation among office-based primary care pediatricians increased (Tang et al., 2018).

- Allow for equitable reimbursement for comprehensive health services, including psychosocial, behavioral health, dental, optical, and nutrition services.
- Eliminate the 5-year eligibility restriction on the use of Medicaid for documented immigrant adolescents, opening up health insurance access to adolescents from immigrant families.[16]

While they are important, categorical funding streams such as Medicaid, with their own unique eligibility requirements, have sometimes stifled the development of multidimensional interventions. To finance the provision of comprehensive, adolescent-friendly health services, federal and state policy makers should adapt eligibility requirements to allow a blending of existing funding mechanisms across sectors at the local level. Blended funding mechanisms, such as those that combine educational and health collaborative efforts, help maximize existing funding, and develop additional, sustainable funding to meet funding gaps, such as for school-based mental health support (Brindis and Sanghvi, 1997), have been adopted by several states, localities, and organizations (Trust for America's Health, 2018). By decategorizing siloed but overlapping government-funded programs, communities can maximize the provision of interrelated services to respond to adolescents' health needs. In addition to this blending and braiding of services, collaborative efforts are needed to help maximize existing funding, and additional, sustainable, and integrated funding needs to be developed to meet major gaps in the field of adolescent health.

RECOMMENDATION 7-2: Improve access to comprehensive, integrated, coordinated health services for adolescents.

Adolescents have distinct health care needs that span the health care system. To provide youth with the supports they need for healthy development, the health care system should provide comprehensive, integrated, and coordinated health services for all adolescents. If full integration is not possible, then authentic collaboration is recommended. State and federal agencies, health systems, and health care providers should collaborate to provide integrated care for adolescents, linking physical and mental health providers as well as other vital support services to the health sector. For

---

[16]Lack of insurance coverage limits access to care for undocumented adolescents and even for U.S.-born children of undocumented immigrant parents (DeCamp and Bundy, 2012; Ku and Matani, 2001), and legally documented immigrants must live in the United States for 5 years before they are entitled to apply for Medicaid (National Conference of State Legislatures, 2017). Many undocumented minors also need assistance accessing health care services. To meet the needs of these youth, states could adopt policies such as those implemented in New York State.

example, federal and state health agencies, health systems, and insurers can continue to support preventive health visits for adolescents, as well as assignment to a medical home that can provide integrated services (physical and behavioral health).

Creating effective linkages is a means to reduce the problem of stovepiped services, with increasing system coordination through inter-agency collaboration as the most viable approach. Policies that support the coordination and continuity of care, such as improving services to transition adolescents to adult care, need to be implemented universally. With help from federal agencies and designated funding, health care providers, public and private health organizations, and community agencies should work to develop or enhance coordinated, linked, and interdisciplinary adolescent health services. This includes funding community outreach efforts to attract and retain adolescents and their families in the health care system. Adolescents need not only community outreach to enroll in health insurance and create linkages to a medical home, but also tailored follow-up services to assure continuity of services and compliance with necessary medical care.

Finally, to better understand effective methods for delivering coordinated care, federal research agencies (such as the National Institutes of Health) and other research funders should encourage and replicate pilot programs and interventions that aim to decrease fragmentation and alleviate the complicated maze of services for adolescents and their families.

As part of a comprehensive, integrated, and coordinated health system for adolescents, health care providers and health organizations should implement policies and practices that support adolescents' emerging sense of agency and independence. To prepare for adulthood, adolescents need to learn how to independently navigate the health system and make their own decisions about their health. Health care providers can support this growth by progressively empowering adolescents to meaningfully participate in their health care, in line with their maturity level.

Creating opportunities for adolescents to develop their sense of agency around health is particularly important for socially marginalized adolescents (Patton et al., 2016). Youth who are in the foster care or justice system or experiencing homelessness may be especially vulnerable to risk factors for poor health. In addition, there is a growing recognition that complex health problems will often require multiple interventions of varying intensity and length. These interventions may need to be further tailored for specific subgroups of adolescents who may need different levels of intervention. Such interventions will require an expansion and enhancement of efforts that actively engage adolescents, including increasing their level of knowledge, access, skill development, and personal motivation. Taking this tailored approach, and building upon adolescents' growing sense of agency, are important means for increasing health equity among the adolescent population.

Likewise, health care providers, public and private health organizations, health insurers, and state governments should ensure that all adolescents receive confidential care for sensitive services. Health care providers, for example, should adhere to confidentiality guidelines developed by the American Medical Association, American Academy of Pediatrics, American Academy of Family Physicians, and the Society for Adolescent Health and Medicine, among others (English et al., 2012). Since the Health Insurance Portability and Accountability Act (HIPAA) of 1996[17] defers to state laws on key issues of confidentiality for minors (English et al., 2010), state lawmakers play a key role in ensuring the privacy rights of adolescents. At a minimum, policies and ethical guidelines should enable adolescents who are minors to give their own consent for health services and to receive those services on a confidential basis when necessary to protect their health. In addition, states should enact stronger regulations that promote confidential access to sensitive services, such as those adopted in Maine, New York, Wisconsin, and Hawaii.[18]

However, none of these statutes will solve the problem in its entirety, and alternative pathways for privacy protection, either through laws or health insurance and billing policies, will need to be explored. State departments of insurance, which are charged with protecting consumers and regulating insurers' business practices within the state (English et al., 2010), may play a key role in protecting confidentiality for minors who use private insurance. For example, they can ensure that explanations of benefits (EOBs) are not sent to the primary policyholder for sensitive services that may have been delivered to an adolescent.

RECOMMENDATION 7-3: Increase access to behavioral health care and treatment services.

Mental health services must be equitably accessible to reduce health disparities among adolescents. A key priority is to increase both access to and utilization of behavioral health care and treatment services. The need to provide behavioral health care to adolescents is pressing: rates of depression, substance abuse, and other behavioral and mental health disorders are increasing among young people. Because of the early onset of many common mental health disorders (Patton et al., 2014) and the consequent impairment experienced later in life (Copeland et al., 2015), it is important

---

[17] HIPAA was passed by Congress in 1996. HIPAA does the following: provides the ability to transfer and continue health insurance coverage for millions of American workers and their families when they change or lose their jobs; reduces health care fraud and abuse; mandates industrywide standards for health care information on electronic billing and other processes; and requires the protection and confidential handling of protected health information.

[18] See English et al. (2010) for a discussion of existing statutes.

to consider implementing preventive interventions in early childhood and adolescence, but availability of behavioral health services remains limited.

Availability of services is constrained by both a lack of sufficient providers nationwide and a maldistribution of the behavioral health workforce. Across the country, there are more than 5,000 areas identified as suffering from a shortage of mental health professionals, and more than one-half of U.S. counties, mostly in rural areas, have no practicing psychiatrists or social workers (Kaiser Family Foundation, 2018). Moreover, this shortage is projected to worsen: in 2015, HRSA estimated that an additional 250,000 behavioral health providers will be needed to meet demand by 2025 (Health Resources and Services Administration, 2015). Young people, who are already an underserved population in behavioral health, will feel this shortage keenly.

Currently, the lack of sufficient resources, including providers and funding, and the insufficient integration between behavioral and primary health care prevent many adolescents and their families in need of services from receiving behavioral health care. To address adolescents' needs for mental and behavioral health services, policy makers and insurers should ensure that behavioral health services are widely available and accessible to all adolescents.

Federal agencies and behavioral health education institutions should work together to grow the behavioral health workforce available to adolescents, particularly those in underserved areas. They can do this, for example, by expanding HRSA's Behavioral Health Workforce Education and Training Program, which partners with universities and nonprofit organizations to train behavioral health professionals and paraprofessionals with an emphasis on medically underserved populations and integrative care (Kepley and Streeter, 2018). While this program shows promise for increasing the number of behavioral health providers serving youth, it needs to be greatly expanded to meet adolescents' growing need for integrated behavioral health care. At the same time, HRSA should work to recruit undergraduate students into behavioral health careers by expanding the National Health Service Corps' scholarship program to include mental and behavioral health providers. The diversity of the future behavioral health workforce is also important to consider in such efforts.

In addition, federal, state, and local policy makers should develop and implement behavioral health programs for prevention, screening, and treatment that better meet the needs of all adolescents, especially programs serving vulnerable groups such as youth in foster care or in detention. Moreover, adolescents should actively participate in program development and implementation. Adolescents' engagement in planning and shaping the types of behavioral health services, location, and other elements is key in helping to assure that services are more responsive to their needs and less stigmatized (see Box 7-7 for examples of youth engagement in health programming).

RECOMMENDATION 7-4: Improve the training and distribution and increase the number of adolescent health care providers.

Clearly, there is a need to better prepare health care professionals to feel competent and comfortable caring for adolescents. Significant work is needed to develop a workforce that is comfortable and competent in serving

---

BOX 7-7
Examples of Youth Engagement

The Zuni Youth Enrichment Project (ZYEP), established to serve the children of Zuni Pueblo, New Mexico, through recreational and cultural programming, engages adolescents and young adults as leaders and mentors in its programs. ZYEP offers year-long sports, after-school, and community programming, including summer camps. Zuni adolescents and young adults serve as camp counselors and coaches of sports teams for younger children in their community. ZYEP prepares its adolescent and young-adult counselors for camp through intensive wilderness retreats, where they learn leadership skills, reflect on their life experiences, and discuss how they can support Zuni children. Counselors and coaches are also encouraged to incorporate Zuni language, culture, and tradition in their programming. Engaging adolescents as leaders gives them "a chance for them to be mentors and positive role models, [and] also to see themselves as the leaders they could be" (Notah Begay III Foundation, 2018).

From 2003 through 2006, researchers from the University of California, San Francisco, the Alameda County School-Based Health Center Coalition, and the nonprofit organization Youth in Focus partnered to incorporate student-led research into the evaluation of the school-based health centers. Nineteen student research teams, made up of youth from diverse economic and ethnic backgrounds, were developed to conduct research on specific health topics at their schools. The teams identified challenges facing the student population and advocated for changes in programming to meet student needs. For example, one student research team identified stress as a serious concern in their schools. With guidance from the university researchers, they surveyed the student population concerning their stress load. The survey showed that stress affected many students, even though few turned to the Alameda County School-Based Health Center Coalition for counseling and mental health services. The student research team presented its findings to the coalition's staff and executive board as well as the school board, and eventually recommended the creation of a peer counseling program to address mental health issues in school. Their recommendations inspired the creation of a peer advocate program at the school, which trains students to be advocates and health educators for other students (Soleimanpour et al., 2008).

the health care needs of teens, and in helping them feel welcomed and safe to disclose their concerns. Moreover, with very few physicians and psychiatrists specializing in adolescent health care, there is a pressing need to both increase the number of adolescent medicine specialists and strengthen the skills and competencies of all health care providers who interact with adolescents. To create an adolescent-friendly health system, the training, distribution, and number of adolescent health care providers across the nation must be improved.

Training of health providers is needed at all levels addressing health issues that are particularly relevant to adolescents. These issues include consent and confidentiality requirements, coercive sex, STIs, diagnosis and treatments, behavioral health, sexual orientation, cultural beliefs, immunizations, health promotion and education, counseling techniques, management of victims of violence, and provision of services to special populations of adolescents, such as youth in foster care. New training programs in adolescent health will need to prepare specialists, researchers, and educators in all relevant health disciplines to work with both the general adolescent population and selected groups that require special and/or more intense services. Regulatory bodies for health professions in which an appreciable number of providers offer care to adolescents—such as the American College of Obstetrics and Gynecology, American Academy of Family Medicine, American Academy of Pediatrics, American Academy of Physician Assistants, and state boards of nursing and social work—should include a minimum set of competencies in adolescent health care and development into their licensing, certification, and accreditation requirements. In addition, all pediatricians and primary care providers should have a minimum level of competency in adolescent medicine. Both public- and private-sector funding supporting improved interdisciplinary training and capacity-building among those delivering adolescent health care services will also be needed.

In addition to strengthening the competency of the health care workforce, efforts should be made to increase the number of board-certified adolescent medicine specialists nationwide. As experts in adolescent health care, adolescent medicine physicians are well trained to care for this population (Gilbert et al., 2018). Despite the need for adolescent health care specialists, the field remains small. To address this undersupply, public agencies and private organizations should work together to expand the number of training sites for board-certified adolescent medicine fellowships across multiple academic training centers. At present, there are only 26 training programs in adolescent medicine in the entire country (Society for Adolescent Health and Medicine, 2018). The HRSA, medical and nursing schools, and other key stakeholders should work together to create new pathways for medical students and other health professionals to become adolescent health specialists. More specifically:

- HRSA's Maternal and Child Health Bureau should fund adolescent medicine fellowships within medical schools across the country to increase the number of adolescent medicine fellowships nationwide.
- HRSA should also add an adolescent health care focus to the National Health Service Corps to bring providers to geographically underserved areas.
- Congress should appropriate funds to HRSA to assess the number, type, and distribution of adolescent health care providers needed to support optimal adolescent health across the country and expand accordingly its Leadership Education in Adolescent Health Program, which prepares health professionals to become leaders in adolescent and young adult health.
- Existing adolescent medicine training sites should offer 1-year clinical training programs in adolescent medicine for those wishing to enhance their expertise in adolescent medicine without becoming board certified.
- Pediatric residency programs should expand their adolescent medicine offerings to increase pediatricians' proficiency in adolescent health. For example, residency programs could extend the length of the mandatory adolescent medicine rotation or create a combined pediatrics/adolescent medicine residency.

Increasing the diversity of the adolescent health care workforce is also critical to achieving an adolescent-friendly health care system. A previous National Academies report, *In the Nation's Compelling Interest: Ensuring Diversity in the Health-Care Workforce*, found that a more diverse health care workforce increases access to care for minority patients, improves patient choice and satisfaction, results in better patient-provider communication, and ultimately can produce better quality of care for all Americans (Institute of Medicine, 2004). Because the current generation of adolescents is the most diverse in U.S. history and evidence shows that adolescents value providers who share their cultural backgrounds, it is even more imperative that the health care system, and systems that train and prepare the health care workforce, strive to increase the diversity of the adolescent health care workforce.

Like the previous National Academies panel, this committee endorses the reduction of barriers to entry for underrepresented minorities to the health professions by reformulating admissions practices so that they consider each applicant comprehensively and the reduction of financial barriers to participation in training through public and private investment.

RECOMMENDATION 7-5: Improve federal and state data collection on adolescent health and well-being, and conduct adolescent-specific health services research and disseminate the findings.

In addition to the efforts the committee recommends to improve service delivery and access to adolescent-friendly health care, the committee recommends improving data collection on adolescent health and well-being and conducting research and disseminating findings on effective adolescent health care practices.

First, efforts should be made to improve federal and state data collection on adolescent health and well-being. The current system for collecting data on adolescents' health has three gaps:

1. what data are collected,
2. collection of data on the "whole" adolescent, and
3. how the data are used.

The gaps in what data are collected are obvious. Data on key adolescent health indicators among subgroups of adolescents are lacking nationally. On average, data at the subpopulation level are available for about one-third of the 21 health objectives for adolescents identified by *Healthy People 2010* (Knopf et al., 2007). Data are particularly limited for low-income, sexual minority, immigrant, and foster care and justice-involved youth (Knopf et al., 2007), although some progress has been made.[19] This lack of data impedes national efforts to improve health outcomes for all adolescents and ameliorate health inequities. The Federal Interagency Forum on Child and Family Statistics should work with federal agencies and, when possible, states to organize and disseminate data on the health of and health services for adolescents, including developmental and behavioral health. These data should encompass adolescents generally, with subreports further broken down by age, selected population characteristics, and other circumstances.

Second, the data that are collected on adolescents is frequently uncoordinated and siloed into granular topic areas. By focusing singularly on one or two topic areas of interest, current data collection systems fail to recognize the interrelated nature of adolescent health. This also hinders researchers' efforts to understand the impact of the social determinants of health on adolescents. Moreover, current data systems are not set up to build a profile of an individual adolescent. However, existing data systems can be built upon to include cross-sectional data. For example, data on an adolescents' social and behavioral determinants of health could be collected during visits with

---

[19]For example, the 2017 Youth Risk Behavior Survey included a pilot question on transgender identity. See https://www.cdc.gov/healthyyouth/disparities/smy.htm.

their health care provider and recorded in their electronic health record. Including social determinants of health data in electronic health records is essential for improving health care quality, efficiency, and access (Institute of Medicine, 2014).

A previous report from the Institute of Medicine recommended that information on 11 domains of social and behavioral health be collected in patient's electronic health records (Institute of Medicine, 2014). These domains include neighborhood median income, depression, education, financial resource strain, intimate partner violence, physical activity, social connections and social isolation, and stress (Institute of Medicine, 2014). Pediatric, internal, and adolescent medicine practices nationwide could incorporate these measures into adolescents' electronic health records.

Finally, there are gaps in the ways in which data are used. It is not enough to have reliable, detailed data on adolescent health. To improve the health of adolescents, data must be used to assess whether existing programs and services are working. State and local health agencies should work with community-level adolescent service providers to identify opportunities for improvement in their programs. The spirit of this quality improvement process should be constructive and collaborative, not punitive.

Federal health agencies and private foundations should prepare a research agenda for improving adolescent health services. The agenda should include

- assessing existing service models to identify promising, evidence-based options, and scale and implement models that work;
- developing new models for providing adolescent-friendly health services that are accessible, acceptable, appropriate, effective, and equitable;
- piloting projects to develop and test innovative approaches for incorporating neurodevelopmental and socio-behavioral sciences in the delivery of health care to adolescents; and
- evaluating the effectiveness of collaborations that bring different sectors together, as well as those that work at the individual, family, community, and policy levels simultaneously.

To complement this research agenda, accelerated sharing of research findings across federal health agencies, private foundations, and the research community is needed. Federal health agencies can promote the widespread dissemination, transfer, and application of knowledge about adolescent development and health and other services for adolescents with their partners. For example, federal health agencies could work with philanthropic partners and other stakeholders to develop learning collaboratives for adolescent health services models. Such collaboratives could provide the support, training, and technical assistance needed to successfully implement an adolescent-friendly health services model. In addition, private foundations could support the improvement of adolescent health services by funding the development and dissemination of information to policy makers on the cost-effectiveness of prevention programs.

8

Child Welfare System

This chapter addresses the child welfare system, one of two legal systems that regulate the lives of adolescents and their families. The other system is the juvenile justice system, addressed in Chapter 9, which exercises jurisdiction over juveniles charged with delinquent acts. The purpose of the child welfare system is to protect children at risk of abuse or neglect from their parents or guardians (or from whomever the state defines as a perpetrator). Box 8-1 provides a glossary of child welfare terms used in this report.

There is a third statutory category as well, which establishes court jurisdiction over children who are alleged to be truant, ungovernable, or in need of supervision. Children determined to be in this category are classified as having committed *status offenses*. Because many states define status offenses as grounds for involvement by the child welfare system, status offenses are also covered in this chapter.[1]

This chapter proceeds as follows. We set the stage by revisiting a key scientific theme explored in this report: the biological mechanisms through which child maltreatment can get "under the skin" to change the trajectory of child and adolescent development. We then present a brief overview of the child welfare system focused on older youth in care, augmenting the 2014 report, *New Directions in Child Abuse and Neglect Research* (Insti-

---

[1] Youth who are truant or who run away from home or placement may also "cross over" into the juvenile justice system for violations of court orders controlling their behavior so information on status offenses is also relevant for a complete understanding of the relationship between the child welfare and juvenile justice systems.

BOX 8-1
Glossary of Child Welfare Terms as Used in This Report

Child Welfare System

In this report, we use the term *"child welfare system"* to refer to the full range of services provided by a public agency, from reporting and investigation through reunification, placement, placement monitoring, adoption, and all other dispositions. In common parlance, the term "foster care system" is sometimes used even more broadly to be interchangeable with the term "child welfare system," but we do not do so here. Likewise, while the term "child protection system" is sometimes used as another name for the full system, we do not use it that way here, since "child protection" has a second, more narrow usage, referring to the front end of the child welfare system—namely, reporting, investigating, and recordkeeping of allegations of abuse and neglect.

Foster Care

Foster care is one type of placement, most specifically referring to placement in a family-like setting but also sometimes used more generally to refer to out-of-home placement. In this report, we follow the latter, broader usage, since "aging out of foster care" is a common phrase denoting an important transition, even if the youth's last placement was a group home or independent living program and not with a foster family.

Foster Care System

The *foster care system* refers to the portion of the child welfare system involving out-of-home placements, since only a subset of children in the child welfare system go into placements.

Public Benefits System

The *public benefits system*, though it is sometimes referred to as the "welfare system," covers a separate area of services entirely from the child welfare system. Federal funding for the child welfare system is embedded in the Social Security Act in the same sections that deal with public assistance benefits (as is discussed more fully in the text), and this may cause some to confuse the two. While families may be involved with both the public benefits and child welfare systems, here we address the latter, the legal system responding to allegations of abuse and neglect and the services that follow.

tute of Medicine and National Research Council, 2014), followed by a summary of the federal laws that specifically address the needs of adolescents
in the child welfare system, including key provisions of the 2018 Family
First Preventive Services Act. We then review developmental research on
the effects of involvement in the child welfare system on youth outcomes,
including mental health and educational outcomes and outcomes related
to the permanence of placement and aging out of care. Next, the chapter
reviews promising programs and program components for youth involved
in the child welfare system. Finally, it concludes with a blueprint for a
developmentally informed child welfare system.

CHILD MALTREATMENT AND THE ADOLESCENT BRAIN

There is a growing body of evidence that abuse and neglect—common
precursors to involvement in the child welfare system—have effects on the
adolescent brain. The majority of prospective research in this area has been
conducted during early childhood, but there is a growing body of research
on adolescence, and a sizable body of retrospective studies with adults that
make use of their recollections of childhood abuse (see Chapter 3).

In a review of the brain imaging literature, McCrory and colleagues
(2012) concluded that several structural and functional brain differences
are associated with early adversity such as abuse and neglect. Specifically,
they report on brain structural differences in three regions: the corpus
callosum, cerebellum, and prefrontal cortex. These brain regions are important because they help the brain share information from one hemisphere
to the other (corpus callosum), are responsible for higher brain functions
such as thought and action (cerebellum), and are involved in planning, self-
regulation, and decision making (prefrontal cortex). Further, their review
of the literature suggests functional differences in brain regions associated
with emotional and behavioral regulation, including the amygdala and
anterior cingulate cortex.[2] These brain differences may represent adaptations to early experiences of heightened stress that lead to an increased risk
of psychopathology during adolescence and beyond.

One study of adolescents focused on neglect during childhood and
examined its association with brain structure and cognitive performance
(Hanson et al., 2013). The authors examined the brain's white matter
(myelinated axions) and neurocognitive performance in early adolescent
children who had previously experienced neglect, as compared to adolescents raised in typical environments. They found that the microstructure of
prefrontal white matter differed between the two groups, with adolescents

---

[2] See Chapters 2 and 3 for a more detailed discussion of these brain regions and the ways
trauma can affect them and the pathways among them.

who had suffered childhood neglect showing more diffuse organization, which was related to neurocognitive deficits that they displayed relative to the comparison youth.

A long-term longitudinal study of female victims of sexual abuse, who were assessed at six points in time, from childhood through late adolescence and emerging adulthood, compared these young women with others who had no history of sexual abuse, and it too suggests that early experiences may modify an individual's biological response to stress (Trickett et al., 2010). In that study, cortisol levels, which are a biological marker of the ability to regulate stress, declined in young women who had experienced sexual abuse starting in adolescence, with significantly lower levels of cortisol evident by emerging adulthood among female victims. According to the authors, the experience of childhood abuse might disrupt the neurobiology of stress management, whereby victims of child abuse show a decline in their ability to release hormones responsible for effective stress regulation later in development, perhaps due to over-release of stress regulatory responses earlier in development, at the time when they were exposed to abuse.

Research also suggests that the timing of maltreatment may be important for brain development and may lead to different effects across childhood and adolescence (Pechtel and Pizzagalli, 2011). For example, in young adulthood, retrospective reports of childhood sexual abuse indicated that sexual abuse that occurred at ages 3 to 5 and ages 11 to 13 was associated with reduced hippocampal volume in young adults, while childhood sexual abuse that occurred at ages 9 to 10 was associated with reduced corpus callosum in young adults, and childhood sexual abuse that occurred at ages 14 to 16 was associated with attenuated frontal cortex (Andersen et al., 2008). As reviewed in Chapters 2 and 3, these brain regions are important for emotion regulation and memory (hippocampus), sharing of information between brain hemispheres (corpus callosum), and behavioral control, decision making, and planning (prefrontal cortex). The developmental differences, identified by Anderson and colleagues (2008), may reflect the fact that brain regions develop at different rates at distinct times in development and, accordingly, youth may be vulnerable to different degrees and for different outcomes based on the timing of maltreatment.

Similarly, a recent study on the impact of maltreatment on the brain volume of the amygdala, thalamus, and caudate by Pechtel and colleagues (2014) found timing to be important. When asked to recall specific periods of maltreatment during their childhood, Pechtel and colleagues (2014) found that exposure to childhood maltreatment (e.g., parental and peer verbal abuse, physical maltreatment, and non-verbal emotional abuse) was associated with increased volume in the right amygdala, which is important for emotion processing and regulation (Pechtel et al., 2014). Moreover, when moderate maltreatment occurred at ages 10 to 11, this exposure contributed to increased volume in the right amygdala.

There is some evidence that interventions delivered during early childhood can normalize some dimensions of brain function, including diurnal cortisol patterns (Fisher et al., 2007), although the potential benefit of interventions on neurobiological functioning for adolescents in the child welfare system has not yet been examined. Nonetheless, combined with the documented findings on adolescent brain plasticity presented in Chapter 3, interventions delivered during adolescence to improve brain and neurodevelopmental functioning may hold promise for adolescents who are or have been in the child welfare system.[3]

INTRODUCTION TO THE CHILD WELFARE SYSTEM

It is critical to understand that the child welfare system was not developed with adolescents at the center of the legislation. In 1962, Dr. Henry Kempe and his colleagues published their influential article, *The Battered Child Syndrome* (Kempe et al., 1962). In addition to describing characteristics of the injuries abused children suffer, the Kempe article identified other characteristics of the "battered child":

> The battered child syndrome may occur at any age, but, in general, the affected children are younger than 3 years. In some instances the clinical manifestations are limited to those resulting from a single episode of trauma, but more often the child's general health is below par, and he shows evidence of neglect including poor skin hygiene, multiple soft tissue injuries, and malnutrition. One often obtains a history of previous episodes suggestive of parental neglect or trauma. A marked discrepancy between clinical findings and historical data as supplied by the parents is a major diagnostic feature of the battered child syndrome. (Kempe et al., 1962, pp. 105–106)

The American Medical Association subsequently led a successful campaign to pass reporting laws in all states by 1967 so that physicians would be freed from confidentiality restrictions to report abuse and there would be a system in place to receive the reports. This led in 1974 to the first federal law governing the child welfare system, the Child Abuse Prevention and Treatment Act (CAPTA). These early origins make clear that, from the

---

[3] As an adolescent moves from a harmful environment to a safe one—such as from an abusive home into a supportive foster family—an opportunity is provided to leverage the power of observational research to prospectively examine how a supportive context can promote resilience and the generation of new and adaptive brain connections (this would require data collection on each youth before and after the new placement).

child welfare system's genesis, the physically abused infant/toddler was the paradigm that guided the system's processes and procedures.

Federal Child Welfare Legislation

Primary responsibility for protecting children from abuse and neglect rests at the state level, generally with county- or state-operated child welfare agencies governed by state law. However, the federal government has played an important role in funding and guiding state child welfare agencies, beginning with the enactment of CAPTA in 1974. CAPTA and all subsequent child welfare federal legislation have been codified as part of the Social Security Act provisions governing income maintenance. Federal mandates are imposed upon states in exchange for federal reimbursement for a portion of their child welfare funding. To be eligible for federal reimbursement for various aspects of the child welfare system, children must meet the eligibility guidelines for income maintenance.

In 1980, the Adoption Assistance and Child Welfare Act created title IV-E, an open-ended source of matching funds for foster care and adoption assistance for eligible poor children. However, the same law capped funding for prevention services. This meant that states were reimbursed no matter how high their placement or adoption costs for poor children but had only limited reimbursement available for prevention services. The most recent federal law, the Family First Prevention Services Act of 2018 (discussed below) has begun to change this funding paradigm, allowing matching funds to be used for preventive services, not just placement services, and removing the eligibility requirement linked to public assistance eligibility for those prevention services.

The intersectionality between poverty and abuse and neglect continues to plague the system and creates disparities in the system, as discussed throughout this chapter and in detail in Chapter 4. Reports of child maltreatment have increased far beyond the numbers imagined when the systems were first designed. When Congress held hearings before passing CAPTA, senators were warned that up to 60,000 children could be victims of child abuse and neglect nationally. In 2015, 4 million reports of abuse or neglect were made to state reporting systems (Children's Bureau, 2017). In that year, the rate of such reports for children under age 1 was 24 out of 1,000 children; the rate for youth ages 11 and older was less than 7 per 1,000. Consequently, the child welfare system and its resources remain focused on younger children. This committee's assignment is to envision how the child welfare system can be *re-envisioned* to support the needs of adolescents as well, given their developing cognitive, social, and emotional assets and development.

Status Offenses

Just as Congress was staking out a federal role to support states in preventing child abuse and neglect, states were also reforming their juvenile justice systems (as discussed in Chapter 9). One element of those reforms was to separate out noncriminal behavior such as truancy, running away, and "ungovernability" and assigning jurisdiction over these cases to the child welfare system. Illinois, the site of the country's first juvenile court in 1899, along with New York State, again led the way in the 1960s to establish jurisdiction over two categories of youth: minors in need of services (MINS) and children in need of services (CHINS). In 1967, a presidential commission recommended the Illinois and New York model, and most states created separate laws and procedures to govern status offenses. In 1976, the Institute for Judicial Administration—American Bar Association Juvenile Justice Standards Project emphasized the use of voluntary services to address status offenses rather than court involvement, a practice commonly referred to as "diversion." Many states continue to encourage diversion rather than court filing. The services utilized to serve children and families in these cases are often the same services available for older youth in foster care.

Congress dramatically furthered the noncriminal distinction of the status offender system with the Juvenile Justice and Delinquency Prevention Act (JJDPA) in 1974, the same year CAPTA was passed to govern the child welfare system. Under JJDPA, youth adjudicated due to status offenses could not be held in secure detention. JJDPA was amended in 1980 to create a "bootstrapping" provision: if youth adjudicated as status offenders violated a valid court order, they could be detained in detention facilities, thus funneling them into the juvenile delinquency system. In October 2018, Pew Charitable Trusts issued state-by-state statistics showing that nearly one-quarter of all incarcerated youth never committed a crime: they were incarcerated for a status offense (Pew Charitable Trusts, 2018). These are youth who were runaways, truant, or adjudged "ungovernable," and then violated a court order designed to address their adolescent behavior problem, the latter violation ultimately placing them in a juvenile facility.

Noncriminal misconduct is not unusual among adolescents, of course, and it can even be part of a normal developmental pathway to adulthood. Acknowledging this, and to reduce the unnecessary funneling of adolescents into the justice system, the American Law Institute has adopted a *Restatement* that recommends four principles to guide the courts in these cases.[4] This *Restatement* is consistent with federal and state law, as well as best

---

[4]Restatement of the Law: Children and the Law, Preliminary Draft No. 5 (September 5, 2018), Sections 3.00, 3.10, 3.20 and 3.30, pp. 19–63.

practices in responding to noncriminal misconduct by children, and the committee also endorses it (see the blueprint outlined at the end of this chapter).

Foster Care and Out-of-Home Services

Foster care is the term often used for a broad array of out-of-home services, including placement in a home with strangers, with relatives through kinship care, in congregate care facilities such as group homes, or in larger settings and inclusive of supervised independent living. Non-therapeutic group homes and supervised independent living are available almost exclusively to adolescents, but younger children with specific needs may also be placed in congregate care settings, including therapeutic group homes. According to the Adoption and Foster Care Analysis and Reporting System, on any given day approximately 443,000 children are in foster care. These figures have grown steadily from under 400,000 in 2012 to the present levels, although a slight decline in those entering foster care occurred from 2016 to 2017 (U.S. Department of Health and Human Services, 2018).

Historically and up to the present day, two defining aspects of the child welfare system have been the focus on young children and the focus on the prevention of serious physical abuse. These foci are coupled with a funding scheme that has provided unlimited funds for out-of-home placement of these endangered children. The result is a system that is under-resourced for efforts to prevent out-of-home placement (which requires support services) and for providing support to families, particularly families with adolescents. As described in Chapter 3, this approach is ill-suited to help adolescents involved in the child welfare system flourish, given their more advanced decision-making skills, their need for a balance of autonomy and healthy relationships, and their ability to use technology to seek solutions, relative to younger children. In addition, insufficient services are available to address acting-out behaviors that may bring adolescents before a court for status offenses, specifically services needed to address the underlying and presenting problems of these youth and their families.

In 2014, the United States spent $29.1 billion on child welfare services. This amount of spending has been roughly constant over the past 10 years, although the share provided by state and local governments has increased and now stands at 57 percent. Of the $29 billion, roughly one-half (46%) is spent on out-of-home placement, 15 percent on in-home preventive services, 19 percent on adoption and legal guardianship costs, and 15 percent on child protective services. Only 2 percent of the total is spent on services and assistance for older youth (Child Trends, 2016, p. 11). The low percentage of total cost expended on in-home prevention and services for older youth spotlights the challenge of properly serving adolescents in the child welfare system while avoiding adjudication for status offenses.

Over the past two decades, Congress has gradually reversed some of the harmful consequences of earlier laws to better serve the needs of adolescents by focusing attention on family reunification, prioritizing placement with kin over strangers, and including a specific focus on older youth and services for those aging out of foster care. There is a renewed emphasis on permanency for all children, not just younger children. Although additional innovations are needed to best serve adolescents in the child welfare system, these statutory changes are significant advances that align with the developmental assets and challenges that adolescents face, and are the subject of our review of Congressional initiatives further below.

Disparities in the Child Welfare System

Before describing recent legal changes, it is important to draw attention to statistics showing that poor children and children of color are disproportionately referred to the child welfare system. Black children represent 13 percent of the U.S. population but 23 percent of children identified by the child welfare system as victims. For non-Hispanic Whites the shares are 52 percent (population) and 46 percent (child welfare system), respectively, while for Asian Americans they are 5 percent and 1 percent, for Latinx they are 21 percent and 24 percent, and for Native Americans 0.9 percent and 1.3 percent (Children's Bureau, 2016). Moreover, a recent analysis of nationally representative data finds that LGBT youth are overrepresented in the child welfare system generally, in foster care, and in other out-of-home placements (Fish et al., 2019).

In general, both disproportionate need and differential treatment by both community members and the child welfare system play important roles in explaining these disparities. Research on the sources of these disparities has been summarized elsewhere (Annie E. Casey Foundation, 2011). As described in Chapter 4, observational data and experimental research data show that community reporters are more likely to report children of color to child welfare authorities. Although some studies suggest that this pattern is attributable to personal bias, others are consistent with a more systematic source of discrimination such as increased maltreatment surveillance in communities of color (Chaffin and Bard, 2006).

A second important source of systemic disparity lies in families of color being offered fewer in-home services that might prevent the placement of a child or adolescent in foster care (Annie E. Casey Foundation, 2011). As a result, children of color are both more likely to be removed from a home and more likely to remain in their placement longer, without permanent resolution.

To reduce such disparities, one should first consider policies and practices that ensure that families of color have access to the same levels of in-home preventative services as other at-risk families. A second and more involved policy response would require evaluation and determination of the appropriate level of surveillance in a community. Both under- and over-surveillance are problematic. Establishing guidelines and protocols regarding appropriate levels of surveillance would improve the overall efficiency and benefit of surveillance systems and likely reduce disparities.

As noted in Chapters 4 and 9, dual involvement in the child welfare system and the juvenile justice system is common, with the same adolescents disproportionately represented in both systems.[5] Some have argued that the disproportionate share of minority adolescents in the child welfare system is one of the main drivers of the disproportionate share of minority adolescents in juvenile detention. Child welfare involvement is an especially important avenue or pathway to the juvenile justice system for female adolescents (Ryan et al., 2007), who often pass through the status offense system. As child welfare system innovations and legislative initiatives are launched, attention to strategies to reduce disparities will continue to be front and center.

ALIGNING THE CHILD WELFARE SYSTEM WITH THE NEEDS OF ADOLESCENTS

A child welfare system traditionally focused on child safety, permanency, and well-being is not aligned with the needs and capacities of adolescents as they develop their identities and begin to shape their own futures. The help and support they require differs markedly from the protective cocoon needed by the developing child. Cognitively, the adolescent brain is maturing, and adolescents are capable of more abstract thinking and problem solving than they were in childhood, including an understanding of cause and effect, perspective-taking, having a sense of agency, and increased planning/future orientation skills. These developing skills enable them to be active participants in planning for their future. Socially, adolescents have typically developed a network of relationships with other adolescents and young adults, in contrast to their more singular focus on their own family and parents during early childhood. These peer-based social connections often take center stage in adolescents' lives, impacting their well-being as well as providing important social connections that may not be currently available in their relationships with parents or other caregivers.

---

[5]Children involved in both child protective services and juvenile justice are referred to as *crossover youth*. Roughly 30 percent of children in the child welfare system have future involvement in juvenile justice system as well (https://www.ncbi.nlm.nih.gov/pubmed/16233913/), but there do not appear to be any national statistics. All statistics come from individual studies of local areas.

As noted in Chapter 1, adolescents are also astute users of technology, both to communicate with their peers and to seek information. These skills can be leveraged to help adolescents in decision making around career, housing, and health solutions. In addition, adolescents have greater awareness of their own and others' feelings and emotions than they did just a few years prior, enabling them to understand the perspective of others and contribute as productive members of society. Together, the higher-level cognitive, social, and emotional capacities that adolescents develop provide them with a toolkit of skills they can use to actively participate in creating their own futures, and to participate in and play a lead role in decision making about their education, residential and custodial situations, and treatment and health care needs.

There is a challenge, however, in reconciling the emerging capabilities of adolescents with the historical definitions of safety, permanency, and well-being that are in the child welfare system due to its origin in ensuring protection of young children. Concerns in the child welfare system about safety and prevention of death are relatively fewer for adolescents than for infants and young children; adolescents are better equipped emotionally, cognitively, and behaviorally to protect themselves in ways that young children simply cannot. Rather, the safety issues that are of a more central concern to adolescents in the child welfare system are issues related to maintaining their own health, including addressing medical concerns, preventing homelessness, and avoiding violent victimization by partners or gangs (e.g., Keller et al., 2007). However, mental health needs typically emerge in adolescence as well, and addressing them requires access to proper behavioral health professionals and community-based services that are not a primary focus for younger children in the child welfare system.

The needs of adolescents are associated with the challenge of making a successful transition to adulthood rather than the paramount need for a stable and permanent family placement. Their need for family connections and supportive adults continues even after adults are no longer legally "responsible" for supporting or protecting them. There is nothing magical about age 18 or even age 21 as a marker of adulthood, and few children outside the child welfare system are expected to be "independent" once they reach the age of majority. At the same time, the successful transition to adulthood does require that older youth have experience with making their own decisions that are developmentally appropriate.

There is no clear metric or measure of "well-being" that can be used across counties and states to determine whether the child welfare system is effective in improving youth well-being. However, it is clear that the definition of well-being as an outcome measure has to be adapted to the evolving developmental needs of welfare-involved youth as they mature from infancy to childhood to adolescence. For adolescents, well-being includes having family and supportive adults available for love and guidance, having self-efficacy and confidence, having a sense of meaning and purpose, overcoming distress or dysfunction from mental health problems that might have resulted from earlier trauma and maltreatment, achieving educational success, and making healthy decisions around their own substance use and sexual behaviors. Metrics such as those would be very different from the ones used in monitoring early childhood development, and the child welfare system has not established them as developmentally appropriate metrics of well-being.

Given the cognitive, social, and emotional skills of adolescents, our society is missing an opportunity to nurture well-being in adolescents when the child welfare system does not fully incorporate their more advanced developmental needs and abilities into its aims and methods. Fortunately, the major federal statutory changes that have been mandated and implemented in the past 20 years have begun to make headway in this area, although much more needs to be done, and implementation at the local level is far from consistent. Four such federal statutory changes are summarized next.

Recent Congressional Initiatives Focusing on the Needs of Adolescents

Fortunately, recent federal statutory initiatives aimed at addressing the needs, skills, and assets of adolescents in foster care have filled some of the gaps in a system originally designed for younger children. These adolescent-specific provisions include provisions authorizing assistance and support in developing a transition plan that is personalized at the direction of the child (Fostering Connections to Success and Increasing Adoptions Act of 2008), facilitating age-appropriate experiences for adolescents (Preventing Sex Trafficking and Strengthening Families Act of 2014), permitting federal support for youth to age 23 through a range of services, including housing (called "Chafee services"), and permitting states to provide eligibility for education and training vouchers to age 26 (Family First Prevention Services Act of 2018). These legislative initiatives are generally aligned with the developmental capacities and needs of adolescents while recognizing that adolescents continue to need protection and stability.

When implemented successfully, these statutory improvements can help support adolescents in learning skills such as how to secure and maintain employment, handle finances, and independently navigate social systems such as health and mental health care, education, and housing support. Adolescents' ability to navigate social media and the internet can be an asset in this regard, helping them to locate housing, education, and health and mental health care options if proper data are provided to them and resources are available in the community. In addition, given their increased cognitive and social skills, adolescents are capable of being active participants in their own permanency decisions—something that younger children cannot do, at least not to the same extent.

The Foster Care Independence Act of 1999

In its statutory "findings" written into the Foster Care Independence Act of 1999, also known as the "Chafee Act" (creating the John H. Chafee Foster Care Independence Program), Congress emphasized its concern for this vulnerable group of former children in foster care:

(1) States are required to make reasonable efforts to find adoptive families for all children, including older children, for whom reunification with their biological family is not in the best interests of the child. However, some older children will continue to live in foster care. These children should be enrolled in an Independent Living program designed and conducted by State and local government to help prepare them for employment, postsecondary education, and successful management of adult responsibilities.

(2) Older children who continue to be in foster care as adolescents may become eligible for Independent Living programs. These Independent Living programs are not alternative to adoption for these children. Enrollment in Independent Living programs can occur concurrent with continued efforts to locate and achieve placement in adoptive families for older children in foster care.

(3) About 20,000 adolescents leave the Nation's foster care system each year because they have reached 18 years of age and are expected to support themselves.

(4) Congress has received extensive information that adolescents leaving foster care have significant difficulty making a successful transition to adulthood; this information shows that children aging out of foster care show high rates of homelessness, non-marital childbearing, poverty, and delinquent or criminal behavior; they are also frequently the target of crime and physical assaults.

(5) The Nation's State and local governments, with financial support from the Federal Government, should offer an extensive program of education, training, employment, and financial support for young adults leaving foster care, with participation in such program beginning several years before high school graduation and continuing, as needed, until the young adults emancipated from foster care establish independence or reach 21 years of age.[6]

---

[6]Pub. L. 106–169, § 101(a)(1)-(5).

Congress's decision to allow states to extend care to age 21, launched nearly 20 years ago, marked a critical first step in recognizing the particular developmental needs of adolescents by mandating programming to support independent living skills of older children and adolescents in foster care as they strive for self-sufficiency often referred to as "Chafee services." As noted below, the intent of these provisions has evolved in subsequent legislative mandates to recognize the interest of adolescents in acquiring the experiences they need for a successful transition to adulthood while maintaining connections to loving and supportive adults.

The Fostering Connections to Success and Increasing Adoptions Act of 2008

Approximately 10 years after the foregoing law was passed, a second law was enacted that provided additional supports for adolescents and young adults in foster care and recognized their more advanced cognitive abilities and needs, relative to younger children, as well as their employment needs. The Fostering Connections to Success and Increasing Adoptions Act of 2008 permits states to elect to continue federally supported foster care assistance to youth up to age 21 if the youth are in school, working, or meet other requirements. In addition, at least 90 days before a youth reaches age 18 (or up to age 21 if the state has chosen to extend foster care), the state must "provide the child with assistance and support in developing a transition plan that is personalized at the direction of the child, includes specific options on housing, health insurance, education, local opportunities for mentors and continuing support services, and work force supports and employment services and is as detailed as the child may elect."[7]

Recognizing that "independent living" is not a realistic goal for many young adults, Congress adjusted the goal for youth exiting care as "Another Planned Permanent Living Arrangement" (AAPLA) or "Other Planned Permanent Living Arrangement" (OPPLA). This change recognizes that adolescents at age 18 or even 21 are not "independent" and is consistent with the large body of developmental research that highlights the growth in autonomy-seeking and decision-making capacities of adolescents, while recognizing that adolescents in foster care need loving and supportive adults and continue to have specific and substantial educational and health/health care needs that the child welfare system can address.

---

[7]Pub. L. 110–351, § 202; 42 U.S.C. § 675(5)(H). (The committee is unaware of any data on the quality and efficacy of the provisions states provide youth within the last 90 days of leaving foster care.)

The Preventing Sex Trafficking and Strengthening Families Act of 2014

A third legislative change in the child welfare system was the Preventing Sex Trafficking and Strengthening Families Act of 2014. This act recognized that "typical adolescent experiences" are important stepping stones to a successful transition to adulthood (e.g., going to a friend's house, attending prom, taking a school trip, traveling with a sports team or participating in clubs, driving, and part-time employment). Participation in experiences such as these help adolescents develop interests, skills, and supportive and lasting relationships. However, because of real and perceived constraints, foster youth are often denied the chance to partake in these activities, which are important for their successful transition to adulthood. Consequently, the social and professional growth of youth as they age out of foster care may in turn be limited, thus leaving them ill-prepared and potentially vulnerable to experiencing negative outcomes, such as homelessness, unemployment, and poverty. One reason for these poorer life outcomes may be their lack of "normal" adolescent experiences (although research is needed to rigorously test this potential linkage).

The 2014 law promotes well-being and normalcy for youth in the foster care system by directing contracted providers, state child welfare agencies, and courts to facilitate experiences that are age- and developmentally appropriate and that support normalcy and promote permanency, particularly for those youth who are most likely to remain in foster care until age 18. The law establishes a "reasonable and prudent parent" standard for youth participation in activities, and thereby protects foster parents from liability so long as this "reasonable and prudent parent" standard is satisfied. As with the previous legal changes, the 2014 law recognized the differential challenges and opportunities for adolescents in the child welfare system, relative to young children, and aimed to support their healthy social development in the foster care system.

The 2018 Family First Prevention Services Act (FFPSA)

Most recently, Congress recognized the developmental challenges and needs faced by older adolescents in the foster care system with the Family First Prevention Services Act (FFPSA) of 2018. For many years, researchers, child advocates, and an increasing number of state and local policy makers have been focused on reducing the number of children in group care and expanding access to family-based placements. FFPSA represents the first major contribution to this effort at the federal level, restricting federal funding to most group care settings and imposing robust requirements on the limited group care settings that can continue to draw down federal dollars.

Both before and after the passage of FFPSA, Title IV-E funds could be used to fund placements in a "family foster home," defined as a home with 24-hour care for six or fewer children (with some exceptions), or a "child care institution," defined as an institution for up to 25 children that is not a detention center.[8] Under FFPSA, a child's Title IV-E eligibility ends after 2 weeks of placement in a child care institution. Thus, placements in settings with more than six children lasting longer than 2 weeks generally are ineligible for federal funding once these provisions go into effect in each state.

FFPSA created several exceptions to this funding restriction to meet the needs of older youth and youth with special needs, consistent with adolescents' developmental skills and the tasks that they face in child welfare, in particular their emerging capacity to be self-sufficient. First, the act permits federal reimbursement for supervised independent living placements for youth ages 18 and older, allowing states with extended foster care to continue to offer an array of developmentally appropriate placements. It also exempts group care settings providing "high-quality residential care and supportive services" to youth who have been or are at risk of being victims of sex trafficking.[9] Specialized settings for pregnant and parenting youth also retain Title IV-E eligibility beyond the 2-week cutoff.[10]

In addition to these exceptions, FFPSA created an entirely new placement type—Qualified Residential Treatment Programs—not subject to the 2-week cap.[11] These programs must be designed to accommodate children with serious emotional or behavioral disorders, use a trauma-informed treatment model, incorporate family members proactively, and provide discharge planning and aftercare, among other requirements. The statute also provides that, prior to placement in a Qualified Residential Treatment Program, a child must receive an individualized assessment to identify his or her strengths and needs and to determine whether placement is consistent with his or her short- and long-term goals.

There is concern that limiting congregate care in the child welfare system may push more youth into the juvenile justice system or encourage overdiagnosis of behavioral health conditions in order to meet the congregate care exception. The 2018 statute attempted to avoid these potential pitfalls by requiring states to provide an "assurance of nonimpact on the juvenile justice system" and by imposing protocols to prevent inappropriate diagnoses.[12]

---

[8] Facilities that house more than 25 children are not eligible for federal Title IV-E reimbursement. See https://www.acf.hhs.gov/sites/default/files/cb/title_iv_e_review_guide.pdf.

[9] FFPSA § 50741(a)(2)(D).

[10] FFPSA § 50741(a)(2)(B).

[11] FFPSA § 50741(a)(2)(A).

[12] FFPSA § 50741(d); 50743.

FFPSA directly impacts older adolescents, who are overrepresented in group care, by increasing the capacity of systems to support their successful transition to adulthood through modifications to the Chafee Foster Care Independence Program. First, by changing the name to the Chafee Successful Transition to Adulthood, the law recognized that support should be provided to help youth transition to *adulthood*, rather than overemphasizing "independence." As described in Chapter 2, the latest adolescent brain development research shows that the developmental period from adolescence through emerging adulthood features the creation of new neural pathways and the enhancement of connections between brain systems and neural networks. This period of growth provides one of the greatest opportunities for the brain to heal from past maltreatment and trauma. For adolescents in the child welfare system, attaining independence gradually while maintaining connections to loving and supportive adults is key to maximizing the opportunities for brain development and resilience, increasing autonomy within a safe nurturing environment.

FFPSA provides states with extended foster care programs the option to extend Chafee supports and services to youth until age 23, and it extends eligibility for education and training vouchers to age 26.[13] The education and training vouchers have a 5-year time limit, but this time does not have to be used consecutively. However, only 25 states and the District of Columbia currently offer extended foster care to youth over age 18 (National Conference of State Legislatures, 2017). Given the growing body of research on poor outcomes for older youth, FFPSA requires a report on the experiences and outcomes of older youth in care by October 2019 based upon the National Youth in Transitions database.[14]

Finally, agencies are now required to provide youth who have aged out with official documentation showing they were previously in care. This allows young adults to establish eligibility for special categories of benefits targeted at former foster youth, including Medicaid and financial aid for postsecondary education and training. Under the Affordable Care Act (ACA), if an adolescent previously received Medicaid while in foster care and remained in foster care until at least age 18, he or she will continue to be eligible for Medicaid until age 26. However, the ACA does not require states to continue Medicaid benefits for foster care youth over the age of 18 if they lived in a different state while in foster care.

---

[13] FFPSA § 50753. Also see Juvenile Law Center, "Extended Foster Care," at https://jlc.org/issues/extended-foster-care.
[14] FFPSA § 50753.

An Unfinished Policy Transition

Taken together, these four statutes provide a suite of developmentally appropriate supports and legal provisions to help adolescents flourish and successfully transition to adulthood. However, despite the recent changes, many of these provisions are optional or are not implemented comprehensively in every jurisdiction in a state, or both (Juvenile Law Center, 2018b). As a result, society is missing an opportunity to help launch child welfare-involved youth into adulthood with sufficient skills, resources, and the connections to loving and supportive adults that all adolescents need to become productive, healthy, and thriving members of our society. The child welfare system has not changed sufficiently, and as a result, youth still want to exit the system before the maximum age of services in their state or do not receive the comprehensive, individualized service array that they need to successfully launch to adulthood.

As is described in the remaining sections of this chapter, additional system-level changes and broader uptake of the optional components of recent laws would further promote resilience and positive outcomes for adolescents involved in the child welfare system. To contextualize a blueprint for a future child welfare system that effectively supports the healthy development of adolescents, next we provide a brief review of the skills and capacities of adolescents in child welfare, alongside a description of the challenges they face and promising solutions.

DEVELOPMENTAL RESEARCH ON ADOLESCENTS IN THE CHILD WELFARE SYSTEM: CHALLENGES AND PROMISING SOLUTIONS

The known effects of maltreatment and trauma on the developing brain (see Chapter 3), together with the opportunity for recovery created by the development of new brain pathways and structural changes during adolescence, represent a challenge for the child welfare system that recent changes in federal law are helping to address. In this section, we present an overview of the challenges and promising solutions across multiple domains, including mental health, education, and placement permanency, and conclude with a section on common elements of evidence-based programs shown to improve the health and well-being of adolescents in the child welfare system.

Mental Health Challenges and Promising Solutions

As a result of the psychological impacts of abuse and neglect, as well as their impacts on the brain and other body systems (see Chapter 3), it is not surprising that adolescents who have been in the child welfare system have elevated mental health symptoms. In fact, mental health is perhaps the most widely studied outcome for adolescents in the child welfare system.

The National Survey of Child and Adolescent Well-Being (NSCAW), a landmark study that documented mental health outcomes for youth in the child welfare system over a 17-year period, provides compelling evidence of elevated mental health symptoms among youth with child-welfare system involvement in the United States. The NSCAW made use of a nationally representative sample of more than 6,000 children and families who were studied by public child protective services programs in the United States between 1997 and 2014. The information collected was gathered from youth, their parents, other caregivers, caseworkers, teachers, and administrative records. The resulting dataset has made possible a large number of technical reports and peer-reviewed publications to date (Institute of Medicine and National Research Council, 2014).

Analyses using the NSCAW dataset indicate that emotional and behavioral problems are present in more than 50 percent of the children in the sample (Burns et al., 2004). Specifically, for adolescents ages 11 to 14, the prevalence of clinical-level mental health symptoms was 65.7 percent (versus 46.8% for 6–10-year-olds and 32.3% for 2–5-year-olds). Numerous other publications using the NSCAW dataset have documented the prevalence of specific mental health problems in adolescents with child welfare system involvement (e.g., Orton et al., 2009; Southerland et al., 2009).

The findings from the NSCAW study are consistent with those from other studies that have found elevated mental health problems for adolescents in the child welfare system. Using a sample of adolescents ages 12 to 17 in the public-use file of the 2000 National Household Survey on Drug Abuse (n = 19,430, including 464 adolescents with a history of foster care placement), Pilowsky and Wu (2006) found that adolescents involved with foster care had a higher rate than other adolescents of past-year psychiatric symptoms. In particular, adolescents involved in foster care had more disruptive behavior disorder symptoms, suicide ideation and suicide attempts, and depression and anxiety symptoms, as well as more past-year substance use disorders, than those never placed in foster care. Conversely, some studies have found no differences between clinical-level depression for youth entering foster care and published norms, as measured in the Children's Depression Inventory for children between ages 8 and 16 (Allen et al., 2000).

In terms of criminal offenses, arrests of adolescents ages 18 to 21 in foster care occurred at more than four times the national rate for individuals ages 18 to 24 (RTI International, 2008). Similarly, between the ages of 17 and 24, 46 percent of former foster youth tracked in the NSCAW experienced at least one arrest; these arrests were evenly distributed across drug, nonviolent, and violent crimes (Cusick et al., 2012).

The negative mental health outcomes experienced by adolescents with a history of involvement in the child welfare system often extend to the next generation. Females exiting foster care are at heightened risk for multiple pregnancies (relative to their age-matched female counterparts), and they are also at higher risk than their male counterparts exiting foster care of maltreating their own children (Dworsky and DeCoursey, 2009; Kerr et al., 2009; Leve et al., 2013). The heightened rates of parenting for females exiting foster care (relative to their male counterparts) may play a role in the apparent sex difference in maltreatment rates. Caution is warranted in making conclusions about sex differences in maltreatment rates, however, because mothers more often retain custody of their child as compared to fathers. It is also important to consider that, although adolescents with child welfare system involvement have higher rates of mental health problems, this does not mean that the child welfare system causes mental health problems. As discussed earlier in this chapter, it is highly likely that many of these young people had mental health problems when they entered care due to the maltreatment and trauma they experienced earlier in life and the associated impacts on neurobiological and socio-emotional development.

The aforementioned studies document the significant need for mental health services for adolescents of all ages in the child welfare system, as well as a need for enhanced health literacy. Unfortunately, among early adolescent youth in the child welfare system, being Black and living at home significantly reduced the likelihood of receiving mental health services (Burns et al., 2004). This might reflect the stigma often associated with help-seeking behaviors, as well as underlying biases in the delivery of effective mental health services to all youth, regardless of race, income, or ethnicity. A study of differences in mental health service use among Latinx, Black, and White youth ages 17 and older in foster care examined their rates of mental health service use both while in foster care and upon exit from the foster care system, and found that Latinx youth had the lowest rate of service use before and after foster care exit (Villagrana, 2017). Specifically, Latinx youth were slightly less likely to use mental health services (33.9% of them using it) than Black (35%) and White (39.9%) youth while in foster care, and were also the least likely to use mental health services (41%) upon exit from foster care as compared to Black (50%) and White youth (50%).

However, Villegas and Pecora (2012) found that the race and ethnicity of foster families and children were less predictive in determining mental health outcomes or the need for mental health services later in life. Factors such as gender, age of entrance into foster care, number of placements, and maltreatment (prior to and while in foster care) were predictive of future mental health service needs. There is, however, a lack of data on this topic. Given that racial and ethnic minorities account for a significant portion of all children in the child welfare system, additional research is needed.

Despite the documentation of poorer mental health and increased behavior problems for adolescents who have been in the child welfare system, as well as disparities in access to services and outcomes, a range of interventions and programs have shown positive results. This suggests that resiliency is possible during adolescence when the right supports and services are provided. In their systematic review of interventions for foster and kinship families, Dickes and colleagues (2018) identified 17 unique studies of psychosocial interventions for this population, delivered between 1992 and 2015. The selection of these studies required that they all have been published in peer-reviewed journals, had more than 20 participants, and used a quasi-random or random allocation of participants to control for experimental conditions.

More than one-half (10) of the included studies in the review by Dickes and colleagues focused on adolescents who were between ages 9 and 18. The most common aim of the intervention across studies was to improve youth behavior outcomes, including their mental health. In fact, 88 percent of the studies reported improvements in behavior problems for youth in the intervention condition, whose problems ranged from externalizing behavior to aggression, oppositional behavior, and substance use. For example, the Middle School Success Program, an intervention for girls in foster care delivered across 9 months during the transition to middle school that included youth skill development and parenting support groups, resulted in increases in prosocial behavior, which led to reductions in externalizing and internalizing symptoms, which in turn led to reduced substance use 3 years later (Kim and Leve, 2011).

Another successful program, the Fostering Healthy Futures (FHF) intervention, combined one-on-one mentoring with therapeutic skills groups to promote well-being of foster youth ages 9 to 11 with a history of maltreatment by identifying and addressing mental health needs as well as preventing risk-taking and promoting competence and improve the overall well-being. The intervention was delivered over 30 weeks during the school year. Further, immediately following the intervention, FHF participants reported an improved quality of life, followed by a reduction in mental health therapy 6 months post-intervention (Taussig and Culhane, 2010).

Educational Challenges and Promising Solutions

Adolescents involved in the child welfare system often show worse educational outcomes than other adolescents; challenges related to educational disruptions, course credit transfer, lack of appropriate school placement and services, and transitions to higher education are commonplace. A study using the NSCAW data showed that connections to employment and education were associated with a lower risk for arrest (Cusick et al., 2012), suggesting a potential opportunity for child welfare policy and practice to improve outcomes for adolescents in care by promoting employment and education success.

Further, research suggests that educational challenges can continue to be a problem for youth when they leave the child welfare system. One study of pregnant or parenting foster care alumni in Chicago, for example, found that only 44 percent of females and 27 percent of males possessed a high school diploma or equivalent when they exited care (Dworsky and DeCoursey, 2009). More recently, a study of more than 600 youth in foster care indicated that 71 percent of youth had attained a high school credential by age 19, and half of foster youth had enrolled in a college (the vast majority of which were 2-year colleges) by age 19 or 20 (Okpych et al., 2017). Some of the predictors of high school completion were residing in rural or suburban counties (as compared to urban counties), completing 11th grade, reading proficiency, a lack of substance use problems, and a lack of prior sexual abuse.

Importantly, a study of foster youth's and their child welfare workers' perceptions of the youth's educational preparedness at age 19 found that one-half of the sample had enrolled in college by age 20, with enrollment in 2-year colleges being more common than enrollment in 4-year colleges (Torres-Garcia et al., 2019). Further, caseworkers' perceptions of the youth's educational readiness significantly predicted their odds of entering college by age 20, suggesting a potential opportunity for caseworkers to help advise youth in terms of selecting a college or career option that best matches their skills and interests.

Because educational attainment continues to be a significant factor in obtaining successful employment, adolescents aging out of the foster care system are ill-equipped to compete. Westat Inc. (1991), the largest study, found that 51 percent of former foster care youth were unemployed 2.5 to 4 years after they had transitioned out of care, and 62 percent were not able to maintain a job for a full year. According to Courtney and Piliavin (1998), 39 percent of former foster care youth were not employed within 1 to 1.5 years after aging out of the system. Barth (1990) found that 25 percent were unemployed 1 to 10 years after leaving foster care.

However, there is hope in the child welfare system's ability to turn these educational trajectories around, including by supporting youth in foster care to attend school and complete homework. For example, Treatment Foster Care Oregon is a program delivered to adolescents with a history of serious juvenile delinquency who are placed in out-of-home care by the juvenile justice system (Chamberlain, 2003). It includes a focus on school engagement by supporting youth to complete 30 minutes of homework each day and through use of a school report card whereby each teacher indicates the student's homework and assignments for the day, which is shared with the youth's foster parent, to increase parental knowledge and engagement in the youth's education. One study of this program found that the intervention had protective educational effects for girls ages 13 to 17; it increased school attendance and homework completion, which then reduced subsequent juvenile justice involvement as measured by days spent in locked settings (Leve and Chamberlain, 2007).

A second program, the Better Futures model, also showed potential educational benefit for older adolescents in foster care. This program is focused on improving postsecondary preparation and participation for youth in foster care with mental health challenges. In a small randomized controlled trial, 67 adolescents were assigned to participate in a Summer Institute, individual peer coaching, and mentoring workshops. Researchers found that, compared to the control group, adolescents in the intervention group had greater rates of improvement in postsecondary participation, postsecondary and transition preparation, hope, self-determination, and mental health empowerment. They also showed positive trends in the areas of mental health recovery, quality of life, and high school completion (Greenen et al., 2015).

These programs and the encouraging body of evidence on their effects provide great hope for improving educational outcomes for adolescents in the child welfare system, particularly when combined with the policy changes described above pertaining to the extension to age 26 of education and training vouchers for child welfare-involved youth.

Placement Permanency and Aging Out of Care: Challenges and Promising Solutions

As noted earlier, one of the primary goals of the child welfare system is to keep children safely at home or else reunify them promptly, either with their biological family, their kin or, if necessary, with new supportive, loving adults. The goal is to ensure a permanent home and caregiving solution for youth who have entered the child welfare system. This section discusses challenges and promising solutions to placement permanency as well as necessary supports for adolescents aging out of care without a permanent placement. Importantly, youth who have been involved in the foster care system emphasize the importance of including system-involved youth in permanency planning as well as the need to identify, initiate, and maintain supportive relationships with adults. (These youth perspectives appear in Box 8-2.)

BOX 8-2
Youth Perspectives: Permanency Planning and
Relationships with Supportive Adults

Youth Fostering Change (YFC) is an advocacy program for youth who are currently or formerly involved in the child welfare system. YFC youth, in discussing the need to engage youth in permanency planning meetings and dependency court hearings reported that in their experience:

- Meetings were scheduled without our consideration.
- There were a lot of meetings, and we sometimes had to miss school to attend.
- The meeting's purpose was not always clearly explained to us.
- No prep from our team before the meetings, so we could not meaningfully participate.
- Transportation was not reliable or available for us to get to the meetings.
- The meeting outcomes didn't reflect what we want or need.
- We did not know who would attend, and this affected our willingness to participate. (Juvenile Law Center, 2018a, p. 10)

YFC participants also stated the importance of identifying, initiating, and maintaining relationships with supportive adults and kin. In recounting their experiences in the foster care system, YFC youth reported:

- We lost connections with supportive adults who were in our lives before care.
- Constantly moving placements caused us to lose contact or limited our ability to build lasting relationships.
- We struggled to build and maintain connections with supportive adults due to mistrusting others because of our experiences.
- We did not get the emotional or logistical support to connect to supportive adults.
- We did not always know who the supportive adults were in our lives or how they could help us.
- We aged out of care without any supportive adult connections.
- When we had help building and maintaining connections with supportive adults, it helped us grow and created opportunities for us. (Juvenile Law Center, 2018a, p. 16)

Placement Permanency

A two-pronged approach would support the goal of permanency for adolescents in the system: including effective supports for child welfare-involved parents with an open case in order to prevent an episode of maltreatment; and providing intervention services once documented maltreatment has occurred and a child is removed from the home. Distressingly, within 12 to 24 months of initial placement, approximately one-third to two-thirds of foster placements fail (Wulczyn et al., 2007). In addition to youth problem behavior, other factors, such as the age at placement, history of residential treatment, and number of prior placements, are predictive of placement failure (Oosterman et al., 2007). Similarly, Fisher and colleagues (2005) found that placement instability gives rise to further instability.

Placement transitions in foster care can also result from bureaucratic, administrative, and policy-led decisions. These can include changes in county contracts with foster care providers, as well as (for a child already in foster care) the subsequent removal from the birth parents of a sibling, which necessitates a new move for the previously placed sibling whose placement cannot accommodate the additional sibling. Moreover, even positive changes, such as reunification with birth parents or adoption, represent caregiver transitions that can be stressful. Thus, by the time a child reaches adolescence, if he or she remains involved in the child welfare system, there is a high likelihood that he or she will have experienced prior failed placements and have had multiple caregivers during childhood.

Regardless of the cause, caregiver transitions have the potential to compromise typical development, which can have sustained effects into adolescence and beyond. For example, when Rubin and colleagues (2007) studied placement instability among NSCAW children, they found that more than 25 percent did not achieve stable placement (rather than multiple placements or a temporary placement) within 18 months in out-of-home care. Placement instability was associated with a 63 percent rise in problem behaviors. Chamberlain and colleagues (2006) also found an association between problem behaviors in youth ages 5 to 12 and placement disruptions.

Although the evidence is clear that having multiple caregiver transitions, placement disruptions, and multiple home placements is harmful to the developing child, there is research evidence that interventions and programs from early childhood to adolescence can reduce the number of placement transitions a child experiences, thus promoting well-being for adolescents with a history of child welfare system involvement. In early childhood, the Multidimensional Treatment Foster Care for Preschoolers Program (TFCO-P) uses a behavior-management approach to train, supervise, and support foster caregivers to provide positive adult support and consistent limit setting through weekly parenting groups, individual therapy, family therapy, and 24/7 on-call support for 6 to 9 months. This program has been shown to improve placement stability across a 2-year period and mitigate the effect of multiple placements on later placement failures (Fisher et al., 2005).

In early adolescence, the KEEP-SAFE intervention showed a similar positive effect on improving placement stability. In a randomized controlled trial of 700 children ages 5 to 12 in the KEEP-SAFE Program, caregivers were assigned to either regular foster care services or the KEEP-SAFE parenting intervention (Chamberlain et al., 2008). The KEEP-SAFE intervention included 16 weeks of caregiver training focused on supervision and applying behavior management strategies. Like TFCO-P, KEEP-SAFE was found to improve placement stability and mitigate the risks often associated with mitigating the risk-prior multiple placements (Price et al., 2008). Further, adolescents in the intervention group were more likely to be either reunified with their biological parents or permanently placed with relatives or an adoptive family within the first year of placement.

Finally, in the Middle School Success study described earlier, the intervention resulted in fewer placement changes at a 12-month follow-up for middle school-age girls relative to children in a foster care as-usual condition (Kim and Leve, 2011). Thus, there is great potential to improve placement stability during early childhood and into adolescence for youth in the child welfare system, and ameliorate the negative behavioral and educational effects that are often associated with transitions in child welfare placements. Nonetheless, despite the positive effect of these intervention programs on placement permanency, most children are still not in permanent placements—that is, adopted or reunified—within 1 year of placement in foster care.

Aging Out of Care

For older adolescents in the child welfare system, "placement permanency" takes on a different meaning. Many foster youth who age out of care suddenly are often left without supportive family relationships and important life skills, which can result in negative outcomes that continue into adulthood: they are at high risk of becoming homeless after turning 18 and are less likely than other youth to graduate from high school, go to college, or get a job. The Jim Casey Youth Opportunities Initiative estimates that the lifetime social cost to taxpayers and communities is $300,000 for every youth who ages out of the system (Annie E. Casey Foundation, 2013).

This problem is compounded by the increasing number of youth aging out of foster care. Each year, more than 20,000 youth age out of foster care and lose their system of support overnight (U.S. Department of Health and Human Services, 2015). The John H. Chafee Foster Care program for successful transition to adulthood reports that in fiscal year 2017, 19,000 youth aged out of care. In addition, the percentage of exits due to aging out increased, from 7 percent in 2000 to 10 percent in 2012. Promoting normalcy (consistent with the 2018 FFPSA) has the potential to improve this trend in two ways: it can increase the opportunities to achieve permanency as well as improve a youth's readiness to leave the system as a young adult who is prepared for adulthood and connected to supportive and loving adults.

Studies of children who have aged out of foster care are scarce, but findings are consistently disturbing. For example, in a representative sample of foster youth in California, over one-third of aged-out 19-year-olds experienced homelessness and more than 40 percent couch-surfed (Courtney et al., 2016). In Washington State, analysis of administrative data showed that 28 percent of youth experienced a homeless episode within 12 months of aging out of foster care. Further, not all youth were equally vulnerable to homelessness; youth who were Black, had experienced prior housing instability, or were parents were at the highest risk of homelessness (Shah et al., 2016). A systematic review of the intersection between foster care involvement and homelessness found that most studies focus on either foster care or homelessness, rather than examining overlapping needs (Zlotnick et al., 2012).

According to Westat (1991), 25 percent of foster care alumni have experienced homelessness for one or more nights. Further, a study by Courtney and Piliavin (1998) found that 27 percent of men and 10 percent of women had been incarcerated one or more times within 12 to 18 months of leaving foster care. Another study by Barth (1990) showed that 35 percent of foster care alumni have experienced homelessness or housing instability. This study also found that 35 percent of foster care alumni have spent time in jail or prison.

A study with the NSCAW data emphasized the important role families play in encouraging housing stability, while critiquing the child welfare system's current focus on preparing foster youth for independent living (Fowler et al., 2017). In that study, youth reported on their experiences of housing problems at 18- and 36-month follow-ups. The data indicate that adolescents who reunited with their families after being placed in out-of-home care were less likely to experience homelessness, while youth who aged out of care experienced similar rates of homelessness as youth investigated by child welfare but who were never placed outside their homes. Exposure to independent living services and extended foster care was not predictive of homelessness prevention, but reunification with family had a positive effect.

Teenage girls in foster care are twice as likely to be parents by age 19 as non-foster care teens (17.2% to 8.2%) (Stotland and Godsoe, 2006). These teen mothers are also even more at risk of homelessness than other children in foster care when they age out:

> The vast majority of such women are unmarried and receive little or no support from their children's fathers, who tend to be poor themselves. Friends and relatives who have a spare couch for one person may balk when that person brings along a toddler and a crying baby. Landlords who rent individual rooms and studios prefer single tenants to those with

children. The cost of basic necessities for their children, such as diapers and baby formula, drains away what little income former wards may have to pay for housing.

> Most disturbingly, examining the connection between homelessness and foster care reveals a generational cycle of foster care placement. Homeless parents in New York City who grew up in foster care are almost twice as likely as parents without such a history to have their children placed in the system. Similarly, a nationwide survey of homeless families in shelters showed that 77 percent of parents with a foster care history had at least one child who was or had been in foster care, as compared with 27 percent of parents without such a history. (Stotland and Godsoe, 2006, p. 55)

Many young people are emancipated from foster care to "independent" living. There is a natural push toward independence during adolescence and emerging adulthood; however, prioritizing *interdependence* and connecting young people with a consistent and supportive network are vital to healthy development. In a mixed-methods study, where data were collected from 404 youth transitioning from foster care who were interviewed nine times between ages 17 and 19, McCoy and colleagues (2008) found that youth, especially those with externalizing behavior problems, left their foster care placements before required—typically abruptly and because they were dissatisfied with their experiences within the foster care system. While some returned to the homes of their biological families, those that chose to remain in the system often lived in their own apartments.

Young people who are ready to live on their own need a range of housing options that can help them move toward independence in settings that support their needs and connect them with a network of family, mentors, and supportive peers. Supportive caregivers and social workers can help adolescents by providing advice on choosing safe and stable housing. Similarly, housing managers can help adolescents by creating materials that outline resident responsibilities using multiple communication platforms that are easily accessible.

A qualitative study that included focus groups with older adolescents in foster care echoed the potential value of connecting youth considering emancipation with supportive, non-parental adults from within the adolescent's existing social system (Greeson et al., 2015). In that study, coded transcriptions on the focus groups suggested that these young people were cautiously optimistic about the potential of child welfare-based natural mentoring interventions (using relationships within their existing social network) to promote their social and emotional well-being.

Overall, these findings highlight the developmental importance of families and supportive caregivers in promoting housing stability in the transition to adulthood, while also indicating that fundamental improvements are needed in the approaches the child welfare system is using to provide foster youth with the skills they need to secure housing and employment or education as they exit adolescence and enter young adulthood.

FLOURISHING FOR CHILD WELFARE-INVOLVED ADOLESCENTS

As indicated by the research reviewed above and elsewhere in this report, the evidence is clear that the experience of maltreatment during childhood can have lasting effects on the developing brain and behavior systems and can also precipitate instability in caregiving and family relationships. It is equally clear, however, that adolescence can be a period of resilience. The right supports and interventions for youth currently or previously involved in the child welfare system can help change the life trajectory for a child welfare system-involved adolescent.

A number of reviews have been conducted over the past decade that describe effective interventions for youth who have been involved in the child welfare system (see Dickes et al., 2018; Fisher et al., 2016; Leve et al., 2012). Most recently, a meta-analysis was conducted to identify effective components of maltreatment interventions (van der Put et al., 2018), and a systematic review was conducted of effective program components of psychosocial interventions for youth in foster or kinship care (Kemmis-Riggs, et al., 2018). Together, these last two reviews suggest a set of core supports that can be beneficial in improving outcomes for youth in the child welfare system.

To examine interventions aimed at preventing or reducing child maltreatment, van der Put and colleagues' (2018) literature search yielded 121 independent studies (N = 39,044). From these studies, 352 effect sizes were extracted (most studies examined more than one outcome). The overall effect size was significant, suggesting intervention benefits, although it was small in magnitude for both preventive interventions (d = 0.26, p < .001) and curative interventions (d = 0.36, p < .001). The most effective approaches and techniques included cognitive behavioral therapy, home visitation, parent training, family-based/multisystemic interventions, and substance abuse prevention.

Preventive interventions found larger effect sizes with short-term interventions (0–6 months), interventions aimed at increasing parental self-confidence, and professionally delivered interventions. Increased follow-up duration was also a factor in increased effect sizes, indicating that the positive effects of preventive interventions often appear later in development, possibly due to brain plasticity during adolescence. Larger effect sizes were found in curative interventions that sought to improve parenting skills and increase access to social and/or emotional support.

To examine interventions focused on youth in foster care, a systematic review was conducted to examine the components in foster and kinship care interventions, with the aim of exploring their potential benefits to youth and caregiver well-being. Seventeen studies published between 1990 and 2016 and describing 14 interventions were identified that each used a randomized or quasi-randomized trial focused on psychosocial outcomes for youth in foster care (Kemmis-Riggs et al., 2018). Effective interventions often included aims that were clearly defined, targeted domains and developmental stages, coaching, and role play. Further, interventions that were developed to reduce the effects of maltreatment and relationship disruption were often found to be successful. Behavioral problems were often successfully addressed by interventions that provided consistent discipline coupled with positive reinforcement, trauma psychoeducation, and skills development (e.g., problem solving). Parent–child relationships were often improved through interventions that aimed to develop empathy, sensitivity, and parental responses attuned to adolescent's needs. Together, these recent meta-analysis and research review studies suggest that there are both specific programs and more general attributes of programs that can help adolescents in the child welfare system thrive.

RECOMMENDATIONS

A challenge for the child welfare system is to extend the knowledge acquired from individual programs and program components to implement system-level change. In order to do so, the committee outlines below recommendations for improving the child welfare system to better support the process and outcomes of adolescent development. These recommendations center on adolescents within the child welfare system as needing services and supports that vary from their younger counterparts and as involved partners in decisions affecting their own housing, health/mental health, and education. Taken together, the recommendations constitute a blueprint for achieving an adolescent-oriented and developmentally appropriate child welfare system. Box 8-3 summarizes this blueprint for an adolescent-oriented and developmentally appropriate child welfare system. We next focus on the six recommendations of the blueprint and discuss them in turn.

RECOMMENDATION 8-1: Reduce racial and ethnic disparities in child welfare system involvement.

As described above, conditional on underlying risk, there is evidence that families of color are more likely to be referred to child protective services. Two proximate causes are the unequal provision of in-home preventative services and higher levels of surveillance for families of color. Thus, to

---

BOX 8-3
Blueprint for a Developmentally Informed
Child Welfare System for Adolescents

Recommendation 8-1: Reduce racial and ethnic disparities in child welfare system involvement.
   A. State and local departments of child welfare should implement policies and practices that ensure that families of color have access to the same levels of in-home preventative services as other at-risk families.
   B. State and local departments of child welfare should establish guidelines and protocols regarding appropriate levels of surveillance in communities to improve the overall efficiency and benefit of surveillance systems, a practice also expected to reduce disparities. Responsible agencies should actively monitor implementation of these guidelines.

Recommendation 8-2: Promote broad uptake by the states of federal programs that promote resilience and positive outcomes for adolescents involved in the child welfare system.
   A. All states should adopt the existing federal option to provide extended care to youth until age 21 and Chafee services to age 23 and provide comprehensive aftercare support to youth as they transition out of the child welfare system.
   B. All states should ensure that child welfare system-involved youth are eligible for education and training vouchers until they reach age 26 and should facilitate and support youths' application process.
   C. All states should ensure that youth who have experienced foster care are eligible for Medicaid until age 26.

Recommendation 8-3: Provide services to adolescents and their families in the child welfare system that are developmentally informed at the individual, program, and system levels.
   A. State and local departments of child welfare should implement policies and practices that incorporate a developmental approach to service provision and case management for adolescents with child welfare system involvement, prioritizing family connections and supportive adults, and taking maximum advantage of adolescents' increasing cognitive and social capacities.
   B. State and local departments of child welfare should adjust the type and structure of services and the level of adolescent involvement in decision making related to their housing, education, and services to best align with adolescents' developmental capabilities and needs.
   C. Recognizing the growing capacity of adolescents for self-direction, case managers and courts should ensure that adolescents have the opportunity to fully participate in developing and implementing their service and transition plans, while maintaining critical ties with caring adults. To this end, adolescents should be viewed as respected partners in decision making regarding their placements, education, and support services.

continued

BOX 8-3 Continued

Recommendation 8-4: Conduct research that reflects all types and ages of adolescents in the child welfare system.
   A. The federal government, state and local child welfare agencies, and philanthropic institutions should fund research on service characteristics and outcomes for the full range of adolescents in the child welfare system in order to better design and evaluate services specifically for adolescents, depending upon their age, child welfare system history, and placement situation.
   B. Individual and program successes identified through this research should be scaled to system-level change for adolescents in the child welfare system.

Recommendation 8-5: Foster greater collaboration between the child welfare, juvenile justice, education, and health systems.
   A. Child welfare, juvenile justice, education, and health agencies should collaborate to create an integrated data system that links information to track, evaluate, and provide an effective and integrated set of services to adolescents across these systems.
   B. State and local child welfare and education agencies should collaborate to minimize educational disruptions for child welfare system-involved youth. This includes insuring proper transfer of credits, appropriate school placement and services, and school transportation services when continuation in the original school is desired.
   C. An arrest, court petition, delinquency finding, or other involvement in the juvenile justice system should not disqualify an otherwise eligible child from remaining in or re-entering foster care for the full period of eligibility.

Recommendation 8-6: Provide developmentally appropriate services for adolescents who engage in noncriminal misconduct without justice system involvement.
   A. The primary strategy for states and localities for addressing noncriminal misconduct (status offenses) by adolescents should be the provision of services to the youths and their families on a voluntary basis, wholly outside the legal system.
   B. States should end the practice of treating a violation of a court order by an adolescent adjudicated as a child in need of services (CHINS) as contempt of court and, thus, as a legal basis for initiating a juvenile delinquency proceeding.
   C. If adolescents are referred to the juvenile justice system for noncriminal misconduct, the disposition should be limited exclusively to placement in a community-based program that emphasize the provision of services and keeps the child at home.

reduce such disparities, state and local departments of child welfare should implement policies and practices that ensure that families of color have access to the same levels of in-home preventative services as other families. A second and more involved policy response would require evaluation and determination of the appropriate level of surveillance in a community. Both under- and over-surveillance are problematic. To reduce disparities, state and local departments of child welfare should establish guidelines and protocols regarding appropriate levels of surveillance in communities to improve the overall efficiency and benefit of surveillance systems, a practice also expected to reduce disparities. Responsible agencies should actively monitor implementation of these guidelines.

RECOMMENDATION 8-2: Promote broad uptake by the states of federal programs that promote resilience and positive outcomes for adolescents involved in the child welfare system.

As described above, a number of recent statutory changes embrace a developmentally informed approach to child welfare system practices and policies. However, many of these provisions are optional or not implemented rigorously or systematically. As a result, we are missing an opportunity to help launch child welfare system-involved youth into adulthood with sufficient skills, resources, and the connections to supportive adults that all adolescents need to become productive, healthy, and thriving members of our society. To better promote resilience and positive outcomes for adolescents involved in the child welfare system, all states should adopt the existing federal option to provide extended care to youth until age 21 and Chafee services to age 23 and provide comprehensive aftercare support to youth as they transition out of the child welfare system. In addition, all states should ensure that all youth who have experienced foster care are eligible for Medicaid until they reach age 26. Further, all states should ensure that child welfare system-involved youth are eligible for education and training vouchers until they reach age 26 and should facilitate and support youths' application process.

RECOMMENDATION 8-3: Provide services to adolescents and their families in the child welfare system that are developmentally informed at the individual, program, and system levels.

Adolescents' ability to problem solve, plan for the future, take the perspective of others, and weigh risks and benefits of actions increases dramatically across the span of adolescence. At the same time, their need for close relationships with caring adults and peers remains vital. Intervention and intervention practices discussed in this chapter offer promise in terms of the plasticity of adolescent development and the ability of intervention programs delivered during adolescence to improve socio-emotional outcomes. However, these interventions—and the child welfare system itself—have yet to incorporate a developmental approach to service provision and case management for adolescents with child welfare system involvement. Thus, state and local departments of child welfare should implement policies and practices that incorporate a developmental approach to service provision and case management for adolescents with child welfare system involvement, prioritizing family connections and supportive adults and taking maximum advantage of adolescents' increasing cognitive and social capacities. Further, state and local departments of child welfare should adjust the type and structure of services and the level of adolescent involvement in decision making related to their housing, education, and services to best align with adolescents' developmental capabilities and needs.

In light of the research evidence on the positive benefits of developing and maintaining a positive relationship with an adult (a family member, caregiver, mentor, or social support provider), services and programs should ensure that every system-involved youth is connected with a qualified and caring adult with ready access to advice and support from the responsible agency. Adolescents in the child welfare system also benefit when they remain engaged in the education system. Recognizing the growing capacity of adolescents for self-direction, case managers and courts should ensure that adolescents have the opportunity to fully participate in developing and implementing their service and transition plans, while maintaining critical ties with caring adults. To this end, adolescents should be involved as respected partners in decision making regarding their placements, education, and support services.

RECOMMENDATION 8-4: Conduct research that reflects all types and ages of adolescents in the child welfare system.

Most studies of adolescents who are involved in the child welfare system contain a heterogeneous set of participants ranging from those entering their first foster care placement to those who are 3 months into their fifth foster care placement, for example. Further, over the course of any given study (or intervention, in the case of intervention studies), adolescents may exit from care, terminate one placement and be placed in a new foster home, or be reunified with their parents. For the child welfare system to serve adolescents in a developmentally informed manner, services and programs must be designed specifically for adolescents, and those services must be evaluated. There is currently insufficient research on services designed specifically for adolescents, and the research that does exist generally does not span the full spectrum of adolescents involved in child welfare and is not reflective of the racial and ethnic composition of child welfare youth. Thus, the federal government, state and local child welfare agencies, and philanthropic institutions should fund research on service characteristics and outcomes for the full range of adolescents in the child welfare system in order to better design and evaluate services specifically for adolescents, depending upon their age, child welfare system history, and placement situation.

Although there is a general consensus that the child welfare system must be guided by trauma-informed and developmentally appropriate services, the effectiveness of such services has only been evaluated at the individual program level. Current child welfare system services are neither focused on adolescents nor delivered systemwide. The most effective approaches and techniques evaluated at the individual or program level have included cognitive behavioral therapy, home visitation, parent training, family-based/multisystemic interventions, and substance abuse prevention.

In order to make real progress and improve the well-being of adolescents in the child welfare system, successful programs and interventions delivered only at the individual level or the research-study level need to be delivered and implemented across the child welfare system, in sustainable ways. Further, individual and program successes identified through this research should be scaled to system-level change for adolescents in the child welfare system.

RECOMMENDATION 8-5: Foster greater collaboration between the child welfare, juvenile justice, education, and health systems.

Most adolescents in the child welfare system have experiences across multiple systems, including education, justice, status offense, and health and mental health care, yet most child welfare systems do not yet have access to an integrated data system that links information across systems while maintaining confidentiality. This is important, because effective services and best practices often require outreach to multiple systems. In addition, with the increased incorporation of predictive analytic tools, child welfare systems may have the ability to tailor services based on additional information about youth most in need of intensive services (and those in need of lighter or more targeted services), based on the constellation of their behaviors and outcomes across multiple systems (see Chapter 4). To best serve youth, child welfare, juvenile justice, education, and health agencies should collaborate to create an integrated data system that links information to track, evaluate, and provide an effective and integrated set of services to adolescents across these systems. However, an arrest, court petition, delinquency filing or other involvement in the juvenile justice system should not disqualify an otherwise eligible child from remaining in or re-entering foster care for the full period of eligibility.

Moreover, as described above, adolescents involved in the child welfare system often show worse educational outcomes than other adolescents, which is partly related to educational disruptions, problems with credit transfers, and a lack of appropriate school placement and services. They also show poorer physical health outcomes. Data from a nationally representative sample of noninstitutionalized children in the United States show that children placed in foster care are twice as likely to have asthma and three times as likely to have hearing problems and vision problems as those without foster care histories (Turney and Wildeman, 2016). State and local child welfare agencies, education agencies, and health care providers need to work together to ensure that child welfare system-involved youth are provided with appropriate health care and educational opportunities and are not hindered in pursuing their education by poor health or their involvement with the child welfare system. State and local child welfare and education agencies should collaborate to minimize educational disruptions for child welfare system-involved youth. This includes insuring proper transfer of credits, appropriate school placement and services, and school transportation services when continuation in the original school is desired.

An arrest, court petition, delinquency finding, or other involvement in the juvenile justice system should not disqualify an otherwise eligible child from remaining in or re-entering foster care for the full period of eligibility.

RECOMMENDATION 8-6: Provide developmentally appropriate services for adolescents who engage in noncriminal misconduct without justice system involvement.

Troubling behavior by children, such as truancy and running away, is often symptomatic of underlying issues in school or at home, but the court system is generally ill-equipped to resolve these issues. The state has a general interest in ensuring that a child and family receive supportive services, because a child's noncriminal misconduct can pose a danger to the child and others. However, the primary strategy for states and localities for addressing noncriminal misconduct (status offenses) should be the provision of services on a voluntary basis, wholly outside the legal system.

Drawing on the proposed "restatement of the law" relating to child welfare under consideration by the American Law Institute, the committee recommends that any legal response to noncriminal misconduct by children should draw a clear distinction between this misconduct and conduct that would be a crime if committed by an adult. Legal intervention for a CHINS is not intended to be punitive and instead should be focused solely on ensuring that a child and family receive needed services. Although noncriminal misconduct *can* lead to delinquent acts, for most children this behavior does not escalate to more serious misconduct. Thus, states should end the practice of treating a violation of a court order by an adolescent adjudicated as a CHINS as contempt of court and, thus, as a legal basis for initiating a juvenile delinquency proceeding.

When courts do become involved, the noncriminal misconduct of a child is most effectively addressed through community-based programs that emphasize the provision of services and keep the child at home. Courts should minimize the risk of a child's involvement with the juvenile justice system. Of particular concern is the practice in some states of treating a violation of a court order in a CHINS petition as criminal contempt of court and thus the basis for a juvenile delinquency proceeding. If adolescents are referred to the juvenile justice system for noncriminal misconduct, the disposition should be limited exclusively to placement in a community-based program that emphasizes the provision of services and keeps the child at home. This practice should be ended whenever possible. Similarly, children who are arrested should not be disqualified from child welfare services, but placement stability and the option of re-entry should remain available to them.

9

Justice System

In the United States, as in most other societies, the rate at which young people engage in antisocial behavior begins to increase substantially around the time of puberty, often increasing by a factor of 10 and peaking during late adolescence or early adulthood (Moffitt, 1993). Although a small share of people engage in antisocial behavior at every life stage, from early childhood through late adulthood, for the majority of people the rate of criminal behavior declines steadily as they enter their 20s and 30s. The scientific study of adolescent development—particularly in neuroscience— may explain this pattern among the majority of people: that the parts of the brain sensitive to sensation seeking and peer influence are particularly active in puberty, while the executive functioning regions are not fully formed until the early 20s (see, e.g., Steinberg, 2014).

These patterns highlight the possible tensions between the different aims of the juvenile justice system, the criminal justice system, and the social service agencies and education system. Our society aims to help teens navigate this life stage in a way that promotes their successful maturation and helps them avoid events that can set back their future prospects. At the same time, our society wishes to ensure public safety by preventing violence and other types of crimes, a goal that is in many ways congruent with the goal of promoting adolescent well-being because so much of the crime committed by youth—particularly the most serious violent crimes—is against other young people (see, e.g., Cook and Laub, 1998). Moreover, a growing body of research highlights the adverse effects on education, mental health, and other outcomes from growing up in a community where violence is common (Sharkey, 2010; Sharkey and Elwert, 2011; Sharkey

295

and Faber, 2014). However, the goals of the three systems may also be in tension, to the extent that interventions designed to prevent future crime by offending adolescents—namely detention—can harm the future prospects of many youth who would not have re-offended even in the absence of the intervention.

The fact that not all teens are the same—that most would not re-offend, while a small share are "life-course persistent" in their criminal activity— means that ideally our social systems could individualize and tailor their treatment of youth. In the justice system, for example, this would amount to creating an analog of what is known as "precision medicine" and would provide services that enhance the prospects of successful development and reduce the risk of future offending rather than interrupting positive development or making it more likely that youth will re-offend. But society's track record in making such behavioral predictions and in redirecting future trajectories in the desired way is not impressive.

The potential tensions among these different goals can be seen in society's shifts over time in policies and practices pertaining to antisocial behavior by adolescents. As early as the late 19th century, it was recognized that juveniles are developmentally different from adults, which led to the first juvenile justice system being founded in 1899. These early reformers believed that young people were less capable of understanding the criminality of their actions and therefore required the guidance of the court rather than punishment (Institute of Medicine and National Research Council, 2001). In the years since the creation of the juvenile court, the pendulum of the juvenile justice system has swung back again, from paternalistic to punitive, with changes in due process and supervision that illustrate the tensions between punishment and rehabilitation. The current context for juvenile justice policy is based on advances in neurobiological science and adolescent development research. As awareness grows about adolescent development in general, and adolescent brain development in particular, there remains a persistent challenge to simultaneously support the healthy development of juveniles and preserve public confidence in public safety.

Chapter 2 of this report describes the scientific basis for our understanding that although adolescents may develop some adult-like cognitive abilities by late adolescence (roughly age 16), the cognitive control capacities needed for inhibiting risk-taking behaviors continue to develop through young adulthood (age 25) (McCormick et al., 2016). Furthermore, in comparison to adults, youth demonstrate a greater capacity for growth, may be more amenable to treatment, and may be more receptive to interventions that address deficiencies in their social environments (Scott and Grisso, 1997). The landmark report *Reforming Juvenile Justice: A Developmental Approach* (National Research Council, 2013) detailed the specific application of developmental science to the juvenile justice system. The purpose of this chapter is to not repeat the work of that report, but to summarize key aspects of juvenile justice reform and relevant research over the past 5 years, and to identify opportunities for continued reforms.

The committee needed to address an important question regarding the scope of this chapter. In Chapter 1, we noted that, developmentally speaking, adolescence encompasses young adults as well as teenagers, and it might therefore be appropriate and within the committee's charge to address the interactions of young adults with the criminal justice system. After all, the number of 18–25-year-olds in the criminal justice system (roughly 3.2 million arrests in 2010) far exceeds the number of youth under age 18 in the juvenile justice system (roughly 1.6 million arrests in 2010). However, the committee decided to focus on the juvenile justice system for the same reasons we focused almost entirely on secondary schools in Chapter 6. First, like the education system, the juvenile justice system is designed for adolescents and should be grounded firmly in developmental knowledge. By contrast, higher education (including technical education) and the criminal justice system are designed to address all ages and to effectuate much more complex social purposes. Second, this committee was not constituted to take on the challenges of reforming criminal justice and higher education, notwithstanding the observation that young adults ages 18 to 25 may sensibly be characterized as adolescents from a developmental point of view.

Moreover, other National Academies' studies have recently addressed these two topics. For example, many important issues regarding young adults in the criminal justice system were addressed recently in the National Research Council's report on *The Growth of Incarceration in the United States: Exploring Causes and Consequences,* which focused primarily on the adult criminal justice system (National Research Council, 2014a). The developmental significance of higher education and criminal justice for young adults was also addressed in the 2014 National Academies report, *Investing in the Health and Well-Being of Young Adults* (Institute of Medicine and National Research Council, 2015).

Although this report focuses primarily on the juvenile justice system, we touch on two developmentally significant issues regarding the criminal justice system. One is the prosecution of younger adolescents (under 18) in the criminal courts, and the other is a renewed policy interest in correctional programs focusing specifically on the needs of young adults.

DEVELOPMENTALLY INFORMED JUVENILE JUSTICE: PROGRESS REPORT

A developmental approach to juvenile justice recognizes that delinquency occurs during a developmental stage when adolescents are more likely to exercise poor judgment, take risks, and pursue thrills, elements of adolescence that do not uniformly result in delinquent behavior. A juvenile justice system centered on a developmental approach will respond to delinquent behavior with individualized, developmentally appropriate treatment and services that address the three guiding principles of the system—promoting accountability, preventing re-offending, and treating youth fairly—with an emphasis on rehabilitation. These points are outlined further in Box 9-1, but their three core goals and associated practices may be distilled as follows (National Research Council, 2013, p. 121):

1. *Promoting Accountability*: Focus youth on repairing the social injury or damage, understanding how the behavior has affected other people, and take responsibility for their action.
2. *Preventing Re-offending*: Provide a diverse array of activities, supports, and opportunities for normal growth (e.g., emotional, physical, intellectual) in environments that are appropriate to the ages and stages of the youth involved, and engage family and neighborhood.
3. *Fairness*: Ensure youth participate in all proceedings, are represented by properly trained counsel, and are treated fairly and with dignity; intensify efforts to reduce racial/ethnic disparities; and develop strategies to reduce perceptions of bias or discrimination.

This developmental approach is critical to an effective juvenile justice system due to the distinctions between adolescents and adults. The key differences are that youth often lack the capacity for self-regulation in emotionally charged situations, have a heightened sensitivity to external influences such as peer pressure and immediate incentives, and show less ability to make decisions that require a future orientation (Icenogle et al., 2019). Another important feature is that adolescents are more keenly aware of injustices, and the appearance of unfairness will reinforce this perception. The literature suggests that "juveniles may be more likely to accept responsibility for less serious offenses early in the process if they perceive delinquency proceedings to be fair and transparent and any sanctions imposed to be proportionate to their offenses" (National Research Council, 2013, p. 130). As a result, the treatment of adolescents by the legal system may either reinforce a predisposition toward delinquent behavior or, alternatively, encourage respect and discourage re-offending. Hallmarks of a developmental approach, as outlined by the 2013 and 2014 National Academies' reports are shown in Box 9-1.

Contributing to perceptions of unfairness in the justice system is the disproportionate representation of minorities at every stage. Young people of color "are more likely than White youth to be stopped, arrested, and subsequently referred to court by police" (National Research Council, 2013, p. 221). As a result, "Black youth perceive a high degree of police-instigated

---

BOX 9-1
Hallmarks of a Developmentally Appropriate Justice System

Drawing from previous National Academies' reports, the committee highlights the following hallmarks of a developmental approach for justice reform (National Research Council, 2013, 2014b):

Accountability without criminalization
- Preserving youth opportunities to become productive adults

Alternatives to justice system involvement
- Providing services to prevent re-offending with minimal engagement with the formal justice system

Individualized response based on assessment of needs and risks
- Placing less emphasis on categories of offending
- Placing more emphasis on the malleable factors that may contribute to antisocial behavior in each case

Confinement only when necessary for public safety
- Restricting residential placements to the most serious youth
- Restricting periods of residential placements to the time needed to provide intensive services

A genuine commitment to fairness
- Ensuring that youth are represented by properly trained counsel
- Ensuring that youth understand the proceedings and can participate meaningfully

Sensitivity to disparate treatment
- Working to reduce the effects of discrimination by reducing unnecessary system involvement and confinement

Family engagement
- Aggressively seeking to work with all families
- Keeping a focus on addressing cognitive errors

---

discrimination, especially when they live in more racially integrated neighborhoods" (National Research Council, 2013, p. 113). Moreover, the structural and social contexts in which young people live are also relevant to understanding the disproportionate representation of minorities in the juvenile justice system. Neighborhoods that are economically disadvantaged often lack the public resources and supports necessary for youth to thrive. Health care facilities, high-performing school systems, recreation centers, and other community resources are critical for positive youth development, and studies suggest that youth are more likely to be arrested when raised in neighborhoods lacking these services (National Research Council, 2013, pp. 224–225). An essential purpose for a developmentally informed juvenile justice system is to reduce racial disparities to improve the fundamental integrity of the system and promote a sense of fairness among youth.

Further, the research led the 2013 committee to conclude that predominantly punitive policies and programs are ineffective for the majority of youth, as they neither foster prosocial development nor reduce recidivism. For far too many youth, juvenile incarceration has likely increased their risk of re-offending (National Research Council, 2013, p. 136), of dropping out of high school, and of involvement in the adult criminal justice system (Aizer and Doyle, 2015). Moreover, harsh sentences and lengthy confinement may adversely affect the developmental trajectories of many youth with no discernible benefit to public safety. A developmentally appropriate system will seek to individualize treatment based on the characteristics of the youth concerned: their maturity, needs, circumstances, role in the offense, and past criminal record. Developmental knowledge regarding rehabilitation does not displace the specific corrective aims of the justice system, but rather is relevant to any prevailing penal philosophy.

A great deal of progress has been made toward achieving a developmentally appropriate justice system in the past two decades. This section reviews recent scientific evidence that confirms the need for developmentally appropriate reforms and the adoption of developmentally appropriate policies and practices at the state and local levels.

Affirming the Scientific Consensus

Over the past 15 years, developmental science has greatly transformed the juvenile justice system. New evidence from developmental neuroscience has affirmed and strengthened findings from the psychological sciences. For example, the use of functional magnetic resonance imaging (fMRI) has revealed that the maturation of structural connectivity within the prefrontal cortex is paralleled by increases in functional connectivity and changes in important activation patterns. Specifically, this maturation is paralleled by increases in the extent to which different regions coactivate during particular tasks and by changes in patterns of activation during tasks that measure working memory, planning, and the inhibition of responses—all of which are important for impulse control and for thinking ahead (Casey, 2015; Luna et al., 2010; Stevens et al., 2007).

Such findings of structural and functional differences between adolescent and adult brains, which are plausibly linked to differences in the ability to control impulses and respond to peer pressure, suggest that these aspects of adolescent immaturity are not merely reflective of juveniles' poor choices or different values. Rather, they suggest that they are at least partly due to factors that are not entirely under their individual control. To illustrate this with a familiar example, while driving a car, adolescents and adults may both estimate the risks of reckless driving, such as receiving a ticket or getting into an accident, in a similar fashion. However, while they are cognitively able to estimate and understand the risk the same way, adolescents tend to weigh the potential rewards (in this case, the thrill of driving fast) more heavily than adults would. In short, the adolescents would be more likely to engage in the reckless behavior despite understanding the risks. It is during this time in early adolescence that the brain develops the affective neural systems that are tied to reward sensitivity (e.g., the ventral striatum and anterior insula), which helps explain the age differences clearly evident in sensation seeking and risk taking.

Of course, identifying the neurobiological underpinnings of differences in capabilities and capacities by age does not mean that these differences are immutable. As discussed in Chapters 2 and 3, adolescence is a period of heightened plasticity, a time when the brain is especially malleable and responsive to experiences. The neuroscientific evidence, rather, bolsters the argument that adolescents—including young adults in their 20s—are neurologically less mature than adults. This adds strength to the understanding that adolescent wrongdoing is unlikely to reflect irreparable depravity.

Taken together, recent scientific evidence about adolescents' behavior and thinking, as well as the development of their brain structure and function, affirms the need for a developmental approach to juvenile justice as outlined in the 2013 and 2014 National Academies' reports. It also affirms the need for developmentally appropriate practices for older adolescents involved in the criminal justice system. That is, the normative development of youth's brains, behaviors, and environmental influences require different responses to their misbehavior than what is required for adults. Moreover, this heightened developmental predilection for change and responsiveness to intervention means we can also reduce delinquency by supporting programs and interventions targeted to at-risk youth rather than merely responding with punitive punishment and incarceration.

Such a response furthers the public safety goals of the justice system while simultaneously promoting (as compared with detention) the goal of helping the youth themselves and, given the high costs of youth incarceration, potentially even reducing government expenditures at the same time. The cascade of neuroscientific evidence gathered within the past 5 years complements and corroborates the behavioral science that has long guided our common understanding that young people are fundamentally different from adults (Steinberg, 2017).

Adoption of Developmentally Appropriate Policies and Practices

As the scientific evidence continues to mount, a growing number of states and localities have adopted a developmental approach to juvenile justice, according to a 2015 assessment prepared by the MacArthur Foundation:

Family and juvenile courts in 18 states are now more likely to hear cases formerly processed in the adult system, to evaluate a youth's competency to stand trial, and to consider the youth's development and maturity in sentencing. Fourteen states have increased the use of diversion and community-based programs, resulting in fewer youth being incarcerated. Ten states have raised their standards for youth placement facilities, increased mental and behavioral health services, and taken steps to keep young offenders closer to their own communities. Nine states have increased juveniles' access to counsel and in other ways made the legal process fairer for adolescents. Eight states have stopped automatically referring adolescents to the juvenile justice system because they are truant, defiant, or act out in school. (MacArthur Foundation, 2015, p. 14)

Some states have broadly reformed their juvenile justice systems. For example, beginning in 2013, Georgia rewrote its juvenile code; in 2015, Nevada enacted legislation to address age of jurisdiction and use of solitary confinement; and in the same year, Kentucky made changes to reduce the use of secure confinement and increase the use of community-based options. Hawaii also enacted legislation to reduce secure confinement, strengthen community supervision, and target resources to programs and practices proven to reduce recidivism (Durnan et al., 2018). Table 9-1 provides additional examples of recent state legislative reforms consistent with a developmental approach.

While it is clear that a developmental approach to the juvenile justice system has been widely embraced and is having a discernible impact on law and practice in many states, progress is uneven. Sustained effort and attention are needed to accelerate advances and to prevent an erosion of gains, which would likely have negative consequences for adolescents involved in the justice system. Indeed, recent calls for a "re-balancing" (Davis, 2018) of efforts away from diversion and interventions for youth toward short-term safety concerns reflect a misunderstanding and misapplication of the scientific consensus on adolescent development and behavior. As noted above and detailed in *Reforming Juvenile Justice: A Developmental Approach* (National Research Council, 2013, pp. 119–120, 135), a developmental approach to juvenile justice recognizes the following:

1. The developing adolescent brain functions in such a way that predisposes adolescents to risk-taking behavior, and psychosocial influences on decision making during adolescence distinguish juvenile choices from those of adults and indicate that, at a quite fundamental level, the determinants of criminal involvement among juveniles generally differ from the determinants of adult criminality, making juveniles less culpable than adults for criminal choices.

TABLE 9-1 Examples of State-level Legislation Consistent with a Developmental Approach to Juvenile Justice

State	Year	Category	Brief Description
California	2018	Expansion of services to include young adults	*Act No. 2018-1007:* Expands on the Transitional Age Youth Pilot Program to allow youth from Alameda, Butte, Napa, Nevada, Santa Clara, and Ventura counties between the ages of 18 to 21 to participate in the Deferred Entry of Judgement Pilot Program. The program allows eligible youth convicted of felonies to receive additional services, including developmentally appropriate educational and vocational programs and mental health services, including cognitive behavioral therapy.
Connecticut	2016	Conditions of confinement	*Act No. 16-186:* Requires the Department of Children and Families and the Department of Corrections to limit the use of seclusion and restraint on adolescents under the age of 20 and to submit a yearly report that explains the frequency and reasons for using seclusion and restraint.
Hawaii	2018	Expansion of services to include young adults	*Act No. 208:* For the creation of Kawailoa Youth and Family Wellness Centers at youth correction facilities in Hawaii. The program is available for youth up to age 24. The wellness centers should include programs for substance abuse treatment, mental health treatment, vocational training, crisis centers, and family counseling services.
Indiana	2018	Truancy and school disciplinary actions	*Act No. 151-2018:* Allows students to participate in evidence-based plans to improve behavior. The plan must attempt to reduce out-of-school suspension and disciplinary actions. Limits referrals to law enforcement or arrests on school property.
Montana	2017	Juvenile sex offenders	*Act No. 208:* Revises juvenile sex offender laws so that juvenile offenders do not have to register as sex offenders if they do not have a history of sexual offenses and if they are not considered a threat to the public.

continued

TABLE 9-1 Continued

State	Year	Category	Brief Description
New Hampshire	2018	Conditions of confinement	*Act No. 2017-180:* Prohibits the use of handcuffs and shackles on minors being escorted or held in a court facility that is occupied by members of the public. Prevents prosecutors, law enforcement officers, or other state or municipal employees from advising juveniles or their parent or guardian to waive the right to counsel.
Oregon	2017	Conditions of confinement	*Act No. 257:* Prohibits use of physical restraints on juveniles during in court proceedings unless the youth has a history of dangerous behavior or there is a serious risk of the youth harming themselves or others. Prohibits use of physical restraints in transportation of youth, youth offenders, young persons, wards, and children by Department of Human Services or the Oregon Health Authority unless there is a serious risk of the youth harming themselves or others. Prevents the use of restraints as a substitute for supervision or as a punishment.
Oregon	2017	Conditions of confinement	*Act No. 134:* Prevents adolescents under the age of 18 from being incarcerated in a Department of Corrections institution.
South Dakota	2016	Sentencing	*Act No. 121:* Prohibits adolescents under the age of 18 from receiving a life sentence without parole.
Texas	2017	Truancy and school disciplinary actions	*Act No. 691:* Establishes a pilot program in certain public high schools that places students in Junior Reserve Officers' Training Corps programs to avoid placing them in a juvenile justice alternative education program.
Vermont	2016	Sentencing	*Act No. 22:* Prohibits courts from sentencing a person to life imprisonment without the possibility of parole if the person was under age 18 when the offense was committed.

TABLE 9-1 Continued

State	Year	Category	Brief Description
Virginia	2018	Truancy and school disciplinary actions	*Act No. 585:* Prevents students from being expelled for truancy alone. Prevents students in preschool through the third grade from being suspended for more than 3 days or expelled unless their actions resulted in a physical injury to others or there was a credible threat of harm to another.
Virginia	2015	Comprehensive services for at-risk youth	*Act No. 406:* Establishes interagency programmatic and fiscal policies for the Office of Comprehensive Services for At-Risk Youth and Families to support the purposes of the Comprehensive Services Act (Section 2.2-5200 et seq.). The Comprehensive Services Act requires that a collaborative system of services and funding be established to address the needs of at-risk youth and their families.
Washington	2017	Truancy and school disciplinary actions	*Act No. 291:* Procedures implemented to promote school attendance and reduce truancy. Requires that multiple steps be taken to address the underlying issues leading to multiple unexcused absences before involving the justice system.

SOURCE: National Conference of State Legislatures (2019), Juvenile Justice Bills Tracking Database. See http://www.ncsl.org/research/civil-and-criminal-justice/ncsls-juvenile-justice-bill-tracking-database.aspx.

2. Criminal punishments can have a lasting negative effect on youth by disrupting psychosocial development, limiting employment and educational opportunities, and hampering their ability to develop relationships with noncriminal affiliates, thus making the transition to noncriminal adult life extremely difficult if not impossible.

3. Given that only a small percentage of youth will continue to offend into adulthood unless justice system interventions themselves impede or prevent a successful transition to law-abiding adult life, the goal of reducing crime and increasing public safety will be furthered by ensuring that interventions holding young offenders accountable for their misdeeds do not have the unwanted effect of increasing the risk of reoffending and otherwise impeding successful maturation.

4. Developmental science indicates that adolescence is a period during which youth progress toward acquiring skills and capacities necessary to successfully assume adult roles through interaction between the individual and the social environment, and juvenile justice interventions that genuinely aim to reduce recidivism will seek to provide opportunity structures that can promote young offenders' development into productive adults.

This scientific understanding of adolescence, then, suggests that overly harsh punishments that mimic criminal punishments may have the opposite effect of reducing crime and promoting public safety, and are particularly harmful for youth. According to the same National Research Council (2013, p. 185) report:

> [A]ccountability practices in juvenile justice should be designed specifically for juvenile justice rather than being carried over from the criminal courts and should be designed to promote healthy social learning, moral development, and legal socialization during adolescence. If designed and implemented in a developmentally informed way, procedures for holding adolescents accountable for their offending can promote positive legal socialization, reinforce a prosocial identity, and facilitate compliance with the law. However, unduly harsh interventions and negative interactions between youth and justice system officials can undermine respect for the law and legal authority and reinforce a deviant identity and social disaffection.

Since the publication of the 2013 report, the committee has found no evidence contrary to this position and no evidence that suggests that reforms to align the juvenile justice system with a developmental approach have resulted in increased crime or public safety concerns. In fact, crime rates among juveniles ages 10 to 17 have declined by 72 percent since 1996, and the number of youth in residential placement has declined from approximately 105,000 in 1997 to 45,500 in 2016 (U.S. Department of Justice, 2018).

These statistics thus confirm the previous committee's findings that scientific understanding of adolescent development aligns with the goals of the juvenile justice system—holding youth accountable, being fair, and preventing re-offending—which all serve to improve public safety. Moreover, in a study of the adverse consequences of juvenile detention, Aizer and Doyle (2015) find particularly harmful effects on those adolescents who are still enrolled in school, which—when combined with the fact that school enrollment rates are much higher among adolescents than adults—supports the idea that detention has more severe consequences for adolescents than adults. In short, a developmentally appropriate juvenile justice system acknowledges the potential of youth and helps them become successful, law-abiding members of their communities, promoting public safety more effectively than a punitive approach.

REDUCING RACIAL DISPARITIES

More than 10 years after its expiration, Congress reauthorized the Juvenile Justice and Delinquency Prevention Act (JJDPA) in late 2018. Among many other reforms, Congress embraced a developmentally in-formed juvenile justice system as an overarching goal of federal policy: the reauthorization bill amended the JJDPA to require federal and state policies and plans to "reflect the science of adolescent development."

Reducing racial and ethnic disparities within the juvenile justice system, a problem often referred to as "disproportionate minority contact," has been an explicit federal policy priority for decades. This history was sum-marized in the 2013 National Academies' report as follows:

> Congress first gave attention to racial disparities in 1988 when it amended the Juvenile Justice and Delinquency Prevention Act (JJDPA) of 1974 (P.L. 93-415, 42 U.S.C. 5601 *et seq.*) to require states that received formula funds from the Office of Juvenile Justice and Delinquency Prevention (OJJDP) to ascertain the proportion of minority youth detained in secure detention facilities, secure correctional facilities, and lockups compared with the general population and, if the number of minority youth was disproportionate, to develop and implement plans to reduce the dispro-portionate representation (Section 223(a)(23)). In 1992, the JJDPA was amended. Disproportionate minority confinement was made a core re-quirement, and 25 percent of a state's formula funds could be withheld if states did not comply. In 2002, Congress again modified the disproportion-ate minority confinement requirement and mandated states to implement juvenile delinquency prevention efforts and system improvement efforts designed to reduce, without establishing or requiring numerical standards or quotas, the disproportionate number of juvenile members of minority groups who come into contact with the juvenile justice system (P.L. 107-273, Sec. 12209). Thus the disproportionate minority contact (DMC) core requirement was broadened from "confinement" to "contact," and states were required to implement strategies aimed at reducing disproportional-ity. (National Research Council, 2013, pp. 211–212)

The 2018 reauthorization bill amends the JJDPA to strengthen each of the act's core protections, including greater specificity and structure for the states' obligation to decrease racial and ethnic disparities. This is an important revision because despite a decades-long mandate to reduce racial and ethnic disparities, inequities within the juvenile justice system continue to persist and are growing (see also the discussion in Chapter 4). While the overall number of youth in detention has declined, the racial disparity has worsened: in 2013, Black youth were 4.3 times more likely to be incarcerated than White youth, up from 3.7 times as likely in 2003 (National Center for Juvenile Justice, 2017).

As noted in Chapter 4, disparities in the treatment of adolescents, as defined by race and ethnicity, seem to increase at every stage of the process, from arrest, to decision to prosecute and removal to adult court, to sentencing, to type of confinement (DeLone and DeLone, 2017; Fader et al., 2014; Sickmund et al., 2014). Moreover, recent data also indicate that LGBTQ youth, and particularly LGBTQ youth of color, are overrepresented in the juvenile justice system (Dank et al., 2015; Hunt and Moodie-Mills, 2012; Irvine and Canfield, 2016; Majd et al., 2009; Wilson et al., 2017). LGBTQ adolescents represent 5 to 7 percent of the overall adolescent population, yet represent 13 to 15 percent of those currently in the juvenile justice system (Hunt and Moodie–Mills, 2012; Majd et al., 2009).

Root Causes of Disparities

While there has been much debate among scholars as to the root causes of these disparities, most emphasize some combination of differential selection and treatment by the justice system (possibly attributable to implicit or explicit bias) and differential offending by White and minority youth (differences in the actual extent of engaging in law-breaking behaviors), likely the result of disparities in the social conditions children grown up in (National Research Council, 2013). Differential selection suggests that a combination of differential enforcement and differential processing by the juvenile justice system leads to more minority youth being arrested, convicted, and subsequently confined than White youth (Piquero, 2008). Differential offending, conversely, is viewed as contributing to disproportionality through differences in rates at which racial or ethnic groups engage in different types of criminal behavior (National Research Council, 2013).

The idea that racial disparities, particularly in violent crime, are largely attributable to persistent structural disadvantages disproportionately concentrated in Black communities was first theorized by Sampson and Wilson (1995) and, in a recent review, was validated. Although they specifically analyzed data related to adults, Sampson and colleagues (2018) argue that a general thesis of racial invariance can be applied in the juvenile context. As they frame it, this thesis is "the assertion that racial disparities in rates of violent crime ultimately stem from the very different social ecological contexts in which Blacks and Whites reside, and that concentrated disadvantage predicts crime similarly across racial groups" (Sampson et al., 2018, p. 14). The authors find that (1) large racial disparities in violent crime and ecological contexts (e.g., concentrated poverty, family disruption) continue to exist, (2) structural ecological factors are strong predictors of violent crime and account for a substantial proportion of racial disparities, and (3) the predictive power of these factors transcends racial boundaries. That is, the societal contexts in which youth find themselves—resulting from, in part, the failure of youth-serving systems, such as education, child welfare, and health care, to create positive, supportive environments for youth—lead to disparities in rates of engaging in or being victimized by crime.

The increase in racial disparities in recent years is particularly troubling given the system's goal of promoting fairness and the federal mandate to reduce racial and ethnic disparities. A possible explanation for the increase in disparate treatment over time is the decline in serious offenses, the type that allows less discretion in decisions to prosecute and sentence. As the number of less serious offenses increases as a proportion of the total, there may be more discretion for practitioners at every stage of the process, potentially resulting in more biased decisions (Arnold et al., 2018; National Council on Crime and Delinquency, 2007). Other possible explanations include (1) disparities in access to alternatives to incarceration, (2) disparities in the selection of alternatives to incarceration due to a family's inability or perceived inability to participate in a placement alternative, which depends on the parental or family involvement, (3) disparities in offending driven by widening social inequalities and structural disadvantages, and (4) disparities in the selection of youth referred to the juvenile justice system from other adolescent-serving systems, such as schools[1] (Hager, 2015; Mears and Cochran, 2015). Box 9-2 further discusses the relationship between school discipline practices and disproportionate juvenile justice system-involvement for minority youth.

The existing literature is insufficient to draw conclusions about the relative contribution of differential offending, differential enforcement and process, and structural inequalities to these disparities, it is clear that this lack of progress in reducing disparities within the juvenile justice system leads to negative outcomes for youth and the system itself (Aizer and Doyle, 2015; National Research Council, 2014; Pew Charitable Trusts, 2015). Ensuring that youth *perceive* that they have been treated fairly contributes to social learning, moral development, and legal socializing[2] during adolescence (Office of Juvenile Justice and Delinquency Prevention, 2012). Reducing racial and ethnic disparities in the administration of juvenile justice, thus,

---

[1] Similar trends have appeared in the education field, as progress in narrowing test-score gaps between Black and White students has stalled. It is possible that both trends share similar underlying causes. This potential connection could be an important area for future research.

[2] "Legal socialization" is the product of accumulated interactions with legal authorities, and personal experiences with justice system actors, thus shaping a person's views about the system.

BOX 9-2
Relationship Between School Disciplinary
Policies and the Juvenile Justice System

One explanation for the recent increase in racial disparities in the juvenile justice system is the existence of disparities in the ways youth are selectively referred to the juvenile justice system from other adolescent-serving systems. Since the 1990s, school disciplinary practices have increasingly resulted in removing students from the classroom, placing them on a pathway into the juvenile justice system. A disproportionate number of Black, Native American, Latinx, and youth with disabilities are suspended or expelled from school as a result of discretionary disciplinary infractions, like willful disobedience, while similar disproportionality is not evident for defined offenses that are predicated on objective acts, such as drug use. In addition, disparities are evident in the number of Black, Native American, and Latinx youth who are referred to law enforcement for minor offenses, such as truancy (American Bar Association, 2018).

Once students are in the juvenile justice system, they can become trapped in a harmful cycle that pulls them further away from an educational system meant to help them, and there is growing evidence that even when other factors are held constant, every school suspension makes the next suspension, expulsion, dropout, or arrest more likely (American Bar Association, 2018; Fabelo et al., 2011; Morgan et al., 2014).

Given the disproportionate filtering of students into the juvenile justice system from schools, one strategy to reduce disparities in the juvenile justice system is to invest in alternative school disciplinary strategies, such as the use of multitiered systems of support (MTSS) (Child Trends, 2018; Ricks and Esthappan, 2018). Two

---

is critical to achieving a fair juvenile justice system and promoting positive adolescent development.

Theories of legitimacy suggest that those who perceive the justice system to be more legitimate are more likely to comply with the law (National Academies of Sciences, Engineering, and Medicine, 2018; Tyler, 1990), although questions remain as to the causal connection between changes in treatment and changes in compliance (Nagin and Telep, 2017). The experiences of others, or vicarious experiences, may also influence attitudes. Indeed, Black youth consistently report more negative attitudes toward the police than White youth (Hurst et al., 2000; Peck, 2015). These experiences likely lead minority youth to perceive the justice system as biased.

Moreover, the formation of attitudes toward the justice system over the course of adolescence and early adulthood varies dramatically by race and ethnicity. Black youth, for example, often have a negative view of the justice system based on personal experiences or events they have witnessed. Latinx and White youth report similar attitudes toward the justice system

promising MTSS models include Integrated School Supports (ISS) and Positive Behavioral Intervention Supports (PBIS), both of which work with parents, schools, and other community stakeholders to address the specific needs of the students and schools they serve. Evaluations of these models conducted by the American Institutes for Research (AIR), MDRC, and ICF International have resulted in mixed reviews that range from null to positive, with no negative findings. While these strategies hold promise for ending the pathway from school discipline to justice system involvement and, ultimately, reducing the disproportionate number of youth of color coming into contact with the juvenile justice system, ongoing evaluations are needed to monitor program outcomes and implementation fidelity if these programs are to be successful in supporting adolescent development and academic success (Child Trends, 2018).

Another program that has shown promise in reducing racial disparities in the juvenile justice system is the Philadelphia Police School Diversion Program. This program, which was started by the Philadelphia Police Department in 2014, allows students with no prior criminal history who have been arrested for misdemeanor crimes the chance to avoid being officially charged with a criminal offense. Rather than enter the justice system, these adolescents are moved into a diversion program designed to help them change their behaviors and life trajectory. A key component of the program is the assignment of a social worker and provision of academic support, mentoring, social and emotional competency building, and other services. Since the program began in 2014, there has been a 54 percent drop in arrests in the city's schools. The program is currently participating in a 3-year outcomes evaluation with funding provided by the Office of Juvenile Justice and Delinquency Prevention. Results from this evaluation will be available in 2020 (Office of Juvenile Justice and Delinquency Prevention, 2017).

during adolescence, but White youth, over time, have been found to view the system more positively than Latinx youth. These results suggest that attitude differences emerge through the course of adolescence. Indeed, White youth are the only group whose attitudes about the system become more positive as they age (Fine and Cauffman, 2015).

Reducing Racial Disparities in the Justice System

Given the disproportionate representation of minority youth in the juvenile justice system, the dovetailing of attitudes about the justice system between White and non-White youth likely represents recognition and awareness among youth of racial bias in the system. In such a climate— where youth recognize the biases undergirding a system purporting to dole out impartial, fair justice—it is all the more important to continue to affirm a commitment to accounting for, acknowledging, and tackling disproportionate minority contact.

Critical to this accounting is the continued collection of data on disparities in the system, which, as noted above, has been strengthened under the
JJDPA reauthorization act. As part of its core requirements, the Office of
Juvenile Justice and Delinquency Prevention is mandated to provide grants
and training to local justice system actors with the aim of reducing racial
and ethnic disparities. States receiving funding must identify, assess, evaluate, and monitor disparities. Understanding where disparities exist within
the system, thus, is an important first step to resolving the problem of disproportionate minority contact and is imperative for building the legitimacy
of the system. However, such an understanding can only be achieved if
states are required to furnish specific, rigorous metrics on race and ethnicity.

Of course, it is not simply enough to collect data about the disparities within the juvenile justice system. Remarkably little progress has been
made despite more than 20 years of research and policy focus on this issue.
The 2013 National Academies' report cited earlier noted that the lack of
progress in this area was partly due to several deficits: a lack of motivation, insufficient cross-system collaboration, inadequate resources, deeply
rooted structural biases, and the extreme difficulties of disentangling the
many complex, multilevel, and interrelated contributing factors (National
Research Council, 2013, p. 213).

In the same report, the committee urged that "reform efforts to reduce
racial/ethnic disparities should pay special attention to the arrest and detention stages at the front end of the system" (National Research Council,
2013, p. 239). It is also critical for school systems to invest in developmentally appropriate alternatives to punitive and discretionary school disciplinary practices as they are more likely to result in a referral to the
juvenile justice system (National Research Council, 2013, pp. 239–240).
This committee supports those recommendations.

Because racial and ethnic disparities within the juvenile justice system
may also result from disparities in rates of engaging in or being victimized by different types of criminal behavior, policies that prioritize some
groups for extra prevention programming to reduce criminal involvement
or delinquency may be appropriate. For instance, if there are differences
in group rates of offending due to differences in family, neighborhood, or
school social conditions, evidence-based interventions that are targeted,
implemented upstream, and preventive in focus may have positive effects
on individual and social behaviors. Practitioners and communities have a
greater chance of creating positive behavioral and environmental changes
if they select interventions based on the characteristics and circumstances
of the participating individual, group, or community and follow established
implementation and evaluation frameworks, such as those included in
Office of Juvenile Justice and Delinquency Prevention's Model Programs

Guide.[3] In short, because the factors that drive human behaviors (including delinquent and criminal behaviors) are rooted in social and structural conditions that different racial groups experience differently, the most successful solutions will address changes to both the systems' policies and the individuals and communities that they serve.

It is important to note that there is no inherent trade-off between reducing racial and ethnic disparities and promoting public safety. It is possible to improve outcomes for youth without harming public safety. To achieve this goal, it is critical to understand the root causes of disparities in the justice system and implement policies and practices that target these inequalities while continuing to hold youth accountable.

OPPORTUNITIES FOR CONTINUED JUVENILE JUSTICE REFORMS

Developmental science can inform policy and practice in the juvenile justice system in a number of key areas. Drawing on this scientific evidence base, in this section we first discuss opportunities for increasing family engagement when youth are involved in the juvenile justice system. Next, we discuss opportunities to create greater procedural fairness in the system, including interactions with the police, legal representation for youth, and juvenile fines and fees. Finally, we discuss several ways in which additional reforms can ameliorate the harmful effects of justice system involvement on the youth's future prospects, including restricting access to juvenile records, avoiding overuse of sex offender classification, and curtailing use of solitary confinement.

Family Engagement

As described elsewhere in this report, parental engagement and support are critical to adolescents' success in academic settings, autonomy development, relational competence, and a host of other domains. In fact, several recent psychological and neuroscientific studies have demonstrated that parents continue to matter for adolescents' decision making, in contrast to common assumptions that parents begin to "matter less" as peers "matter more" to adolescents (Guassi et al., 2018; Welborn et al., 2016). It is no surprise, then, that parental engagement for youth who are involved in the justice system has been shown to have positive effects both on young people's desistance from crime and on their mental health outcomes. A robust body of evidence has shown that a supportive parent-child rela-

---

[3] The Model Programs Guide (MPG) contains a searchable database of evaluated and rated interventions and implementation guides. For more information, see https://www.ojjdp.gov/mpg/.

tionship is an important protective factor in desistence from crime among youthful offenders, suggesting that parents play a key role in helping adolescents navigate the justice system (Hoeve et al., 2008, 2009). According to the National Research Council (2014b, p. 23), a developmentally informed system would "aggressively seek to work with all families and family-focused organizations based on the understanding that they are necessary and critical partners."

Because young people generally lack an understanding of their legal rights, responsibilities, and courtroom procedures, they often find it difficult to navigate the complexity of the justice system without assistance (Goodwin-DeFaria and Marinos, 2012; Grisso et al., 2003; Miner-Romanoff, 2014; Redding and Fuller, 2004). As a result of children's well-recognized dearth of legal knowledge, a foundational expectation of the juvenile justice system is that parents have the necessary legal knowledge to partner with the system and guide their children through the justice process (Rozzell, 2013). However, few resources are available to teach parents to help their youth navigate the juvenile justice process, including information related to their family's rights and duties during the process (Davies and Davidson, 2001; Feierman et al., 2011).

Youth most at-risk for juvenile justice system involvement, including youth from low socioeconomic status backgrounds and youth of color (Woolard et al., 2008), may have parents who are not well equipped to navigate the juvenile justice system. Latinx parents and low-income parents may be especially deferential to authorities, leading them to capitulate to the knowledge of legal authorities after their adolescent has been arrested (Gaitan, 2004; Harding, 2006; Holloway et al., 1995). Additionally, non-English-speaking parents, because of cultural and linguistic barriers, may not have a clear understanding of probation requirements. Studies have found that parents with less knowledge of the juvenile justice system were less likely to participate in their child's legal proceedings. Further, their adolescents were more likely to report engaging in re-offending behavior. This suggests that a lack of legal knowledge may limit parental participation in the legal process and perhaps even contribute to a youth's prolonged or more serious involvement with the justice system, such as having probation extended because the original terms were not met (Cavanagh and Cauffman, 2017). Thus, given that youth are more likely to complete their probationary terms and desist from crime when their parents are included in the legal process, legal education for the parents and caregivers of justice-involved youth is key to encouraging parental engagement (Burke et al., 2014; Cavanagh and Cauffman, 2017; Vidal and Woolard, 2016).

Parental engagement may also have positive effects on incarcerated youths' mental health. As discussed previously, youth in the justice system are disproportionately likely to have been diagnosed with a mental illness or experience poor mental health, and incarceration accentuates these problems (Cauffman et al., 2007; Grisso, 2004; Potter and Jenson, 2003; Teplin et al., 2002). One method for promoting successful adaptation to incarceration for youth is to facilitate early and continued parent-adolescent visits. In a study of serious offenders who were adolescent males, Monahan and colleagues (2010) found that parental visitation was associated with better mental health during a juvenile's initial adjustment to incarceration, and that more visits from parents were associated with increasingly rapid declines in depressive symptoms over time.[4] The authors argued that "to the extent that the positive effects of parental visits on depressive symptoms became stronger over time, allowing parental visits as soon as youth become incarcerated may produce earlier declines in depressive symptoms among incarcerated adolescents" (Monahan et al., 2010, p. 7).

To facilitate such parental visits, juvenile facilities should limit the use of restrictions on visitation rights as punishment. Further, policies should be put in place to assist families in overcoming barriers to prison visitation, such as geographic distance and lack of resources. Box 9-3 discusses the "Close to Home" initiative in New York, which increased opportunities for parents, caregivers, and other relatives to stay connected to their children. This model is being replicated across the country in programs such as Philadelphia's Safely Home Philly initiative.

The justice system can also draw lessons from other systems to build strategies for engaging parents in improving outcomes for their children. For example, the education system has long attempted to improve parent engagement with varying degrees of success. A recent experimental effort focused on student absenteeism shows promise for scalability within the education system and transferability to the justice system, namely: addressing parental cognitive errors. This randomized experiment underscored the importance of tailoring interventions to target parents by demonstrating that correcting the false assumptions parents hold can bring about significant changes in student behavior (Rogers and Feller, 2018).

Similarly, there is evidence that family engagement is useful in reducing recidivism for adults, which has implications for the juvenile justice system (Cavanagh and Cauffman, 2017). The study also suggests that the impacts could be even larger for adolescents when parents are provided with critical information that is regular, timely, and in context. More evidence on the effectiveness of parent legal education, and on what are the most effective types, is needed.

---

[4]The study also found that the quality of the parent-adolescent relationship did not moderate the effect of parental visitation on youth mental health, suggesting that the mere presence of a parent has positive effects on the incarcerated youth's adjustment to confinement.

BOX 9-3
New York's Close to Home Initiative

New York's Close to Home initiative began in 2012 with two primary objectives: removing New York City youth from large, inefficient, and often dangerous facilities far from their homes, and integrating New York City youth back into the city's communities. The foundation for Close to Home included the passage of a string of reforms, such as the merging of the New York City Department of Justice and New York City Administration for Children's Services, to create the Division of Youth and Family Justice. This new division was able to leverage the Administration for Children's Services' valuable community relationships and services to engage stakeholders and implement evidence-based programs.

Close to Home was further helped by the Brooklyn for Brooklyn Initiative and other program models that were able to demonstrate the value of working with youth and families using small community-based programs. These models provided solid evidence that justice-involved youth can be successful and productive members of society if consistently provided with the right tools during and after system involvement.

Close to Home uses the Risk-Needs-Responsivity framework and the Positive Youth Development framework, along with seven core principles to guide their work. The principles are as follows:

1. *Public Safety*—such as intensive supervision of youth during and after program release
2. *Accountability*—including using data to inform decision making
3. *Evidence-Based and Evidence-Informed Treatment*—so that services can be targeted to individual risk factors
4. *Educational Continuity and Achievement*—to support youth in the attainment of educational success
5. *Community Integration*—such as through ongoing relationships with caring adults and other members of the community
6. *Family Engagement and Collaboration*—involving parents in the rehabilitation process
7. *Permanency*—including services designed to support youth when they return to their community.

Close to Home evaluation results show that the program is improving youth outcomes. For example, in 2016, 79 percent of youth in the Close to Home program and 93 percent of middle school students enrolled in the program's Passages Academy were advanced to the next grade level. While this success is encouraging, Close to Home is using the evaluation data and feedback from community stakeholders to improve the program's future implementation (Annie E. Casey Foundation, 2018).

Procedural Fairness

Procedural fairness[5] refers to whether the justice system is impartial and equitable, whether litigants feel respected and have a fair opportunity to be heard, and whether the fact-finding procedures are neutral and trustworthy (National Academies of Sciences, Engineering, and Medicine, 2018). The fairness of this process for juveniles is affected by their developmental immaturity, which influences their ability to exercise their rights and participate competently. As a result, the Supreme Court has articulated constitutional protections specific to juveniles because they are less likely than adults to understand their rights (for example to an attorney and to remain silent) and more likely to succumb to pressure or to an inducement to waive their rights. Juveniles are also more likely than adults to confess to crimes (Grisso, 1980, 1981; National Research Council, 2013). Areas of particular interest are interactions with police, especially police interactions, and legal representation.

Interactions with Police

Police/youth interaction has substantially increased as a result of the police presence in our nation's schools, making the impact of those interactions on youth perceptions or behavior of particular interest (National Center for Education Statistics, 2018; Travis and Coon, 2005). The National Academies' 2013 report concluded that "negative observations and contacts that youth have with police may produce cynicism and undermine legal socialization" (National Research Council, 2013, p. 194). However, in examining police/adult interactions, the National Academies found that "the research base is currently insufficient to draw conclusions about whether procedurally just policing causally influences either perceived legitimacy or cooperation" (National Academies of Science, Engineering, and Medicine, 2018, p. 248), while also acknowledging that negative encounters could be a far more consequential influence on youth perceptions than positive encounters. Minority youth, who tend to experience a significant share of police attention, are more likely to hold critical opinions of the police and adopt protective responses, such as avoidance and resistance, compared to other youth (National Research Council, 2013).

The implications for procedural fairness are considerable in light of the extensive research that adolescents are vulnerable to intimidating encounters with law enforcement, particularly during questioning under circumstances that can be coercive, such as when they are isolated from adult support (Feld,

---

[5] "Procedural fairness" and "procedural justice" are terms used interchangeably in the literature and in this chapter as well.

2006). For example, one study found that only 8 percent of defendants ages 14 and under remained silent during an interrogation (Viljoen et al., 2005). It appears the younger the adolescent, the more susceptible they are, as demonstrated by a laboratory study that found children under 15 were more likely to confess than older teens (Grisso et al., 2003). The Supreme Court has long recognized this disadvantage, holding in 1967 that "the empirically based premise that juveniles, because of their developmental immaturity, are more vulnerable to coercion and less likely to understand or to exercise their interrogation rights has led courts to examine the confessions of juveniles with 'special caution'."[6] The Court recently extended that protection to include circumstances when police question youth in a closed schoolroom.[7]

There has been considerable litigation in recent years on the validity of juvenile confessions. This litigation has focused on doubts concerning their reliability (the potential for false confessions) and voluntariness (whether the juvenile was unduly pressured), as well as on whether juveniles understand their rights (to remain silent and to be represented by counsel) and make a "knowing" decision when they waive them. At a minimum, defendants need to understand the basic protections provided by the *Miranda* decision, but research shows that adolescents under age 15 do not have the ability to comprehend those rights (Grisso, 1980). Based on its review of the literature regarding the capacity of adolescents to understand their rights and the consequences of waiving them, the committee believes that adolescents under age 15 should not be permitted to waive the right to an attorney or the right to remain silent without prior consultation with an attorney. A *per se* rule is indicated in this context, as declared by the American Law Institute in its *Restatement of the Law: Children and the Law*.[8]

Legal Representation

"The right to representation by counsel is not a formality. It is not a grudging gesture to a ritualistic requirement. It is the essence of justice."[9] With these words the Supreme Court articulated a constitutional protection that it has repeatedly upheld—that due process demands representation by an attorney whenever a juvenile is in legal proceedings where the juvenile's liberty is at stake.[10] As previously discussed, juveniles younger than 15 lack the requisite cognitive capacity to knowingly waive their right to counsel, and they certainly lack the requisite knowledge to represent their own

---

[6] In re Gault, 387 U.S. at 45.

[7] J. D. B. v. North Carolina, 564 U.S. 261 (2011).

[8] American Law Institute, Restatement of the Law: Children and the Law, Section 14.22 (approved at Annual Meeting, May, 2018).

[9] Kent v. United States, 383 U.S. 541, 561 (1966).

[10] In re Gault, (387 U.S. 1 (1967)).

interests. Yet many states allow youth to make decisions about their pleas and sentences without the guidance or support of a lawyer (Feld, 1989). For example, one recent study of court proceedings in various states found that up to 90 percent of juveniles waive their right to counsel and enter into plea agreements, without consulting an attorney and without warnings regarding the consequences (National Juvenile Defender Center, 2016).

One element of procedural fairness is voice, such as when a person is able to fully participate in the legal proceedings. This is the role an attorney plays in juvenile proceedings; giving a platform to the adolescent client's voice in the courtroom. The role of the juvenile defender is to insist on fair and lawful juvenile court proceedings, guarantee that the child's voice is heard at every stage of the process, and safeguard the child's due process and equal protection rights (National Juvenile Defender Center, 2016). Procedural fairness is virtually unachievable without skilled lawyers advocating for their young clients. While statutes and judicial precedents in most states permit juveniles to waive counsel in delinquency proceedings, this practice has been widely criticized by legal commentators, and a systematic review of rulings by state appellate courts over the past decade indicates that trial court rulings permitting waiver tend to be reversed, especially in cases involving felony offenses or significant periods of confinement.[11] In the committee's view, waiver of counsel should rarely, if ever, be permitted, in accord with the position taken by the Council of the American Law Institute in 2018.[12]

Procedural fairness can also be enhanced by creating legal teams that include social workers, housing specialists, and other critical services. In addition to improving procedural fairness, a recent 10-year comparison study found that the use of interdisciplinary legal teams in adult court cases in the Bronx, New York City, significantly reduced incarceration and saved taxpayer dollars, without harming public safety (Anderson et al., forthcoming).

Juvenile Fines and Fees

Courts can sentence offenders to fines, fees, restitution, and surcharges. These monetary sanctions act as a "fee-for-service," aimed at recouping the costs of the justice system (Harris, 2016). If outstanding legal fees are not paid regularly, offenders may be called to court hearings and warrants may be issued for their arrest for violation of court orders, if they fail to

---

[11] This systematic review of state appellate rulings was conducted for the American Law Institute's Restatement of Law: Children and the Law by the Co-Reporter's for the Project in the summer of 2018. See Reporter's Note for Section 15.21. American Law Institute, Restatement of the Law: Children and the Law, Section 15.21 (approved by Council, September, 2018).

[12] American Law Institute, Restatement of the Law: Children and the Law, Section 15.21 (approved by Council, September, 2018).

pay or appear before the court. Moreover, if fines and fees are not paid in full, offenders cannot regain certain rights lost upon conviction, such as the right to vote and have their records sealed. In this way, indigent defendants often remain under the supervision of the court long after their original sentences (Harris, 2016).

Although most research to date on the effects of financial penalties has focused on the adult criminal justice system, a recent study by Piquero and Jennings (2017) looked at the effects fines and fees have on recidivism rates in the juvenile justice system. According to their analysis of data collected from 1,167 youth from Allegheny County, Pennsylvania, non-White youth with a history in the juvenile justice system were more likely to have higher total amounts of fines and fees when their case closed and were at higher risk of recidivism than White youth. Similar disparities have been found in relation to fines and fees in the criminal justice system.[13]

While fines and fees may be used to improve youth outcomes by reducing recidivism rates and increasing youth understanding of empathy and accountability, excessive fees that do not consider one's ability to pay can have long-lasting effects on youth, their families, and society. For instance, youth, and sometimes parents, who receive penalties for failure to pay may suffer negative effects on employability, which in turn can make it difficult to avoid re-entering the justice system (Feierman et al., 2016; Harris, 2016).

Although more research is needed on the outcomes associated with the current systems of fines and fees for juveniles at the national, state, and local levels, Piquero and Jennings (2017) encourage policy makers to consider currently available evidence and improve current policies to return the juvenile justice system to its mission of providing justice for victims and encouraging the rehabilitation of youth offenders so that they may become positive and productive members of their communities (Piquero and Jennings, 2017).

Reducing Harm

Harm after exiting the justice system may result from system interventions that impede or prevent a successful transition to a law-abiding adult life by making it difficult for youth to productively re-enter their communities. We have previously discussed the cardinal aim of reducing secure placements in correctional settings unless necessary for public protection

---

[13] According to a recent report by the U.S. Commission on Civil Rights (2017), families of color with low-income levels are more likely to receive financial penalties in the criminal court system. Further, even fines and fees imposed for minor crimes can increase family debt, creating substantial difficulties for families with limited incomes (U.S. Commission on Civil Rights, 2017).

and then only for periods of days or months, not years. Much progress has been made in recent years. In this section, we discuss three additional practices that should be used only when essential to protect public safety, if at all: allowing access to records of justice system involvement, using sex offender registries, and allowing solitary confinement.

Access to Juvenile Offense Records

As previously discussed, much of adolescent delinquent behavior is influenced by developmental factors, and therefore, when given access to supportive resources, most youth will mature out of criminal activity. In fact, research clearly indicates that only a small number of adolescent offenders persist in their offending beyond their mid to late 20s (Mulvey et al., 2014). This pattern among adolescents of criminal involvement and disengagement suggests that society's goal of reducing crime will be furthered by interventions that hold young people accountable for their misdeeds while not increasing the risk of re-offending or otherwise hindering positive development and maturation (National Research Council, 2013).

While it is well recognized that the declared ethos of juvenile court system has traditionally been "to hide youthful errors from the full gaze of the public and bury them in the graveyard of the forgotten past" (Juvenile Law Center, 2016, p. 3), in practice easy access to juvenile records is now commonplace in most jurisdictions (Juvenile Law Center, 2014a, 2014b). During the first generation of the juvenile court period (1899–1967), the general practice was to seal records (close them to public view) or expunge them (physically destroy them). However, these practices were abandoned in many states during the last two decades of the 20th century as a more punitive model of juvenile justice was widely embraced. As a result, state statutes are now quite complicated. As of 2014, record information was completely confidential in only nine states—that is, they allowed no public access to juvenile records, regardless of the seriousness of the offense, the number of offenses, or the age of the child (Juvenile Law Center, 2013). At the other end of the spectrum, seven states categorically make all juvenile records public, although there are some exceptions in each of these states. In the remaining 33 states and the District of Columbia, access to the records typically turns on the age of the juvenile, the nature of the offense, the number of offenses, or the amount of time since the adjudication; a blunt distinction is often drawn between felonies and less serious offenses.

In recent years, the pendulum has begun to swing back in the direction of confidentiality. According to the most recent data, 42 states offer juveniles a chance to expunge or seal their records after a certain period (Juvenile Law Center, 2018b; National Conference of State Legislatures, 2018). However, of these states, only 12 provide automatic sealing or expungement of these records. If the principle is accepted that the only overriding justification for allowing access to records of juvenile offending is to protect public safety, there is no justification for allowing access to the records in connection with employment, occupational licensing, and other purposes unrelated to law enforcement.

Among the most contested questions in the continuing debate about access to juvenile records is whether delinquency adjudications should count as "criminal convictions" for purposes of mandatory sentencing enhancements for re-offending. Many legal commentators have argued that these records should not be used for this purpose, because findings of delinquency in most states do not have the degree of reliability that criminal convictions have due to the informality of juvenile court proceedings and the weakness of procedural safeguards, including the lack of a right to a jury trial, and because enhancing later sentences based on a juvenile offense is disproportionate to the juvenile's culpability (Feld, 2003). It is also doubtful that automatically enhancing a later sentence without regard to the circumstances of the offense can be defended on public safety grounds, but more individualized use by sentencing judges might be defensible as an element of a general policy that allows prior offending to be taken into account in criminal sentencing.

Use of Juvenile Records in Risk Assessment

A related issue is whether and in what way juvenile offending should be considered in statistical risk assessments. Predictive decisions are made routinely in the justice system, and particularly in cases involving adolescents, including whether to place a youth in detention after being charged with an offense, whether to place an adjudicated delinquent in a secure facility, whether to transfer a juvenile charged with a serious offense to the criminal court for trial on the ground that retaining the youth in the juvenile system would not adequately protect public safety, and, if the youth is prosecuted in the criminal court, whether incarceration is required for public protection. The parallel assessment in the context of juvenile dispositions is whether the services provided to the juvenile will reduce the risk of re-offending.

These are exactly the sort of prediction tasks that human beings have enormous difficulty with, since they require thinking probabilistically, drawing inferences, and making attributions (see, e.g., Kahneman, 2011). As a consequence, a large body of research in psychology shows that on average, statistical models are typically able to formulate such predictions much more accurately than human beings (Dawes 1971, 1979; Dawes et al., 1989; Grove et al., 2000; Meehl, 1954).

Research on risk assessment tools has examined a variety of factors to determine predictive accuracy and reliability, such as including a history of arrest as a juvenile (Bechtel et al., 2011). This has prompted considerable debate and ongoing research as to the utility of these assessment tools, with some critical of the potential for inherent biases (Harcourt, 2015) and others praising objectivity as potentially increasing fairness (Flores et al., 2016).

The likely consequence of human misprediction in the justice system is that judges detain many low-risk people while releasing many high-risk ones, and more generally they detain more people overall than necessary to achieve a given level of crime reduction (Kleinberg et al., 2018). The well-documented biases that affect human cognition may also lead judges and other human decision makers to consciously or subconsciously predict in ways that adversely affect disadvantaged groups. These same challenges to human cognition may affect other criminal justice decisions, as well as efforts to prioritize and target social services, educational services, and other remediation programs that too often do not have adequate capacity to serve everyone who might potentially benefit.

Risk prediction models have the potential, if properly regulated, to improve the quality of predictions and hence justice system decisions (Kleinberg et al., forthcoming; see also Goel et al., 2019). For example in a study of the adult justice system in New York City, Kleinberg and colleagues (2018) show that basing pretrial release decisions on statistical predictions rather than judges' predictions would allow for the current jail population to be reduced by more than 40 percent with no increase in either crime or skipped court appearances, by limiting detention to those who are truly high-risk. Moreover, these gains can be achieved while simultaneously reducing racial disparities in pretrial detention relative to the status quo. However, these outcomes are not guaranteed. Risk tools, like any technology, can be misused, which is a particular concern in the context of the criminal justice and juvenile justice systems in the United States, where over-representation of racial and ethnic minority groups remains a longstanding problem in urgent need of repair. Putting the proper regulatory and legal systems in place to deal with these new tools, which would require approaches quite different from the legal systems required to regulate human decision making (Kleinberg et al., forthcoming), is critical to help ensure that this new technology is used in helpful ways.

This discussion highlights the potential benefits from making juvenile records available for risk prediction by judges and other criminal justice officials; but of course there are also potential costs. However, if these records are made available to the general public, rather than being restricted to use by judges and other officials, they are likely (all else equal) to hamper adolescents' ability to attend college, get a job, complete occupational license, or secure housing, among other critical life events. Making juvenile records widely available would compound the consequences of justice system involvement. However, making records available for the purposes of better risk prediction and hence justice system decisions and targeting of social services has the potential to accomplish the opposite, reducing the prevalence of justice system involvement. More research is urgently needed to better understand the tradeoffs involved here and how society can best manage them. It does seem well within our capability to allow proper uses for risk assessment while restricting access to these records for purposes of education, employment, and other purposes unrelated to the prevention of crime.

Sex Offender Registries

Perhaps the most severe version of juvenile offense information preventing future life opportunities is sex offender registration for non-violent offenses committed as a juvenile.

In 2006, Congress enacted the Sex Offender Registration and Notification Act (SORNA), which established minimum guidelines for registrations with which states must comply.[14] SORNA was the first federal legislation that explicitly covered juvenile sex offenders, including those who were either at least 14-years-old and adjudicated delinquent for sex offenses involving aggravating circumstances or convicted in criminal court. In 2011, the Department of Justice clarified that states were not required to publicly disclose the names of juvenile sex offenders. However, many states nonetheless require younger juveniles to register (even for less serious offenses) and provide public notification (Najdowski et al., 2016). Thirty-eight states have some form of juvenile sex offender registration and notification laws. Moreover, six states require *lifetime* registration of juvenile offenders.[15] Many jurisdictions have implemented policies for juveniles adjudicated delinquent that mirrored the practices used for adult offenders (Sandler et al., 2017). In those states that require registration, adolescents are sometimes directed to register as sex offenders for behaviors that are not violent, including sexting and engaging in consensual sexual relationships with similar-aged peers (Higgins, 2010). In these cases, youth exploring sexual identities—a normative process of adolescence—are unfairly required to register as sex offenders. While some states have adopted laws and policies to protect this behavior—typically through "Romeo-and-Juliet" provisions that allow for relationships between adolescents within specified age ranges—those provisions often do not protect juveniles from registration in cases involving same-sex relationships.

---

[14]Under SORNA, a "sex offense" includes offenses having "an element involving a sexual act or contact with another"; "video voyeurism"; having possession of, producing, or distributing child pornography; and "any conduct that by its nature is a sex offense against a minor."

[15]The six states that require lifetime registration of juvenile sex offenders are California, Florida, Montana, South Carolina, Virginia, and Washington.

An increasing number of legal scholars have questioned the constitutionality of requiring juveniles to register as sex offenders for these non-violent behaviors, based on both the Supreme Court's decisions in *Roper v. Simmons*,[16] *Graham v. Florida*,[17] and *Miller v. Alabama*,[18] as well as research findings on the profoundly negative impact on the life outcomes of juveniles. Studies show that juveniles registered as sex offenders suffer shame, ostracism, and depression in the short term, and long-term effects have been documented in mental health, education, employment, homelessness, and relationship disruptions (Chaffin, 2008; Levenson and Cotter, 2005; Mercado et al., 2008; Tewksbury and Lees, 2006). In 2013, Pittman and Parker published the results of 300 interviews that contained consistent accounts of the irreparable harm experienced by youth and their families due to the juvenile sex offender registries. They reported pervasive harassment, stigmatization, isolation, and suicidality (Human Rights Watch, 2013).

Research has demonstrated that rates of re-offending are as low as 5 percent among juveniles adjudicated as sex offenders (Bureau of Justice Statistics, 2003; Hanson et al., 2014; Zgoba et al., 2016; Zimring, 2004), substantially lower than the re-offending rates of those adjudicated or convicted of violent, property, and drug crimes (Durose et al., 2014; Sample and Bray, 2006). In addition to the extremely low rate of recidivism, there appears to be little relationship between early offending and offending as an adult. One study noted that 85 percent of juvenile sex offenders did not re-offend as adults and that 92 percent of adult sex offenders had not offended as juveniles (Jennings et al., 2009). The recidivism and re-offense rates also show no connection with whether or not youth were registered as sex offenders. To date, no demonstrated reductions in sexual offenses has been attributable to registering as a sex offender (Agan, 2011) or to the existence of sex offender registries themselves (Letourneau et al., 2010).

The foregoing findings led Jennings and colleagues (2015) to conclude that "in light of these empirical consistencies, it appears that community notification and registration policies seem to overly penalize and misidentify sex offender recidivists, especially among juvenile sex offenders, and may be doing more harm than good" (Jennings et al., 2015). The data suggest that there would be little risk to public safety if sex offender registration were to be eliminated for non-violent juveniles.

---

[16] Roper v. Simmons, 543 U.S. 551, 618 (2005) (Scalia J., dissenting).
[17] Graham v. Florida, 560 U.S. 48 (2010).
[18] Miller v. Alabama, 132 S. Ct. 2455 (2012).

Solitary Confinement

The practice of placing incarcerated individuals alone in a cell for an extended period of time is most commonly termed *solitary confinement* but is also known as "room confinement," "seclusion," "isolation," or "segregation." While current data are insufficient to estimate the prevalence of the use of solitary confinement for juveniles, a 2010 national study reported that more than one-third of the roughly 100,000 youth placed in juvenile residential facilities spent time in solitary confinement (Sedlak and McPherson, 2010). The Office of Juvenile Justice and Delinquency Prevention has reported that, in 2014, nearly one-half of juvenile detention facilities and training schools used practices that confined youth alone for more than 4 hours at a time (Hockenberry et al., 2016). A 2017 report details the persistent use of solitary confinement for up to 23 hours per day in some facilities (Feierman et al., 2017). While high-quality research about the effects of solitary confinement on outcomes like safety within a detention facility is quite limited, some correctional administrators apparently believe that isolation increases the safety and security of the facilities (Feierman et al., 2017).

Social science research to date has provided very little assessment of what, if any, benefits solitary confinement provides for facility safety, but the research is quite clear that the practice poses a number of demonstrated harms to juveniles. As discussed in Chapter 3, positive interactions with peers facilitate psychosocial maturity and growth in adolescents; therefore, confining youth alone for extended periods of time inhibits their ability to interact with peers and deprives them of a developmentally appropriate environment. Moreover, given the heightened plasticity of the adolescent brain, negative environments and adverse experiences, such as being held in solitary confinement, will result in significant trauma (Haney, 2003) and adversely affect adolescent brain development (see, e.g., Cauffman et al., 2018; Tottenham and Galván, 2016). Indeed, extensive research in rodents shows that solitary and barren housing has detrimental effects on dendritic morphology, which further suggests that solitary confinement has impacts on brain development at the neuronal level (see, e.g., Beery and Kaufer, 2014; Hyer and Glasper, 2017; Medendorp et al., 2018).

Although there is little systematic evidence specifically demonstrating the harmful effects of solitary confinement on youth, studies of incarcerated adults consistently demonstrate that those who experience solitary confinement are at greater risk for mental illness and suicide (Grassian, 2006). According to the National Research Council's 2014 report, *The Growth of Incarceration in the United States: Exploring Causes and Consequences*, "an extensive empirical literature indicates that long-term isolation or solitary confinement in prison settings can inflict emotional damage. The overwhelming majority of studies document the painful and potentially damaging nature of long-term prison isolation (Lobel and Akil, 2018)" (National Research Council, 2014a, p. 187). Indeed, considering that many incarcerated youth prior to incarceration experienced trauma or suffered from an undiagnosed mental illness (Vermeiren et al., 2006), youth are likely to be particularly vulnerable to the harmful effects of solitary confinement, and it is likely that solitary confinement exacerbates their pre-existing conditions (Rademacher, 2016). Though studies have not specifically examined the effects of solitary confinement on juveniles' well-being and development, the committee concludes that this practice is at least as harmful to adolescents as it is for adults, and probably more so.

Recognizing these ill effects, the Obama Administration banned the use of solitary confinement for juveniles in federal prisons (The White House, 2016), and the criminal justice reform legislation known as the First Step Act, passed and enacted in late 2018, also includes a ban on solitary confinement for juveniles in federal prisons. A broad array of professional associations have condemned youth solitary confinement, including the American Academy of Child and Adolescent Psychiatry, the American Correctional Association, the American Medical Association, the American Psychological Association, the American Public Health Association, the National Commission on Correctional Health Care, the National Task Force on Children Exposed to Violence, the Council of Juvenile Correctional Administrators, and the National Council of Juvenile and Family Court Judges (Feierman et al., 2017). Thirty states and the District of Columbia have eliminated the use of the practice for punitive reasons, although 25 states still allow the solitary confinement of juveniles for other purposes, including safety concerns (Lowenstein Center for the Public Interest, 2016). Many of these states permit indefinite extensions of limits on the amount of time a juvenile may be held in solitary confinement (Feierman et al., 2017).

Of the youth experiencing solitary confinement while detained, it is likely that youth of color, youth identifying as LGBTQ, and youth with disabilities are disproportionately represented. While no national database tracks the placement of juveniles in solitary confinement by race, data regarding use of the practice in adult facilities suggest that individuals of color are subject to disparate treatment within facilities, including disparate exposure to solitary confinement (Feierman et al., 2017). According to a 2015 survey of 48 jurisdictions conducted by Yale Law School, approximately 7 percent of individuals housed in solitary confinement in adult facilities identified as transgender, even though they accounted for less than 1 percent of the incarcerated population (Association of State Correctional Administrators and Yale Law School, 2016). Youth with disabilities may also be disproportionately placed in detention and other correctional facilities. Qualitative evidence suggests that individuals with physical disabilities and transgender youth may be placed in solitary confinement because of a lack of adequate accommodations in general housing or because correctional facility staff deem solitary confinement necessary to protect these youth from the general population (American Civil Liberties Union, 2017; Feierman et al., 2017).

While little research has been conducted on effective alternatives to solitary confinement, a number of jurisdictions are adopting changes in policy and practice designed to protect both the safety of individuals and the facilities as a whole (National Institute of Justice, 2016). For example, the Vera Institute of Justice has been working on two separate projects with adult corrections officials in 13 states: Illinois, Louisiana, Maryland, Minnesota, Nebraska, Nevada, New Mexico, North Carolina, Oregon, Pennsylvania, Utah, Virginia, and Washington. The goals of the institute's Segregation Reduction Project and Safe Alternatives to Segregation Initiative are to help states reduce the use of solitary confinement and develop effective alternatives in adult facilities. Strategies largely fall into three categories: using specialty units; designing policies and coordinating staff and training (training examples include de-escalation and behavioral intervention techniques); and programming for offenders (Zyvoloski, 2018). One example of specialized units is the New York City Clinical Alternative to Punitive Segregation (CAPS) unit. This treatment unit, which was established for inmates with serious mental illnesses, provides alternatives to solitary confinement, including group therapy, medication, and other therapeutic interventions to reduce injury caused by self-harm and altercations with inmates and prison staff (Glowa-Kollisch et al., 2016). Researchers who studied the intervention found that participation in the program is effective at reducing self-harm and injury and may be cost-effective when health, hospitalization, and fees associated with legal actions are considered.

Although research on effective alternatives continues to be developed, the lifelong harm to youth has led many policy makers, courts, and correctional administrators to agree that solitary confinement for juveniles should be immediately reduced and ultimately eliminated (see Box 9-4). In 2016, the National Council of Juvenile and Family Court Judges passed a resolution to eliminate the solitary confinement of juveniles, listing a series of alternatives such as having clear facility policies that limit room confinement; engaging in staff training in verbal and nonverbal de-escalation strategies; developing behavior management programs; increasing the staff-to-youth ratios; providing mental health professionals to assess youth in crises; and establishing less restrictive alternative housing settings (National Council of Juvenile and Family Court Judges, 2016). It is worthy of note that the Council of Juvenile Correctional Administrators (2015, p. 4) issued a toolkit to reduce the use of isolation in juvenile facilities, stating, "There is no research showing the benefits of using isolation to manage youths'

BOX 9-4
Youth Perspectives: Solitary Confinement

The Juvenile Law Center's Juveniles for Justice class of 2017–2018 recently shared their experiences with the juvenile justice system in *Broken Bridges: How Juvenile Placements Cut Off Youth from Communities and Successful Futures* (Juvenile Law Center, 2018a). Their experiences with solitary confinement are as follows (Juvenile Law Center, 2018a, pp. 17–18):

Qilah: "While I was in placement, often the whole group would get punished for behavior of one person. One time, I was placed in solitary confinement for one day for defending myself when a staff person threw a walkie talkie in my face. Another time at a holding facility, I was put in solitary for about 3–4 days. When I was in solitary, there was only a metal chair in the room and a table nailed to the floor. A person brought me food throughout the day and brought me a pen and paper for me to write to my family."

Ange: "In general, you can't talk to anyone or look at anyone (in a silly way) or you would get in trouble. I was placed in isolation rooms for being considered a 'threat' because I moved too quickly while talking to staff."

Hid: "I was in solitary for one week once, and the room was cushion—a sponge-like substance. They put me there because someone in the cafeteria was looking at me and I felt threatened. They thought that we both might get into a fight because we were staring at each other, so we were both put into solitary. They only checked on me when it was time for meals, and they brought my class work to me, otherwise there was nothing for me to do and no one for me to interact with. I slept, looked at the wall, worked out in the room, and I ate—that's it, for a whole week. At first, I didn't think it would affect me, but after being in the room with nothing to do for even a few minutes it started to bother me. It made me feel weak because there was nothing I could do to get out. There was only really me, the walls, and the floor."

Jaheem: "At the detention center, if there was a fight everyone would be on lock down for some hours or a full day. It depended on the situation, like if a youth was in a unit fight, we would all be on lock down for 24 hours. We also would not be able to see our families if a lockdown happened. This was upsetting because it felt as if we were all being punished for someone else's behavior. This was also frustrating because if I had court the same day the lockdown happened, my court date got pushed back, sometimes almost a month. It shouldn't be that if one youth acts out in a facility, we are all punished even when we did not cause any trouble."

behavior." Urgent research is needed to identify effective alternatives to solitary confinement, so that detention facilities will be able to scale back or even eliminate the use of this practice without having adverse effects on the facilities' safety and functioning.

A DEVELOPMENTALLY INFORMED CRIMINAL JUSTICE SYSTEM

As noted in Chapter 1, the committee regards the period of adolescence as extending into the twenties from a developmental standpoint, but we have chosen to focus attention concerning the justice system on early, middle, and late adolescents (ages 10 to 17). This is the age group termed "juveniles," the young people whom the juvenile justice system has traditionally served. Historically, one of the most contested (and frequently litigated) issues in the entire field of juvenile justice was the practice of trying many, if not most, older "juveniles" (those between ages 15 and 17) in *criminal* courts. This longstanding dispute revolves around two age-related issues: (1) the maximum jurisdictional age of the juvenile court (typically 18, but sometimes 16 or 17), which classifies *all* 16–17-year-olds as "adults" and subjects them to severe criminal punishments; and (2) the transfer age—the age at which a juvenile otherwise within the jurisdiction of the juvenile court may be transferred to the criminal court for trial as an adult (typically age 14 but widely varying according to the offense charged as well as prior offending).

As a result of developmentally driven reforms in recent years, it is now generally accepted that the maximum age of juvenile court jurisdiction should not be lower than 18 (National Conference of State Legislatures, 2018). The recently emerging discussion is whether the jurisdictional age should be raised even higher than 18, thereby conferring juvenile court jurisdiction in some classes of cases involving young adults ages 18 to 21, based on the developmental argument that the adolescent brain continues to mature into the mid-twenties. This issue will be briefly addressed later in the chapter.

Transfer Age and Effects of Transfer to Criminal Courts

For the purposes of this report, the central age-related issue concerns the "transfer age"—specifically, the circumstances under which adolescents *younger than 18* should be subject to criminal prosecution and punishment instead of being retained in the juvenile court. That issue is the main focus of the remainder of this chapter.

Since the juvenile court was first created more than a century ago, juvenile judges have had authority to "transfer" older juveniles (those ages 14 to 17) to the criminal court for trial as adults. Typically, these decisions have been individualized judicial determinations based on the juvenile's age and maturity, seriousness of the offense charged, danger to public safety, and "amenability" to the treatment and services offered in the juvenile system. In the 1990s, in direct response to a spike in youth violence, many states revised the transfer procedures to *require* criminal prosecution in specified categories of cases involving older adolescents charged with more serious offenses, or to tighten the criteria or shift the burden of proof to the juvenile. All states made some type of change designed to facilitate criminal prosecution of adolescents under age 18 (Office of Juvenile Justice and Delinquency Prevention, 1997).

To summarize the current structure of transfer statutes, criminal court jurisdiction may be established in three basic ways: by statutory exclusions from juvenile court jurisdiction or "automatic transfer" (offenses determined by law as requiring criminal court jurisdiction); by traditional judicial decisions after a hearing waiver (allowing the judge to transfer a case from juvenile to criminal court or allowing the criminal courts to transfer a case to juvenile court); or by prosecutorial decisions to file criminal charges (also known as "direct file") (National Research Council, 2013, p. 52; National Conference of State Legislatures, 2019). The minimum age for transfer is 14 in most states, but it varies according to the seriousness of offense. In recent years, there has been a modest trend to restore juvenile court jurisdiction and return discretion to the judges.

The consequences of transferring a juvenile to criminal court can be severe. Available sentences are much lengthier than typical juvenile court dispositions and can expose the juvenile to mandatory periods of incarceration. Adolescents tried as adults are also at risk of being incarcerated in adult facilities, where they are at greater risk of sexual and physical victimization; although adolescents under age 18 constitute a small minority of inmates in adult facilities, they constitute 21 percent of all victims of substantiated incidents of sexual violence (Beck and Harrison, 2008). The extraordinarily high stakes in transfer proceedings are magnified by the fact that Black youth are more likely to be sentenced to adult prison with longer terms than White youth (Lehmann et al., 2017).

The practice of placing youth in adult facilities continues due to a belief that housing juveniles tried as adults in juvenile facilities poses a risk to other youth in those juvenile facilities (Bechtold and Cauffman, 2014; Burke, 2005). However, empirical evidence shows that youth incarcerated in adult facilities do not commit more institutional offenses than youth incarcerated in juvenile facilities and might not pose a greater threat than youth tried in juvenile court (Bechtold and Cauffman, 2014).

Conversely, as noted by the National Research Council (2013, p. 134), "prisons have been characterized as developmentally toxic settings for adolescents" adversely affecting adolescents' development of psychosocial maturity, a critical developmental skill for desistance from crime (also see Dmitrieva et al., 2012). Youth confined in adult settings have less access to rehabilitation and education programs than do youth in juvenile facilities (Arya, 2007). This is illustrated by the cost differential between juvenile and adult facilities. For example, in Chicago, the per diem cost of housing a juvenile at the Juvenile Temporary Detention Center is more than three times the per diem cost of doing so in the Cook County Jail due to the services and programs provided (Circuit Court of Cook County Illinois, 2018; Joint Criminal Justice Reform Committee, 2014). Even youth housed in residential treatment facilities for adults, environments that are focused on rehabilitation, experience decreases in psychosocial maturity over time (Hahn et al., 2007).

While it is clear that placing adolescents in adult prisons has harmful effects on their development, well-being, and health, it is possible that these concerns are mitigated or offset by the incapacitative effect of confinement and by reducing the risk of further offending upon release. As previous National Research Council reports (National Research Council, 2013, 2014) concluded, youth transferred to the adult criminal justice system fare worse than those who remain in the juvenile justice system (Austin et al., 2000; Task Force on Community Preventive Services, 2007). It also concluded that they are at greater risk of reoffending upon release (Bishop and Frazier, 2000; Mulvey and Schubert, 2011; Redding, 2008).

A number of researchers have found that adolescents who are transferred to the adult system are more likely to re-offend, likely to do so at a greater rate, and likely be rearrested for more serious offenses, on average, than those retained in the juvenile justice system (Bishop and Frazier, 2000; Bishop et al., 1996; Kupchik et al., 2003; Mulvey and Schubert, 2012; Winner et al., 1997). Zane and colleagues (2016) conducted a meta-analysis of the specific deterrent effects of juvenile transfer and found that judicial waiver, in particular, may increase recidivism among transferred youths relative to nontransferred youths (Zane et al., 2016). However, the results might not be conclusive, because their research design does not account for omitted variable or selection bias. That is, while it is plausible that the adult system could have adverse effects on youth outcomes, another plausible explanation for finding increased recidivism rates in the transferred population could be that criminal justice system actors have prioritized the highest-risk juveniles for transfer into the adult system, thereby driving the divergent pattern of recidivism rates.

Other recent studies have used regression discontinuity designs to overcome this concern about selection bias, and these provide more robust evidence. Hansen and Waddell (2014) in an analysis of adult prosecutions of juveniles in Oregon, found some evidence that harsher punishments do deter crime. Loeffler and Grunwald (2015) similarly found that processing juveniles in the adult system may not uniformly increase offending and may reduce offending in some circumstances. However, these studies do not provide definitive conclusions as to the impact of transfers on recidivism. Further, since they rely on a minimum age cutoff for eligibility for transfer to adult courts, they do not tell us anything about the effects of criminal prosecution on older youths (those between ages 18 and 26) (Loeffler and Chalfin, 2017; National Research Council, 2013).

In sum, the scientific evidence on the effects of transfer on juveniles' outcomes appears to be mixed. There is strong evidence of the negative effects of transfer on adolescents' development and well-being; however, evidence as to the effects of transfer on recidivism is still emerging. This still-developing body of evidence on transfer does little to inform debates as to the proper maximum age of juvenile court adjudication or the mechanisms by which juveniles should or should not be prosecuted in criminal courts. Given that punishing adolescents for criminal behavior in the same way that adults are punished has a long-lasting or enduring negative effect, this committee reaffirms the National Research Council's 2013 report findings, which clearly stated that transfer decisions should be guided by the principles of proportionality and individualization with consideration given to the maturity, needs, and circumstances of the individual offender (National Research Council, 2013).

Blended Sentencing

A related controversial issue is whether juvenile courts should have the authority to impose adult sentences for youth who have been charged as adults while being tried in juvenile court. This practice, often referred to as "blended sentencing," can occur in juvenile or criminal courts after the waiver or transfer of youth and is most often used for serious juvenile offenders. Blended sentencing generally takes three forms: (1) the court sentences the youth to a juvenile disposition or an adult sentence; (2) the court sentences youth to a juvenile disposition along with a suspended criminal sentence, conditional upon nonoffending; and (3) the court sentences youth to a juvenile sentence disposition with extended juvenile jurisdiction, usually up to age 21, at which time there is a hearing to determine whether an adult sentence is appropriate or whether the youth has been successfully rehabilitated.

Blended sentencing is a creative effort to use the threat of a criminal sentence as leverage to facilitate compliance with juvenile court dispositional requirements. Data are not yet available to compare outcomes between cases in which similarly situated youth are retained in juvenile court with juvenile dispositions alone and cases in which the youth were transferred to criminal court outright. For the moment, the most policy-relevant questions are whether the juvenile procedures for blended sentencing conform with constitutionally required safeguards and whether the placements are developmentally appropriate. In the committee's judgment, juveniles (offenders younger than 18) sentenced to terms of confinement (whether by juvenile judges or criminal court judges) should be placed in juvenile correctional settings when younger than 18, should be entitled to all of the services they would have received if they had received a juvenile disposition, and, upon turning 18, should be entitled to placement in facilities and services available to young adult offenders. Their sentences should also be subject to formal review on an individualized basis to determine whether their criminal sentences should be adjusted in light of their mitigated culpability and prospects for successful adjustment in the community.

The scientific evidence is clear that a developmentally appropriate response to adolescent misbehavior recognizes the need to hold young people accountable and that adolescents' developmental immaturity also requires that sanctions imposed on adolescents should be different from those imposed on adult offenders. "Juvenile offenders as a class are less culpable than their adult counterparts and the decision to prosecute a juvenile as an adult is one that should be made with careful deliberation on an individualized basis" (Listenbee et al., 2012, p. 189; National Research Council, 2013, p. 136).

Programs for Young Offenders in the Criminal Justice System

Since the introduction of the concept of "emerging adults" (Arnett, 2000)—a category that covers the period of development between the ages of 18 and 25—researchers, practitioners, and policy makers have debated the implications for the criminal and juvenile justice systems. Some have advocated extending the age of the juvenile justice system to 21 with a gradually diminishing "immaturity discount" for young people ages 21 to 25 in the adult system (Gupta-Kagan, forthcoming; Perker and Chester, 2017; Schiraldi et al. 2015). Others have proposed creating a third system for this age group (Rocque et al., 2017). Scott and colleagues (2016) rejected "raising the age of juvenile court jurisdiction or creating a third type of court" and argued instead for developmentally informed sentencing and correctional programming in criminal courts. Predictably some have questioned the very formulation of this developmental stage in the first place (Côté, 2014).

This debate prompted the National Institute of Justice to assemble a study group of 33 experts to review the literature on a range of issues related to the justice system and emerging adults (Loeber et al., 2013). They examined criminal career patterns, special categories of offenders, influences, risk and needs assessments, prevention, interventions, and the border between the juvenile and criminal justice systems. A key finding of their work is that 40 to 60 percent of juvenile delinquents stop offending by early adulthood, consistent with the "age-crime curve" theory, which demonstrates that most antisocial behavior peaks in late adolescence and declines rapidly in early adulthood. Indeed, the 2015 National Academies' report, *Investing in the Health and Well-Being of Young Adults,* concluded that "one of the most important characteristics of young adults involved with the justice system is that, left on their own, most would soon desist from criminal behavior" (Institute of Medicine and National Research Council, 2015).

In 2016, the National Institute of Justice conducted an environmental scan to capture the range of developmentally informed correctional programming serving emerging adults in the justice system that might promote accountability and reduce reoffending. The resulting report (Hayek, 2016) documented approximately 45 programs newly focused on the emerging adult developmental stage, which fell into seven categories: young adult courts, probation and parole programs, district attorney-led programs, community-based partnerships, hybrid partnerships, prison-based programs, and advocacy and research programs. The common elements were a grounding in developmental science; significant collaboration across the justice system (e.g., courts, police, and prosecution) and across the system of care (e.g., mental health, substance abuse, education, social services) in partnership with community-based service providers; and case management to address the "intensity of services required to alter the trajectory for those involved in the justice system" (Hayek, 2016, p. 5). As an example, the report highlighted Roca, Inc., an innovative program in Massachusetts that tries to change the trajectory of the lives of young adults involved in the justice system (see Box 9-5).

Examples from Europe are instructive for states considering the challenges of addressing the needs of young adults within the existing adult system to improve outcomes and increase public safety. Twenty-eight out of 35 European countries have special provisions for emerging adults in their justice systems (Matthews et al., 2018). Germany, in particular, began developing a "minimum intervention" approach in 1923, where services, diversion, and nonpunitive approaches are emphasized. A specialized court has been established for youth between the ages of 14 and 21, which is required to limit confinement to violent offenses and, even then, the facilities are designed to encourage self-respect, promote education, and support rehabilitation. The living conditions are "normalized" with services such as "professional woodworking, metal working, culinary instruction and farming, with no use of solitary confinement or strip searching" (Matthews et al., 2018, p. 11). Across the European countries, the systems incorporate emerging adults, emphasize informal approaches and rehabilitation, and restrict or rely less upon incarceration than in the United States without compromising protection of the community.

BOX 9-5
Roca Inc.
A Program in Chelsea, Springfield, Lynn,
and Boston, Massachusetts

Roca Inc. was founded in Chelsea, Massachusetts, in 1988 and initially focused on addressing teen pregnancy to reduce child poverty. Since 1988, Roca's mission has evolved and taken on numerous social issues to reduce poverty and incarceration. Its intervention model is designed to work with youth at multiple stages in their developmental cycle and to provide them with continuous access to those services as they mature. The program seeks to solve the underlying challenges that may lead young men and women to make choices that could potentially pull them into the justice system.

Roca Inc. engages local stakeholders in this process and offers assistance that is individualized to meet the most pressing needs of each participating youth. Services offered include education, life skills, and career assistance. The outcomes of program participants are encouraging, with a 2017 study finding that 76 percent of male participants held jobs for at least 3 months and that 84 percent of males did not re-offend, while for females 97 percent held a job for at least 3 months and 89 percent delayed pregnancy. However, little is currently known about the degree to which ROCA itself has affected these outcomes, although there is a large-scale randomized trial currently under way (Urban Institute, 2014).

OPPORTUNITIES FOR CROSS-SYSTEM COLLABORATION

For youth who do become involved with the justice system, it is important that they receive the resources and services needed for positive development and rehabilitation so that their contact with the justice system is beneficial. All adolescents have the potential to thrive and flourish if given the proper supports, particularly those aimed at improving educational and physical and mental health outcomes. When youth are provided with these opportunities, the justice system can be a pathway toward positive developmental trajectories. To this end, increased coordination and collaboration between the education, health, justice, and child welfare systems is necessary to ensure that involvement with the justice system is rare, just, not harmful and, ideally, beneficial. This section discusses the role of the health and education systems in supporting justice-involved youth (see Chapter 8 for a discussion of needed collaboration between the child welfare and justice systems).

Collaboration with the Education System

Providing high-quality education in secure settings presents unique challenges for administrators, teachers, and staff who are responsible for the education, rehabilitation, and welfare of the young people in their care. The more than 2,500 residential facilities housing juveniles in the United States need support from federal, state, and local educational agencies and their communities to improve services for detained youth. Key to these supports are efforts to foster facility environments that prioritize education and provide the conditions for learning, to recruit and retain qualified educators, and to provide rigorous and relevant curricula aligned with state academic and career and technical education standards (U.S. Department of Education, 2014).

The education of youth in juvenile justice facilities presents a number of challenges that previous research suggests might benefit from better collaboration between the juvenile justice and education systems. For example, previous estimates suggest that while perhaps 40 percent of youth in juvenile detention require special education services (Coffey and Gemignani, 1994), many of these developmental deficits have not previously been diagnosed (see, e.g., Macomber et al., 2010). Similarly, estimates from juvenile detention facilities in Cook County, Illinois, suggest that 66 percent of male youth and 74 percent of female youth met clinical criteria for at least one mental health disorder (Teplin et al., 2002). Too little is currently known about the quality of the screening methods used in both juvenile justice and education systems to identify special education or mental health needs, the legal or other barriers to successfully sharing information across systems about what is learned about what youth need, or what the consequences would be for youth from developing better screening and information sharing across systems. Deficiencies in these areas make it difficult to capitalize on opportunities to help youth successfully desist from delinquency and re-engage with school.

We also know from previous research that most of the general challenges of successfully educating adolescents are even more challenging within the juvenile justice system, so there may be important benefits from enhanced efforts by public school systems to support education within the juvenile justice context. For example, previous research on public K–12 systems suggests that, all else being equal, teachers on average prefer to work in schools serving more advantaged student populations (Engel et al., 2014). This means successfully staffing schools serving juvenile justice populations—who come disproportionately from economically and educationally disadvantaged backgrounds—will be particularly difficult, and may also be one reason for the high rates of teacher turnover reported in schools serving juvenile detention facilities.[19] Education systems may have an important role to play in supporting or incentivizing the supply of high-quality teachers to juvenile justice facilities, and in helping such facilities do a better job identifying the most effective teacher candidates for those positions. However, too little is currently known about how to make improvements on either the supply or the demand side of this teacher labor market in general (Jacob, 2007).

For those educators currently serving justice-involved populations, there is a need to improve professional development opportunities, given the unique challenges of education within that environment. Evidence is now accumulating about how to successfully provide professional development to improve student learning and teacher-student interactions generally (e.g., see Allen et al., 2011), and there may be value in ensuring that education systems provide these best-practice professional development opportunities for teachers within juvenile justice settings.

Similarly, there may be benefits as well from having the juvenile justice system support to the greatest degree possible the educational efforts of schools serving youth in the justice system. Youth in juvenile detention settings should be provided with psychosocial supports that position them to benefit as much as possible from educational opportunities during and following detention. Heller and colleagues (2017) show that juvenile justice staff can successfully provide these types of supports during nonschool time in ways that improve youth outcomes inside detention facilities and also reduce recidivism.

Collaboration with the Health System

The prevalence of justice-involved adolescents exhibiting physical or mental health problems is high. These youth have significantly higher rates of tuberculous, sexually transmitted infections (STIs), alcohol use (74%), and illegal drug use (85%) (American Academy of Pediatrics, 2011). Recent results from the Survey of Youth in Residential Placement indicate that at least 50 percent of youth in juvenile facilities have experienced anxiety, anger, and loneliness, and approximately 1 in 5 have previously attempted suicide (American Academy of Pediatrics, 2011). Moreover, according to the National Center for Mental Health and Juvenile Justice (2007), justice-involved youth are more likely to have experienced one or more traumas before entering the justice system, increasing their chances of having disruptive behavioral issues, such as oppositional defiant disorder.

Given the prevalence of health needs within the population of justice-involved youth, ensuring that the justice system provides necessary health

---

[19] Office of Juvenile Justice and Delinquency Prevention (1994).

screenings and subsequent care is critical. Failure to provide adequate screenings and services can result in long-term health issues for adolescents, thus increasing their chances of re-offending in youth or as adults (Barnert et al., 2017; DiClemente and Wingood, 2017).

The most recent standards issued by the National Commission on Correctional Health Care require that youth in accredited facilities undergo a comprehensive health assessment within 7 days of arrival including, for example, a review of immunization records, TB screening, exposure to trauma, suicidal or violent behavior, and substance abuse (American Academy of Pediatrics, 2011). However, health screenings and care are not standard across juvenile facilities and often vary by state. For example, Pajer and colleagues (2007) found that the responsibility for conducting health screenings and care is inconsistent across facilities. Based on an analysis of self-report data, 62 percent of health screenings in U.S. juvenile detention facilities are conducted by the detention center staff. Those not conducted by staff may be assigned to either a contract provider (28%), private provider (3%), or public provider (7%) (Pajer et al., 2007).

Given the high percentage of detention center staff responsible for conducting screenings in juvenile facilities, adolescents will likely have better health outcomes if staff are trained to identify and respond to mental health issues when they surface. According to the Substance Abuse and Mental Health Services Agency (SAMHSA), all juvenile justice staff should be provided with continuous training in topics such as cultural sensitivity, administering and interpreting screening instruments, identifying reading difficulties, interpersonal communication, and counseling techniques (Center for Substance Abuse Treatment, 2000). The National Center for Mental Health and Juvenile Justice (2007) further recommends that the juvenile justice system provide trauma-informed services that include follow-up screenings and connection to trauma-specific services when needed.

It is important to note that screening for and responding to health issues is needed at every stage in the juvenile justice process, including the time during which youth are transitioning out of the system. Recent research suggests that individuals who were incarcerated in adolescence tend to have high-risk sexual behaviors, adult depressive symptoms, and an increased risk for suicide (Abram et al., 2017; Barnert et al., 2017; DiClemente and Wingood, 2017). Community-based re-entry programs that encourage collaborative partnerships among systems, families, and communities may help youth during this transition as they return to their schools, neighborhoods, and families, reducing the chances that they will re-offend in the future and improving their employment and health outcomes (Mears and Travis, 2004; Youth.gov, 2018).

RECOMMENDATIONS

Given the resounding scientific evidence about the neurobiological and socio-behavioral development of adolescents, it is clear that both the juvenile justice and criminal justice systems need to adopt policies and practices that support the positive development of all young people. While the juvenile justice system has embraced a wave of developmentally motivated reforms in this area in recent years, much more needs to be done to tackle the continued racial disparities in the system and to ensure that those youth that do become system-involved receive the necessary supports to achieve their full potential. Similar reform efforts that recognize the unique developmental needs of older adolescents and young adults are emerging within the criminal justice system. It is important that these efforts be guided by the science of adolescent development and the core principles of a developmental approach.

As noted above, the previous National Academies' reports on juvenile justice outlined recommendations for needed reforms to ensure that the juvenile justice system accounts for and attends to the developmental needs of youth. This committee reaffirms those recommendations, and offers several additional recommendations to promote a developmentally informed justice system, including continued opportunities within the juvenile justice system and emerging opportunities in the criminal justice system. Box 9-6 outlines these recommendations. Taken together, they constitute a blueprint for achieving a developmentally appropriate justice system.

RECOMMENDATION 9-1: Reduce disparities based on race, ethnicity, gender, ability status, and sexual orientation or gender identity and expression among adolescents involved in the justice system.

Given increasing racial disparities in the justice system, and growing evidence as to disparities related to ethnicity, gender, ability status, and sexual orientation, Congress should ensure proper implementation of the recently reauthorized JJDPA, including oversight of state efforts to monitor and reduce racial and ethnic disparities with an increased focus on research and data collection. The Office of Juvenile Justice and Delinquency Prevention (OJJDP), in accordance with requirements laid out in the JJDPA, should require at a minimum that all states furnish specific, rigorous metrics on the race and ethnicity of youth involved in the justice system.

School systems should leverage available federal, state, and local funding to implement evidence-based programs to improve social and structural conditions to reduce racial disparities and student referrals to the justice system. Law enforcement officials and other institutions and community organizations should undertake prevention programming designed to

---

BOX 9-6
Blueprint for Achieving a Developmentally
Appropriate Justice System

Recommendation 9-1: Reduce disparities based on race, ethnicity, gender, ability status, and sexual orientation or gender identity and expression among adolescents involved in the justice system.
  A. Congress should ensure proper implementation of the Juvenile Justice and Delinquency Prevention Act (JJDPA), including oversight of state efforts to monitor and reduce racial and ethnic disparities with an increased focus on research and data collection.
  B. The Office of Juvenile Justice and Delinquency Prevention (OJJDP), in accordance with requirements laid out in the JJDPA, should require at a minimum that all states furnish specific, rigorous metrics on the race and ethnicity of youth involved in the justice system.
  C. School systems should leverage available federal, state, and local funding to implement evidence-based programs to improve social and structural conditions to reduce racial disparities and student referrals to the justice system.
  D. Law enforcement officials and other institutions and community organizations should undertake prevention programming designed to reduce justice system involvement by disadvantaged groups, based on social and structural inequities differentially experienced by those groups.

Recommendation 9-2: Ensure that youth maintain supportive relationships while involved in the justice system and receive appropriate guidance and counsel from legal professionals and caregivers.
  A. Juvenile facilities should amend policies that curtail visitation rights as punishment, and states and localities should implement policies and practices to assist families in overcoming barriers to prison visitation so that youth can remain connected to parents, caregivers, and other relatives.
  B. Probationary programs should connect parents and caregivers with community and educational resources that can teach them how to help their child succeed and avoid future interactions with the justice system.
  C. State legislatures and courts should ensure that justice-involved youth are provided with competent counsel throughout the legal process.
  D. State legislatures and courts should ensure that adolescents under the age of 15 are not allowed to waive the right to an attorney or the right to remain silent without prior consultation with an attorney.

Recommendation 9-3: Implement policies that aim to reduce harm to justice-involved youth in accordance with knowledge from developmental science.
  A. Congress and state legislatures should enact legislation to eliminate the use of sex offender registries for non-violent juveniles.

continued

BOX 9-6 Continued

    B. Given the robust evidence of the harmful effects of solitary confinement, the federal government or philanthropic organizations should fund research on effective alternatives to solitary confinement so that detention facilities will be able to scale back or eliminate the use of this practice as soon as practicable.

Recommendation 9-4: Implement developmentally appropriate and fair policies and practices for adolescents involved in the criminal justice system.
    A. Legislatures should restore judicial discretion in decision making about transferring juveniles to or from criminal courts.
    B. Prosecutors and courts should be guided by the principles of proportionality and individualization with consideration given to the maturity, needs, and circumstances of the individual offender when making transfer decisions.
    C. Judges sentencing juveniles in criminal courts should place these youth in juvenile correctional settings rather than adult correctional facilities. These youth should be entitled to all of the services they would have received if they had received a juvenile disposition and, upon turning 18, should be entitled to placement and services available to young adult offenders. Courts should conduct formal review of youths' criminal sentences on an individualized basis to determine whether the sentences should be adjusted in light of their mitigated culpability and prospects for successful adjustment in the community.

Recommendation 9-5: For those youth in the custody of the justice system, ensure that policies and practices are implemented to prioritize the health and educational needs of adolescents and avoid causing harm.
    A. Correctional programming for adolescents and young adults in the criminal justice system should promote accountability and reduce re-offending through developmentally appropriate services in both correctional facilities and residential and community settings, including mental health, substance abuse, education, and social services.
    B. Researchers, in partnership with practitioners, should urgently examine and evaluate effective alternatives to solitary confinement that promote the healthy development of individual youth and protect the safety of all in the facility.
    C. State and local educational agencies should work in partnership with their justice system counterparts to ensure that rigorous and relevant curricula for adolescents are delivered in residential facilities and that these curricula are aligned with career and technical education standards and meet the needs of all youth, including those with disabilities and English learners.

reduce justice-system involvement by disadvantaged groups, based on social and structural inequities differentially experienced by those groups.

RECOMMENDATION 9-2: Ensure that youth maintain supportive relationships while involved in the justice system and receive appropriate guidance and counsel from legal professionals and caregivers.

Developmental science is clear that supportive relationships are critical for positive youth development and play a protective role. Given this understanding, juvenile facilities should amend policies that curtail visitation rights as punishment, and states and localities should implement policies and practices to assist families in overcoming barriers to prison visitation so that youth can remain connected to parents, caregivers, and other relatives.

The juvenile justice system is complex, and many caregivers and juveniles do not have the specialized knowledge required to successfully navigate the system. Probationary programs should connect parents and caregivers with community and educational resources that can teach them how to help their child succeed and avoid future interactions with the justice system. State legislatures and courts should ensure that justice-involved youth are provided with competent counsel throughout the legal process and ensure that adolescents under the age of 15 are not allowed to waive the right to an attorney or the right to remain silent without prior consultation with an attorney.

RECOMMENDATION 9-3: Implement policies that aim to reduce harm to justice-involved youth in accordance with knowledge from developmental science.

Extensive evidence demonstrates that harm after exiting the juvenile justice system may result from system interventions that impede or prevent a successful transition to adulthood by making it difficult for youth to productively re-enter their communities. The 2014 National Academies committee noted, "States and local jurisdictions should enact laws and policies to keep official records of a juvenile's encounters with the justice system strictly confidential, except in extraordinary circumstances involving a compelling need to protect public safety, so as to fully preserve the youth's opportunities for successful integration into adult life (p. 19)." This committee reaffirms that recommendation.

In response to laws that criminalize non-violent sexual exploration (such as sexting) and evidence questioning the efficacy of sex offender registries, especially for juveniles, Congress and state legislatures should enact legislation to eliminate the use of sex offender registries for non-violent juveniles.

Given the robust evidence of the harmful effects of solitary confinement, the federal government or philanthropic organizations should fund research on effective alternatives to solitary confinement so that detention facilities will be able to scale back or eliminate the use of this practice as soon as practicable.

> **RECOMMENDATION 9-4: Implement developmentally appropriate and fair policies and practices for adolescents involved in the criminal justice system.**

The committee's recognition that development occurs through the mid-twenties informs its call for the criminal justice system to implement developmentally appropriate and fair policies and practices for adolescents involved in the criminal justice system. To this end, legislatures should restore judicial discretion in decision making about transferring juveniles to or from criminal courts. Prosecutors and courts should be guided by the principles of proportionality and individualization with consideration given to the maturity, needs, and circumstances of the individual offender when making transfer decisions.

Judges sentencing juveniles in criminal courts should place these youth in juvenile correctional settings rather than adult correctional facilities. These youth should be entitled to all of the services they would have received if they had received a juvenile disposition and, upon turning 18, should be entitled to placement and services available to young adult offenders. Courts should conduct formal review of youths' criminal sentences on an individualized basis to determine whether the sentences should be adjusted in light of their mitigated culpability and prospects for successful adjustment in the community.

> **RECOMMENDATION 9-5: For those youth in the custody of the justice system, ensure that policies and practices are implemented to prioritize the health and educational needs of adolescents and avoid causing harm.**

For those youth in the custody of the justice system, ensure that policies and practices are implemented to prioritize the health and educational needs of adolescents and avoid causing harm. Correctional programming for adolescents and young adults in the criminal justice system should promote accountability and reduce re-offending through developmentally appropriate services in both correctional facilities and residential and community settings, including mental health, substance abuse, education, and social services.

Researchers, in partnership with practitioners, should urgently examine and evaluate effective alternatives to solitary confinement that promote the healthy development of individual youth and protect the safety of all in the facility.

State and local educational agencies should work in partnership with their justice system counterparts to ensure that rigorous and relevant curricula for adolescents are delivered in residential facilities and that these curricula are aligned with career and technical education standards and meet the needs of all youth, including those with disabilities and English learners.

10

The Scientific Opportunity

This report has been inspired by important and exciting advances in the science of adolescent development that have been achieved in the 21st century, and the committee has no doubt that the scientific findings summarized in this report provide a firm foundation for resolute action by governments at all levels and by all stakeholders committed to the well-being of adolescents. However, for each advance, new questions and scientific opportunities arise. Although this report is focused on the implications and applications of current knowledge for changes in policy and practice, it is well to take note of some key priorities for future research as well as the limitations in existing data that will need to be addressed to move the field forward.

Until the early years of the 21st century, leading scholars of adolescence subscribed to the view that by adolescence the brain had developed all of the functional capacity that it has in adulthood. It was believed that life experience was the primary distinction between adolescents and adults with respect to a host of human functions and behaviors—including domains such as self-regulation, cognitive judgment, and decision making. The emergence of developmental neuroscience has profoundly challenged that idea, pointing instead to ongoing fundamental changes in the adolescent brain— changes that continue beyond the teenage years and into the mid-twenties. Thus, one of the biggest shifts in scientific thinking about adolescence during the 21st century has been a recognition that fundamental neurobiological mechanisms, involving their connections with each brain domain as well as with the environment, continue to develop.

Moreover, our ability to measure and understand these neurobiological processes in adolescents, and in humans generally, has grown at a remarkable pace, undergirded by advances in magnetic resonance imaging (MRI) scanning tools and techniques for processing and analyzing genetic material. Along with these technical advances has come a wave of research using these new methods and a proliferation of data and new knowledge.

We now understand that brain development does not end in early childhood, and it is never "too late" to change the trajectory of development. The adolescent brain is plastic and resilient. Compensatory mechanisms of recovery can often redirect development and change the trajectories of brain circuits and body systems. In short, our understanding of adolescence has grown by leaps and bounds, and the application of this knowledge has the potential to change developmental trajectories of adolescents who might otherwise have been left behind.

To capitalize on these gains in knowledge from neuroscience, it is critical to better integrate our understanding of adolescent development within a model that also incorporates the social-contextual influences experienced by contemporary youth, and particularly the challenges faced by disadvantaged youth, including the effects of growing up in an impoverished and dangerous neighborhood and the impact of bias and discrimination. Now is the time to pursue this work because of the surging public interest in brain development and the potential to guide the next generation of research on adolescent social and behavioral development. In sum, future research must embed neurobiology within a social-contextual framework that is inclusive and representative of today's youth.

DATA LIMITATIONS

Although our knowledge about adolescence is growing rapidly, considerable gaps remain in pertinent data bearing on adolescent outcomes across sectors. Regarding health outcomes, for example, a 2007 review lamented the scarcity of data regarding specific health status or health objectives (e.g., increase the proportion of adolescents who engage in regular physical activity) for different adolescent populations, and recommended a "national adolescent data-priority agenda to develop strategies for improving health data regarding adolescent sub-populations" (Knopf et al., 2007, p. 335). This data gap has important implications for both researchers and policy makers, because inadequate outcome measures hamper our ability to design effective policies to address disparities. Below we discuss multiple reasons why measuring and assessing disparities in adolescent development is challenging, and why consideration of new methods and processes to overcome these limitations are needed.

First, a substantial proportion of the current developmental research categorizes adolescent subjects in fairly gross ways (for example, by gender and race/ethnicity but not by nativity or sexual orientation) and rarely allows analyses of intersections among groups. This makes it difficult to examine comparable measures across multiple groups of adolescents.

Second, studies typically aim to measure different outcomes at different points in time, thereby precluding a comprehensive profile of youth at a particular point in time. In addition, even if the data source collects information on a diverse set of variables, the sample may be incomplete; for example, many adolescent surveys (e.g., the Centers for Disease Control and Prevention's (CDC's) Youth Risk Behavior Survey or YRBS) are limited to school-enrolled adolescents, thereby leaving out many at-risk adolescents who have already left school. Further, the CDC's work depends on partnerships with state school districts to collect these data, leading to variation in the modules included in the survey. For example, a state might be hesitant to collect data on issues pertaining to reproductive health and may only selectively collect data on other topics that are perceived to be less controversial in nature.

Third, even when more comprehensive data are available, the surveys tend to focus on problem behaviors, rather than indicators of positive youth development. For example, documenting declining rates in smoking tells little about the assets and strengths of young people.

Fourth, differences in the wording of survey questions among national sources of data (such as the National Health Survey, YRBS, and Medical Expenditure Panel Survey) may result in different profiles of the health status of youth depending upon the data source—for example, whether the adolescent or a parent completes the survey—or depending on the site of data collection (e.g., at school, at home, in a health care setting, at a youth detention center).

Fifth, because some groups of adolescents, including Native Americans, comprise a relatively small share of the population, a general population-wide survey is insufficient to measure their outcomes accurately. In some cases, as with respect to sexual orientation and gender identity, researchers may fail to collect information on these characteristics altogether, and some youth may be uncomfortable or feel unsafe disclosing this information.

Sixth, some adolescent outcomes that researchers believe to be important in terms of influencing adult outcomes are not easily collected. For example, while academic test scores of adolescents are widely available and relatively straightforward to collect, consistently collected measures of adolescent emotional well-being or conduct, both of which have been found to be highly predictive of future adult circumstances, are not (Layard et al., 2014).

Seventh, national datasets currently do not collect information on the perceptions and experiences of young adolescents regarding equity, disparities, and racism.

RECOMMENDATIONS FOR FUTURE RESEARCH

The previous chapters show that our understanding of adolescence has grown markedly in recent years. Advances in neuroscience coupled with deepening knowledge from the social and behavioral sciences have solidified our understanding of adolescence as a period of opportunity. But, as noted in Chapter 4, we also know that many youth are hindered in their development by persistent and worsening inequities in many domains, including family income and wealth and neighborhood resources. To harness the promise of adolescence, our nation will need to grapple with these two underlying realities: This critical period of life is ripe with opportunity for learning, growth, and development, which can be utilized not only to launch extraordinary career trajectories but also to remediate previous developmental setbacks during childhood. Yet persistent inequities in social and environmental conditions curtail opportunity for many adolescents.

These realities amount to a compelling scientific challenge as well as a political one. To understand how we can help all adolescents flourish, we need to connect these two bodies of research—deepened understanding of developmental processes must also encompass a richer understanding of the impact of the social environment. This will require a major commitment by our research establishment. Sketching out a research portfolio was not one of the committee's core assignments (we were asked only to offer a handful of research recommendations), but we think it well within our charge to comment on the need to undertake a major investment in connecting developmental research on adolescence with the burgeoning research on social equity. This short chapter will set forth a few broad suggestions.

In undertaking this research effort, it is important to recognize that adolescents themselves have the capacity to make meaningful contributions to the design and execution of research. Future research funding can invest in youth expertise and agency by engaging youth in the research process. If we aim to use research to improve the conditions of youth's lives, we must support opportunities to involve youth in identifying the issues that are most pressing for them and provide them with the skills to investigate those issues. An existing example of this is Youth Participatory Action Research (YPAR), an approach that empowers youth by equipping them with skills to systematically study issues in their communities (Cammarota and Fine, 2008; Ozer, 2016). Inherent in this approach is a belief in the capability of youth to rigorously investigate social challenges and take action to address them (Berg et al., 2009). YPAR exploits the developmental opportunities afforded during adolescence (e.g., cognitive flexibility, openness to exploration) in order to create mutually beneficial change for youth and for society. Funding to support YPAR work is essential for advancing our knowledge of adolescent development in a manner that includes adolescents as critical stakeholders.

Moreover, to effect change, evidence must be translated into policy and practice. To this end, implementation studies should identify factors that can contribute to or impede effective and timely uptake and replication of adolescent research. Using implementation methodology, investigations should also examine system capacity for replicating evidence-based practices by, for example, identifying training needs of professional staff and community members and providing adequate reimbursement, and other system incentives to ensure replication of evidence-based practices with fidelity.

Future research investments in adolescence should support efforts that: (1) deepen our knowledge of the processes of adolescent development and the effectiveness of interventions, (2) examine the socio-environmental contexts that offer opportunities for flourishing, and (3) seek to understand and combat inequities that curtail the promise of adolescence for all youth.

Deepen Understanding of Developmental Processes and the Effectiveness of Interventions

Research seeking to deepen our understanding of the developmental processes of adolescence should consider the timing, type, and effectiveness of interventions for adolescents. These are the key questions: Given the rapid development of areas of the brain responsible for planning and decision making during adolescence, do interventions that rely on cognitive control (e.g., cognitive behavioral therapy) vary in effectiveness across the span of adolescence? Are there more effective windows within adolescence to deliver such interventions, where the adolescent brain is "ready" to benefit from the intervention? Do the most effective types of interventions therefore vary across adolescence? Is brain development a better indicator than chronological age of readiness as to when an adolescent can optimize the benefit from specific educational curricula?

Of course, in answering these questions it will be necessary to understand nature and correlates of individual variation in adolescent behavior and development, as age is an imprecise measure and brain maturation varies as much across ages as it does within ages (Galván, 2014). Current policy discussions applying the science of adolescence (using psychological and behavioral measures as well as neurobiological ones) have largely been based on group data due to methodological constraints necessitating inference based on a large sample of research participants. However, advances in policy and practice necessitate greater understanding of whether generic guidelines about maturation can be established. A key question, as posed by Galván (2014, p. 264) is "whether individual variation [is] so great as to. preclude the establishment of a biological benchmark for adult-like maturity and judgment."

Future research funding should also support

- studies that enact holistic approaches to understanding adolescent outcomes characterized by the consideration of achievement, health, and other outcome domains simultaneously;
- studies that demonstrate the specific social conditions and supports linked to epigenetic mechanisms that activate processes related to resilience and positive outcomes for young people, despite challenging circumstances;
- studies that identify, substantiate, and implement interventions that build locus of control and agency in adolescents and that promote resilience, for example by delivering specified curricula to youth and their caregivers, as was done in the Strong African American Families study (see Brody et al., 2017); and
- studies specifically designed to test optimal timing of interventions, posing questions such as "What are the trajectories of true developmental change in connectivity within and between neural networks implicated in cognitive control and emotional processing? Are these trajectories of change steeper or quicker during some periods than others potentially providing key windows for input and intervention?" (Fuligni et al., 2018, p. 151).

Examine Socio-Environmental Contexts

A large and rigorous knowledge base from developmental and intervention studies shows that adolescents (including both their brains and their behaviors) are influenced by their context, including their families, peers, schools, neighborhoods, and socio-cultural systems. Yet these influences on adolescent development have been neglected or obscured in much of the neurobiological research on adolescents to date, possibly because we lack good measures for assessing context—especially through the lenses of young people themselves. It is critical that future research better integrate our understanding of adolescent development within a model that incorporates social contexts and environmental influences experienced by today's youth.

Important considerations in this context are whether adolescents (and their developing brains) are more sensitive to some features of the social environment than others and whether some adolescents may flourish in particular contexts while others may struggle in that same context

(Fuligni et al., 2018). The role of technology and digital media as a context for development provides one example of an area ripe for further exploration along these lines. Research in this area is burgeoning, but critics of this work have raised serious concerns about the quality of the evidence base. If it is the case that some adolescents are adversely affected by exposure to digital technology and media, it appears that others are unaffected, and still others benefit from it. A high priority for research is identifying characteristics of youth who are most at risk for deleterious consequences, as well as practices that moderate the potential outcomes (George and Odgers, 2015; Orben and Przybylski, 2019; Seabrook et al., 2016; Twenge et al., 2019).

Understanding how the social and environmental context (and factors within that context) can offer opportunities for flourishing outcomes or for worsened outcomes for youth and emerging adults is critical. Studies should focus on:

- Understanding the policy impact of laws and policies that improve or impede adolescent health, well-being, safety, and security;
- Ascertaining what social and economic policies may improve opportunities for youth to thrive and test whether their effectiveness differs by race/ethnicity or context; and
- Identifying what interventions might ameliorate and (or) enrich the outcomes of youth who have experienced childhood deprivation, oppression, or other negative experiences (such as poverty, trauma, separation, or displacement).

In conducting investigations of this type, it is also important to consider the need to replicate effects behaviorally. For example, if a specific brain region or channel of connectivity between brain systems is discovered through a lab-based functional MRI study, before researchers move to assess intervention implications it is important that their next step be to replicate these effects behaviorally in the youths' social context. In other words, just because a brain pathway appears to light up when doing a task in a scanner, this does not prove that the same pathway will light up in the real everyday world, when peers, family, and other contextual factors are present.

Understand and Reduce Inequity

Understanding—as well as reducing—inequalities in the lives of adolescents is critical to ensuring that all adolescents have the opportunity to flourish. Our growing knowledge about disparities in adolescent outcomes, and the sources of those disparities, has the potential to inform the development of policies and practices designed to achieve equity and help all adolescents flourish and thrive. This goal should be fundamental for all future research on adolescence.

In conducting this research, issues of inclusion and exclusion will be particularly salient. Much of the recent knowledge on adolescents—specifically that derived from MRI studies—has not been representative of contemporary youth. Individuals included in MRI studies have historically been individuals participating in federally sponsored research, often through a university medical facility. As a result, most of these studies have not been fully representative of individuals living in poverty, including ethnically diverse participants, those without medical providers, and those from rural areas. In order to better understand and combat inequities, future research endeavors will need to make efforts to remedy this bias through, for example, direct recruitment efforts and outreach to underrepresented communities.

Future research on adolescence should prioritize studies addressing:

- discrimination and marginalization, with a focus on both neurobiological consequences as well as structural strategies (school, community, state policies and practices) that reduce the conditions in which discrimination and marginalization are prevalent, and that buffer individuals from such experiences;
- youth who historically have been underrepresented, or who are most vulnerable (e.g., youth of color; immigrants; sexual and gender minorities; religious minorities; out-of-home youth or those experiencing homelessness, foster care, or unstable housing); and
- ways in which intersecting axes of oppression shape youth development, particularly against a backdrop of social stratification and oppression, where relationships between identity, experience, and behavior may not operate the same way for all youth.

INVESTMENTS IN RESEARCH ON ADOLESCENCE

Our new understanding of adolescence implies that the adolescent infrastructure should encompass basic and applied research aiming to inform policies and practices that nurture positive development for all children and youth from birth to adulthood. The changes in the brain, body, and behavior that occur during adolescence mark this as a distinct developmental period during which adolescents make critical advances in learning, development, and maturation, but are also susceptible to risk. Interventions made during this period hold promise for supporting positive developmental trajectories and remediating past developmental challenges and have the potential to *prevent* negative trajectories. Investments in this period, thus, can support all adolescents to achieve flourishing trajectories and arrive at adulthood ready to thrive.

Creating positive impact through opportunities not only improves trajectories relevant to multiple outcomes, but also can provide high-impact cost-effective prevention of the elevated risk for negative trajectories during this period (Dahl et al., 2018). Thus, return on investment is not only the measurable positive impact of interventions, but also the savings from preventing later negative impacts that are costly in human as well as economic terms. For example, improving developmental trajectories in early adolescence (e.g., through health, education, and social development) can be an effective strategy for preventing many of the behavioral and emotional health problems that typically emerge in late adolescence—including the increasing rate of substance use, depression, anxiety, suicide, and school failure.

Much like precision medicine or the precision education contemplated in earlier chapters, investments can be targeted to maximize benefits for those most in need. As knowledge of adolescent development continues to increase, it will "lead to greater precision in understanding developmental risk factors and identifying the timing, mechanistic targets, and best contexts to improve adolescent trajectories" (Dahl et al., 2018, p. 447). Recent developmental neuroscience findings, for instance, suggest fundamentally different maturation processes may underlie the dysregulation that precedes anxiety and psychotic spectrum disorders (Tromp et al., 2019; Jalbrzikowski et al., 2019; Meyer and Lee, 2019). Such knowledge—including understanding how factors such as sex, genetic differences, early life adversity, and environment and context influence development—can be used to match interventions to specific developmental stages of adolescence, ultimately optimizing the value of the investment.

CONCLUSION

Marked increases in our understanding of adolescence has the potential to help all adolescents flourish. Yet, data limitations hamper our ability to understand adolescent outcomes across sectors. To benefit from recent gains in scientific understanding, these gaps will need to be addressed in combination with efforts that deepen our understanding of adolescent development, the socio-environmental contexts in which young people live, and the inequities that hinder opportunity for all adolescents.

References

CHAPTER 1

Ananat, E. O. (2011). The wrong side(s) of the tracks: The causal effects of racial segregation on urban poverty and inequality. *American Economic Journal: Applied Economics*, 3(2), 34–66.

Anderson, M., and Jiang, J. (2018). *Teens, Social Media & Technology 2018*. Washington, DC: Pew Research Center. Available: http://www.pewinternet.org/2018/05/31/teens-social-media-technology-2018/.

Anderson, M., and Perrin, A. (2018). *Nearly One-in-Five Teens Can't Always Finish Their Homework Because of the Digital Divide*. Washington, DC: Pew Research Center, October 16. Available: https://www.pewresearch.org/fact-tank/2018/10/26/nearly-one-in-five-teens-cant-always-finish-their-homework-because-of-the-digital-divide/.

Arnett, J. J., and Cravens, H. (2006). G. Stanley Hall's Adolescence: A centennial reappraisal: Introduction. *History of Psychology*, 9(3), 165–171.

Bachman, J. G., Johnston, L. D., and O'Malley, P.M. (1980). *Monitoring the Future: Questionnaire Responses from the Nation's High School Seniors, 1976*. Ann Arbor: Institute for Social Research, University of Michigan.

_____. (2014). *Monitoring the Future: Questionnaire Responses from the Nation's High School Seniors*. Ann Arbor: Institute for Social Research, University of Michigan. Available: http://www.monitoringthefuture.org/datavolumes/2012/2012dv.pdf.

Blakemore, S. J., Burnett, S., and Dahl, R. E. (2010). The role of puberty in the developing adolescent brain. *Human Brain Mapping*, 31(6), 926–933.

Boyd, D. (2014). *It's Complicated: The Social Lives of Networked Teens*. New Haven, CT: Yale University Press.

Caron, C. (2018). In "Rainbow Wave," LGBT candidates are elected in record numbers. *The New York Times*, November 7. Available: https://www.nytimes.com/2018/11/07/us/politics/lgbt-election-winners-midterms.html.

Casey, B. J., Jones, R. M., Levita, L., Libby, V., Pattwell, S. S., Ruberry, E. J., Soliman, F., and Somerville, L. H. (2010). The storm and stress of adolescence: Insights from human imaging and mouse genetics. *Developmental Psychobiology*, 52(3), 225–235.

Chetty, R., Grusky, D., Hell, M., Hendren, N., Manduca, R., and Narang, J. (2017). The fading American dream: Trends in absolute income mobility since 1940. *Science, 356*(6336), 398–406.

Child Trends. (2014.) *Immigrant Children.* Available: https://www.childtrends.org/indicators/immigrant-children.

_____. (2015). *Volunteering: Indicators of Child Well-Being.* Available: https://www.childtrends.org/indicators/volunteering.

Cohen, C. J., Kahne, J., Bowyer, B., Middaugh, E., and Rogowski, J. (2012). *Participatory Politics: New Media and Youth Political Action.* Oakland, CA: Youth and Participatory Politics Research Network. Available: http://ypp.dmlcentral.net/sites/all/files/publications/YPP_Survey_Report_FULL.pdf.

Colby, S. L., and Ortman, J. M. (2014). Projections of the size and composition of the U.S. population: 2014–2060. *Current Population Reports*, P25-1143. Available: https://www.census.gov/content/dam/Census/library/publications/2015/demo/p25-1143.pdf.

Costello, C. R., McNiel, D. E., and Binder, R. L. (2016). Adolescents and social media: Privacy, brain development, and the law. *Journal of the American Academy of Psychiatry and the Law, 44*, 313–321.

Dejonckheere, M., Nichols, L. P., Moniz, M. H., Sonneville, K. R., Vydiswaran, V. V., Zhao, X., Guetterman, T. C., and Chang, T. (2017). MyVoice national text message survey of youth aged 14 to 24 years: Study protocol. *JMIR Research Protocols, 6*(12), 1–12.

DeSilver, D. (2018). A record number of women will be serving in the new Congress. *Fact Tank, Pew Research Center.* December 18. Available: http://www.pewresearch.org/fact-tank/2018/12/18/record-number-women-in-congress.

File, T. (2014). Young-adult voting: An analysis of presidential elections, 1964-2012. *Current Population Survey Reports*, P20-572. Washington, DC: U.S. Census Bureau.

Finlay, A., Wray-Lake, L., and Flanagan, C. (2010). Civic engagement during the transition to adulthood: Developmental opportunities and social policies at a critical juncture. In L. R. Sherrodd, J. Torney-Purta, and C. A. Flanagan (Eds.), *Handbook of Research on Civic Engagement in Youth* (pp. 277–305). Hoboken, NJ: John Wiley & Sons.

Fisher, D.R. (2012). Youth political participation: Bridging activism and electoral politics. *Annual Review of Sociology, 38*, 119–137.

Fontenot, K., Semega, J., and Kollar, M. (2018). *Income and Poverty in the United States: 2017. Current Population Reports*, P60-263. Available: https://www.census.gov/content/dam/Census/library/publications/2018/demo/p60-263.pdf.

Fredrickson, B. L., and Losada, M. F. (2005). Positive affect and the complex dynamics of human flourishing. *American Psychologist, 60*(7), 678–686.

Fuhrmann, D., Knoll, L. J., and Blakemore, S.J. (2015). Adolescence as a sensitive period of brain development. *Trends in Cognitive Sciences, 19*(10), 558–566.

Galván, A. (2014). Insights about adolescent behavior, plasticity, and policy from neuroscience research. *Neuron, 83*, 262–265.

Giedd, J. N., Blumenthal, J., Jeffries, N. O., Castellanos, F. X., Liu, H., Zijdenbos, A., Paus, T., Evans, A. C., and Rapoport, J. L. (1999). Brain development during childhood and adolescence: A longitudinal MRI study. *Nature Neuroscience, 2*(10), 861–863.

Hall, G. S. (1904). *Adolescence: Its Psychology and Its Relations to Physiology, Anthropology, Sociology, Sex, Crime, Religion, and Education (Vols. I & II).* New York: D. Appleton and Co.

Hammack, P. (2018, June 6). *The New Queer Teenager: Sexual and Gender Identity Diversity in the Twenty-First Century.* Presentation to the Committee on the Neurobiological and Socio-behavioral Science of Adolescent Development and Its Applications. Available: https://sites.nationalacademies.org/cs/groups/dbassesite/documents/webpage/dbasse_188002.pdf.

Institute of Medicine and National Research Council. (2014). *Investing in the Health and Well-being of Young Adults*. Washington, DC: The National Academies Press.

Ismail, F. Y., Fatemi, A., and Johnston, M.V. (2017). Cerebral plasticity: Windows of opportunity in the developing brain. *European Journal of Paediatric Neurology, 21*(1), 23–48.

Ito, M., Horst, H., Bittanti, M., Boyd, D., Herr-Stephenson, B., Lange, P. G., Pascoe, C. J., and Robinson, L. (2008). *Living and Learning with New Media: Summary of Findings from the Digital Youth Project*. John D. and Catherine T. MacArthur Foundation Reports on Digital Media and Learning. Available: https://mitpress.mit.edu/books/living-and-learning-new-media.zz.

Keyes, C. M. (2002). The mental health continuum: From languishing to flourishing in life. *Journal of Health and Social Behavior, 43*(2), 207–222.

Langer, G., and Siu, B. (2018). Election 2018 exit poll analysis: Voter turnout soars, Democrats take back the House, ABC News projects. ABC News, November 7. Available: https://abcnews.go.com/Politics/election-2018-exit-poll-analysis-56-percent-country/story?id=59006586.

Lee, S. J. (2009). Online communication and adolescent social ties: Who benefits more from Internet use? *Journal of Computer-Mediated Communication, 14*, 509–531.

Lenroot, R. K., and Giedd, J. N. (2006). Brain development in children and adolescents: Insights from anatomical magnetic resonance imaging. *Neuroscience & Biobehavioral Reviews, 30*(6), 718–729.

Madden, M., Fox, S., Smith, A., and Vitak, J. (2007). *Digital Footprints*. Washington, DC: PEW Internet and American Life Project. Available: http://www.pewinternet.org/2007/12/16/digital-footprints/.

Modell, J. (1991). *Into One's Own: From Youth to Adulthood in the United States, 1920–1975*. Berkeley: University of California Press.

National Academies of Sciences, Engineering, and Medicine. (2016). *Preventing Bullying Through Science, Policy, and Practice*. Washington, DC: The National Academies Press.

Nussbaum, M. (2003). Capabilities as fundamental entitlements: Sen and social justice. *Feminist Economics, 9*(2/3), 33–59.

_____. (2011). *Creating Capabilities*. Cambridge, MA: Harvard University Press.

Oliver, M., and Shapiro, T. (2006). *Black Wealth, White Wealth*. New York, NY: Routledge.

Orben, A., and Przybylski, A.K. (2019). The association between adolescent well-being and digital technology use. *Nature Human Behaviour, 3*, 173–182.

Owens, A. (2016). Inequality in children's contexts: Income segregation of households with and without children. *American Sociological Review, 81*(3), 549–574.

Patton, G. C., Sawyer, S. M., Santelli, J. S., Ross, D. A., Afifi, R., Allen, N. B., Arora, M., Azzopardi, P., Baldwin, W., Bonell, C., Kakuma, R., Kennedy, E., Mahon, J., McGovern, T., Mokdad, A. H., Patel, V., Petroni, S., and Reavley, N. (2016). Our future: A Lancet commission on adolescent health and wellbeing. *The Lancet Commissions, 387*, 2423–2478.

Piketty, T., and Saez, E. (2014). Inequality in the long-run. *Science, 344*, 838–843.

Quillian, L. (2014). Does segregation create winners and losers? Residential segregation and inequality in educational attainment. *Social Problems, 61*(3), 402–426.

Reardon, S. F., and Bischoff, K. (2011). Income inequality and income segregation. *American Journal of Sociology, 116*(4), 1092–1153.

Schlegel, A., and Barry, H. III. (1991). *Adolescence: An Anthropological Inquiry*. New York: Free Press.

Schwartz, S. E. O., Rhodes, J. E., Liang, B., Sanchez, B., Spencer, R., Kremer, S., and Kanchewa, S. (2014). Mentoring in the digital age: Social media use in adult-youth relationships. *Children and Youth Services Review, 47*, 205–213.

Sen, A. (1993). Capability and well-being. In N. Nussbaum and A. Sen (Eds.), *The Quality of Life* (pp. 30–53). Oxford: Clarendon Press.

_____. (1999). *Development as Freedom*. New York: Knopf.

Smith, A. (2013). *Civic Engagement in the Digital Age*. Washington, DC: Pew Charitable Trusts. Available: http://pewinternet.org/Reports/2013/Civic-Engagement.aspx.

Spear, L. P. (2010). *The Behavioral Neuroscience of Adolescence*. New York: W. W. Norton.

Steinberg, L. (2014). *Age of Opportunity: Lessons from the New Science of Adolescence*. New York: First Mariner Books.

Subrahmanyam, K., and Greenfield, P. (2008). Online communication and adolescent relationships. *The Future of Children, 18*(1), 119–146.

Syvertsen, A. K., Wray-Lake, L., Flanagan, C.A., Wayne Osgood, D., and Briddell, L. (2011). Thirty-year trends in U.S. adolescents' civic engagement: A story of changing participation and educational differences. *Journal of Research on Adolescence, 21*(3), 586–594.

Uhls, Y. T., Ellison, N. B., and Subrahmanyam, K. (2017). Benefits and costs of social media in adolescence. *Pediatrics, 140*(Suppl. 2), S67–S70.

U.S. Census Bureau. (2012). Population by sex, age, nativity, and U.S. citizenship status: 2012. *Current Population Survey, Annual Social and Economic Supplement*. Washington, DC: U.S. Census Bureau.

_____. (2018a). *Annual Estimates of the Resident Population by Sex, Age, Race, and Hispanic Origin for the United States: April 1, 2010 to July 1, 2017*. Available: https://factfinder.census.gov/bkmk/table/1.0/en/PEP/2017/PEPASR6H.

_____. (2018b). *Annual Estimates of the Resident Population by Single Year of Age and Sex for the United States: April 1, 2010 to July 1, 2017*. Available: https://factfinder.census.gov/bkmk/table/1.0/en/PEP/2017/PEPSYASEXN.

Weinstein, E. (2018). The social media see-saw: Positive and negative influences on adolescents' affective well-being. *New Media & Society, 20*(10), 3597–3623.

Worthman, C. M., and Trang, K. (2018). Dynamics of body time, social time and life history at adolescence. *Nature, 554*(7693), 451–457.

Wray-Lake, L., and Hart, D. (2012). Growing social inequalities in youth civic engagement? Evidence from the National Election Study. *PS: Political Science and Politics 45*, 456–461.

CHAPTER 2

Arnett, J. J. (2015). Identity development from adolescence to emerging adulthood: What we know and (especially) don't know. In K. C. McLean and M. Syed (Eds.), *Oxford Handbook of Identity Development* (pp. 53–64). New York, NY: Oxford University Press.

Aubert-Broche, B., Fonov, V. S., García-Lorenzo, D., Mouiha, A., Guizard, N., Coupé, P., and Collins, D. L. (2013). A new method for structural volume analysis of longitudinal brain MRI data and its application in studying the growth trajectories of anatomical brain structures in childhood. *Neuroimage, 82*, 393-402.

Auchus, R. J., and Rainey, W. E. (2004). Adrenarche—physiology, biochemistry and human disease. *Clinical Endocrinology, 60*(3), 288–296.

Barbaro, N., Boutwell, B.B., Barnes, J.C., and Shackelford, T.K. (2017). Genetic confounding of the relationship between father absence and menarche. *Evolution and Human Behavior, 38*(3), 357–365.

Bartal, I. B. A., Decety, J., and Mason, P. (2011). Empathy and pro-social behavior in rats. *Science, 334*(6061), 1427–1430.

Becht, A. I., Nelemans, S. A., van Dijk, M. P. A., Branje, S. J. T., Van Lier, P. A. C., Denissen, J. J. A., and Meeus, W. H. J. (2017). Clear self, better relationships: Adolescents' self-concept clarity and relationship quality with parents and peers across 5 years. *Child Development, 88*(6), 1823–1833.

Belsky, J. (2007). Childhood experiences and reproductive strategies. In *Oxford Handbook of Evolutionary Psychology* (pp. 237–257). New York: Oxford University Press.

Belsky, J., Steinberg, L., and Draper, P. (1991). Childhood experience, interpersonal development, and reproductive strategy: An evolutionary theory of socialization. *Child Development, 62*(4), 647–670.

Bergevin, T. A., Bukowski, W. M., and Karavasilis, L. (2003). Childhood sexual abuse and pubertal timing: Implications for long-term psychosocial adjustment. In C. Hayward (Ed.), *Gender Differences at Puberty* (pp. 187–216). New York, NY: Cambridge University Press.

Berkman, E. T., Livingston, J. L., and Kahn, L. E. (2017). Finding the "self" in self-regulation: The identity-value model. *Psychological Inquiry, 28*(2–3), 77–98.

Bjork, J. M., and Pardini, D. A. (2015). Who are those "risk-taking adolescents"? Individual differences in developmental neuroimaging research. *Developmental Cognitive Neuroscience, 11*, 56–64.

Blakemore, S. J., and Mills, K. L. (2014). Is adolescence a sensitive period for sociocultural processing? *Annual Review of Psychology, 65*, 187–207.

Blakemore, S. J., Burnett, S., and Dahl, R. E. (2010). The role of puberty in the developing adolescent brain. *Human Brain Mapping, 31*(6), 926–933.

Booth, A., Johnson, D.R., Granger, D. A., Crouter. A. C., and McHale, S. (2003). Testosterone and child and adolescent adjustment: The moderating role of parent-child relationships. *Developmental Psychology, 39*(1), 85–98.

Boskey, E. R. (2014). Understanding transgender identity development in childhood and adolescence. *American Journal of Sexuality Education, 9*(4), 445–463.

Brewer, M. B., Gonsalkorale, K., and van Dommelen, A. (2013). Social identity complexity: Comparing majority and minority ethnic group members in a multicultural society. *Group Processes and Intergroup Relations, 16*(5), 529–544.

Bronk, K. C. (2014). Purpose across the lifespan. In *Purpose in Life* (pp. 69–89). Dordrecht, Netherlands: Springer.

Brooks-Gunn, J., and Ruble, D. N. (1982). The development of menstrual-related beliefs about behaviors during early adolescence. *Child Development, 53*, 1567–1577.

Brooks-Gunn, J., Newman, D.L., Holderness, C., and Warren, M.P. (1994). The experience of breast development and girls' stories about the purchase of a bra. *Journal of Youth and Adolescence, 23*, 539–565.

Brummelman, E., and Thomaes, S. (2017). How children construct views of themselves: A social-developmental perspective. *Child Development, 88*(6), 1763–1773.

Burrow, A. L., and Hill, P. L. (2011). Purpose as a form of identity capital for positive youth adjustment. *Developmental Psychology, 47*(4), 1196–1206.

Caballero, A., and Tseng, K.Y. (2016). GABAergic function as a limiting factor for prefontal maturation during adolescence. *Trends in Neuroscience, 39*(7), 441–448.

Cance, J. D., Ennett, S. T., Morgan-Lopez, A. A., Foshee, V.A., Talley, A.E. (2013). Perceived pubertal timing and recent substance use among adolescents: A longitudinal perspective. *Addiction, 108*(10), 1845–1854.

Casey, B. J. (2015). Beyond simple models of self-control to circuit-based accounts of adolescent behavior. *Annual Review of Psychology, 66*, 295–319.

Casey, B. J., and Caudle, K. (2013). The teenage brain: Self control. *Current Directions in Psychological Science, 22*(2), 82–87.

Casey, B. J., Galván, A., and Somerville, L.H. (2016). Beyond simple models of adolescence to an integrated circuit-based account: A commentary. *Developmental Cognitive Neuroscience, 17*(Suppl. 1), 128–130.

Castellanos-Ryan, N., Parent, S., Vitaro, F., Tremblay, R.E., and Seguin, J.R. (2013). Pubertal development, personality, and substance use: A 10-year longitudinal study from childhood to adolescence. *Journal of Abnormal Psychology, 122*(3), 782–796.

Causadias, J. M., and Umaña-Taylor, A. J. (2018). Reframing marginalization and youth development: Introduction to the special issue. *American Psychologist, 73*(6), 707–712.

Cheon, B. K., Im, D., Harada, T., Kim, J., Mathur, V. A., Scimeca, J. M., Parrish, T. B., Park, H. W., and Chiao, J.Y. (2011). Cultural influences on neural basis of intergroup empathy. *Neuroimage, 57*(2), 642–650.

Chumlea, W. C., Schubert, C. M., Roche, A. F., Kulin, H. E., Lee, P. A., Himes, J. H., and Sun, S. S. (2003). Age at menarche and racial comparisons in US girls. *Pediatrics, 111*, 110–113.

Cole, D. A., Maxwell, S. E., Martin, J. M., Peeke, L. G., Seroczynski, A. D., Tram, J. M., and Maschman, T. (2001). The development of multiple domains of child and adolescent self-concept: A cohort sequential longitudinal design. *Child Development, 72*(6), 1723–1746.

Costello E.J., Sung, M., Worthman, C., Angold, A. (2007). Pubertal maturation and the development of alcohol use and abuse. *Drug and Alcohol Dependence, 88*(Suppl. 1), S50–S59.

Crenshaw, K. (1990). Mapping the margins: Intersectionality, identity politics, and violence against women of color. *Stanford Law Review, 43*, 1241.

Crone, E. A., and Dahl, R. E. (2012). Understanding adolescence as a period of social–affective engagement and goal flexibility. *Nature Reviews Neuroscience, 13*(9), 636–350.

Crone, E. A., and Steinbeis, N. (2017). Neural perspectives on cognitive control development during childhood and adolescence. *Trends in Cognitive Sciences, 21*(3), 205–215.

Cservenka, A., Herting, M. M, Mackiewicz Seghete, K. L., Hudson, K. A., and Nagel, B. J. (2013). High and low sensation seeking adolescents show distinct patterns of brain activity during reward processing. *NeuroImage, 66*, 184–193.

Cunningham, W. A., Johnson, M. K., Raye, C. L., Gatenby, J. C., Gore, J. C., and Banaji, M. R. (2004). Separable neural components in the processing of Black and White faces. *Psychological Science, 15*, 806–813.

Daddis, C. (2011). Desire for increased autonomy and adolescents' perceptions of peer autonomy: "Everyone else can; why can't I?" *Child Development, 82*(4), 1310–1326.

Damon, W., Menon, J., and Cotton Bronk, K. (2003). The development of purpose during adolescence. *Applied Developmental Science, 7*(3), 119–128.

Davey, G. C., Yücel, M., and Allen, N. B. (2008) The emergence of depression in adolescence: Development of the prefrontal cortex and the representation of reward. *Neuroscience and Biobehavioral Reviews, 32*(1), 1–19.

Davidow, J. Y., Foerde, K., Galván, A., and Shohamy, D. (2016). An upside to reward sensitivity: The hippocampus supports enhanced reinforcement learning in adolescence. *Neuron, 92*(1), 93–99.

Davis, E. M., Peck, J. D., Peck, B. M., and Kaplan, H. B. (2015) Associations between early alcohol and tobacco use and prolonged time to puberty in boys. *Child: Care, Health and Development, 41*(3), 459–466.

Dawes, M.A., Dorn, L.D., Moss, H.B., Yao, J.K., Kirisci, L., Ammerman, R.T., and Tarter, R.E. (1999). Hormonal and behavioral homeostasis in boys at risk for substance abuse. *Drug and Alcohol Dependence, 55*(1–2), 165–176.

de Vries, A. L., Steensma, T. D., Doreleijers, T. A., and Cohen-Kettenis, P. T. (2011). Puberty suppression in adolescents with gender identity disorder: A prospective follow-up study. *Journal of Sexual Medicine, 8*(8), 2276–2283.

Dean, C. (2017). The role of identity in committing acts of violent extremism–and in desisting from them. *Criminal Behaviour and Mental Health, 27*(4), 281–-285.

Diemer, M. A., and Rapa, L. J. (2016). Unraveling the complexity of critical consciousness, political efficacy, and political action among marginalized adolescents. *Child Development*, 87(1), 221–238.

Diemer, M. A., Wang, Q., Moore, T., Gregory, S. R., Hatcher, K. M., and Voight, A. M. (2010). Sociopolitical development, work salience, and vocational expectations among low socioeconomic status African American, Latin American, and Asian youth. *Developmental Psychology*, 46(3), 619–635.

Diemer, M. A., McWhirter, E. H., Ozer, E. J., and Rapa, L. J. (2015). Advances in the conceptualization and measurement of critical consciousness. *The Urban Review*, 47(5), 809–823.

Diemer, M. A., Rapa, L. J., Park, C. J., and Perry, J. C. (2017). Development and validation of the Critical Consciousness Scale. *Youth & Society*, 49(4), 461–483.

Dorn, L. D., and Biro, F. M. (2011). Puberty and its measurement: A decade in review. *Journal of Research on Adolescence*, 21, 180–195.

Dorn, L. D., Kolko, D. J., Susman, E. J., Huang, B., Stein, H., Music, E., and Bukstein, O. (2009). Salivary gonadal and adrenal hormone differences in boys and girls with and without disruptive behavior disorders: Contextual variants. *Biological Psychology*, 81(1), 31–39.

Dreyfuss, M., Caudle, K., Drysdale, A. T., Johnston, N. E., Cohen, A. O., Somerville, L. H., Galván, A., Tottenham, N., Hare, T. A., and Casey, B. J. (2014). Teens impulsively react rather than retreat from threat. *Developmental Neuroscience*, 36, 220–227.

Dumontheil, I. (2014). Development of abstract thinking during childhood and adolescence: The role of rostrolateral prefrontal cortex. *Developmental Cognitive Neuroscience*, 10, 57–76.

Dumontheil, I., Burgess, P.W., and Blakemore, S.-J. (2008). Development of rostral prefrontal cortex and cognitive and behavioural disorders. *Developmental Medicine and Child Neurology*, 50(3), 168–181.

Ellis, B. J., and Garber, J. (2000). Psychosocial antecedents of variation in girls' pubertal timing: Maternal depression, stepfather presence, and marital and family stress. *Child Development*, 71(2), 485–501.

Erikson, E. (1968). *Identity: Youth and Crisis*. New York, NY: Norton.

Fang, C. Y., Egleston, B. L., Brown, K. M., Lavigne, J. V., Stevens, V. J., Barton, B. A., Chandler, D. W., and Dorgan, J. F. (2009). Family cohesion moderates the relation between free testosterone and delinquent behaviors in adolescent boys and girls. *Journal of Adolescent Health* 44(6), 590–597.

Flanagan, C. A., and Christens, B. D. (2011). Youth civic development: Historical context and emerging issues. *New Directions for Child and Adolescent Development*, 134, 1–9.

Flannery, J., Berkman, E., and Pfeifer, J. (2018). Teens aren't just risk machines—there's a method to their madness. *The Conversation*, February 6. Available: https://theconversation.com/teens-arent-just-risk-machines-theres-a-method-to-their-madness-89439.

Freire, P. (1970). *Pedagogy of the Oppressed*. New York: Herder and Herder.

Fuhrmann, D., Knoll, L. J., and Blakemore, S. J. (2015) Adolescence as a sensitive period of brain development. *Trends in Cognitive Sciences*, 19(10), 558–566.

Fuligni, A. J. (2018, June 6). *Neurobiological Change and Sociocultural Experience during Adolescence*. PowerPoint presented to the Committee on Neurobiological and Sociobehavioral Science of Adolescent Development and Its Applications. The National Academy of Sciences, Washington, DC.

Fuligni, A.J., and Telzer, E.H. (2013). Another way family can get in the head and under the skin: The neurobiology of helping the family. *Child Development Perspectives*, 7(3), 138–142.

Fuligni, A. J., and Tsai, K. M. (2015). Developmental flexibility in the age of globalization: Autonomy and identity development among immigrant adolescents. *Annual Review of Psychology, 66*, 411–431.

Fuligni, A. J., Dapretto, M., and Galván, A. (2018). Broadening the impact of developmental neuroscience on the study of adolescence. *Journal of Research on Adolescence, 28*(1), 150–153.

Furrow, J. L., King, P. E., and White, K. (2004). Religion and positive youth development: Identity, meaning, and prosocial concerns. *Applied Developmental Science, 8*(1), 17–26.

Galambos, N. L., Almeida, D. M., and Petersen, A. C. (1990). Masculinity, femininity, and sex roles in early adolescence: Exploring gender intensification. *Child Development, 61*(6), 1905–1914.

Galván, A. (2010). Adolescent development of the reward system. *Frontiers in Human Neuroscience, 4*, 1–9.

Galván, A., Hare, T. A., Parra, C. E., Penn. J., Voss, H., Glover, G., and Casey, B. J. (2006) Earlier development of the accumbens relative to orbitofrontal cortex might underlie risk–taking behavior in adolescents. *Journal of Neuroscience, 26*(25), 6885–6892.

García Coll, C., Lamberty, G., Jenkins, R., McAdoo, H. P., Crnic, K., Wasik, B. H., and Vásquez García, H. (1996). An integrative model for the study of developmental competencies in minority children. *Child Development, 67*(5), 1891–1914.

Gaylord-Harden, N. K., Barbarin, O., Tolan, P. H., and McBride Murry, V. M. (2018). Understanding development of African American boys and young men: Moving from risks to positive youth development. *American Psychologist, 73*(6), 753–767.

Ge, X., Kim, I. J., Brody, G. H., Conger, R. D., Simons, R. L., Gibbons, F. X., and Cutrona, C. E. (2003). It's about timing and change: Pubertal transition effects on symptoms of major depression among African American youths. *Developmental Psychology, 39*, 430–439.

Gentile, B., Grabe, S., Dolan-Pascoe, B., Twenge, J. M., Wells, B. E., and Maitino, A. (2009). Gender differences in domain-specific self-esteem: A meta-analysis. *Review of General Psychology, 13*(1), 34–45.

Giedd, J. N. (2015) The amazing teen brain. *Scientific American, 312*(6), 32–37.

Ginwright, S., Cammarota, J., and Noguera, P. (2006). *Beyond Resistance! Youth Activism and Community Change: New Democratic Possibilities for Practice and Policy for America's Youth*. New York, NY: Routledge.

Gogtay, N., Giedd, J. N., Lusk, L., Hayashi, K. M., Greenstein, D., Vaituzis, A. C., Nugent, T. F., Herman, D. H., Clasen, L. S., Toga, A. W., Rapoport, J. L., and Thompson, P. M. (2004). Dynamic mapping of human cortical development during childhood through early adulthood. *Proceedings of the National Academy of Sciences of the United States of America, 101*(21), 8174–8179.

Gold, P. W., and Chrousos, G. P. (2002). Organization of the stress system and its dysregulation in melancholic and atypical depression: High vs low CRH/NE states. *Molecular Psychiatry, 7*(3), 254–275.

Gonzales, R. G. (2016). *Lives in Limbo: Undocumented and Coming of Age in America*. Oakland, CA: University of California Press.

Graber, J. A., Nichols, T. R., and Brooks-Gunn, J. (2010). Putting pubertal timing in developmental context: Implications for prevention. *Developmental Psychobiology, 52*, 254–262.

Graham, S. (2018). Race/ethnicity and social adjustment of adolescents: How (not if) school diversity matters. *Educational Psychologist, 53*(2), 64–77.

Grumbach, M. M. (2002). The neuroendocrinology of human puberty revisited. *Hormone Research in Pediatrics, 57*(Suppl. 2), 2–14.

Grumbach, M. M., and Styne, D. M. (2003). Puberty: ontogeny, neuroendocrinology, physiology, and disorders. In P. R. Larsen, H. M. Kronenberg, S. Melmed, and K. S. Polonsky (Eds), *Williams Textbook of Endocrinology* (10th ed., pp. 1115–1286). Philadelphia, PA: W. B. Saunders.

Guerry, J. D., and Hastings, P. D. (2011). In search of HPA axis dysregulation in child and adolescent depression. *Clinical Child and Family Psychology Review, 14*(2), 135–160.

Gunnar, M. R., Wewerka, S., Frenn, K., Long, J. D., and Griggs, C. (2009). Developmental changes in hypothalamus-pituitary-adrenal activity over the transition to adolescence: normative changes and associations with puberty. *Development and Psychopathology, 21*(1), 69–85.

Guyer, A. E., Silk, J. S., and Nelson, E. E. (2016). The neurobiology of the emotional adolescent: From the inside out. *Neuroscience & Behavioral Reviews, 70,* 74–85.

Hammack, P. L. (2018, June). *The New Queer Teenager: Sexuality and Gender Identity Diversity in the Twenty-First Century*. Presentation to the Committee on the Neurobiological and Socio-behavioral Science of Adolescent Development and Its Applications. Available: https://sites.nationalacademies.org/cs/groups/dbassesite/documents/webpage/dbasse_188002.pdf.

Hare, T. A., Tottenham, N., Galván, A., Voss, H. U., Glover, G. H., and Casey, B. J. (2008) Biological substrates of emotional reactivity and regulation in adolescence during an emotional go-nogo task. *Biological Psychiatry, 63*(10), 927–934.

Harter, S. (2012). *The Construction of the Self: Developmental and Sociocultural Foundations* (2nd ed.). New York: Guilford Press.

Hartley, C. A., and Somerville, L. H. (2015). The neuroscience of adolescent decision-making. *Current Opinion in Behavioral Sciences*, *5*, 108.

Hauser, T. U., Iannaccone, R., Walitza, S., Brandeis, D., and Brem, S. (2015). Cognitive flexibility in adolescence: Neural and behavioral mechanisms of reward prediction error processing in adaptive decision making during development. *NeuroImage, 104,* 347–354.

Havelock J. C., Auchus R. J., and Rainey, W. E. (2004). The rise in adrenal androgen biosynthesis: adrenarche. *Seminars in Reproductive Medicine, 22*(4), 337–347.

Hope, E. C., and Spencer, M. B. (2017). Civic engagement as an adaptive coping response to conditions of inequality: An application of phenomenological variant of ecological systems theory (PVEST). In N. J. Cabrera and B. Leyendecker (Eds.), *Handbook on Positive Development of Youth Minority Children and Youth* (pp. 421–435). New York, NY: Springer Science + Business Media.

Hope, M. O., Assari, S., Cole-Lewis, Y. C., and Caldwell, C. H. (2017). Religious social support, discrimination, and psychiatric disorders among Black adolescents. *Race and Social Problems, 9*(2), 102–114.

Hutcheon, E. J., and Wolbring, G. (2012). Voices of "disabled" postsecondary students: Examining higher education "disability" policy using an ableism lens. *Journal of Diversity in Higher Education, 5*, 39.

Ismail, F. Y., Fatemi, A., and Johnston, M.V. (2017). Cerebral plasticity: Windows of opportunity in the developing brain. *European Journal of Paediatric Neurology, 21*(1), 23–48.

Johnson, M. H., Grossmann, T., and Kadosh, K. C. (2009). Mapping functional brain development: Building a social brain through interactive specialization. *Developmental Psychology 45*, 151.

Jolles, D. D., and Crone, E. A. (2012). Training the developing brain: A neurocognitive perspective. *Frontiers in Human Neuroscience, 6*, 1.

Jones, D. J., Loiselle, R., and Highlander, A. (2018). Parent–adolescent socialization of social class in low-income White families: Theory, research, and future directions. *Journal of Research on Adolescence, 28*(3), 622–636.

Kiang, L., Yip, T., and Fuligni, A. J. (2008). Multiple social identities and adjustment in young adults from ethnically diverse backgrounds. *Journal of Research on Adolescence, 18*(4), 643–670.

Kleibeuker, S. W., De Dreu, C. K., and Crone, E. A. (2012). The development of creative cognition across adolescence: Distinct trajectories for insight and divergent thinking. *Developmental Science, 16*(1), 2–12.

_____. (2016). Creativity development in adolescence: Insight from behavior, brain, and training studies. *New Directions for Child and Adolescent Development, 73*.

Klimstra, T. A., Hale, W. W., Raaijmakers, Q. A., Branje, S. J., and Meeus, W. H. (2010). Identity formation in adolescence: Change or stability? *Journal of Youth and Adolescence, 39*(2), 150–162.

Knifsend, C. A., and Juvonen, J. (2013). The role of social identity complexity in inter-group attitudes among young adolescents. *Social Development, 22*(3), 623–640.

_____. (2014). Social identity complexity, cross-ethnic friendships, and intergroup attitudes in urban middle schools. *Child Development, 85*(2), 709–721.

Kroger, J., and Marcia, J. E. (2011). The identity statuses: Origins, meanings, and interpretations. In S. J. Schwartz, K. Luyckx, and V. L. Vignoles (Eds.), *Handbook of Identity Theory and Research* (pp. 31–53). New York, NY: Springer.

Kreukels, B. P., and Cohen-Kettenis, P. T. (2011). Puberty suppression in gender identity disorder: The Amsterdam experience. *Nature Reviews Endocrinology, 7*(8), 466–472.

Kuhn, D. (2006). Do cognitive changes accompany developments in the adolescent brain? *Perspectives on Psychological Science, 1,* 59.

_____. (2009). Adolescent thinking. In R. M. Lerner and L. Steinberg (Eds.), *Handbook of Adolescent Psychology: Individual Bases of Adolescent Development* (pp. 152–186). Hoboken, NJ: John Wiley & Sons Inc.

Lee, J. S., McCarty, C. A., Ahrens, K., King, K. M., Vander Stoep, A., McCauley, E. A. (2014). Pubertal timing and adolescent substance initiation. *Journal of Social Work Practice in the Addictions, 14*(3), 286–307.

Lee, J. M., Wasserman, R., Kaciroti, N., Gebremariam, A., Steffes, J., Dowshen, S., Harris, D., Serwint, J., Abney, D., Smitherman, L., Reiter, E., and Herman-Giddens, M. E. (2016). Timing of puberty in overweight versus obese boys. *Pediatrics, 137*(2), 1–10.

Lenroot, R. K., and Giedd, J. N. (2006). Brain development in children and adolescents: Insights from anatomical magnetic resonance imaging. *Neuroscience and Biobehavioral Reviews, 30*(6), 718–729.

Levin, I. P., and Hart, S. S. (2003). Risk preferences in young children: Early evidence of individual differences in reaction to potential gains and losses. *Journal of Behavioral Decision Making, 16*(5), 397–413.

Lieberman, M. D., Hariri, A., Jarcho, J. M., Eisenberger, N. I., and Bookheimer, S. Y. (2005). An fMRI investigation of race-related amygdala activity in African American and Caucasian American individuals. *Nature Neuroscience, 8,* 720–722.

Lomniczi, A., Wright, H., Castellano, J. M., Sonmez, K., and Ojeda, S.R. (2013). A system biology approach to identify regulatory pathways underlying the neuroendocrine control of female puberty in rats and nonhuman primates. *Hormones and Behavior, 64*(2), 175–186.

Luginbuhl, P. J., McWhirter, E. H., and McWhirter, B. T. (2016). Sociopolitical development, autonomous motivation, and education outcomes among low income Latina/o adolescents. *Journal of Latina/o Psychology, 4,* 53–59.

Marceau, K., Abar, C., and Jackson, K. (2015). Parental knowledge is a contextual amplifier of associations of pubertal maturation and substance use. *Journal of Youth Adolescence, 44*(9), 1720–1734.

Marceau, K., Ram, N., Houts, R. M., Grimm, K., and Susman, E. J. (2011). Individual differences in boys' and girls' timing and tempo of puberty: Modeling development with nonlinear growth models. *Developmental Psychology, 47*, 1389–1409.

Marshall, W. A., and Tanner, J. M. (1969). Variations in pattern of pubertal changes in girls. *Archives of Disease in Childhood, 44*(235), 291–303.

Matchock, R. L., Dorn, L. D., Susman, E. J. (2007). Diurnal and seasonal cortisol, testosterone, and DHEA rhythms in boys and girls during puberty. *Chronobiology International, 24*(5), 969–990.

McAdams, D. P. (2013). The psychological self as actor, agent, and author. *Perspectives on Psychological Science, 8*(3), 272–295.

McDowell, M. A., Brody, D. J., and Hughes, J. P. (2007). Has age at menarche changed? Results from the National Health and Nutrition Examination Survey (NHANES) 1999–2004. *Journal of Adolescent Health, 40*, 227–231.

McElhaney, K. B., Allen, J. P., Stephenson, J. C., and Hare, A. L. (2009). Attachment and autonomy during adolescence. In R. M. Lerner and L. D. Steinberg (Eds.), *Handbook of Adolescent Psychology, Volume 1: Individual Bases of Adolescent Development* (3rd ed.). Hoboken, NJ: Wiley.

McKnight, P. E., and Kashdan, T. B. (2009). Purpose in life as a system that creates and sustains health and well-being: An integrative, testable theory. *Review of General Psychology, 13*(3), 242–251.

McMasters, L. E., Connolly, J., Pepler, D., and Craig, W. M. (2002). Peer to peer sexual harassment in early adolescence: A developmental perspective. *Development and Psychopathology, 14*, 91–105.

McWhirter, E. H., and McWhirter, B. T. (2016). Critical consciousness and vocational development among Latina/o high school youth: Initial development and testing of a measure. *Journal of Career Assessment, 24*(3), 543–558.

Meca, A., Ritchie, R. A., Beyers, W., Schwartz, S. J., Picariello, S., Zamboanga, B. L., and Crocetti, E. (2015). Identity centrality and psychosocial functioning: A person-centered approach. *Emerging Adulthood, 3*(5), 327–339.

Meeus, W., Van De Schoot, R., Keijsers, L., Schwartz, S. J., and Branje, S. (2010). On the progression and stability of adolescent identity formation: A five-wave longitudinal study in early-to-middle and middle-to-late adolescence. *Child Development, 81*(5), 1565–1581.

Melmed, S., Polonsky, K. S., Larsen, P. R., and Kronenberg, H. M. (2015). *Williams Textbook of Endocrinology*. Philadelphia, PA: Elsevier Health Sciences.

Mendle, J., and Ferrero, J. (2012). Detrimental psychological outcomes associated with pubertal timing in adolescent boys. *Developmental Review, 32*(1), 49–66.

Mendle, J., Harden, K. P., Brooks-Gunn, J., and Graber, J. A. (2010). Development's tortoise and hare: Pubertal timing, pubertal tempo, and depressive symptoms in boys and girls. *Developmental Psychology, 46*, 1341–1353.

Mendle, J., Leve, L. D., Van Ryzin, M., Natsuaki, M. N., and Ge, X. (2011). Associations between early life stress, child maltreatment, and pubertal development among girls in foster care. *Journal of Research on Adolescence, 21*(4), 871–880.

Mendle, J., Leve, L. D., Van Ryzin, M., and Natsuaki, M. N. (2014). Linking childhood maltreatment with girls' internalizing symptoms: Early puberty as a tipping point. *Journal of Research on Adolescence, 24*(4), 689–702.

Mendle, J., Ryan, R. M., and McKone, K. M. (2016). Early childhood maltreatment and pubertal development: Replication in a population-based sample. *Journal of Research on Adolescence, 26*(3), 595–602.

Meyza, K. Z., Bartal, I. B. A., Monfils, M. H., Panksepp, J. B., and Knapska, E. (2017). The roots of empathy: Through the lens of rodent models. *Neuroscience & Biobehavioral Reviews, 76,* 216–234.

Mills, K. L., and Tamnes, C. K. (2014). Methods and considerations for longitudinal structural brain imaging analysis across development. *Developmental Cognitive Neuroscience, 9,* 172–190.

Mills, K. L., Goddings, A. L., Clasen, L. S., Giedd, J. N., and Blakemore, S. J. (2014). The developmental mismatch in structural brain maturation during adolescence. *Developmental Neuroscience, 36*(3–4), 147–160.

Mills, K. L., Goddings, A. L., Herting, M. M., Meuwese, R., Blakemore, S. J., Crone, E. A., and Tamnes, C. K. (2016). Structural brain development between childhood and adulthood: Convergence across four longitudinal samples. *Neuroimage, 141,* 273–281.

Moore, S. M. (1995). Girls' understanding and social constructions of menarche. *Journal of Adolescence, 18,* 87–104.

Mrazek, A. J., Harada, T., and Chiao, J. Y. (2015). Cultural neuroscience of identity development. *The Oxford Handbook of Identity Development, 1,* 423.

Mueller, S. C., Cromheeke, S., Siugzdaite, R., and Nicolas Boehler, C. (2017). Evidence for the triadic model of adolescent brain development: Cognitive load and task-relevance of emotion differentially affect adolescents and adults. *Developmental Cognitive Neuroscience, 26,* 91–100.

Murty, V., Calabro, F., and Luna, B. (2016). The role of experience in cognitive development: Integration of executive, memory, and mesolimbic systems. *Neuroscience and Biobehavioral Reviews, 70,* 46–58.

Mustanski, B. S., Viken, R. J., Kaprio, J., Pulkkinen, L., and Rose, R. J. (2004). Genetic and environmental influences on pubertal development: Longitudinal data from Finnish twins at ages 11 and 14. *Developmental Psychology, 40*(6), 1188.

Natsuaki, M. N., Leve, L. D., and Mendle, J. (2011). Going through the rites of passage: Timing and transition of menarche, childhood sexual abuse, and anxiety symptoms in girls. *Journal of Youth and Adolescence, 40*(10), 1357–1370.

Natsuaki, M. N., Samuels, D., and Leve, L. D. (2014). Puberty, identity, and context: A biopsychosocial perspective on internalizing psychopathology in early adolescent girls. *Oxford Handbook of Identity Development,* 389–405.

Nigg, J. T., and Nagel, B. J. (2016). Commentary: Risk taking, impulsivity, and externalizing problems in adolescent development. *Journal of Child Psychology and Psychology, and Allied Sciences, 57*(3), 269–370.

Noll, J. G., Trickett, P. K., Long, J. D., Negriff, S., Susman, E. J., Shalev, I., Li, J. C., and Putnam, F. W. (2017). Childhood sexual abuse and early timing of puberty. *Journal of Adolescent Health, 60*(1), 65–71.

Oberfield, S. E., Mayes, D. M., and Levine, L. S. (1990). Adrenal steroidogenic function in a black and Hispanic population with precocious pubarche. *Journal of Clinical Endocrinology and Metabolism, 70*(1), 76–82.

Ochsner, K. N., and Gross, J. J. (2005). The cognitive control of emotion. *Trends in Cognitive Sciences, 9,* 242.

Østby, Y., Tamnes, C. K., Fjell, A. M., Westlye, L. T., Due-Tønnessen, and Walhovd, K. B. (2009). Heterogeneity in subcortical brain development: A structural magnetic resonance imaging study of brain maturation from 8 to 30 years. *Journal of Neuroscience, 29*(38), 11772–11782.

Oyserman, D., and Destin, M. (2010). Identity-based motivation: Implications for intervention. *The Counseling Psychologist, 38*(7), 1001–1043.

Pattwell, S. S., Bath, K. G., Casey, B. J., Ninan, I., and Lee, F. S. (2011). Selective early-acquired fear memories undergo temporary suppression during adolescence. *Proceedings of the National Academy of Sciences of the United States of America, 108*(3), 1182–1187.

Pattwell, S. S., Duhoux, S., Hartley, C. A., Johnson, D. C., Jing, D., Elliott, M. D., Ruberry, E. J., Powers, A., Mehta, N., Yang, R. R., Soliman, F., Glatt, C. E., Casey, B. J., Ninan, I., and Lee, F. S. (2012). Altered fear learning across development in both mouse and human. *Proceedings of the National Academy of Sciences of the United States of America, 109*(40), 16318–16323.

Paus, T., Keshavan, M., and Giedd, J. N. (2008). Why do many psychiatric disorders emerge during adolescence? Nature reviews. *Neuroscience, 9,* 947.

Peña, E. V., Stapleton, L. D., and Schaffer, L. M. (2016). Critical perspectives on disability identity. *New Directions for Student Services, 154,* 85–96.

Peper, J. S., and Dahl, R. E. (2013). Surging hormones: Brain-behavior interactions during puberty. *Current Directions in Psychological Science, 22*(2), 134–139.

Peter, D., and Gazelle, H. (2017). Anxious solitude and self-compassion and self-criticism trajectories in early adolescence: Attachment security as a moderator. *Child Development, 88*(6), 1834–1848.

Petersen, J. L., and Hyde, J. S. (2009). A longitudinal investigation of peer sexual harassment victimization in adolescence. *Journal of Adolescence, 32*(5), 1173–1188.

Pew Research Center (2015). *Support for Same-Sex Marriage at Record High, but Key Segments Remain Opposed.* June. Available: http://www.pewresearch.org/wp-content/uploads/sites/4/2015/06/6-8-15-Same-sex-marriage-release1.pdf.

_____ (2018). *The Age Gap in Religion Around the World.* June 13. Available: https://www.pewforum.org/2018/06/13/the-age-gap-in-religion-around-the-world/

_____ (2019). *Religion's Relationship to Happiness, Civic Engagement and Health Around the World.* January 31. Available: https://www.pewforum.org/2019/01/31/religions-relationship-to-happiness-civic-engagement-and-health-around-the-world/

Pfeifer, J. H., and Allen, N. B. (2012). Arrested development? Reconsidering dual-systems models of brain function in adolescence and disorders. *Trends in Cognitive Sciences, 16*(6), 322–329.

Pfeifer, J. H., and Berkman, E. T. (2018). The development of self and identity in adolescence: Neural evidence and implications for a value-based choice perspective on motivated behavior. *Child Development Perspectives, 12*(3), 158–164.

Phelps, E. A., O'Connor, K. J., Cunningham, W. A., Funayma, E. S., Gatenby, J. C., and Gore, J. C. (2000). Performance on indirect measures of race evaluation predicts amygdala activity. *Journal of Cognitive Neuroscience, 12,* 1–10.

Phinney, J. S., Kim-Jo, T., Osorio, S., Vilhjalmsdottir, P. (2005). Autonomy and relatedness in adolescent-parent disagreements: Ethnic and developmental factors. *Journal of Adolescent Research, 20,* 8–39.

Poteat, V. P., and Russell, S. T. (2013). Understanding homophobic behavior and its implications for policy and practice. *Theory into Practice, 52*(4), 264–271.

Quinlan, R. J. (2003) Father absence, parental care, and female reproductive development. *Evolution and Human Behavior, 24*(6), 376–390.

Rembeck, G. I., Moller, M., and Gunnarsson, R. K. (2006). Attitudes and feelings towards menstruation and womanhood in girls at menarche. *Acta Pediatrica, 95,* 707–714.

Rivas-Drake, D., Seaton, E. K., Markstrom, C., Quintana, S., Syed, M., Lee, R. M., and the Ethnic and Racial Identity in the 21st Century Study Group. (2014). Ethnic and racial identity in adolescence: Implications for psychosocial, academic, and health outcomes. *Child Development, 85*(1), 40–57.

Romans, S. E., Martin, J. M., Gendall, K., and Herbison, G. P. (2003). Age of menarche: The role of some psychosocial factors. *Psychological Medicine, 33*(5), 933–939.

Romer, D., Betancourt, L. M., Bordsky, N. L., Giannetta, J. M., Yang, W., and Hurt, H. (2011). Does adolescent risk taking imply weak executive function? A prospective study of relations between working memory performance, impulsivity, and risk taking in early adolescence. *Developmental Science, 14*(5), 1119–1133.

Romer, D., Reyna, V. F., and Satterthwaite, T. D. (2017). Beyond stereotypes of adolescent risk taking: Placing the adolescent brain in environmental context. *Developmental Cognitive Neuroscience, 27,* 14–19.

Ruble, D. N., and Brooks-Gunn, J. (1982). The experience of menarche. *Child Development, 53,* 1557–1566.

Rudolph, M. D., Miranda-Domínguez, O., Cohen, A. O., Breiner, K., Steinberg, L., Bonnie, R. J., Scott, E. S., Taylor-Thompson, K., Chein, J., Fettich, K. C., Richeson, J. A., Dellarco, D. V., Galván, A., and Casey, B. J. (2017). At risk of being risky: The relationship between "brain age" under emotional states and risk preference. *Developmental Cognitive Neuroscience, 24,* 93.

Russell, S. T., and Fish, J. N. (2017) Mental health in lesbian, gay, bisexual, and transgender (LGBT) youth. *Annual Review of Clinical Psychology, 12,* 465–487.

Russell, S. T., Chu, J. Y., Crockett, L. J., and Lee, S. A. (2010). Interdependent independence: The meanings of autonomy among Chinese American and Filipino American adolescents. In S. T. Russell, L. J. Crockett, and R. K. Chao (Eds.), *Asian American Parenting and Parent-Adolescent Relationships* (pp. 101–116). New York, NY: Springer.

Santos, C. E., and Toomey, R. B. (2018). Integrating an intersectionality lens in theory and research in developmental science. *New Directions for Child and Adolescent Development, 2018*(161), 7–15.

Sapolsky, R. M. (2000). Glucocorticoids and hippocampal atrophy in neuropsychiatric disorders. *Archives of General Psychiatry, 57*(10), 925–935.

Satterthwaite, T. D., Vandekar, S., Wolf, D. H., Ruparel, K., Roalf, D. R., Jackson, C., and Davatzikos, C. (2014). Sex differences in the effect of puberty on hippocampal morphology. *Journal of the American Academy of Child & Adolescent Psychiatry, 53*(3), 341–350.

Saxe, R. R., Whitfield-Gabrieli, S., Scholz, J., and Pelphrey, K. A. (2009). Brain regions for perceiving and reasoning about other people in school-aged children. *Child Development, 80*(4), 1197–1209.

Scherf, K. S., Smyth, J. M., and Delgado, M. R. (2013). The amygdala: An agent of change in adolescent neural networks. *Hormones and Behavior, 64*(2), 298–313.

Schwartz, S. J., Dunkel, C. S., and Waterman, A. S. (2009). Terrorism: An identity theory perspective. *Studies in Conflict & Terrorism, 32*(6), 537–559.

Schwartz, S. J., Côté, J. E., and Arnett, J. J. (2005). Identity and agency in emerging adulthood: Two developmental routes in the individualization process. *Youth & Society, 37*(2), 201–229.

Schwartz, S. J., Beyers, W., Luyckx, K., Soenens, B., Zamboanga, B. L., Forthun, L. F., and Whitbourne, S. K. (2011). Examining the light and dark sides of emerging adults' identity: A study of identity status differences in positive and negative psychosocial functioning. *Journal of Youth and Adolescence, 40*(7), 839–859.

Selemon, L. D. (2013). A role for synaptic plasticity in the adolescent development of executive function. *Translational Psychiatry, 3,* e238.

Shedd, C. (2015). *Unequal City: Race, Schools, and Perceptions of Injustice.* New York, NY: Russell Sage Foundation.

Shulman, E. P., Smith, A. R., Silva, K., Icenogle, G., Duell, N., Chein, J., and Steinberg, L. (2016). The dual systems model: Review, reappraisal, and reaffirmation. *Developmental Cognitive Neuroscience, 17*, 103–117.

Simonneaux, V., Ancel, C., Poirel, V.J., and Gauer, F. (2013). Kisspeptins and RFRP-3 act in concert to synchronize rodent reproduction with seasons. *Frontiers in Neuroscience, 7*, 1–22.

Sisk, C. L., and Foster, D. L. (2004). The neural basis of puberty and adolescence. *Nature Neuroscience, 7*, 1040–1047.

Smart, J., and Smart, D. (2007). Models of disability. The psychological and social impact of illness and disability, 75–100.

Spear, L. P. (2013). Adolescent neurodevelopment. *Journal of Adolescent Health, 52*(2 Suppl 2), S7–13.

Spencer, M. B. (1995). Old issues and new theorizing about African-American youth: a phenomenological variant of the ecological systems theories. In R. L. Taylor, (Ed.), *Black Youth: Perspectives on Their Status in the United States* (pp. 37–70). New York: Praeger.

Stattin, H., and Magnusson, D. (1990). *Pubertal Maturation in Female Development.* Hillsdale, NJ: Erlbaum.

Steinbeis, N., and Crone, E. A. (2016). The link between cognitive control and decision-making across child and adolescent development. *Current Opinion in Behavioral Sciences, 10*, 28–32.

Steinberg, L. (2005). Cognitive and affective development in adolescence. *Trends in Cognitive Sciences 9*, 69.

_____. (2008). A social neuroscience perspective on adolescent risk-taking. *Developmental Review, 28*(1), 78–106.

_____. (2014). *Age of Opportunity: Lessons from the New Science of Adolescence.* Boston, MA: Houghton Mifflin Harcourt.

Steinberg, L., Graham, S., O'Brien, L., Woolard, J., Cauffman, E., and Banich, M. (2009). Age differences in future orientation and delay discounting. *Child Development, 80*(1), 28–44.

Steinberg, L., Icenogle, G., Shulman, E. P., Breiner, K., Chein, J., Bacchini, D., and Fanti, K. A. (2018). Around the world, adolescence is a time of heightened sensation seeking and immature self-regulation. *Developmental science, 21*(2), e12532.

Steingraber, S. (2007). *The Falling Age of Puberty in U.S. Girls: What We Know, What We Need to Know.* San Francisco, CA: Breast Cancer Fund. Available: http://gaylesulik. com/wp-content/uploads/2010/07/falling-age-of-puberty.pdf.

Stroud, L. R., Papandonatos, G. D., Williamson, D. E., and Dahl, R. E. (2004). Applying a nonlinear regression model to characterize cortisol responses to corticotropin-releasing hormone challenge. *Annals of the New York Academy of Sciences, 1032*(1), 264–266.

Stubbs, M. L. (2008). Cultural perceptions and practices around menarche and adolescent menstruation in the United States. *Annals of New York Academy of Sciences, 1135*, 58–66.

Suárez-Orozco, C., Motti-Stefanidi, F., Marks, A., and Katsiaficas, D. (2018). An integrative risk and resilience model for understanding the adaptation of immigrant-origin children and youth. *American Psychologist, 73*(6), 781–796.

Sumner, R., Burrow, A. L., and Hill, P. L. (2018). The development of purpose in life among adolescents who experience marginalization: Potential opportunities and obstacles. *American Psychologist, 73*(6), 740–752.

Sung, S., Simpson, J. A., Griskevicius, V., Kuo, S. I. C., Schlomer, G. L., and Belsky, J. (2016). Secure infant-mother attachment buffers the effect of early-life stress on age of menarche. *Psychological Science, 27*(5), 667–674.

Syed, M. (2017). Advancing the cultural study of personality and identity: Models, methods, and outcomes. *Current Issues in Personality Psychology*, 1, 65–72.

Syed, M., Santos, C., Yoo, H. C., and Juang, L. P. (2018). Invisibility of racial/ethnic minorities in developmental science: Implications for research and institutional practices. *American Psychologist*, 73(6), 812.

Sylvia Rivera Law Project. (2012). *Fact Sheet: Transgender & Gender Nonconforming Youth in School*. Available: https://srlp.org/resources/fact-sheet-transgender-gender-nonconforming-youth-school/.

Smetana, J. G. (2011). *Adolescents, Families, and Social Development: How Teens Construct Their Worlds*. Hoboken, NJ: John Wiley & Sons.

Tamnes, C. K., Walhovd, K. B., Engvig, A., Gyrdeland, H., Krosgrud, S.K., Østby, Y., Holland, D., Dale, A. M., and Fjell, A. M. (2014). Regional hippocampal volumes and development predict learning and memory. *Developmental Neuroscience, 36*, 161–174.

Tamnes, C. K., Herting, M. M., Goddings, A. L., Meuwese, R., Blakemore, S. J., Dahl, R. E., and Mills, K. L. (2017). Development of the cerebral cortex across adolescence: A multisample study of inter-related longitudinal changes in cortical volume, surface area, and thickness. *Journal of Neuroscience*, 37(12), 3402–3412.

Tang, C. S., Yeung, D. Y., and Lee, A. M. (2003). Psychosocial correlates of emotional responses to menarche among Chinese adolescent girls. *Journal of Adolescent Health, 33*, 193–201.

Telzer, E. H., Masten, C. L., Berkman, E. T., Lieberman, M. D., and Fuligni, A. J. (2010). Gaining while giving: An fMRI study of the rewards of family assistance. *Social Neuroscience, 5*, 508–515.

Telzer, E. H., Humphreys, K. L., Shapiro, M., and Tottenham, N. (2013). Amygdala sensitivity to race is not present in childhood but emerges over adolescence. *Journal of Cognitive Neuroscience*, 25(2), 234–244.

Terasawa, E., and Fernandez, D. L. (2001). Neurobiological mechanisms of the onset of puberty in primates. *Endocrine Reviews*, 22(1), 111–151.

Thomas, A. J., Barrie, R., Brunner, J., Clawson, A., Hewitt, A., Jeremie-Brink, G., and Rowe-Johnson, M. (2014). Assessing critical consciousness in youth and young adults. *Journal of Research on Adolescence*, 24(3), 485–496.

Tolman, D. L., and McClelland, S. I. (2011). Normative sexuality development in adolescence: A decade in review, 2000-2009. *Journal of Research on Adolescence*, 21(1), 242–255.

Trickett, P. K., and Putnam, F. W. (1993). Impact of child sexual abuse on females: Toward a developmental, psychobiological integration. *Psychological Science*, 4(2), 81–87.

Tsai, K. M., Telzer, E. H., and Fuligni, A. J. (2012). Continuity and discontinuity in perceptions of family relationships from adolescence to young adulthood. *Child Development, 84*, 471–484.

Turner, P. K., Runtz, M. G., and Galambos, N. L. (1999). Sexual abuse, pubertal timing, and subjective age in adolescent girls: A research note. *Journal of Reproductive and Infant Psychology*, 17(2), 111–118.

Tymula, A., Rosenberg Belmaker, L. A., Roy, A. K., Ruderman, L., Manson, K., Glimcher, P. W., and Levy, I. (2012). Adolescents' risk-taking behavior is driven by tolerance to ambiguity. *Proceedings of the National Academy of Sciences of the United States of America*, 109(42), 17135–17140.

Umaña-Taylor, A. J., Quintana, S. M., Lee, R. M., Cross Jr, W. E., Rivas-Drake, D., Schwartz, S. J., and Ethnic and Racial Identity in the 21st Century Study Group. (2014). Ethnic and racial identity during adolescence and into young adulthood: An integrated conceptualization. *Child Development*, 85(1), 21–39.

van den Bos, W., Rodriguez, C. A., Schweitzer, J. B., and McClure, S. M. (2015). Adolescent impatience decreases with increased frontostriatal connectivity. *Proceedings of the National Academy of Sciences of the United States of America, 112*(29), E3765–E3774.

Vandekar, S. N., Shinohara, R. T., Raznahan, A., Roalf, D. R., Ross, M., DeLeo, N., Ruparel, K., Verma, R., Wolf, D. H., Gur, R. C., Gur, R. E., and Satterthwaite, T. D. (2015). Topologically dissociable patterns of development of the human cerebral cortex. *Journal of Neuroscience, 35*(20), 599–609.

Velez, G., and Spencer, M. B. (2018). Phenomenology and intersectionality: Using PVEST as a frame for adolescent identity formation amid intersecting ecological systems of inequality. *New Directions for Child and Adolescent Development, 2018*(161), 75–90.

Verkuyten, M., and Martinovic, B. (2012). Social identity complexity and immigrants' attitude toward the host nation: The intersection of ethnic and religious group identification. *Personality and Social Psychology Bulletin, 38*(9), 1165–1177.

Vijayakumar, N., de Macks, Z. O., Shirtcliff, E. A., and Pfeifer, J. H. (2018). Puberty and the human brain: Insights into adolescent development. *Neuroscience & Biobehavioral Reviews, 92*, 417–436.

Wagner, I. V., Sabin, M., and Kiess, W. (2015). Influences of childhood obesity on pubertal development. In W. Kiess, M. Wabitsch, C. Maffeis, and A. M. Sharma (Eds.), *Metabolic Syndrome and Obesity in Childhood and Adolescence, Pediatric Adolescent Medicine* (pp. 110–125). Basel, Switzerland: Karger. Available: https://www.karger.com/Article/Abstract/368112.

Wahlstrom, D., Collins, P., White, T., and Luciana, M. (2010). Developmental changes in dopamine neurotransmission in adolescence: Behavioral implications and issues in assessment. *Brain and Cognition, 72*(1), 146–159.

Walker, E. F., Sabuwalla, Z., and Huot, R. (2004). Pubertal neuromaturation, stress sensitivity, and psychopathology. *Development and Psychopathology, 16*(4), 807–824.

Watkins, D. J., Sánchez, B. N., Téllez-Rojo, M. M., Lee, J. M., Mercado-García, A., Blank-Goldenberg, C., Peterson, K. E., and Meeker, J. D. (2017). Phthalate and bisphenol A exposure during in utero windows of susceptibility in relation to reproductive hormones and pubertal development in girls. *Environmental Research, 159*, 143–151.

Watts, R. J. (2018, June). *Powerful Youth, Powerful Communities: The Youth Development Benefits of Community Organizing.* Presentation to the Committee on the Neurobiological and Socio-behavioral Science of Adolescent Development and Its Applications. Available:; https://sites.nationalacademies.org/cs/groups/dbassesite/documents/webpage/dbasse_188004.pdf.

Watts, R. J., Diemer, M. A., and Voight, A. M. (2011). Critical consciousness: Current status and future directions. *New Directions for Child and Adolescent Development, 2011*(134), 43–57.

Webster, G. D., Graber, J. A., Gesselman, A. N., Crosier, B. S., and Schember, T. O. (2014). A life history theory of father absence and menarche: A meta-analysis. *Evolutionary Psychology, 12*(2), 273–294.

Westling, E., Andrews, J. A., Hampson, S. E., Peterson, M. (2008). Pubertal timing and substance use: The effects of gender, parental monitoring and deviant peers. *Journal of Adolescent Health, 42*(6), 555–563.

Wierenga, L., Langen, M., Ambrosino, S., van Dijk, S., Oranje, B., and Durston, S. (2014). Typical development of basal ganglia, hippocampus, amygdala and cerebellum from age 7 to 24. *Neuroimage, 1*(96), 67–72.

Williams, J. L., and Hamm, J. V. (2017). Peer group ethnic diversity and social competencies in youth attending rural middle schools. *The Journal of Early Adolescence, 38*(6), 795–823.

Williams, J. L., Tolan, P. H., Durkee, M. I., Francois, A. G., and Anderson, R. E. (2012). Integrating racial and ethnic identity research into developmental understanding of adolescents. *Child Development Perspectives, 6*(3), 304–311.

Williams, J. L., Anderson, R. E., Francois, A. G., Hussain, S., and Tolan, P. H. (2014). Ethnic identity and positive youth development in adolescent males: A culturally integrated approach. *Applied Developmental Science, 18*(2), 110–122.

Wilson, B. D. M., Choi, S. K., Herman, J. L., Becker, T., and Conron, K. J. (2017). *Characteristics and Mental Health of Gender Nonconforming Adolescents in California: Findings from the 2015-2016 California Health Interview Survey.* Los Angeles, CA: The Williams Institute and UCLA Center for Health Policy Research. Available: http://healthpolicy.ucla.edu/publications/Documents/PDF/2017/gncadolescents-factsheet-dec2017.pdf.

Windham, G. C., Pinney, S. M., Voss, R. W., Sjödin, A., Biro, F. M., Greenspan, L. C., Stewart, S., Hiatt, R. A., and Kushi, L. H. (2015). Brominated flame retardants and other persistent organohalogenated compounds in relation to timing of puberty in a longitudinal study of girls. *Environmental Health Perspectives, 123*(10), 1046–1052.

Wise, L. A., Palmer, J. R., Rothman, E. F., and Rosenberg, L. (2009). Childhood abuse and early menarche: Findings from the Black Women's Health Study. *American Journal of Public Health, 99*(S2), S460–S466.

Yeager, D. S., Bundick, M. J., and Johnson, R. (2012). The role of future work goal motives in adolescent identity development: A longitudinal mixed-methods investigation. *Contemporary Educational Psychology, 37*(3), 206–217.

Yeager, D. S., Henderson, M. D., Paunesku, D., Walton, G. M., D'Mello, S., Spitzer, B. J., and Duckworth, A. L. (2014). *Journal of Personality and Social Psychology, 107*(4), 559–580.

Young, E. A., and Altemus, M. (2004). Puberty, ovarian steroids, and stress. *Annals of the New York Academy of Sciences, 1021*, 124–133.

Zuckerman, M., and Kuhlman, D. M. (2000). Personality and risk-taking: Common biosocial factors. *Journal of Personality, 68*(6), 999–1029.

CHAPTER 3

Adams, S. K., Daly, J. F., and Williford, D. N. (2013). Adolescent sleep and cellular phone use: Recent trends and implications for research. *Health Services Insights, 6*, 99–103.

Allfrey, V. G. (1970). Changes in chromosomal proteins at times of gene activation. *Federation Proceedings 29*, 1447–1460.

Aronen, E. T., Paavonen, E. J., Fjällberg, M., Soininen, M., & Törrönen, J. (2000). Sleep and psychiatric symptoms in school-age children. *Journal of the American Academy of Child & Adolescent Psychiatry, 39*(4), 502–508.

Arora, T., Broglia, E., Thomas, G. N., and Taheri, S. (2014). Associations between specific technologies and adolescent sleep quantity, sleep quality, and parasomnias. *Sleep Medicine, 15*(2), 240–247.

Asarnow, L. D., McGlinchey, E., and Harvey, A. G. (2014). The effects of bedtime and sleep duration on academic and emotional outcomes in a nationally representative sample of adolescents. *The Journal of Adolescent Health: Official Publication of the Society for Adolescent Medicine, 54*, 350–356.

Barnes, J. C., and Meldrum, R. C. (2015). The impact of sleep duration on adolescent development: A genetically informed analysis of identical twin pairs. *Journal of Youth and Adolescence, 44*(2), 489–506.

Baum, K. T., Desai, A., Field, J., Miller, L. E., Rausch, J., and Beebe, D. W. (2014). Sleep restriction worsens mood and emotion regulation in adolescents. *Journal of Child Psychology and Psychiatry, 55*(2), 180–190.

Biessels, G. J., and Reagan, L. P. (2015). Hippocampal insulin resistance and cognitive dysfunction. *Nature Reviews Neuroscience, 16*, 660–671.

Bohacek, J., and Mansuy, I. M. (2015). Molecular insights into transgenerational non-genetic inheritance of acquired behaviours. *Nature Reviews Genetics, 16*, 641–652.

Boyce, W. T., and Ellis, B. J. (2005). Biological sensitivity to context: I. An evolutionary-developmental theory of the origins and functions of stress reactivity. *Development and Psychopathology, 17*, 271–301.

Brody, G. H., Gray, J. C., Yu, T., Barton, A. W., and Beach, S. R. (2017a). Protective prevention effects on the association of poverty with brain development. *JAMA Pediatrics, 171*, 46–52.

Brody, G. H., Yu, T., Chen, E., and Miller, G. E. (2017b). Family-centered prevention ameliorates the association between adverse childhood experiences and prediabetes status in young Black adults. *Preventive Medicine, 100*, 117–122.

Brouwer, J. P., Appelhof, B. C., van Rossum, E. F., Koper, J. W., Fliers, E., Huyser, J., Schene, A. H., Tijssen, J. G., Van Dyck, R., Lamberts, S. W., Wiersinga, W. M., and Hoogendijk, W. J. (2006). Prediction of treatment response by HPA-axis and glucocorticoid receptor polymorphisms in major depression. *Psychoneuroendocrinology, 31*(10), 1154–1163.

Brunello, N., Armitage, R., Feinberg, I., Holsboer-Trachsler, E., Leger, D., and Mendlewicz, J. (2000). Depression and sleep disorders: Clinical relevance, economic burden and pharmacological treatment. *Neuropsychobiology, 43*(3), 107–119.

Cacioppo, J. T., Hawkley, L. C., Norman, G. J., Berntson, G. G. (2011). Social isolation. *Annals of the New York Academy of Sciences, 1231*, 17–22.

Cameron, H. A., and Gould, E. (1996). The control of neuronal birth and survival. In C. A. Shaw (Ed.), *Receptor Dynamics in Neural Development*, pp. 141–157. New York: CRC Press.

Carskadon, M. A., Harvey, K., Duke, P., Anders, T. F., Litt, I. F., and Dement, W. C. (1980). Pubertal changes in daytime sleepiness. *Sleep, 2*(4), 453–460.

Casey, B. J., Jones, R. M., and Hare, T. A (2008). The adolescent brain. *Annals of the New York Academy of Sciences, 1124*(1), 111–126.

Chattarji, S., Tomar, A., Suvrathan, A., Ghosh, S., Rahman, M.M. (2015). Neighborhood matters: Divergent patterns of stress-induced plasticity across the brain. *Nature Neuroscience 18*, 1364–1375.

Clarke, G., and Harvey, A. G. (2013). The complex role of sleep in adolescent depression. *Child and Adolescent Psychiatric Clinics of North America, 21*(2), 385–400.

Classen, C. C., Palesh, O. G., and Aggarwal, R. (2005). Sexual revictimization: A review of the empirical literature. *Trauma, Violence, & Abuse, 6*(2), 103–129.

Copeland, K., Angold, A., and Costello., EJ. (2007). Traumatic events and posttraumatic stress in childhood. *Archives of General Psychiatry, 64*, 577–584.

Culpin, I., Stapinski, L., Miles, O. B., Araya, R., and Joinson, C. (2015). Exposure to socio-economic adversity in early life and risk of depression at 18 years: The mediating role of locus of control. *Journal of Affective Disorders, 183*, 269–278.

Dahl, R. E., and Harvey, A. G. (2007). Sleep disorders. In M. L. Rutter, (Ed.), *Oxford Textbook of Child and Adolescent Psychiatry*. Oxford: Oxford University Press.

Dahl, R. E., and Lewin, D. S. (2002). Pathways to adolescent health sleep regulation behavior. *Journal of Adolescent Health, 31*(6 Suppl), 175–184.

Danielsson, N. S., Harvey, A. G., MacDonald, S., Jansson-Fröjmark, M., and Linton, S. J. (2013). Sleep disturbance and depressive symptoms in adolescence: The role of catastrophic worry. *Journal of Youth and Adolescence, 42*(8), 1223–1233.

Davidow, J. Y., Foerde, K., Galván, A., and Shohamy, D. (2016). An upside to reward sensitivity: The hippocampus supports enhanced reinforcement learning in adolescence. *Neuron, 92*(1), 93–99.

Del Giudice, M., Ellis, B. J., and Shirtcliff, E. A. (2011). The adaptive calibration model of stress responsivity. *Neuroscience and Biobehavioral Reviews 35*, 1562–1592.

Dias, B. G., and Ressler, K. J. (2014). Parental olfactory experience influences behavior and neural structure in subsequent generations. *Nature Neuroscience, 17*(1), 89–96.

Eaton, D. K., McKnight-Eily, L. R., Lowry, R., Perry, G. S., Presley-Cantrell, L., and Croft, J. B. (2010). Prevalence of insufficient, borderline, and optimal hours of sleep among high school students–United States, (2007). *Journal of Adolescent Health, 46*(4), 399–401.

Eckenrode, J., Campa, M. I., Morris, P. A., Henderson, C. R., Jr., and Bolger, K. E. (2017). The prevention of child maltreatment through the nurse family partnership program: Mediating effects in a long-term follow-up study. *Child Maltreatment, 22*, 92–99.

Entringer, S., Buss, C., and Wadhwa, P.D. (2015). Prenatal stress, development, health and disease risk: A psychobiological perspective. 2015 Curt Richter Award Paper. *Psychoneuroendocrinology, 62*, 366–375.

Erickson, K. I., Voss, M. W., Prakash, R. S., Basak, C., and Szabo, A. (2011). Exercise training increases size of hippocampus and improves memory. *Proceedings of the National Academy of Sciences of the United States of America, 108*, 3017–3022.

Fallone, G., Acebo, C., Seifer, R., and Carskadon, M. A. (2005). Experimental restriction of sleep opportunity in children: Effects on teacher ratings. *Sleep, 28*(12), 1561–1567.

Fergusson, D. M., Horwood, J. and Lynskey, M. T. (1997). Childhood sexual abuse, adolescent sexual behaviors and sexual revictimization. *Child Abuse and Neglect, 21*, 789–803.

Fergusson, D. M., Horwood, L. J., Ridder, E. M., and Beautrais, A. L. (2005). Sexual orientation and mental health in a birth cohort of young adults. *Psychological Medicine, 35*(7), 971–981.

Finkelhor, D., Ormrod, R. K., and Turner, H. A. (2007). Polyvictimization and trauma in a national longitudinal cohort. *Development and Psychopathology, 19*(1), 149–166.

Fraga, M. F., Ballestar, E., Paz, M. F., Ropero, S., and Setien, F. (2005). Epigenetic differences arise during the lifetime of monozygotic twins. *Proceedings of the National Academy of Sciences of the United States of America, 102*, 10604–10609.

Freund, J., Brandmaier, A. M., Lewejohann, L., Kirste, I., Kritzler, M., Krüger, A., Sachser, N., Lindenberger, U., and Kempermann, G. (2013). Emergence of individuality in genetically individual mice. *Science, 340*(6133), 756–759.

Gamble, A. L., D'Rozario, A. L., Bartlett, D. J., Williams, S., Bin, Y. S., Grunstein, R. R., and Marshall, N. S. (2014). Adolescent sleep patterns and night-time technology use: Results of the Australian Broadcasting Corporation's Big Sleep Survey. *PloS One, 9*(11), 1–9.

Gee, D. G., Gabard-Durnam, L. J., Flannery, J., Goff, B., and Humphreys, K. L. (2013a). Early developmental emergence of human amygdala-prefrontal connectivity after maternal deprivation. *Proceedings of the National Academy of Sciences of the United States of America, 110*, 15638–15643.

Gee, D. G., Humphreys, K. L., Flannery, J., Goff, B., and Telzer, E. H. (2013b). A developmental shift from positive to negative connectivity in human amygdala-prefrontal circuitry. *Journal of Neuroscience, 33*, 4584–4593.

Gianaros, P. J., Marsland, A. L., Sheu, L. K., Erickson, K. I., Verstynen, T. D. (2013). Inflammatory pathways link socioeconomic inequalities to white matter architecture. *Cerebral Cortex, 23*, 2058–2071.

Giannotti, F., and Cortesi, F. (2009). Family and cultural influences on sleep development. *Child and Adolescent Psychiatric Clinics of North America, 18*(4), 849–861.

Gold, S. M., Dziobek, I., Sweat, V., Tirsi, A., and Rogers, K. (2007). Hippocampal damage and memory impairments as possible early brain complications of type 2 diabetes. *Diabetologia, 50*, 711–719.

Gray, J. D., Rubin, T. G., Hunter, R. G., and McEwen, B. S. (2014). Hippocampal gene expression changes underlying stress sensitization and recovery. *Molecular Psychiatry, 19*, 1171–1178.

Griffiths, B. B., and Hunter, R. G. (2014). Neuroepigenetics of stress. *Neuroscience, 275*, 420–435.

Grillo, C. A., Piroli, G. G., Lawrence, R. C., Wrighten, S. A., and Green, A. J. (2015). Hippocampal insulin resistance impairs spatial learning and synaptic plasticity. *Diabetes, 64*, 3927–3936.

Hair, N. L., Hanson, J. L., Wolfe, B. L., and Pollak, S. D. (2015). Association of child poverty, brain development, and academic achievement. *JAMA Pediatrics, 169*(9), 822–829.

Hale, L., and Guan, S. (2015). Screen time and sleep among school-aged children and adolescents: A systematic literature review. *Sleep Medicine Reviews, 21*, 50–58.

Halfon, N., Larson, K., Lu, M., Tullis, E., and Russ, S. (2014). Lifecourse health development: Past, present and future. *Maternal and Child Health Journal, 18*, 344–365.

Hanson, J. L., Hair, N., Shen, D. G., Shi, F., Gilmore, J. H., Wolfe, B. L., and Pollack, S. D. (2013). Family poverty affects the rate of human infant brain growth. *PLoS One, 8*, e80954.

Hanson, J. L., Nacewicz, B. M., Sutterer, M. J., Cayo, A. A., and Schaefer, S. M. (2015). Behavioral problems after early life stress: Contributions of the hippocampus and amygdala. *Biological Psychiatry, 77*, 314–323.

Harvey, A. G. (2000). Sleep hygiene and sleep-onset insomnia. *The Journal of Nervous and Mental Disease, 188*(1), 53–55.

Herringa, R. J. (2017). Trauma, PTSD, and the developing brain. *Current Psychiatry Reports, 19*(10), 69.

Huber, E., Donnelly, P. M., Rokem, and A., Yeatman, J. D. (2018). Rapid and widespread white matter plasticity during an intensive reading intervention. *Nature Communications, 9*, 2260.

Huber, R., and Born, J. (2014). Sleep, synaptic connectivity, and hippocampal memory during early development. *Trends in Cognitive Science, 18*(3), 141–152.

Hysing, M., Pallesen, S., Stormark, K. M., Jakobsen, R., Lundervold, A.J., and Sivertsen, B. (2015). Sleep and use of electronic devices in adolescence: Results from a large population–based study. *BMJ Open, 5*(1), 1–7.

Iglowstein, I., Jenni, O. G., Molinari, L., and Largo, R. H. (2003). Sleep duration from infancy to adolescence: Reference values and generational trends. *Pediatrics, 111*(2), 302–307.

Ising, M., Horstmann, S., Kloiber, S., Lucae, S., Binder, E. B., Kern, N., Künzel, H. E., Pfennig, A., Uhr, M., and Holsboer, F. (2007). Combined dexamethasone/corticotropin releasing hormone test predicts treatment response in major depression—A potential biomarker? *Biological Psychiatry, 62*(1), 47–54.

Iuculano, T., Rosenberg-Lee, M., Richardson, J., Tenison, C., and Fuchs, L. (2015). Cognitive tutoring induces widespread neuroplasticity and remediates brain function in children with mathematical learning disabilities. *Nature Communications, 6*, 8453.

Jan, J. E., Reiter, R. J., Bax, M. C., Ribary, U., Freeman, R. D., and Wasdell, M. B. (2010). Long-term sleep disturbances in children: A cause of neuronal loss. *European Journal of Paediatric Neurology, 14*(5), 380–390.

Jenni, O. G., and O'Connor, B. B. (2005). Children's sleep: An interplay between culture and biology. *Pediatrics, 115*(1 Suppl), 204–216.

Kaufmann, C. N., Mojtabai, R., Hock, R. S., Thorpe Jr., R. J., Canham, S. L., Chen, L.-Y., and Spira, A. P. (2016). Racial/ethnic differences in insomnia trajectories among U.S. older adults. *The American Journal of Geriatric Psychiatry, 24*(7), 575–584.

Keller, T. A., and Just, M. A. (2009). Altering cortical connectivity: Remediation-induced changes in the white matter of poor readers. *Neuron, 64,* 624–631.

Kesner, R. P. (2007). A behavioral analysis of dentate gyrus function. *Progress in Brain Research, 163,* 567–576.

_____. (2018). An analysis of dentate gyrus function (an update). *Behavioural Brain Research, 354,* 84–91.

King, D. L., Gradisar, M., Drummond, A., Lovato, N., Wessel, J., Micic, G., and Delfabbro, P. (2013). The impact of prolonged violent video-gaming on adolescent sleep: An experimental study. *Journal of Sleep Research, 22*(2), 137–143.

Kleibeuker, S. W., Stevenson, C. E., van der Aar, L., Overgaauw, S., van Duijvenvoorde, A. C., and Crone, E. A. (2017.) Training in the adolescent brain: An fMRI training study on divergent thinking. *Developmental Psychology, 53,* 353–365.

Kraus, N., Hornickel, J., Strait, D.L., Slater, J., and Thompson, E. (2014a). Engagement in community music classes sparks neuroplasticity and language development in children from disadvantaged backgrounds. *Frontiers in Psychology, 5,* 1403.

Kraus, N., Slater, J., Thompson, E. C., Hornickel, J., and Strait, D. L. (2014b). Auditory learning through active engagement with sound: Biological impact of community music lessons in at-risk children. *Frontiers in Neuroscience, 8,* 351.

_____. (2014c). Music enrichment programs improve the neural encoding of speech in at-risk children. *Journal of Neuroscience, 34,* 11913–11918.

Kuo, S. I., Updegraff, K. A., Zeiders, K. H., McHale, S. M., Umana-Taylor, A. J., and De Jesus, S. A. (2015). Mexican American adolescents' sleep patterns: Contextual correlates and implications for health and adjustment in young adulthood. *Journal of Youth and Adolescence, 44,* 346–361.

Louca, M., and Short, M. A. (2014). The effect of one night's sleep deprivation on adolescent neurobehavioral performance. *Sleep, 37*(11), 1799–1807.

Lupien, S. J., Parent, S., Evans, A. C., Tremblay, R. E., Zelazo, and P. D. (2011). Larger amygdala but no change in hippocampal volume in 10-year-old children exposed to maternal depressive symptomatology since birth. *Proceedings of the National Academy of Sciences of the United States of America, 108,* 14324–14329.

Lupien, S. J., Ouellet-Morin, I., Trepanier, L., Juster, R. P., and Marin, M. F. (2013). The DeStress for Success Program: Effects of a stress education program on cortisol levels and depressive symptomatology in adolescents making the transition to high school. *Neuroscience, 249,* 74–87.

Majeno, A., Tsai, K. M., Huynh, V. W., McCreath, H., and Fuligni, A. J. (2018). Discrimination and sleep difficulties during adolescence: The mediating roles of loneliness and perceived stress. *Journal of Youth and Adolescence, 47*(1), 135–147.

McEwen, B. S. (1998). Protective and damaging effects of stress mediators. *New England Journal of Medicine, 338,* 171–179.

McEwen, B. S., and Gianaros, P. J. (2011). Stress- and allostasis-induced brain plasticity. *Annual Review of Medicine, 62,* 431–445.

McEwen, C. A., and McEwen, B. S. (2017). Social structure, adversity, toxic stress, and intergenerational poverty: An early childhood model. *Annual Review of Sociology, 43,* 445–472.

McEwen, B. S., and Morrison, J. H. (2013). The brain on stress: Vulnerability and plasticity of the prefrontal cortex over the life course. *Neuron, 79,* 16–29.

McEwen, B. S., and Stellar, E. (1993). Stress and the individual: Mechanisms leading to disease. *Archives of Internal Medicine, 153*(18), 2093–2101.

McEwen, B. S., and Wingfield, J. C. (2003). The concept of allostasis in biology and biomedicine. *Hormones and Behavior, 43*(1), 2–15.

McEwen, B. S., Bowles, N. P., Gray, J. D., Hill, M. N., and Hunter, R. G. (2015a). Mechanisms of stress in the brain. *Nature, Neuroscience, 18,* 1353–1363.

McEwen, B. S., Gray, J. D., and Nasca, C. (2015b). 60 years of neuroendocrinology: Redefining neuroendocrinology: stress, sex and cognitive and emotional regulation. *Journal of Endocrinology, 226,* T67–T83.

McLaughlin, K. A., Koenen, K. C., Hill, E. D., Petukhova, M., Sampson, N. A., Zaslavsky, A. M., and Kessler, R. C. (2013). Trauma exposure and posttraumatic stress disorder in a national sample of adolescents. *Journal of the American Academy of Child and Adolescent Psychiatry, 52*(8), 815–830.

Mehler, M. F. (2008). Epigenetic principles and mechanisms underlying nervous system functions in health and disease. *Progress in Neurobiology, 86,* 305–341.

Mehler, M. F., and Mattick, J. S. (2007). Noncoding RNAs and RNA editing in brain development, functional diversification, and neurological disease. *Physiological Reviews, 87,* 799–823

Meyer, I. H. (2003). Prejudice, social stress, and mental health in lesbian, gay, and bisexual populations: Conceptual issues and research evidence. *Psychological Bulletin, 129*(5), 674–697.

Miller, G. E., Brody, G. H., Yu, T., and Chen, E. (2014). A family-oriented psychosocial intervention reduces inflammation in low-SES African American youth. *Proceedings of the National Academy of Sciences of the United States of America, 111,* 11287–11292.

Miller, G. W., and Jones, D. P. (2014). The nature of nurture: Refining the definition of the exposome. *Toxicological Sciences, 137*(1), 1–2.

Mindell, J. A., Sadeh, A., Kwon, R., and Goh, D.Y. (2013). Cross-cultural differences in the sleep of preschool children. *Sleep Medicine, 14*(12), 1283–1289.

Minihane, A. M., Vinoy, S., Russell, W. R., Baka, A., Roche, H. M., Tuohy, K. M., and McArdle, H. J. (2015). Low-grade inflammation, diet composition and health: Current research evidence and its translation. *British Journal of Nutrition, 114*(7), 999–1012.

Mitchell, J. A., Rodriguez, D., Schmitz, K. H., and Audrain-McGovern, J. (2013). Sleep duration and adolescent obesity. *Pediatrics, 131*(5), e1428–e1434.

National Academies of Sciences, Engineering, and Medicine. (2017). *Communities in Action: Pathways to Health Equity.* Washington, DC: The National Academies Press.

National Research Council and Institute of Medicine. (2000). *From Neurons to Neighborhoods: The Science of Early Childhood Development.* Washington, DC: The National Academies Press.

National Sleep Foundation. (2006). *Sleep in America Poll.* Washington, DC: National Sleep Foundation.

———— (2010). *Adolescent Sleep Needs and Patterns.* Washington, DC: National Sleep Foundation.

Obradovic, J., and Boyce, W. T. (2009). Individual differences in behavioral, physiological, and genetic sensitivities to contexts: Implications for development and adaptation. *Developmental Neuroscience, 31*(4), 300–308.

Obradovic, J., Bush, N. R., Stamperdahl, J., Adler, N. E., and Boyce, W. T. (2010). Biological sensitivity to context: The interactive effects of stress reactivity and family adversity on socioemotional behavior and school readiness. *Child Development, 81,* 270–289.

O'Mara S. (2005). The subiculum: What it does, what it might do, and what neuroanatomy has yet to tell us. *Journal of Anatomy, 207*(3), 271–282.

Owens, S., Hunte, H., Sterkel, A., Johnson, D. A., and Johnson-Lawrence, V. (2017). Association between discrimination and objective and subjective sleep measures in the MIDUS adult sample. *Psychosomatic Medicine, 79*(4), 469.

Paavonen, E. J., Raikkonen, K., Lahti, J., Komsi, N., Heinonen, K., and Pesonen, A. K. (2009). Short sleep duration and behavioral symptoms of attention-deficit/hyperactivity disorder in healthy 7- to 8-year-old children. *Pediatrics, 123*, e857–e864.

Parthasarathy, S., Carskadon, M. A., Jean-Louis, G., Owens, J., Bramoweth, A., Combs, D., and Hasler, B. P. (2016). Implementation of sleep and circadian science: Recommendations from the Sleep Research Society and National Institutes of Health workshop. *Sleep, 39*(12), 2061–2075.

Peach, H. D., and Gaultney, J. F. (2013). Sleep, impulse control, and sensation-seeking predict delinquent behavior in adolescents, emerging adults, and adults. *Journal of Adolescent Health, 53*(2), 293–299.

Perkinson-Gloor, N., Lemola, S., and Grob, A. (2013). Sleep duration, positive attitude toward life, and academic achievement: The role of daytime tiredness, behavioral persistence, and school start times. *Journal of Adolescence, 36*(2), 311–318.

Petrov, M. E., and Lichstein, K. L. (2016). Differences in sleep between Black and White adults: An update and future directions. *Sleep Medicine, 18*, 74–81.

Putnam, F. W. (2003). Ten-year research update review: Child sexual abuse. *Journal of the American Academy of Child & Adolescent Psychiatry, 42*, 269–278.

Rasgon, N. L., and McEwen, B. S. (2016). Insulin resistance—a missing link no more. *Molecular Psychiatry, 21*, 1648–1652.

Roane, B. M., Johnson, L., Edwards, M., Hall, J., Al-Farra, S., and O'Bryant, S. E. (2014). The link between sleep disturbance and depression among Mexican Americans: A Project FRONTIER study. *Journal of Clinical Sleep Medicine, 10*(04), 427–431.

Roberts, R. E., and Duong, H. T. (2014). The prospective association between sleep deprivation and depression among adolescents. *Sleep, 37*(2), 239–244.

Roffwarg, H. P., Muzio, J. N., and Dement, W. C. (1996). Ontogenetic development of the human sleep-dream cycle. *Science, 152*(3722), 604–619.

Romeo, R. D. (2017). The impact of stress on the structure of the adolescent brain: Implications for adolescent mental health. *Brain Research, 1654*, 185–191.

Romeo, R. R., Christodoulou, J. A., Halverson, K. K., Murtagh, J., and Cyr, A. B. (2018). Socioeconomic status and reading disability: Neuroanatomy and plasticity in response to intervention. *Cerebral Cortex, 28*, 2297–2312.

Saper, C. B., Cano, G., and Scammell, T. E. (2005). Homeostatic, circadian, and emotional regulation of sleep. *Journal of Comparative Neurology, 493*(1), 92–98.

Schwarz, E., and Perry, B. D. (1994). The post-traumatic response in children and adolescents. *Psychiatric Clinics of North America, 17*(2), 311–326.

Shanahan, L., Copeland, W. E., Angold, A., Bondy, C. L., and Costello, E. J. (2014). Sleep problems predict and are predicted by generalized anxiety/depression and oppositional defiant disorder. *Journal of the American Academy of Child & Adolescent Psychiatry, 53*(5), 550–558.

Shonkoff, J. P., and Garner, A. S. (2012). The lifelong effect of early childhood adversity and toxic stress. (Technical Report.) *American Academy of Pediatrics.* Available: http://pediatrics.aappublications.org/content/129/1/e232.full.

Shonkoff, J. P., Boyce, W. T., and McEwen, B. S. (2009). Neuroscience, molecular biology, and the childhood roots of health disparities. *JAMA, 301*, 2252–2259.

Short, M. A., Gradisar, M., Lack, L. C., and Wright, H. R. (2013). The impact of sleep on adolescent depressed mood, alertness and academic performance. *Journal of Adolescence, 36*(6), 1025–1033.

Simpson, T. L., and Miller, W. R. (2002). Concomitance between childhood sexual and physical abuse and substance use problems: A review. *Clinical Psychology Review, 22*(1), 27–77.

Slopen, N., Lewis, T. T., and Williams, D. R. (2016). Discrimination and sleep: A systematic review. *Sleep Medicine, 18*, 88–95.

Steinberg, L. (2008). A social neuroscience perspective on adolescent risk-taking. *Developmental Review, 28*(1), 78–106.

Sterling, P., and Eyer, J. (1988). Allostasis: A new paradigm to explain arousal pathology. In S. Fisher and J. Reason (Eds.), *Handbook of Life Stress, Cognition, and Health* (pp. 629–649). Oxford, England: John Wiley & Sons.

Suglia, S. F., Kara, S., and Robinson, W. R. (2014). Sleep duration and obesity among adolescents transitioning to adulthood: Do results differ by sex? *The Journal of Pediatrics, 165*(4), 750–754.

Szyf, M., McGowan, P., and Meaney, M. J. (2008). The social environment and the epigenome. *Environmental and Molecular Mutagenesis, 49*, 46–60.

Tang, Y. Y., Holzel, B. K., and Posner, M. I. (2015). The neuroscience of mindfulness meditation. *Nature Reviews Neuroscience, 16*, 213–225.

Tasali, E., Leproult, R., Ehrmann, D. A., and Van Cauter, E. (2008). Slow-wave sleep and the risk of type 2 diabetes in humans. *Proceedings of the National Academy of Sciences of the United States of America, 105*, 1044–1049.

Teicher, M. H., Samson, J. A., Anderson, C. M., and Ohashi, K. (2016). The effects of childhood maltreatment on brain structure, function and connectivity. *Nature Reviews Neuroscience, 17*, 652–666.

Telzer, E. H., Fuligni, A. J., Lieberman, M. D., and Galván, A. (2013). The effects of poor quality sleep on brain function and risk taking in adolescence. *Neuroimage, 71*, 275–283.

Telzer, E. H., Goldenberg, D., Fuligni, A. J., Lieberman, M. D., and Galván, A. (2015). Sleep variability in adolescence is associated with altered brain development. *Developmental Cognitive Neuroscience, 14*, 16–22.

Trejo, J. L., Carro, E., and Torres-Aleman, I. (2001). Circulating insulin-like growth factor I mediates exercise-induced increases in the number of new neurons in the adult hippocampus. *Journal of Neuroscience, 21*, 1628–1634.

Trickett, P. K., Noll, J. G., and Putnam, F. W. (2011). The impact of sexual abuse on female development: Lessons from a multigenerational, longitudinal research study. *Development and Psychopathology, 23*(2), 453–476.

Tyler, K. A., Schmitz, R. M., and Ray, C. M. (2017). Role of social environmental protective factors on anxiety and depressive symptoms among Midwestern homeless youth. *Journal of Research on Adolescence, 28*(1), 199–210.

Valk, S. L., Bernhardt, B. C., Trautwein, F. M., Bockler, A., and Kanske, P. (2017). Structural plasticity of the social brain: Differential change after socio-affective and cognitive mental training. *Science Advances, 3*, e1700489.

van der Kolk, B. A., Roth, S., Pelcovitz, D., Sunday, S., and Spinazzola, J. (2005). Disorders of extreme stress: The empirical foundation of a complex adaptation to trauma. *Journal of Traumatic Stress, 18*(5), 389–399.

Verstynen, T. D., Weinstein, A. M., Schneider, W. W., Jakicic, J. M., Rofey, D. L., and Erickson, K. I. (2012). Increased body mass index is associated with a global and distributed decrease in white matter microstructural integrity. *Psychosomatic Medicine, 74*, 682–690.

Wang, C., Weng, J., Yao, Y., Dong, S., Liu, Y., and Chen, F. (2017). Effect of abacus training on executive function development and underlying neural correlates in Chinese children. *Human Brain Mapping, 38*, 5234–5249.

Weng, J., Xie, Y., Wang, C., and Chen, F. (2017). The effects of long-term abacus training on topological properties of brain functional networks. *Scientific Reports, 7*, 8862.

Wolfson, A. R., and Carskadon, M. A. (1998). Sleep schedules and daytime functioning in adolescents. *Child Development, 69*(4), 875–887.

Wong, M. M., and Brower, K. J. (2012). The prospective relationship between sleep problems and suicidal behavior in the National Longitudinal Study of Adolescent Health. *Journal of Psychiatric Research, 46*(7), 953–959.

Woods, H. C., and Scott, H. (2016). # Sleepyteens: Social media use in adolescence is associated with poor sleep quality, anxiety, depression and low self-esteem. *Journal of Adolescence, 51,* 41–49.

Yaribeygi, H., Panahi, Y., Sahraei, H., Johnston, T. P., and Sahebkar, A. (2017). The impact of stress on body function: A review. *EXCLI Journal, 16,* 1057–1072.

Yau, P. L., Castro, M. G., Tagani, A., Tsui, W. H., and Convit, A. (2012). Obesity and metabolic syndrome and functional and structural brain impairments in adolescence. *Pediatrics, 130,* e856–e864.

CHAPTER 4

Adams, S. H., Park M. J., Twietmeyer, L., Brindis, C. D., and Irwin, C. E. Jr. (2017). Association between adolescent preventive care and the role of the Affordable Care Act. *JAMA Pediatrics, 21*(6), 1221–1226.

Aizer, A., and Doyle, J. J. (2015). Juvenile incarceration, human capital, and future crime: Evidence from randomly assigned judges. *Quarterly Journal of Economics, 130*(2), 759–804.

Alegría, M., Vallas, M., and Pumariega, A. (2010). Racial and ethnic disparities in pediatric mental health. *Child and Adolescent Psychiatric Clinics of North America, 19*(4), 759–774.

Alegría, M., Carson, N. J., Gonçalves, M., Keefe, K. (2011). Disparities in treatment for substance use disorders and co-occurring disorders for ethnic/racial minority youth. *Journal of the American Academy of Child & Adolescent Psychiatry, 50*(1), 22–31.

Alegría, M., Lin, J. Y., Green, J. G., Sampson, N. A., Gruber, M. J., and Kessler, R. C. (2012). Role of referrals in mental health service disparities for racial and ethnic minority youth. *Journal of the American Academy of Child and Adolescent Psychiatry, 51*(7), 703–711.

Alliance for Racial Equity in Child Welfare. (2011). *Disparities and Disproportionality in Child Welfare: Analysis of the Research.* Center for the Study of Social Policy, The Annie E. Casey Foundation and the Alliance for Racial Equity in Child Welfare. Available: http://www.aecf.org/m/resourcedoc/AECF-DisparitiesAndDisproportionalityInChild Welfare-2011.pdf.

Anda, R. F., Felitti, V. J., Bremner, J. D., Walker, J. D., Whitfield, C., Perry, B. D., Dube, S. R., and Giles, W. H. (2006). The enduring effects of abuse and related adverse experiences in childhood: A convergence of evidence from neurobiology and epidemiology. *European Archives of Psychiatry and Clinical Neuroscience, 256,* 174.

Arneson, R. (2015). Equity of opportunity. In E. N. Zalta (Ed.), *The Stanford Encyclopedia of Philosphy.* Stanford, CA: Metaphysics Research Lab, Stanford University.

Assari, S., Moazen-Zadeh, E., Caldwell, C. H., and Zimmerman, M. A. (2017). Racial discrimination during adolescence predicts mental health deterioration in adulthood: Gender differences among Blacks. *Frontiers in Public Health, 5,* 104.

Barel, E., Van IJzendoorn, M. H., Sagi-Schwartz, A., and Bakermans-Kranenburg, M. J. (2010). Surviving the Holocaust: A meta-analysis of the long-term sequelae of a genocide. *Psychological Bulletin, 136*(5), 677.

Blair, C., and Raver, C. C. (2012). Child development in the context of adversity: Experiential canalization of brain and behavior. *American Psychologist, 67,* 309–318.

_____. (2016). Poverty, stress, and brain development: New directions for prevention and intervention. *Academic Pediatrics, 16*(3), S30–S36.

Boardman, J. D., and Saint Onge, J. M. (2005). Neighborhoods and adolescent development. *Child, Youth, and Environments, 15*(1), 138–164.

Bombay, A., Matheson, K., and Anisman, H. (2011). The impact of stressors on second generation Indian residential school survivors. *Transcultural Psychiatry, 48*(4), 367–391.

Bond, L., Toumbourou, J. W., Thomas, L., Catalano, R. F., and Patton, G. (2005). Individual, family, school, and community risk and protective factors for depressive symptoms in adolescents: A comparison of risk profiles for substance use and depressive symptoms. *Prevention Science, 6*(2), 73–88.

Boonstra, H. D. (2014). What is behind the declines in teen pregnancy rates? *Guttmacher Policy Review, 17*(3).

Boozer, M. A., Krueger, A. B., Wolkon, S. (1992). Race and school quality since *Brown v. Board of Education*. Washington, DC: Brookings Institution. Available: https://www.brookings.edu/wp-content/uploads/1992/01/1992_bpeamicro_boozer.pdf.

Boustan, L. P. (2013). *Racial Residential Segregation in American Cities*. Cambridge, MA: National Bureau of Economic Research.

Brave Heart, M. Y., and DeBruyn, L. M. (1998). The American Indian holocaust: Healing historical unresolved grief. *American Indian and Alaska Native Mental Health Research, 8*(2), 56–78.

Brody, G. H., Chen, Y. F., Kogan, S. M., Yu, T., Molgaard, V. K., DiClemente, R. J., and Wingood, G. M. (2012a). Family-centered program deters substance use, conduct problems, and depressive symptoms in black adolescents. *Pediatrics, 129*(1), 108–115.

Brody, G. H., Gray, J. C., Yu, T., Barton, A. W., Beach, S. R. H., Galván, A., MacKillop, J., Windle, M., Chen, E., Miller, G. E., and Sweet, L. H. (2017). Protective prevention effects on the association of poverty with brain development. *JAMA Pediatrics, 171*(1), 46–52.

Brody, G. H., Kogan, S. M., and Grange, C. M. (2012b). Translating longitudinal, developmental research with rural African American families into prevention programs for rural african american youth. In R. B. King and V. Maholmes (Eds.), *The Oxford Handbook of Poverty and Child Development* (pp. 553–570). New York, NY: Oxford University Press.

Brody, G. H., Lei, M. K., Chen, E., and Miller, G. E. (2014). Neighborhood poverty and allostatic load in African American youth. *Pediatrics, 134*(5), e1362–e1368.

Brody, G. H., Murry, V. M., Gerrard, M., Gibbons, F. X., Molgaard, V., McNair, L., Brown, A. C., Wills, T. A., Spoth, R. L., Luo, Z., Chen, Y. F., and Neubaum-Carlan, E. (2004). The strong African American families program: Translating research into prevention programming. *Child Development, 75*(3), 900–917.

Browman, A. S., Destin, M. P., Carswell, K. L., and Svoboda, R. C. (2017). Perceptions of socioeconomic mobility influence academic persistence among low socioeconomic status students. *Journal of Experimental Social Psychology, 72*, 45–52.

Browman, A. S., Destin, M., Kearney, M. S., and Levine, P. B. (2019). How economic inequality shapes mobility expectations and behavior in disadvantaged youth. *Nature Human Behaviour, 3*, 214–220.

Brunwasser, S. M., Gillham, J. E., and Kim, E. S. (2009). A meta-analytic review of the Penn resiliency program's effect on depressive symptoms. *Journal of Consulting and Clinical Psychology, 77*(6), 1042–1054.

Bureau of Justice Statistics. (2000). *Monitoring the Future: Sourcebook of Criminal Justice Statistics, 2000*. Washington, DC: U.S. Department of Justice, Office of Justice Programs.

Burgess, D. J., Fu, S. S., and van Ryn, M. (2004). Why do providers contribute to disparities and what can be done about it? *Journal of General Internal Medicine, 19*(11), 1154–1159.

Campbell, C. D., and Evans-Campbell, T. (2011). Historical trauma and Native American child development and mental health: An overview. In M. C. Sarche, P. Spicer, P. Farrell, and H. E. Fitzgerald (Eds.), *Child Psychology and Mental Health. American Indian and Alaska Native Children and Mental Health: Development, Context, Prevention, and Treatment* (pp. 1–26). Santa Barbara, CA: Praeger/ABC-CLIO.

Case, A., and Deaton, A. (2015). Rising morbidity and mortality in midlife among white non-Hispanic Americans in the 21st century. *Proceedings of the National Academy of Sciences of the United States of America, 112*(49), 15078–15083.

Case, A., Lubotsky, D., and Paxson, C. (2002). Economic status and health in childhood: The origin of the gradient. *American Economic Review, 92*(5), 1308–1334.

Center for the Study of Social Policy. (2009). *Race Equity Review: Findings from a Qualitative Analysis of Racial Disproportionality and Disparity for African American Children and Families in Michigan's Child Welfare System.* Washington, DC: Center for the Study of Social Policy.

Centers for Disease Control and Prevention. (2016). Sexual identity, sex of sexual contacts, and health-related behaviors among students grades 9–12, United States 2015. *Surveillance Summaries, 65*(9), 1–202. Available: https://www.cdc.gov/mmwr/volumes/65/ss/ss6509a1.htm.

———. (2017). Quickstats: Suicide rates for teens aged 15–19 years, by sex—United States, 1975-2015. *Morbidity and Mortality Weekly Report, 66*(30), 816.

Chaffin, M., and Bard, D. (2006). Impact of intervention surveillance bias on analyses of child welfare report outcomes. *Child Maltreatment, 11*(4), 301–312.

Charles, K. K., and Hurst, E. (2003). The correlation of wealth across generations. *Journal of Political Economy, 111*(6), 1155–1182.

Chen, W. Y., Corvo, K., Lee, Y., and Hahm, H. C. (2017). Longitudinal trajectory of adolescent exposure to community violence and depressive symptoms among adolescents and young adults: understanding the effect of mental health service usage. *Community Mental Health Journal, 53*(1), 39–52.

Chetty, R., Hendren, N., and Katz, L. F. (2016). The effects of exposure to better neighborhoods on children: New evidence from the Moving to Opportunity Project. *American Economic Review, 106*(4).

Chetty, R., Friedman, N., Hendren, N., Jones, M. R., and Porter, S. P. (2018). *The Opportunity Atlas: Mapping the Childhood Roots of Social Mobility.* Working Paper No. 25147. Cambridge, MA.: National Bureau of Economic Research. Available: https://www.nber.org/papers/w25147.

Chiang, J. J., Bower, J. E., Almeida, D. M., Irwin, M. R., Seeman, T. E., and Fuligni, A. J. (2015). Socioeconomic status, daily affective and social experiences, and inflammation during adolescence. *Psychosomatic Medicine, 77*(3), 256–266.

Child Trends. (2018). *Key Facts about Juvenile Incarceration.* Available: https://www.childtrends.org/indicators/juvenile-detention.

Child Trends Databank. (2018). *High School Dropout Rates.* Available: https://www.childtrends.org/?indicators=high-school-dropout-rates.

Children's Bureau. (2016). *Racial Disproportionality and Disparity in Child Welfare.* Washington, DC: U.S. Department of Health and Human Services, Administration for Children and Families.

Chithambo, T. P., Huey, S. J., Jr., and Cespedes-Knadle, Y. (2014). Perceived discrimination and Latino youth adjustment: Examining the role of relinquished control and sociocultural influences. *Journal of Latina/o Psychology, 2*(1), 54–66.

Coley, R. L., Leventhal, T., Lynch, A. D., and Kull, M. (2013). *Poor Quality Housing Is Tied to Children's Emotional and Behavioral Problems.* Chicago, IL: MacArthur Foundation.

Conger, R. D., Conger, K. J., and Martin, M. J. (2010). Socioeconomic status, family processes, and individual development. *Journal of Marriage and Family, 72*(3), 685–704.

Corcoran, M., and Matsudaira, J. (2009). Is stable employment becoming more elusive for young men? In I. Schoon and R. K. Silberseisen (Eds.), *Transitions from School to Work: Globalization, Individualization, and Patterns of Diversity* (pp. 45–66). The Jacobs Foundation Series on Adolescence. Cambridge, England: Cambridge University Press.

Costello, E. J., Compton, S. N., Keeler, G., and Angold, A. (2003). Relationships between poverty and psychopathology: A natural experiment. *Journal of the American Medical Association, 290*(15), 2023–2029.

Culhane, D. P., Byrne, T., Metraux, S., Moreno, M., Torow, H., and Stevens, M. (2011). *Young Adult Outcomes of Youth Exiting Dependent or Delinquent Care in Los Angeles County.* Supported by the Conrad N. Hilton Foundation. Available: https://www.socalgrantmakers. org/sites/default/files/resources/Foster%20Youth_LA_County_Report.pdf.

Cummings, J. L., and DiPasquale, D. (1999). The low-income housing tax credit: An analysis of the first ten years. *Housing Policy Debate, 10*(2), 251–307.

Cunha, F., and Heckman, J. (2007). The technology of skill formation. *American Economic Review, 97*(2), 31–47.

Cunningham, R. M., Walton, M. A., and Carter, P. M. (2018). The major causes of death in children and adolescents in the United States. *New England Journal of Medicine, 379*(25), 2468–2475.

Currie, J., and Schwandt, H. (2016). Mortality inequality: The good news from a county-level approach. *Journal of Economic Perspectives, 30*(2), 29–52.

Dai, H. (2017). Tobacco product use among lesbian, gay, and bisexual adolescents. *Pediatrics, 139*(4), 1–8.

Dang, M. T., Conger, K. J., Breslau, J., and Miller, E. (2014). Exploring protective factors among homeless youth: The role of natural mentors. *Journal of Health Care for the Poor and Underserved, 25*(3), 1121–1138.

Danziger, S., and Ratner, D. (2010). Labour market outcomes and the transition to adulthood. *Future of Children, 20*(1), 133–158.

Davis, A. N., Carlo, G., Schwartz, S. J., Unger, J. B., Zamboanga, B. L., Lorenzo-Blanco, E. I., Cano, M. A., Baezconde-Garbanati, L., Oshri, A., Streit, C., Martinez, M. M., Pina-Watson, B., Lizzi, K., and Soto, D. (2016). The longitudinal associations between discrimination, depressive symptoms, and prosocial behaviors in U.S. Latino/a recent immigrant adolescents. *Journal of Youth Adolescence, 45*(3), 457–470.

DeCelles, K. A., and Norton, M. I. (2016). Physical and situational inequality on airplanes predicts air rage. *Proceedings of the National Academy of Sciences of the United States of America, 113*(20), 5588–5591.

DeLone, M. A., and DeLone, G. J. (2017). Racial disparities in juvenile justice processing. In C. J. Schreck (Ed.), *The Encyclopedia of Juvenile Delinquency and Justice.* Hoboken, NJ: Wiley & Sons, Inc.

Denham, A. R. (2008). Rethinking historical trauma: Narratives of resilience. *Transcultural Psychiatry, 45*(3), 391–414.

Dettlaff, A. J., Rivaux, S. L., Baumann, D. J., Fluke, J. D., Rycraft, J. R., and James, J. (2011). Disentangling substantiation: The influence of race, income, and risk on the substantiation decision in child welfare. *Children and Youth Services Review, 33*(9), 1630–1637.

Doyle, J. J. Jr. (2007). Child protection and child outcomes: Measuring the effects of foster care. *American Economic Review, 97*(5), 1583–1610.

Dray, J., Bowman, J., Campbell, E., Freund, M., Wolfenden, L., Hodder, R. K., McElwaine, K., Tremain, D., Bartlem, K., Bailey, J., Small, T., Palazzi, K., Oldmeadow, C., and Wiggers, J. (2017). Systematic review of universal resilience-focused interventions targeting child and adolescent mental health in the school setting. *Journal of the American Academy of Child and Adolescent Psychiatry, 56*(10), 813–824.

Dubé, C., Gagné, M.-H., Clément, M.-È., and Chamberland, C. (2018). Community violence and associated psychological problems among adolescents in the general population. *Journal of Child & Adolescent Trauma, 11*(4), 411–420.

Duran, E., Duran, B., Brave Heart, M. Y. H., and Yellow Horse-Davis, S. (1998). Healing the American Indian soul wound. In Y. Danieli (Ed.), *The Plenum Series on Stress and Coping. International Handbook of Multigenerational Legacies of Trauma* (pp. 341–354). New York, NY: Plenum Press.

Edwards, K. M., Probst, D. R., Rodenhizer-Stämpfli, K. A., Gidycz, C. A., and Tansill, E. C. (2014). Multiplicity of child maltreatment and biopsychosocial outcomes in young adulthood: The moderating role of resiliency characteristics among female survivors. *Child Maltreatment, 19*, 188–198.

Elgar, F. J. (2010). Income inequality, trust, and population health in 33 countries. *American Journal of Public Health, 100*(11), 2311–2315.

Eskin, M., Kaynak-Demir, H., and Demir, S. (2005). Same-sex sexual orientation, childhood sexual abuse, and suicidal behavior in university students in Turkey. *Archives of Sexual Behavior, 34*(2), 185–195.

Evans-Campbell, T. (2008). Historical trauma in American Indian/Native Alaska communities: A multilevel framework for exploring impacts on individuals, families, and communities. *Journal of Interpersonal Violence, 23*(3), 316–338.

Fader, J., Kurlychek, M. C., and Morgan, K. A. (2014). The color of juvenile justice: Racial disparities in dispositional decisions. *Social Science Research, 44*, 126–140.

Fast, E., and Collin-Vézina, D. (2010). Historical trauma, race-based trauma and resilience of indigenous peoples: A literature review. *First Peoples Child & Family Review, 5*(1).

Feldman, R. (2015). The adaptive human parental brain: Implications for children's social development. *Trends in Neurosciences, 38*(6), 387–399.

Fergusson, D. M., Horwood, L. J., Ridder, E. M., and Beautrais, A. L. (2005). Sexual orientation and mental health in a birth cohort of young adults. *Psychological Medicine, 35*(7), 971–981.

Fish, J. N., and Baams, L. (2018). Trends in alcohol-related disparities between heterosexual and sexual minority youth from 2007 to 2015: Findings from the youth risk behavior survey. *LGBT Health, 5*(6), 359–367.

Fish, J. N., and Pasley, K. (2015). Sexual (minority) trajectories, mental health, and alcohol use: A longitudinal study of youth as they transition to adulthood. *Journal of Youth and Adolescence, 44*(8), 1508–1527.

Fish, J. N., Pollitt, A. M., Schulenberg, J. E., and Russell, S. T. (2017). Alcohol use from adolescence through early adulthood: An assessment of measurement invariance by age and gender. *Addiction, 112*(8), 1495–1507.

Fish, J. N., Baams, L., Wojciak, A. S., and Russell, S. T. (2019). Are sexual minority youth overrepresented in foster care, child welfare, and out-of-home placement? Findings from nationally representative data. *Child Abuse & Neglect, 89*, 203–211.

Fleming, T. M., Merry, S. N., Robinson, E. M., Denny, S. J., and Watson, P. D. (2007). Self-reported suicide attempts and associated risk and protective factors among secondary school students in new zealand. *The Australian and New Zealand Journal of Psychiatry, 41*(3), 213–221.

Fluke, J., Harden, B. J., Jenkins, M., and Ruehrdanz, A. (2011). *Research Synthesis on Child Welfare: Disproportionality and Disparities*. Washington, DC: Center for the Study of Social Policy.

Font, S. A., Berger, L. M., and Slack, K. S. (2012). Examining racial disproportionality in child protective services case decisions. *Children and Youth Services Review, 34*(11), 2188–2200.

Fontenot, K., Semega, J., and Kollar, M. (2018). *Income and Poverty in the United States: 2017*. Washington, DC: U.S. Census Bureau.

Ford, J. D., and Blaustein, M. E. (2013). Systemic self-regulation: A framework for trauma-informed services in residential juvenile justice programs. *Journal of Family Violence, 28*, 665–677.

Fowler, P. J., Tompsett, C. J., Braciszewski, J. M., Jacques-Tiura, A. J., and Baltes, B. B. (2009). Community violence: A meta-analysis on the effect of exposure and mental health outcomes of children and adolescents. *Development and Psychopathology, 21*(1), 227–259.

Frey, W. (2010). *Census Data: Blacks and Hispanics Take Different Segregation Paths*. Op-Ed. Brookings Institution. Available: https://www.brookings.edu/opinions/census-data-blacks-and-hispanics-take-different-segregation-paths/.

Friedson, M., and Sharkey, P. (2015). Violence and neighborhood disadvantage after the crime decline. *Annals of the American Academy of Political and Social Science, 660*(1), 341–358.

Gershenson, S., Holt, S. B., and Papageorge, N. (2016). Who believes in me? The effect of student-teacher demographic match on teach expectations. *Economics of Education Review, 52*, 209–224.

Gershenson, S., Hart, C. M. D., Lindsay, C. A., and Papageorge, N. W. (2017). *The Long-Run Impacts of Same-Race Teachers*. IZA Institute of Labor Economics. Available: http://ftp.iza.org/dp10630.pdf.

Gay, Lesbian, and Straight Education Network. (2017). *National School Climate Survey*. Available: https://www.glsen.org/article/2017-national-school-climate-survey.

Goldin, C., and Katz, L. F. (2008). *The Race Between Education and Technology*. Cambridge, MA: Belknap Press of Harvard University Press.

Gordon, N. (2018). *Disproportionality in Student Discipline: Connecting Policy to Research*. Brookings Institution. Available: https://www.brookings.edu/research/disproportionality-in-student-discipline-connecting-policy-to-research/.

Gunnar, M., and Quevedo, K. (2007). The neurobiology of stress and development. *Annual Review of Psychology, 58*, 145–173.

Guryan, J., Hurst, E., and Kearney, M. (2008). Parental education and parental time with children. *Journal of Economic Perspectives, 22*(3), 23–46.

Hackman, D. A., Farah, M. J., and Meaney, M. J. (2010). Socioeconomic status and the brain: Mechanistic insights from human and animal research. *Nature Reviews, 11*, 651–659.

Harris, M., and Fallot, R. D. (2001). Envisioning a trauma-informed service system. *New Directions for Mental Health Services, 2001*(89), 3–23.

Heinze, J. E., Cook, S. H., Wood, E. P., Dumadag, A. C., and Zimmerman, M. A. (2018). Friendship attachment style moderates the effect of adolescent exposure to violence on emerging adult depression and anxiety trajectories. *Journal of Youth and Adolescence, 47*(1), 177–193.

Heissel, J. A., Sharkey, P. T., Torrats-Espinosa, G., Grant, K., and Adam, E. K. (2018). Violence and vigilance: The acute effects of community violent crime on sleep and cortisol. *Child Development, 89*(4), e323–e331.

Herringa, R. J. (2017). Trauma, PTSD, and the developing brain. *Current Psychiatry Reports, 19*(10), 69.

Herz, D. C., and Ryan, J. P. (2008a). *Bridging Two Systems: Youth Involved in the Child Welfare and Juvenile Justice Systems*. Washington, DC: Georgetown University, Center for Juvenile Justice Reform.

Herz, D. C. and Ryan, J. P. (2008b). *Exploring the Characteristics and Outcomes of 241.1 Youths in Los Angeles County*. San Francisco, CA: California Courts, The Administrative Office of the Courts.

Hjemdal, O., Aune, T., Reinfjell, T., Stiles, T. C., and Friborg, O. (2007). Resilience as a predictor of depressive symptoms: A correlational study with young adolescents. *Clinical Child Psychology and Psychiatry, 12*(1), 91–104.

Hjemdal, O., Vogel, P. A., Solem, S., Hagen, K., and Stiles, T. C. (2011). The relationship between resilience and levels of anxiety, depression, and obsessive-compulsive symptoms in adolescents. *Clinical Psychology and Psychotherapy, 18*(4), 314–321.

Hodgdon, H. B., Kinniburgh, K., Gabowitz, D., Blaustein, M. E., and Spinazzola, J. (2013). Development and implementation of trauma-informed programming in youth residential treatment centers using the ARC Framework. *Journal of Family Violence, 28*, 679–692.

Hoxby, C. M., and Avery, C. (2012). *The Missing "One-Offs": The Hidden Supply of High-Achieving, Low-Income Students.* Working Paper. Cambridge, MA: National Bureau of Economic Research. Available: https://www.nber.org/papers/w18586.

Hoynes, H., Schanzenbach, D. W., and Almond, D. (2016). Long-run impacts of childhood access to the safety net. *American Economic Review, 106*(4), 903–934.

Hunt, J., and Moodie-Mills, A. (2012). *The Unfair Criminalization of Gay and Transgender Youth: An Overview of the Experiences of LGBT Youth in the Juvenile Justice System.* Washington, DC: Center for American Progress. Available: https://cdn.americanprogress.org/wp-content/uploads/issues/2012/06/pdf/juvenile_justice.pdf.

Irvine, A. (2010). 'We've had three of them': Addressing the invisibility of lesbian, gay, bisexual, and gender-nonconforming youths in the juvenile justice system. *Columbia Journal of Gender and Law, 19*(3), 675–701.

Jussim, L., and Harber, K. (2005). Teacher expectations and self-fulfilling prophecies: Knowns and unknowns, resolved and unresolved controversies. *Personality and Social Psychology Review, 9*(2), 131–155.

Karenian, H., Livaditis, M., Karenian, S., Zafiriadis, K., Bochtsou, V., and Xenitidis, K. (2011). Collective trauma transmission and traumatic reactions among descendants of Armenian refugees. *International Journal of Social Psychiatry, 57*(4), 327–337.

Katz, L. F., Kling, J. R., and Liebman, J. B. (2001). Moving to opportunity in Boston: Early results of a randomized mobility experiment. *Quarterly Journal of Economics, 116*(2), 607–654.

Katz-Wise, S. L., Rosario, M., and Tsappis, M. (2016). Lesbian, gay, bisexual, and transgender youth and family acceptance. *Pediatric Clinics of North America, 63*(6), 1011–1025.

Kearney, M. S., and Levine, P. B. (2016). *Income Inequality, Social Mobility, and the Decision to Drop Out of High School.* Working Paper. Cambridge, MA: National Bureau of Economic Research. Available: https://www.nber.org/papers/w20195.

Kellermann, N. P. (2001). Psychopathology in children of Holocaust survivors: A review of the research literature. *Israeli Journal of Psychiatry Related Science, 38*(1), 36–46.

Kerwin, K., and Hurst, E. (2003). The correlation of wealth across generations. *Journal of Political Economy, 111*(6), 155–182.

Klebanov, K., Brooks-Gunn, J., and Duncan, G. (1994). Does neighborhood and family poverty affect mothers' parenting, mental health, and social support? *Journal of Marriage and Family, 56*(2), 441–455.

Kleinberg, J., Lakkaraju, H., Leskovec, J., Ludwig, J., and Mullainathan, S. (2018a). Human decisions and machine predictions. *Quarterly Journal of Economics, 133*(1), 237–293.

Kleinberg, J., Ludwig, J., Mullainathan, S., and Rambachan, A. (2018b). Algorithmic fairness. *American Economic Association, Papers & Proceedings, 108*, 22–27.

Kleinberg, J., Ludwig, J., Mullainathan, S., and Sunstein, C.R. (forthcoming). Discrimination in the age of algorithms.

Kopel, L. S., Phipatanakul, W., and Gaffin, J. M. (2014). Social disadvantage and asthma control in children. *Paediatric Respiratory Reviews, 15*(3), 256–263.

Kreger, M., Brindis, C., Arons, A., Standish, M., and Guide, R. (2010). *Burden of Asthma on California Schools: Losses in Student Attendance, Achievement, and Revenue.* Paper presented at the 138th APHA Annual Meeting and Exposition, Denver, CO.

Kreger, M., Sargent, K., Arons, A., Standish, M., and Brindis, C. (2011). Creating an environmental justice framework for policy change in childhood asthma: A grassroots to treetops approach. *American Journal of Public Health, 101*(Suppl. 1), S208–S216.

Lafortune, J., Rothstein, J., and Schanzenbach, D.W. (2017). *School Finance Reform and the Distribution of Student Achievement.* Available: https://eml.berkeley.edu/~jrothst/publications/LRS_20170213-complete.pdf.

Lee, E., Larkin, H., and Esaki, N. (2018). Exposure to community violence as a new adverse childhood experience category: Promising results and future considerations. *Families in Society, 98*(1), 69–78.

Lemstra, M., Rogers, M., Thompson, A., Moraros, J., and Buckingham, R. (2012). Risk indicators associated with injection drug use in the Aboriginal population. *AIDS Care: Psychological and Socio-medical Aspects of HIV/AIDS, 24*(11), 1416–1424.

Lochner, L., and Moretti, E. (2004). The effect of education on crime: Evidence from prison inmates, arrests, and self-reports. *American Economic Review, 94*(1), 155–189.

Logan, J. R. (2011). *Separate and Unequal: The Neighborhood Gap for Blacks, Hispanics, and Asians in Metropolitan America.* Providence, RI: Russell Sage Foundation and the American Communities Project of Brown University.

Luthar, S. S., Cicchetti, D., and Becker, B. (2000). The construct of resilience: A critical evaluation and guidelines for future work. *Child Development, 71*(3), 543–562.

Madkins, T. C. (2011). The Black teacher shortage: A literature review of historical and contemporary trends. *Journal of Negro Education, 80*(3), 417–427.

Magnuson, K. A., and Waldfogel, J. (2005). Early childhood care and education: Effects on ethnic and racial gaps in school readiness. *The Future of Children, 15*(1), 169–196.

Magnuson, K. A., Meyers, M. K., Ruhm, C. J., and Waldfogel, J. (2004). Inequality in preschool education and school readiness. *American Education Research Journal, 41*(1), 115–157.

Majd, K., Marksamer, J., and Reyes, C. (2009). *Hidden Injustice: Lesbian, Gay, Bisexual, and Transgender Youth in Juvenile Courts.* San Francisco, CA, and Washington, DC: Legal Services for Children, National Juvenile Defender Center, and National Center for Lesbian Rights. Available: https://www.ncjrs.gov/App/Publications/abstract.aspx?ID=257742.

Manoli, D., and Turner, N. (2014). *Cash-on-Hand & College Enrollment: Evidence from Population Tax Data and Policy Nonlinearities.* Cambridge, MA: National Bureau of Economic Research.

Marshal, M. P., Friedman, M. S., Stall, R., King, K. M., Miles, J., Gold, M. A., Bukstein, O. G., and Morse, J. Q. (2008). Sexual orientation and adolescent substance use: A meta-analysis and methodological review. *Addiction, 103*(4), 546–556.

Marshal, M. P., Dietz, L. J., Friedman, M. S., Stall, R., Smith, H. A., McGinley, J., Thoma, B. C., Murray, P. J., D'Augelli, A. R., and Brent, D. A. (2011). Suicidality and depression disparities between sexual minority and heterosexual youth: A meta-analytic review. *Journal of Adolescent Health, 49*(2), 115–123.

Martin, J. A., Hamilton, B. E., Osterman, M. J., Driscoll, A. K., and Drake, P. (2018). *Births: Final Data for 2016.* Hyattsville, MD: National Center for Health Statistics.

Masten, A. S. (2011). Resilience in children threatened by extreme adversity: Frameworks for research, practice, and translational synergy. *Development and Psychopathology, 23*(2), 493–506.

Maxfield, M. (2013). *The Effects of the Earned Income Tax Credit on Child Achievement and Long-Term Educational Attainment.* East Lansing: Michigan State University.

McInerney, M., and McKlindon, A. (2014). *Unlocking the Door to Learning: Trauma-Informed Classrooms & Transformational Schools Maura.* Available: http://www.vtnea.org/uploads/files/Trauma-Informed-in-Schools-Classrooms-FINAL-December2014-2.pdf.

McKernan, S.-M., Ratcliffe, C., Steuerele, E., and Zhang, S. (2013). *Less than Equal: Racial Disparities in Wealth Accumulation.* Washington, DC: Urban Institute.

McLoyd, V. C. (1998). Socioeconomic disadvantage and child development. *American Psychologist, 53*(2), 185–204.

Mendez, L. M. (2003). Predictors of suspension and negative school outcomes: A longitudinal investigation. *New Directions for Youth Development, 99,* 17–33.

Meredith, L. S., Shadel, W. G., Holliday, S. B., Parast, L., and D'Amico, E. J. (2018). *Influence of Mental Health and Alcohol or Other Drug Use Risk on Adolescent Reported Care Received in Primary Care Settings.* RAND Corporation. Available: https://www.rand.org/pubs/external_publications/EP67497.html.

Meyer, I. H. (1995). Minority stress and mental health in gay men. *Journal of Health Social Behavior, 36*(1), 38–56.

Meyer, I. H. (2003). Prejudice, social stress, and mental health in lesbian, gay, and bisexual populations: Conceptual issues and research evidence. *Psychological Bulletin, 129*(5), 674–697.

Miller, G. E., Chen, E., Armstrong, C. C., Carroll, A. L., Ozturk, S., Rydland, K. J., Brody, G. H., Parrish, T. B., and Nusslock, R. (2018). Functional connectivity in central executive network protects youth against cardiometabolic risks linked with neighborhood violence. *Proceedings of the National Academy of Sciences of the United States of America, 115*(47), 12063–12068.

Mohatt, N. V., Thompson, A. B., Thai, N. D., and Tebes, J. K. (2014). Historical trauma as public narrative: A conceptual review of how history impacts present-day health. *Social Science & Medicine, 106,* 128–136.

Morris, M., and Western, B. (1999). Inequality in earnings at the close of the twentieth century. *American Review of Sociology, 25,* 623–657.

Mowen, T., and Brent, J. (2016). School discipline as a turning point: The cumulative effect of suspension on arrest. *Journal of Research in Crime and Delinquency, 53*(5), 628–653.

Mulvey, K. L., and Killen, M. (2015). Challenging gender stereotypes: Resistance and exclusion. *Child Development, 86*(3), 681–694.

Mulye, T. P., Park, M. J., Nelson, C. D., Adams, S. H., Irwin, C. E., Jr., and Brindis, C. D. (2009). Trends in adolescent and young adult health in the United States. *Journal of Adolescent Health, 45*(1), 8–24.

Musu-Gillette, L., de Brey, C., McFarland, J., Hussar, W., Sonnenberg, W., and Wilkinson-Flicker, S. (2017). *Status and Trends in the Education of Racial and Ethnic Groups, 2017.* Washington, DC: U.S. Department of Education, National Center for Education Statistics. Available: https://nces.ed.gov/pubs2017/2017051.pdf.

National Academies of Sciences, Engineering, and Medicine. (2017). *Communities in Action: Pathways to Health Equity.* Washington, DC: The National Academies Press.

_____. (2019). *A Roadmap to Reducing Child Poverty.* Washington, DC: The National Academies Press.

National Adolescent and Young Health Information Center. (2016). *National Survey of Children's Health* [private data run] (2016). The Child & Adolescent Health Measurement Initiative, University of San Francisco. Available: http://childhealthdata.org/browse/survey/results?q=4556&r=1&g=638.

National Center for Education Statistics. (2017). *Public High School Graduation Rates.* Available: https://nces.ed.gov/programs/coe/indicator_coi.asp.

_____. (2018). *The Nation's Report Card.* Available: https://www.nationsreportcard.gov/.

Needham, B. L. (2012). Sexual attraction and trajectories of mental health and substance use during the transition from adolescence to adulthood. *Journal of Youth and Adolescence, 41*(2), 179–190.

Nord, M. (2009). *Food Insecurity in Households with Children: Prevalence, Severity, and Household Characteristics.* Washington, DC: U.S. Department of Agriculture.

Odgers, C. L. (2015). Income inequality and the developing child: Is it all relative? *American Psychologist, 70*(8), 722–731.

Office of Juvenile Justice and Delinquency Prevention. (2018). *OJJDP Statistical Briefing Book.* Available: http://www.ojjdp.gov/ojstatbb/crime/JAR_Display.asp?ID=qa05260.

Oishi, S., and Kesebir, S. (2015). Income inequality explains why economic growth does not always translate to an increase in happiness. *Psychological Science, 26*(10), 1630–1638.

Oishi, S., Kesebir, S., and Diener, E. (2011). Income inequality and happiness. *Psychological Science, 22*(9), 1095–1100.

Okonofua, J. A., and Eberhardt, J. L. (2015). Two strikes: Race and disciplining of young students. *Psychological Science, 26*(5), 617–624.

Owens, A., Reardon, S. F., and Jencks, C. (2016). Income segregation between schools and school districts. *American Educational Research Journal, 53*(4), 1159–1197.

Owens, E. G. (2017). Testing the school-to-prison pipeline. *Journal of Policy Analysis and Management, 36*(1), 11–37.

Park, I. J., Wang, L., Williams, D. R., and Alegría, M. (2017). Does anger regulation mediate the discrimination-mental health link among Mexican-origin adolescents? A longitudinal mediation analysis using multilevel modeling. *Developmental Psychology, 53*(2), 340–352.

Pascoe, C. J. (2011). *Dude, You're a Fag: Masculinity and Sexuality in High School.* (Second ed.) Oakland, CA: University of California Press.

Perry B. D. 2006. Applying principles of neurodevelopment to clinical work with maltreated and traumatized children: The neurosequential model of therapeutics. In N. B. Webb (Ed.), *Working with Traumatized Youth in Child Welfare* (pp. 27–52). New York, NY: Guilford Press.

Peterson, R., and Krivo, L. J. (2010). *Divergent Social Worlds: Neighborhood Crime and the Racial-Spatial Divide.* New York, NY: Russell Sage Foundation.

Piff, P. K., and Robinson, A. R. (2017). Social class and prosocial behavior: Current evidence, caveats, and questions. *Current Opinion in Psychology, 18*, 6–10.

Pinker, S. (2018). Resilient teens in a dangerous world. *The Wall Street Journal.* Available: https://www.wsj.com/articles/resilient-teens-in-a-dangerous-world-11544628845.

Pokhrel, P., and Herzog, T. A. (2014). Historical trauma and substance use among Native Hawaiian college students. *American Journal of Health Behavior, 38*(3), 420–429.

Poteat, V. P., Scheer, J. R., and Chong, E. S. K. (2016). Sexual orientation-based disparities in school and juvenile justice discipline: A multiple group comparison of contributing factors. *Journal of Educational Psychology, 108*(2), 229–241.

Pumariega, A. J., Atkins, D. L., Rogers, K., Montgomery, L., Nybro, C., Caesar, R., and Millus, D. (1999). Mental health and incarcerated youth: Service utilization in incarcerated youth. *Journal of Child and Family Studies, 8*, 205.

Reardon, S. F. (2011). The widening academic achievement gap between the rich and the poor: New evidence and possible explanations. In G. Duncan and R. J. Murnane (Eds.), *Whither Opportunity? Rising Inequality, Schools, and Children's Life Chances.* New York, NY: Russell Sage Foundation.

Reardon, S. F. (2015). School segregation and racial academic achievement gaps. CEPA Working Paper No. 15-12. CEPA, Stanford University. Available: https://cepa.stanford.edu/sites/default/files/wp15-12v201510.pdf.

Repetti, R. L., Taylor, S. E., and Seeman, T. E. (2002). Risky families: Family social environments and the mental and physical health of offspring. *Psychological Bulletin, 128*(2), 330–366.

Richman, L. S., and Jonassaint, C. (2008). The effects of race-related stress on cortisol reactivity in the laboratory: Implications of the Duke lacrosse scandal. *Annals of Behavioral Medicine: A Publication of the Society of Behavioral Medicine, 35*(1), 105–110.

Riebschleger, J., Day, A., and Damashek, A. (2015). Foster care youth share stories of trauma before, during, and after placement: Youth voices for building trauma-informed systems of care. *Journal of Aggression, Maltreatment & Trauma, 24*(4), 339–360.

Rivaux, S. L., James, J., Wittenstrom, K., Baumann, D., Sheets, J., Henry, J., and Jeffries, V. (2008). The intersection of race, poverty, and risk: Understanding the decision to provide services to clients and to remove children. *Child Welfare, 87*(2), 151–168.

Rovner, J. (2016). *Racial Disparities in Youth Commitments and Arrests*. Washington, DC: The Sentencing Project.

Russell, S. T., and Fish, J. N. (2016). Mental health in lesbian, gay, bisexual, and transgender (LGBT) youth. *Annual Review of Clinical Psychology, 12*, 465–487.

Russell, S. T., Sinclair, K. O., Poteat, V. P., and Koenig, B. W. (2012). Adolescent health and harassment based on discriminatory bias. *American Journal of Public Health, 102*(3), 493–495.

Rutter, M. (2005). Environmentally mediated risks for psychopathology: Research strategies and findings. *Journal of the American Academy of Child and Adolescent Psychiatry, 44*(1), 3–18.

Ryan, C., Russell, S. T., Huebner, D., Dias, R., and Sanchez, J. (2010). Family acceptance in adolescence and the health of LGBT young adults. *Journal of Child and Adolescent Psychiatric Nursing, 23*(4), 205–213.

Ryan, P., Herz, D., Hernandez, P., and Marshall, J. (2007). Maltreatment and delinquency: Investigating child welfare bias in juvenile justice processing. *Children and Youth Services Review, 29*, 1035–1050.

Saewyc, E. M. (2011). Research on adolescent sexual orientation: Development, health disparities, stigma and resilience. *Journal of Research on Adolescence, 21*(1), 256–272.

Saez, E., and Zucman, G. (2014). *Wealth Inequality in the United States since 1913: Evidence from Capitalized Income Tax Data*. Working Paper No. 20625. Cambridge, MA: National Bureau of Economic Research. Available: http://gabriel-zucman.eu/files/Saez-Zucman2014.pdf.

Sampson, R. J. (2012). *Great American City: Chicago and the Enduring Neighborhood Effect*. Chicago: University of Chicago Press.

Sanders, B., Allen, Z., and Maurer, G. (2017). *2017 Telehealth Policy for the National Rural Health Association*. Washington, DC: National Rural Health Association.

Saxbe, D., Lyden, H., Gimbel, S. I., Sachs, M., Del Piero, L. B., Margolin, G., and Kaplan, J. T. (2018). Longitudinal associations between family aggression, externalizing behavior, and the structure and function of the amygdala. *Journal of Research on Adolescence, 28*(1), 134–149.

Seligman, M. E. P., Ernst, R. M., Gillham, J., Reivich, K., and Linkins, M. (2009). Positive education: Positive psychology and classroom interventions. *Oxford Review of Education, 35*(3), 293–311.

Sickmund, M., Sladky, A., and Kang, W. (2014). *Easy Access to Juvenile Court Statistics: 1985–2011*. Washington, DC: U.S. Department of Justice, Office of Juvenile Justice and Delinquency Prevention.

Skiba, R. J., Michael, R. S., Nardo, A. C., and Peterson, R. L. (2002). The color of discipline: Sources of racial and gender disproportionality in school punishment. *The Urban Review, 34*, 317–342.

Skiba, R. J., Mediratta, K., and Rausch, M. K. (Eds.). (2016). *Inequality in School Discipline: Research and Practice to Reduce Disparities*. (Second ed.). New York, NY: Palgrave Macmillan.

Smith, C. A., Ireland, T. O., and Thornberry, T. P. (2005). Adolescent maltreatment and its impact on young adult antisocial behavior. *Child Abuse and Neglect, 29*(10), 1099–1119.

Snyder, T., and Musu-Gillette, L. (2015). *Free or Reduced Price Lunch: A Proxy for Poverty?* Available: https://nces.ed.gov/blogs/nces/post/free-or-reduced-price-lunch-a-proxy-for-poverty.

Southwick, S. M., Bonanno, G. A., Masten, A. S., Panter-Brick, C., and Yehuda, R. (2014). Resilience definitions, theory, and challenges: Interdisciplinary perspectives. *European Journal of Psychotraumatology, 5.*

Steinberg, L. (2014). *Age of Opportunity: Lessons from the New Science of Adolescence*. Boston, MA: Houghton Mifflin Harcourt.

Sue, D. W., Capodilup, C. M., Torino, G. C., Bucceri, J. M., Holder, A. M., Nadal, K. L., and Esquilin, M. (2007). Racial microaggressions in everyday life. *American Psychologist, 62*(4), 271–286.

Task Force Report on Resilience and Strength in African-American Children and Adolescents. (n.d.). *Executive Summary*. Available: https://www.apa.org/pi/families/resources/resilience-rpt-summary.pdf.

Thompson, S. J., Ryan, T. N., Montgomery, K. L., Lippman, A. D. P., Bender, K., and Ferguson, K. (2016). Perceptions of resiliency and coping: Homeless young adults speak out. *Youth and Society, 48*(1), 58–76.

Tlapek, S. M., Auslander, W., Edmond, T., Gerke, D., Schrag, R. V., and Threlfall, J. (2017). The moderating role of resiliency on the negative effects of childhood abuse for adolescent girls involved in child welfare. *Children and Youth Services Review, 73*, 437–444.

Toomey, R. B., and Russell, S. T. (2016). The role of sexual orientation in school-based victimization: A meta-analysis. *Youth and Society, 48*(2), 176–201.

U.S. Department of Education, Office for Civil Rights. (2015). *Protecting Civil Rights, Advancing Equity: Report to the President and Secretary of Education, Under Section 203(b)(1) of the Department of Education Organization Act, FY 13–14*. Available: https://www2.ed.gov/about/reports/annual/ocr/report-to-president-and-secretary-of-education-2013-14.pdf.

U.S. Department of Housing and Urban Development. (2016). *Evidence Matters: Neighborhoods and Violent Crime*. Available: https://www.huduser.gov/portal/periodicals/em/summer16/highlight2.html.

U.S. Government Accountability Office. (2016). *K–12 Education: Better Use of Information Could Help Agencies Identify Disparities and Address Racial Discrimination*. Available: https://www.gao.gov/assets/680/676745.pdf.

Ueno, K. (2010). Mental health differences between young adults with and without same-sex contact: A simultaneous examination of underlying mechanisms. *Journal of Health and Social Behavior, 51*(4), 391–407.

Umaña-Taylor, A. J. (2016). A post-racial society in which ethnic-racial discrimination still exists and has significant consequences for youths' adjustment. *Current Directions in Psychological Science, 25*(2), 111–118.

Vaithianathan, R., Putnam-Hornstein, E., Jiang, N., Nand, P., Maloney, T. (2017). *Developing Predictive Models to Support Child Maltreatment Hotline Screening Decisions: Allegheny County Methodology and Implementation*. Center for Social Data Analytics. Available: https://www.alleghenycountyanalytics.us/wp-content/uploads/2017/04/Developing-Predictive-Risk-Models-package-with-cover-1-to-post-1.pdf.

Valenzuela, J. M., and Smith, L. (2015). Topical review: Provider-patient interactions: An important consideration for racial/ethnic health disparities in youth. *Journal of Pediatric Psychology, 41*(4), 473–480.

Vergolini, L. (2011). Social cohesion in Europe: How do the different dimensions of inequality affect social cohesion. *International Journal of Comparative Sociology, 52*(3), 197–214.

Wagnild, G. M., and Young, H. M. (1993). Development and psychometric evaluation of the resilience scale. *Journal of Nursing Measurement, 1*(2), 165–178.

Wallace, J. M. Jr., Goodkind, S., Wallace, C. M., and Bachman, J. G. (2008). Racial, ethnic, and gender differences in school discipline among U.S. high school students: 1991–2005. *Negro Education Review, 59*(2), 47–62.

Weisz, J. R., Sandler, I. N., Durlak, J. A., and Anton, B. S. (2005). Promoting and protecting youth mental health through evidence-based prevention and treatment. *American Psychologist, 60*(6), 628–648.

White, K., and Borrell, L. N. (2011). Racial/ethnic residential segregation: Framing the context of health risk and health disparities. *Health Place, 17*(2), 438–448.

Wingo, A. P., Ressler, K. J., and Bradley, B. (2014). Resilience characteristics mitigate tendency for harmful alcohol and illicit drug use in adults with a history of childhood abuse: A cross-sectional study of 2024 inner-city men and women. *Journal of Psychiatric Research, 51*(1), 93–99.

Wu, L-T., and Ringwalt, C. L. (2006). Use of alcohol treatment and mental health services among adolescents with alcohol use disorders. *Psychiatric Services, 57*(1), 84–92.

Ziliak, J. P. (2016). *Moderinzing Snap Benefits: Policy Proposal 2016-06.* Washington, DC: The Brookings Institution.

Zolkoski, S. M., and Bullock, L. M. (2012). Resilience in children and youth: A review. *Children and Youth Services Review, 34*(12), 2295–2303.

CHAPTER 5

Ball, H., Wanzer, M. B., and Servoss, T. J. (2013). Parent-child communication on Facebook: Family communication patterns and young adults' decisions to "friend" parents. *Communication Quarterly, 61*(5), 615–629.

Bronfenbrenner, U. (1974). Developmental research, public policy, and ecology of childhood. *Child Development, 45*(1), 1–5.

_____. (1977). Toward an experimental ecology of human development. *American Psychologist, 32*(7), 513–531.

_____. (1979). *The Ecology of Human Development. Experiments by Nature and Design.* Cambridge, MA, and London: Harvard University Press.

Castleman, B. L. (2015). *The 160-Character Solution: How Text Messaging and Other Behavioral Strategies Can Improve Education.* Baltimore, MD: Johns Hopkins University Press.

Daminger, A., Hayes, J., Barrows, A., and Wright, J. (May 2015). *Poverty Interrupted: Applying Behavioral Science to the Context of Chronic Scarcity.* Available: http://www.ideas42. org/wp-content/uploads/2015/05/I42_PovertyWhitePaper_Digital_FINAL-1.pdf.

Dill, L. J. (2017). "Wearing my spiritual jacket": The role of spirituality as a coping mechanism among African American youth. *Health Education & Behavior, 44*(5), 696–704.

Forum for Youth Investment. (2018). *Strategic Convenings: The Secret Sauce in Collaborations Across Departments and Levels of Government.* Washington, DC: Forum for Youth Investment. Available: http://forumfyi.org/strategicconvenings-the-secret-sauce.

Gibbs, J. J., and Goldbach, J. (2015). Religious conflict, sexual identity, and suicidal behaviors among LGBT young adults. *Archives of Suicide Research: Official Journal of the International Academy for Suicide Research, 19*(4), 472–488.

Guo, R. X., Dobson, T., and Petrina, S. (2008). Digital natives, digital immigrants: An analysis of age and ICT competency in teacher education. *Journal of Educational Computing Research, 38*(3), 235–254.

Hope, M. O., Assari, S., Cole-Lewis, Y. C., and Caldwell, C. H. (2017). Religious social support, discrimination, and psychiatric disorders among Black adolescents. *Race and Social Problems, 9*(2), 102–114.

Hussong, A. M., and Jones, D. J. (2018). Parenting adolescents in an increasingly diverse world: Defining, refining, and extending theory and research. *Journal of Research on Adolescence, 28*(3), 568–570.

Hussong, A., Jones, D. J., and Jensen, M. (2018). Synthesizing a special issue on parenting adolescents in an increasingly diverse world. *Journal of Research on Adolescence, 28*(3), 665–673.

Jackson, M. (2019). *Manifesto for a Dream*. Draft manuscript.

Jones, D. J., Loiselle, R., and Highlander, A. (2018). Parent–adolescent socialization of social class in low-income White families: Theory, research, and future directions. *Journal of Research on Adolescence, 28*(3), 622–636.

Kennedy, G. E., Judd, T. S., Churchward, A., Gray, K., and Krause, K. L. (2008). First year students' experiences with technology: Are they really digital natives? *Australasian Journal of Educational Technology, 24*(1), 108–122.

Lansford, J. E., Rothenberg, W. A., Jensen, T. M., Lippold, M. A., Bacchini, D., Bornstein, M. H., Chang, L., Deater-Deckard, D., Di Giunta, L., Kodge, K. A., Malone, P. S., Oburu, P., Pastorelli, C., Skinner, A. T., Sorbring, E., Steinberg, L., Tapanya, S., Uribe Tirado, L. M, Alampay, L. P., and Al-Hassan, S. M. (2018). Bidirectional relations between parenting and behavior problems from age 8 to 13 in nine countries. *Journal of Research on Adolescence, 28*(3), 571–590.

McBride Murry, V. M., and Lippold, M. A. (2018). Parenting practices in diverse family structures: Examination of adolescents' development and adjustment. *Journal of Research on Adolescence, 28*(3), 650–664.

Mullainathan, S., and Datta, S. (2012). Stress impacts good parenting: The behavioral economists' perspective. *Who Knows What: Understanding Vulnerable Children*. 2011 W.K. Kellogg Foundation Annual Report. Available: https://www.wkkf.org/resource-directory/resource/annual-reports/2011-w-k-kellogg-foundation-annual-report.

National Academies of Sciences, Engineering, and Medicine. (2019). *A Roadmap to Reduce Child Poverty*. Washington, DC: The National Academies Press.

National Research Council and Institute of Medicine. (2002). *Community Programs to Promote Youth Development*. Washington, DC: National Academy Press.

Nguyen, A. W., Taylor, R. J., Chatters, L. M., Ahuvia, A., Izberk-Bilgin, E., and Lee, F. (2013). Mosque-based emotional support among young Muslim Americans. *Review of Religious Research, 55*(4), 535–555.

Pearce, L. D., Hayward, G. M., Chassin, L., and Curran, P. J. (2018). The increasing diversity and complexity of family structures for adolescents. *Journal of Research on Adolescence, 28*(3), 591–608.

Pew Research Center. (2014). *Religious Landscape Study: Age Distribution*. Available: https://www.pewforum.org/religious-landscape-study/age-distribution/.

Rogers, T., and Feller, A. (2018). Reducing student absences at scale by targeting parents' misbeliefs. *Nature Human Behaviour, 2*(5), 335–342.

Sameroff, A. J., and Fiese, B. H. (2000). Transactional regulation: The developmental ecology of early intervention. In J. P. Shonkoff and S. J. Meisels (Eds.), *Handbook of Early Interventions* (pp. 135–159). New York, NY: Cambridge University Press.

Sanders, P. W., Allen, G. K., Fischer, L., Richards, P. S., Morgan, D. T., and Potts, R. W. (2015). Intrinsic religiousness and spirituality as predictors of mental health and positive psychological functioning in Latter-day Saint adolescents and young adults. *Journal of Religion and Health, 54*(3), 871–887.

Shilo, G., and Savaya, R. (2012). Mental health of lesbian, gay, and bisexual youth and young adults: Differential effects of age, gender, religiosity, and sexual orientation. *Journal of Research on Adolescence, 22*(2), 310–325.

Stein, G. L., Coard, S. I., Kiang, L., Smith, R. K., and Mejia, Y. C. (2018). The intersection of racial–ethnic socialization and adolescence: A closer examination at stage-salient issues. *Journal of Research on Adolescence, 28*(3), 609–621.

Steinberg, L. (2014). *Age of Opportunity: Lessons from the New Science of Adolescence.* Boston, MA: Houghton Mifflin Harcourt.

Wong, Y. J., Rew, L., and Slaikeu, K. D. (2006). A systematic review of recent research on adolescent religiosity/spirituality and mental health. *Issues in Mental Health Nursing, 27*(2), 161–183.

CHAPTER 6

Acemoglu, D., and Autor, D. (2012). "What does human capital do? A review of Goldin and Katz's *The Race Between Education and Technology.*" *Journal of Economic Literature 50*(2), 426–463.

Acemoglu, D., and Restrepo, P. (2018a). *Artificial Intelligence, Automation and Work.* Working Paper no. 24196. Cambridge, MA: National Bureau of Economic Research.

_____. (2018b). *Modeling Automation.* Working Paper no. 24321. Cambridge, MA: National Bureau of Economic Research.

ACT. (2011). *Breaking New Ground: Building a National Workforce Skills Credentialing System.* Iowa City, IA: ACT. Available: https://files.eric.ed.gov/fulltext/ED515615.pdf.

AEI/Brookings Working Group on Poverty and Opportunity (2015). *Opportunity, Responsibility, and Security: A Consensus Plan for Reducing Poverty and Restoring the American Dream.* Washington, DC: The American Enterprise Institute and the Brookings Institution. Available: https://www.brookings.edu/wp-content/uploads/2016/07/Full-Report.pdf.

Agrawal, A., Gans, J., and Goldfarb, A. (2018). *Prediction Machines: The Simple Economics of Artificial Intelligence.* Boston: Harvard Business Review Press.

Allen, J. P., Pianta, R. C., Gregory, A., Mikami, A. Y., and Lun, J. (2011). An interaction-based approach to enhancing secondary school instruction and student achievement. *Science, 333*(6045), 1034–1037.

Amagir, A., Groot, W., Maassen van den Brink, H., and Wilschut, A. (2018). A review of financial literacy education programs for children and adolescents. *Citizenship, Social and Economics Education, 17*(1), 56–180.

American Academy of Pediatrics. (2014). *Policy Statement: School Start Times for Adolescents.* Available: http://pediatrics.aappublications.org/content/pediatrics/early/2014/08/19/peds.2014-1697.full.pdf.

Anderson, C., and Card, K. (2015). Effective practices of financial education for college students: Students' perceptions of credit card use and financial responsibility. *College Student Journal, 49*(2), 271–279.

Autor, D. H., Lawrence, F., and Kearney, M. S. 2006. Measuring and interpreting trends in economic inequality. *AEA Papers and Proceedings, 96*(2), 189–194.

_____. 2008. Trends in U.S. wage inequality: Revising the revisionists. *The Review of Economics and Statistics, 90*(2), 300–323.

Baay, P. E., van Aken, M. A., van der Lippe, T., and de Ridder, D.T. (2014). Personality moderates the links of social identity with work motivation and job searching. *Frontiers in Psychology, 5,* 1044.

Banaji, M. R., and Greenwald, A. G. (2013). *Blindspot: Hidden Biases of Good People.* New York, NY: Delacorte Press.

Banerjee, A. V., Cole, S., Duflo, E., and Linden, L. (2007) Remedying education: Evidence from two randomized experiments in India. *Quarterly Journal of Economics, 122*(3), 1235–1264.

Banerjee, A., Banerji, R., Berry, J., Duflo, E., Kannan, H., Mukerji, S., Shotland, M., and Walton., M. (2017). From proof of concept to scalable policies: Challenges and solutions, with an application. *Journal of Economic Perspectives, 31*(4), 73–102.

Barrow, L., Schanzenbach, D. W., and Claessens, A. (2015). The impact of Chicago's small high school initiative. *Journal of Urban Economics, 87,* 100–113.

Becker, G. S. (1964). *Human Capital: A Theoretical and Empirical Analysis, with Special Reference to Education.* Chicago, IL: University of Chicago Press

Beebe, D. W. (2011). Cognitive, behavioral, and functional consequences of inadequate sleep in children and adolescents. *Pediatric Clinics, 58*(3), 649–665.

Bei, B., Byrne, M.L., Ivens, C., Waloszek, J., Woods, M.J., Dudgeon, P., Murray, G., Nicholas, C. L., Trinder, J., and Allen, N. B. (2013). Pilot study of a mindfulness-based, multi-component, in-school group sleep intervention in adolescent girls. *Early Intervention in Psychiatry, 7*(2), 213–220.

Belfield, C., Bowden, N., Klapp, A., Levin, H., Shand, R., and Zander, S. (2015). *The Economic Value of Social and Emotional Learning.* Teachers College, Columbia University: Center for Benefit-Cost Studies in Education. Available: http://blogs.edweek.org/edweek/rulesforengagement/SEL-Revised.pdf.

Bergman, P. (Forthcoming). Parent-child information frictions and human capital investment: Evidence from a field experiment. *Journal of Political Economy.*

Beverly, S. G., Sherraden, M., Cramer, R., Williams Shanks, T. R., Nam, Y., and Zhan, M. (2008). Determinants of asset holdings. In S.-M. McKernan and M. Sherraden (Eds.), *Asset Building and Low-Income Families* (pp. 89–151). Washington, DC: Urban Institute Press.

Bitler, Marianne P., Hoynes, H. W., and Domina, T. (2016). *Experimental Evidence on Distributional Effects of Head Start.* NBER Working Paper No. 20434. Cambridge, MA: National Bureau of Economic Research.

Black, W. W., Fedewa, A. L., and Gonzalez, K. A. (2012). Effects of "safe school" programs and policies on the social climate for sexual-minority youth: A review of the literature. *Journal of LGBT Youth, 9*(4), 321–339.

Blackwell, L. S., Trzesniewski, K. H., and Dweck, C. S. (2007). Implicit theories of intelligence predict achievement across an adolescent transition: A longitudinal study and an intervention. *Child Development, 78*(1), 246–263.

Blair, P. Q., and Chung, B. W. (2018). *Job Market Signaling Through Occupational Licensing.* Working Paper no. 24791. Cambridge, MA: National Bureau of Economic Research.

Blattman, C., Jamison, J. C., and Sheridan, M. (2017). Reducing crime and violence: Experimental evidence from cognitive behavioral therapy in Liberia. *American Economic Review, 107*(4), 1165–1206.

Bloom, B. S. (1984). The 2 sigma problem: The search for methods of group instruction as effective as one-on-one tutoring. *Educational Researcher, 13*(6), 4–6.

Blumenfeld, P. C., Soloway, E., Marx, R. W., Krajcik, J. S., Guzdial, M., and Palincsar, A. (1991). Motivating project-based learning: Sustaining the doing, supporting the learning. *Educational Psychologist, 26*(3,4), 369–398.

Blunden, S., and Rigney, G. (2015). Lessons learned from sleep education in schools: A review of dos and don'ts. *Journal of Clinical Sleep Medicine, 11*(6), 671–680.

Bonnar, D., Gradisar, M., Moseley, L., Coughlin, A. M., Cain, N., and Short, M. A. (2015). Evaluation of novel school-based interventions for adolescent sleep problems: Does parental involvement and bright light improve outcomes? *Sleep Health, 1*(1), 66–74.

Borden L. M., Lee, S., and Serido, J. (2008) Changing college students financial knowledge, attitudes, and behavior through seminar participation. *Journal of Family and Economic Issues 29*(1), 23–40.

Bosma, H. A., and Kunnen, E. S. (2001). Determinants and mechanisms in ego identity development: A review and synthesis. *Developmental Review, 21*(1), 39–66.

Bowen C.F., and Jones H. M. (2006). Empowering young adults to control their financial future. *Journal of Family and Consumer Sciences, 98*(1), 33–39.

Brady, S. T., Cohen, G. L., and Walton, G. M. (2017). *Revising the Scarlet Letter of Probation: Reframing Institutional Communications Reduce Shame and Stigma and Enhance Student Success.* Symposium talk presented at the American Educational Research Association Annual Meeting, San Antonio, Texas.

Brady, S. T., Walton, G. M., Cohen, G. L., Fotuhi, O., Gomez, E., and Urstein, R. (2018). *Revising the Scarlet Letter of Academic Probation: Reframing Institutional Messages to Increase Student Success and Reduce Shame and Stigma.* Manuscript in preparation.

Brighouse, H., Ladd, H., Loeb, S., and Swift, A. (2018). Good education policy making: Data-informed but values-driven. *Phi Delta Kappan, 100*(4), 36–39.

Bronfenbrenner, U. 1974. Developmental research, public policy, and the ecology of childhood. *Child Development, 45*(1), 1–5.

_____. 1979. *The Ecology of Human Development. Experiments by Nature and Design.* Cambridge, MA, and London: Harvard University Press.

Bucchianeri, M. M., Arikian, A. J., Hannan, P. J., Eisenberg, M. E., and Neumark-Sztainer, D. (2013). Body dissatisfaction from adolescence to young adulthood: Findings from a 10-year longitudinal study. *Body Image, 10*(1), 1–7.

Byrnes, J. P., Miller, D. C., and Reynolds, M. (1999). Learning to make good decisions: A self-regulation perspective. *Child Development, 70*(5), 1121–1140.

Cabrera, N. L., Milem, J. F., Jaquette, O., and Marx, R. W. (2014). Missing the (student achievement) forest for all the (political) trees: Empiricism and the Mexican American studies controversy in Tucson. *American Educational Research Journal, 51*(6), 1084–1118.

Calzo, J. P., Sonneville, K. R., Haines, J., Blood, E. A., Field, A. E., and Austin, S. B. (2012). The development of associations among body mass index, body dissatisfaction, and weight and shape concern in adolescent boys and girls. *The Journal of Adolescent Health: Official Publication of the Society for Adolescent Medicine, 51*(5), 517–523.

Carlson, J. A., Sallis, J. F., Chriqui, J. F., Schneider, L., McDermid, L. C., and Agron, P. (2013). State policies about physical activity minutes in physical education or during school. *Journal of School Health, 83*(3), 150–156.

Carrell, S. E., Maghakian, T., and West, J. E. (2011). A's from Zzzz's? The causal effect of school start time on the academic achievement of adolescents. *American Economic Journal: Economic Policy, 3*(3), 62–81.

Carter, P. L. (2013). Student and school cultures and the opportunity gap: Paying attention to academic engagement and achievement. In P. L. Carter and K. G. Welner (Eds.), *Closing the Opportunity Gap: What America Must Do to Give Every Child an Even Chance* (pp. 143–155). New York: Oxford University Press.

Carter, P. L., Skiba, R., Arredondo, M. I., and Pollock, M. (2017). You can't fix what you don't look at: Acknowledging race in addressing racial discipline disparities. *Urban Education, 52*(2), 207–235.

Cascio, E. U., and Staiger, D. O. (2012). *Knowledge, Tests, and Fadeout in Educational Interventions.* Working Paper no. 18038. Cambridge, MA: National Bureau of Economic Research.

Casey, B., Jones, R. M., and Somerville, L. H. (2011). Braking and accelerating of the adolescent brain. *Journal Research on Adolescence, 21*(1), 21–33.

Cass, O. (2018). The misguided priorities of our educational system. *New York Times*. Available: https://www.nytimes.com/2018/12/10/opinion/college-vocational-education-students.html.

Cassoff, J., Knäuper, B., Michaelsen, S., and Gruber, R. (2013). School-based sleep promotion programs: Effectiveness, feasibility and insights for future research. *Sleep Medicine Reviews*, 17(3), 207–214.

Cervone, B., and Cushman, K. (2015). *Belonging and Becoming: The Power of Social and Emotional Learning in High Schools*. Cambridge, MA: Harvard Education Press.

Child Trends. (2018). *Racial and Ethnic Composition of the Child Population*. Available: https://www.childtrends.org/indicators/racial-and-ethnic-composition-of-the-child-population.

Chmielewski, A. K., Dumont, H., and Trautwein, U. (2013). Tracking effects depend on tracking type: An international comparison of students' mathematics self-concept. *American Educational Research Journal*, 50(5), 925–957.

Clark, S., Paul, M., Aryeetey, R., and Marquis, G. (2018). An assets-based approach to promoting girls' financial literacy, savings, and education. *Journal of Adolescence, 68*, 94–104.

Community Preventive Services Task Force. (2016). *Obesity: Interventions to Support Healthier Foods and Beverages in Schools*. Available: https://www.thecommunityguide.org/content/obesity-interventions-support-healthier-foods-and-beverages-schools.

Congressional Budget Office. (2018). *The Distribution of Household Income, 2015*. Washington, DC: Congressional Budget Office. Available: https://www.cbo.gov/system/files?file=2018-11/54646-Distribution_of_Household_Income_2015_0.pdf

Converse, P. D., Pathak, J., DePaul-Haddock, A. M., Gotlib, T., and Merbedone, M. (2012). Controlling your environment and yourself: Implications for career success. *Journal of Vocational Behavior, 80*(1), 148–159.

Cook, P. J., Dodge, K., Farkas, G., Fryer, R. G., Guryan, J., Ludwig, J., Mayer, S., Pollack, H., and Steinberg, L. (2015). *Not Too Late: Improving Academic Outcomes for Disadvantaged Youth*. Working Paper 15-01. Northwestern University, Institute for Policy Research.

Costello, E. J., He, J. P., Sampson, N. A., Kessler, R. C., and Merikangas, K. R. (2014). Services for adolescents with psychiatric disorders: 12-month data from the National Comorbidity Survey-Adolescent. *Psychiatric Services, 65*(3), 359–366.

Crosnoe, R., Johnson, M. K., and Elder Jr., G. H. (2004). School size and the interpersonal side of education: An examination of race/ethnicity and organizational context. *Social Science Quarterly, 85*(5), 1259–1274.

Damon, W., Menon, J., and Bronk, K. C. (2003). The development of purpose during adolescence. *Applied Developmental Science, 7*(3), 119–128.

Danner, F., and Phillips, B. (2008). Adolescent sleep, school start times, and teen motor vehicle crashes. *Journal of Clinical Sleep Medicine, 4*(06), 533–535.

Davis, J., Guryan, J., Hallberg, K., and Ludwig, J. (2017). *The Economics of Scale-up*. Working Paper no. 23925. Cambridge, MA: National Bureau of Economic Research.

Dee, T. S. (2004). Teachers, race, and student achievement in a randomized experiment. *Review of Economics and Statistics, 86*(1), 195–210.

Dee, T. S., and Penner, E. K. (2017). The causal effects of cultural relevance: Evidence from an ethnic studies curriculum. *American Educational Research Journal, 54*(1), 127–166.

DeLuca, S., and Rosenblatt, P. (2010). Does moving to better neighborhoods lead to better schooling opportunities? Parental school choice in an experimental housing voucher program. *Teachers College Record, 112*(5), 1443–1491.

Deming, D. J. (2017). The growing importance of social skills in the labor market. *Quarterly Journal of Economics, 132*(4), 1593–1640.

DePaoli, J. L., Atwell, M. N., and Bridgeland, J. (2017). *Ready to Lead: A National Principal Survey on How Social and Emotional Learning Can Prepare Children and Transform Schools.* A Report for CASEL. Civic Enterprises. Available: http://www.casel.org/wp-content/uploads/2017/11/ReadyToLead_ES_FINAL.pdf.

Destin, M., and Oyserman, D. (2010). Incentivizing education: Seeing schoolwork as an investment, not a chore. *Journal of Experimental Social Psychology, 46*(5), 846–849.

Destin, M., Rheinschmidt-Same, M., and Richeson, J. A. (2017). Status-based identity: A conceptual approach integrating the social psychological study of socioeconomic status and identity. *Perspectives on Psychological Science, 12*(2), 270–289.

Destin, M. P., Castillo, C., and Meissner, L. (2018). A field experiment demonstrates near peer mentorship as an effective support for student persistence. *Basic and Applied Social Psychology, 40*(5), 269–278.

Dewald, J. F., Meijer, A. M., Oort, F. J., Kerkhof, G. A., and Bögels, S. M. (2010). The influence of sleep quality, sleep duration and sleepiness on school performance in children and adolescents: A meta-analytic review. *Sleep Medicine Reviews, 14*(3), 179–189.

Dobbie, W., and Fryer, R. G., Jr. (2011). Are high-quality schools enough to increase achievement among the poor? Evidence from the Harlem children's zone. *American Economic Journal: Applied Economics, 3*(3), 158–187.

_____. (2013). Getting beneath the veil of effective schools: Evidence from New York City. *American Economic Journal: Applied Economics, 5*(4), 28–60.

Duflo, E., Dupas, P., and Kremer, M. (2011). Peer effects, teacher incentives, and the impact of tracking: Evidence from a randomized evaluation in Kenya. *American Economic Review, 101*(5), 1739–1774.

Dweck, C. S. (2006). *Mindset: The New Psychology of Success.* New York, NY: Random House.

Eccles, J. S. (2007). Families, schools, and developing achievement-related motivations and engagement. In J. Krusec and P. Hastings (Eds.), *Handbook of Socialization: Theory and Research* (pp. 665–691). New York NY: Guilford Press.

Eccles, J. S., and Roeser, R. W. (2011). Schools as developmental contexts during adolescence. *Journal of Research on Adolescence, 21*(1), 225–241.

Eccles, J. S., Midgley, C., Wigfield, A., Buchanan, C. M., Reuman, D., Flanagan, C., and Mac Iver, D. (1993). Development during adolescence: The impact of stage–environment fit on young adolescents' experiences in schools and in families. *American Psychologist, 48*(2), 90–101.

Egalite, A. J., Kisida, B., and Winters, M. A. (2015). Representation in the classroom: The effect of own-race teachers on student achievement. *Economics of Education Review, 45*, 44–52.

Ellemers, N., Spears, R., and Doosje, B. (2002). Self and social identity. *Annual Review of Psychology, 53*(1), 161–186.

Engel, M., Claessens, A., and Finch, M. A. (2013). Teaching students what they already know? The (mis)alignment between mathematics instructional content and student knowledge in kindergarten. *Educational Evaluation and Policy Analysis, 35*(2), 157–178.

Escueta, M., Quan, V., Nickow, A. J., and Oreopoulos, P. (2017). *Education Technology: An Evidence-based Review.* Working Paper no. 23744. Cambridge, MA: National Bureau of Economic Research.

Esteban-Cornejo, I., Tejero-Gonzalez, C. M., Sallis, J. F., and Veiga, O. L. (2015). Physical activity and cognition in adolescents: A systematic review. *Journal of Science and Medicine in Sport, 18*(5), 534–539.

Fabelo, T., Thompson, M. D., Plotkin, M., Carmichael, D., Marchbanks, M. P., and Booth, E. A. (2011). *Breaking Schools' Rules: A Statewide Study of How School Discipline Relates to Students' Success and Juvenile Justice Involvement.* New York, NY: Council of State Governments Justice Center, Public Policy Research Institute. Available: https://knowledgecenter.csg.org/kc/system/files/Breaking_School_Rules.pdf.

Fairlie, R. W., Hoffmann, F., and Oreopoulos, P. (2014). A community college instructor like me: Race and ethnicity interactions in the classroom. *American Economic Review*, 104(8), 2567–2591.

Fan, W., Williams, C. M., and Wolters, C. A. (2012). Parental involvement in predicting school motivation: Similar and differential effects across ethnic groups. *The Journal of Educational Research*, 105(1), 21–35.

Figlio, D. (2015). *Experimental Evidence of the Effects of the Communities in Schools of Chicago Partnership Program on Student Achievement.* 2015 Evaluation. Chicago, IL: Communities in Schools of Chicago.

FONA (2014). *2014 Trend Insight Report: Purchasing Power of Teens.* Available: https://www.fona.com/wp-content/themes/fona/migrated-files/PurchasingPowerofTeens_TrendInsight_0514_0.pdf.

French, S. E., Seidman, E., Allen, L., and Aber, J. L. (2006). The development of ethnic identity during adolescence. *Developmental Psychology*, 42(1), 1–10.

Friedlaender, D., and Darling-Hammond, L. (2007). *High Schools for Equity: Policy Supports for Student Learning in Communities of Color.* Stanford, CA: School Redesign Network. Available: http://edpolicy.stanford.edu/publications/pubs/100.

Friedline, T. L., Elliott, W., and Nam, I. (2011). Predicting savings from adolescence to young adulthood: A propensity score approach. *Journal of the Society for Social Work and Research*, 2(1), 1–21.

Fryer, R. G. (2014). Injecting charter school best practices into traditional public schools: Evidence from field experiments. *Quarterly Journal of Economics*, 129(3), 1355–1407.

_____. (2017). *Management and Student Achievement: Evidence from a Randomized Field Experiment.* Working Paper no. 23437. Cambridge, MA: National Bureau of Economic Research. Available: https://www.nber.org/papers/w23437.

Fryer, R. G., and Howard-Noveck, M. (forthcoming). High-dosage tutoring and reading achievement: Evidence from New York City. *Journal of Labor Economics.*

Gamoran, A., and Mare, R. D. (1989). Secondary school tracking and educational inequality: Compensation, reinforcement, or neutrality? *American Journal of Sociology*, 94(5): 1146–1183.

Gershenson, S., Hart, C., Lindsay, C., and Papageorge, N.W. (2017). *The Long-Run Impacts of Same-Race Teachers.* IZA DP No. 10630. IZA Institute of Labor Economics. Available: https://www.iza.org/publications/dp/10630.

Goldin, C., and Katz, L. F. (2010). *The Race Between Education and Technology.* Cambridge, MA: Belknap Press.

Goldman-Rakic, P. S. (1995). Architecture of the prefrontal cortex and the central executive. *Annals of the New York Academy of Sciences*, 769(1), 71–84.

Green, J. G., McLaughlin, K. A., Alegría, M., Costello, E. J., Gruber, M. J., Hoagwood, K., and Kessler, R. C. (2013). School mental health resources and adolescent mental health service use. *Journal of the American Academy of Child and Adolescent Psychiatry*, 52(5), 501–510.

Greenough, W. T., Black, J. E., and Wallace, C. S. (1987). Experience and brain development. *Child Development*, 58(3), 539–559.

Gregory, A., Bell, J., and Pollock, M. (2014, March). How educators can eradicate disparities in school discipline: A briefing paper on school-based interventions. *The Discipline
Disparities Research-to-Practice Collaborative.* Bloomington, IN. Available: http://www.
indiana.edu/~atlantic/wp-content/uploads/2014/04/Disparity_Intervention_Full_040414.
pdf.

Gregory, A., Skiba, R.J., and Mediratta, K. (2017). Eliminating disparities in school discipline:
A framework for intervention. *Review of Research in Education, 41*(1), 253–278.

Hafner, M., Stapanek, M., and Troxel, W. M. (2017). *Later School Start Times in the U.S.:
An Economic Analysis.* Santa Monica, CA: RAND Corporation. Available: https://www.
rand.org/pubs/research_reports/RR2109.html.

Halberstadt, A. G., Castro, V. L., Chu, Q., Lozada, F. T., and Sims, C. M. (2018). Preservice
teachers' racialized emotion recognition, anger bias, and hostility attributions. *Contemporary Educational Psychology, 54,* 125–138.

Halpern-Felsher, B. L., and Cauffman, E. (2001). Costs and benefits of a decision: Decision-
making competence in adolescents and adults. *Journal of Applied Developmental Psychology, 22*(3), 257–273.

Hanson, D. (2013). *Assessing the Harlem Children's Zone.* CPI Discussion Paper No. 8.
Washington, DC: Center for Policy Innovation. Available: https://www.heritage.org/
education/report/assessing-the-harlem-childrens-zone.

Harlem Children's Zone. (2009). *Whatever It Takes: A White Paper on the Harlem Children's
Zone.* Available: https://hcz.org/documents-and-publications.

_____. (2010). *The Cradle through College Pipeline: Supporting Children's Development
through Evidence-Based Practices.* Available: https://hcz.org/documents-and-publications/.

Harris, D. N., Ladd, H. F., Smith, M. S., and West, M. R. (2016). *A Principled Federal Role
in PreK–12 Education.* Washington, DC: Brookings Institution. Available: https://www.
brookings.edu/wp-content/uploads/2016/12/gs_20161206_principled_federal_role_
browncenter1.pdf.

Hatzenbuehler, M. L. (2011). The social environment and suicide attempts in lesbian, gay, and
bisexual youth. *Pediatrics, 127*(5), 896–903.

Heaney, R. P., and Weaver, C. M. (2005). Newer perspectives on calcium nutrition and bone
quality. *Journal of the American College of Nutrition, 24*(sup6), 574S–581S.

Heaney, R. P., Abrams, S., Dawson-Hughes, B., Looker, A., Looker, A., Marcus, R., and
Weaver, C. (2000). Peak bone mass. *Osteoporosis International, 11*(12), 985–1009.

Heller, S. B., Shah, A. K., Guryan, J. E., Ludwig, J., Mullainathan, S., and Pollack, H. A.
(2017). Thinking, fast and slow? Some field experiments to reduce crime and dropout in
Chicago. *Quarterly Journal of Economics, 132*(1), 1–54.

Hill, N. E. (2011). Undermining partnerships between African-American families and
schools: Legacies of discrimination and inequalities. In N. E. Hill, T. L. Mann, and H. E.
Fitzgerald (Eds.), *Child Psychology and Mental Health. African American Children and
Mental Health, Vols. 1 and 2: Development and Context, Prevention and Social Policy*
(pp. 199–230). Santa Barbara, CA: Praeger/ABC-CLIO.

Hill, N. E., and Torres, K. (2010). Negotiating the American dream: The paradox of aspirations and achievement among Latino students and engagement between their families and
schools. *Journal of Social Issues, 66*(1), 95–112.

Hill, N. E., and Tyson, D. F. (2009). Parental involvement in middle school: A meta-analytic
assessment of the strategies that promote achievement. *Developmental Psychology, 45*(3),
740.

Hill, N. E., and Wang, M.-T. (2015). From middle school to college: Developing aspirations,
promoting engagement, and indirect pathways from parenting to post high school enrollment. *Developmental Psychology, 51*(2), 224–235.

Hill, N. E., Castellino, D. R., Lansford, J. E., Nowlin, P., Dodge, K. A., Bates, J., and Petit, G. (2004). Parent-academic involvement as related to school behavior, achievement, and aspirations: Demographic variations across adolescence. *Child Development, 75*(4), 1491–1509.

Hill, N. E., Jeffries, J. R., and Murray, K. P. (2017). New tools for old problems: Inequality and educational opportunity for ethnic minority youth and parents. *The ANNALS of the American Academy of Political and Social Science, 674*(1), 113–133.

Hill, N. E., Liang, B., Price, M., Polk, W., Perella J., and Savitz-Romer M. (2018a). Envisioning a meaningful future and academic engagement: The role of parenting practices and school-based relationships. *Psychology in the Schools, 55*, 595–608.

Hill, N. E., Witherspoon, D. P., and Bartz, D. (2018b). Parental involvement in education during middle school: Perspectives of ethnically diverse parents, teachers, and students. *Journal of Educational Research, 111*(1), 12–27.

Hohnen, B., and Murphy, T. (2016). The optimum context for learning: Drawing on neuroscience to inform best practice in the classroom. *Educational & Child Psychology, 33*(1), 75–90.

Hoover-Dempsey, K. V., Ice, C. L., and Whitaker, M. W. (2009). We're way past reading together: Why and how parental involvement in adolescence makes sense. In N. E. Hill and R. K. Chao (Eds.), *Families, Schools and the Adolescent: Connecting Families, Schools, and the Adolescent* (pp. 19-36). New York: Teachers College Press.

Hopkins, N. (2015). *The Path to Baltimore's "Best Prospect" Jobs without a College Degree: Career Credentialing Programs at Baltimore's Community Colleges*. Baltimore, MD: The Abell Foundation. Available: https://www.abell.org/sites/default/files/publications/ed-careercred315.pdf.

Horowitz, E., Sorensen, N., Yoder, N., and Oyserman, D. (2018). Teachers can do it: Scalable identity-based motivation intervention in the classroom. *Contemporary Educational Psychology, 54*, 12–28.

Huber, E., Donnelly, P. M., Rokem, A., and Yeatman, J. D. (2018). Rapid and widespread white matter plasticity during an intensive reading intervention. *Nature Communications, 9*(1), 2260.

Hunt, D. E. (1975). Person-environment interaction: A challenge found wanting before it was tried. *Review of Educational Research, 45*(2), 209–230.

Institute of Medicine. (2007). *Nutrition Standards for Foods in Schools: Leading the Way Toward Healthier Youth*. Washington, DC: The National Academies Press.

_____. (2013). *Educating the Student Body: Taking Physical Activity and Physical Education to School*. Washington, DC: The National Academies Press.

Institute of Medicine and National Research Council. (2014). *Investing in the Health and Well-Being of Young Adults*. Washington, DC: The National Academies Press.

Ioverno, S., Belser, A. B., Baiocco, R., Grossman, A. H., and Russell, S. T. (2016). The protective role of gay–straight alliances for lesbian, gay, bisexual, and questioning students: A prospective analysis. *Psychology of Sexual Orientation and Gender Diversity, 3*(4), 397–406.

Iuculano, T., Rosenberg-Lee, M., Richardson, J., Tenison, C., Fuchs, L., Supekar, K., and Menon, V. (2015). Cognitive tutoring induces widespread neuroplasticity and remediates brain function in children with mathematical learning disabilities. *Nature Communications, 6*, 8453.

Jack, A. A. (2018). *The Privileged Poor: How Elite Colleges Are Failing Disadvantaged Students*. Cambridge, MA: Harvard University Press.

Jackson, C. K., Johnson, C. R., and Persico, C. (2016). The effects of school spending on educational and economic outcomes: Evidence from school finance reforms. *Quarterly Journal of Economics, 131*(1), 157–218.

Jackson, M. (2019). *Manifesto for a Dream.* Draft manuscript.

Jacob, B. A., and Lefgren, L. (2004). The impact of teacher training on student achievement quasi-experimental evidence from school reform efforts in Chicago. *Journal of Human Resources, 39*(1), 50–79.

Jodl, K. M., Michael, A., Malanchuk, O., Eccles, J. S., and Sameroff, A. (2001). Parents' roles in shaping early adolescents' occupational aspirations. *Child Development, 72*(4), 1247–1266.

Johnson, E., and Sherraden, M. (2007). From financial literacy to financial capability among youth. *Journal of Sociology and Social Welfare, 34*(3), 119–146.

Karimli, L., Ssewamala, F. M., Neilands, T. B., and McKay, M. M. (2015). Matched child savings accounts in low-resource communities: Who saves? *Global Social Welfare, 2*(2), 53–64.

Keeley, J. (2011). Learning online in jail: A study of Cook County jail's high school diploma program. B.A. Thesis, University of Chicago.

Keller, T. A., and Just, M. A. (2009). Altering cortical connectivity: Remediation-induced changes in the white matter of poor readers. *Neuron, 64*(5), 624–631.

Kemple, J. J. (2008). *Career Academies: Long-term Impacts on Labor Market Outcomes, Educational, Attainment, and Transitions to Adulthood.* New York, NY: MDRC.

Kerckhoff, A. C. (1995). Institutional arrangements and stratification processes in industrial societies. *Annual Review of Sociology, 21*(1), 323–347.

Kessler, R. C., Petukhova, M., Sampson, N. A., Zaslavsky, A. M., and Wittchen, H. U. (2012). Twelve-month and lifetime prevalence and lifetime morbid risk of anxiety and mood disorders in the united states. *International Journal of Methods in Psychiatric Research, 21*(3), 169–184.

Kett, J. F. (2003). Reflections on the history of adolescence in America. *The History of the Family, 8*(3), 355–373.

Kim, S. W., and Hill, N. E. (2015). Including fathers in the picture: A meta-analysis of parental involvement and students' academic achievement. *Journal of Educational Psychology, 107*(2).

Kimelberg, S. M. (2014). Beyond test scores: Middle-class mothers, cultural capital, and the evaluation of urban public schools. *Sociological Perspectives, 57*(2), 208–228.

Kira, G., Maddison, R., Hull, M., Blunden, S., and Olds, T. (2014). Sleep education improves the sleep duration of adolescents: A randomized controlled pilot study. *Journal of Clinical Sleep Medicine, 10*(7), 787–792.

Kirby, M., Maggi, S., and D'Angiulli, A. (2011). School start times and the sleep–wake cycle of adolescents: A review and critical evaluation of available evidence. *Educational Researcher, 40*(2), 56–61.

Kleibeuker, S. W., Stevenson, C. E., van der Aar, L., Overgaauw, S., van Duijvenvoorde, A. C., and Crone, E. A. (2017). Training in the adolescent brain: An fMRI training study on divergent thinking. *Developmental Psychology, 53*(2), 353.

Klein, J., and Cornell, D. (2010). Is the link between large high schools and student victimization an illusion? *Journal of Educational Psychology, 102*(4), 933–946.

Koepke, S., and J. A. Denissen, J. (2012). Dynamics of identity development and separation-individuation in parent-child relationships during adolescence and emerging adulthood – A conceptual integration. *Developmental Review, 32*(1), 67–88.

Kosciw, J. G., Greytak, E. A., Giga, N. M, Villenas, C., and Danischewski, D. J. (2016). *The 2015 National School Climate Survey.* New York, NY: GLSEN.

Kozlowski, K. P. (2015). Culture or teacher bias? Racial and ethnic variation in student–teacher effort assessment match/mismatch. *Race and Social Problems, 7*(1), 43–59.

Kraus, N., Hornickel, J., Strait, D. L., Slater, J., and Thompson, E. (2014a). Engagement in community music classes sparks neuroplasticity and language development in children from disadvantaged backgrounds. *Frontiers in Psychology, 5*, 1403.

Kraus, N., Slater, J., Thompson, E. C., Hornickel, J., Strait, D. L., Nicol, T., and White-Schwoch, T. (2014b). Auditory learning through active engagement with sound: Biological impact of community music lessons in at-risk children. *Frontiers in Neuroscience, 8*, 351.

Kraus, N., Slater, J., Thompson, E.C., Hornickel, J., Strait, D. L., Nicol, T., and White-Schwoch, T. (2014c). Music enrichment programs improve the neural encoding of speech in at-risk children. *Journal of Neuroscience, 34*(36), 11913–11918.

Kristjánsson, L. Á., Sigfúsdóttir, D. I., and Allegrante, J. P. (2010). Health behavior and academic achievement among adolescents: The relative contribution of dietary habits, physical activity, body mass index, and self-esteem. *Health Education & Behavior, 37*(1), 51–64.

Lareau, A., and Weininger, E. B. (2003). Cultural capital in educational research: A critical assessment. *Theory and Society, 32*(5-6), 567–606.

Leithwood, K., and Jantzi, D. (2009). A review of empirical evidence about school size effects: A policy perspective. *Review of Educational Research, 79*(1), 464–490.

Lindsay, C. A., and Hart, C. M. (2017). Exposure to same-race teachers and student disciplinary outcomes for Black students in North Carolina. *Educational Evaluation and Policy Analysis, 39*(3), 485–510.

Losen, D. J., and Gillespie, J. (2012). *Opportunities Suspended: The Disparate Impact of Disciplinary Exclusion from School.* Los Angeles, CA: Center for Civil Rights Remedies. Available: https://civilrightsproject.ucla.edu/resources/projects/center-for-civil-rights-remedies/school-to-prison-folder/federal-reports/upcoming-ccrr-research/losen-gillespie-opportunity-suspended-2012.pdf.

Losen, D. J., and Skiba, R. J. (2010). *Suspended Education: Urban Middle Schools in Crisis.* Los Angeles, CA: The Civil Rights Project. Available: https://civilrightsproject.ucla.edu/research/k-12-education/school-discipline/suspended-education-urban-middle-schools-in-crisis.

Luthar, S. S., Barkin, S. H., and Crossman, E. J. (2013). I can, therefore I must: Fragility in the upper-middle classes. *Developmental Psychopathology, 25*(4, Pt 2), 1529–1549.

Lyons, A. C. (2004) A profile of financially at-risk college students. *The Journal of Consumer Affairs 38*, 56–80.

Marx, R. W., Blumenfeld, P. C., Krajcik, J. C., Fishman, B., Soloway, E., Geier, R., and Revital, T. (2004). Inquiry-based science in the middle grades: Assessment of learning in urban systemic reform. *Journal of Research in Science Teaching, 41*(10), 1063–1080.

Maurer, T., and Lee, S. (2011) Financial education with college students: Comparing peer-led and traditional classroom instruction. *Journal of Family and Economic Issues 32*(4), 680–689.

McLean, K. C., and Breen, A. V. (2009). Processes and content of narrative identity development in adolescence: Gender and well-being. *Developmental Psychology, 45*(3), 702–710.

McLean, K. C., and Mansfield, C. D. (2012). The co-construction of adolescent narrative identity: Narrative processing as a function of adolescent age, gender, and maternal scaffolding. *Developmental Psychology, 48*(2), 436.

Mindell, J. A., and Williamson, A. A. (2018). Benefits of a bedtime routine in young children: Sleep, development, and beyond. *Sleep Medicine Reviews, 40*, 93–108.

Muralidharan, K., Singh, A., and Ganimian, A. J. (2019). Disrupting education? Experimental evidence on technology-aided instruction in India. *American Economic Review, 109*(4), 1426–1460.

Murphy, M. C., Steele, C. M., and Gross, J. J. (2007). Signaling threat. *Psychological Science, 18*(10), 879–885.

National Academies of Sciences, Engineering, and Medicine. 2018. *Transforming the Financing of Early Care and Education.* Washington, DC: The National Academies Press.

National Center for Education Statistics. (2018). Public High School Graduation Rates. The Condition of Education: Letter from the Commissioner. Available: https://nces.ed.gov/programs/coe/indicator_coi.asp.

National Research Council. (2003). *Engaging Schools: Fostering High School Students' Motivation to Learn.* Washington, DC: National Academies Press.

Norvilitis, J., Szablicki, P. B., and D. Wilson, S. (2003). Factors influencing levels of credit-card debt in college students. *Journal of Applied Social Psychology, 33.*

Nowakowski, R. S. (2006). Stable neuron numbers from cradle to grave. *Proceedings of the National Academy of Sciences of the United States of America, 103*(33), 12219–12220.

Nussbaum, M. (2011). *Creating Capabilites: The Human Development Approach.* Cambridge, MA: The Belknap Press of Harvard University Press.

Nussbaum, M., and Sen, A., (Eds). (1993). *The Quality of Life.* Oxford. Published online through Oxford Scholarship Online.

Office of Head Start. (2017). *Head Start Programs.* Available: https://www.acf.hhs.gov/ohs/about/head-start.

Okonofua, J. A., Paunesku, D., and Walton, G. M. (2016). Brief intervention to encourage empathic discipline cuts suspension rates in half among adolescents. *Proceedings of the National Academy of Sciences of the United States of America, 113*(19), 5221–5226.

Owens, J. (2014). Insufficient sleep in adolescents and young adults: An update on causes and consequences. *Pediatrics, 134*(3). Available: http://pediatrics.aappublications.org/content/pediatrics/134/3/e921.full.pdf.

Owens, J. A., Belon, K., and Moss, P. (2010). Impact of delaying school start time on adolescent sleep, mood, and behavior. *Archives of Pediatrics & Adolescent Medicine, 164*(7), 608–614.

Oyserman, D. (2015). *Pathways to Success Through Identity-Based Motivation.* New York, NY: Oxford University Press.

Oyserman, D., and Destin, M. (2010). Identity-based motivation: Implications for intervention. *The Counseling Psychologist, 38*(7), 1001–1043.

Oyserman, D., Bybee, D., and Terry, K. (2006). Possible selves and academic outcomes: How and when possible selves impel action. *Journal of Personality and Social Psychology, 91*(1), 188.

Page, E. E., and Stone, A. M. (2010, January 25). *From Harlem Children's Zone to Promise Neighborhoods: Creating the Tipping Point for Success.* Paper presented at Family Impact Seminar featuring Kate Shoemaker in Washington, DC. Available: https://www.purdue.edu/hhs/hdfs/fii/wp-content/uploads/2015/07/s_dcfis36report.pdf.

Paschall, M. J., and Bersamin, M. (2017). School-based health centers, depression, and suicide risk among adolescents. *American Journal of Preventive Medicine, 54*(1), 44–50.

Paunesku, D., Walton, G. M., Romero, C., Smith, E. N., Yeager, D. S., and Dweck, C. S. (2015). Mind-set interventions are a scalable treatment for academic underachievement. *Psychological Science, 26*(6), 784–793.

Petanjek, Z., Judaš, M., Šimić, G., Rašin, M. R., Uylings, H. B., Rakic, P., and Kostović, I. (2011). Extraordinary neoteny of synaptic spines in the human prefrontal cortex. *Proceedings of the National Academy of Sciences of the United States of America, 108*(32), 13281–13286.

Pont, S. J., Puhl, R., Cook, S. R., and Slusser, W. (2017). Stigma experienced by children and adolescents with obesity. *Pediatrics,* e20173034.

Porter, M. E., and Rivkin, J. W. (2012). The looming challenge to U.S competitiveness. *Harvard Business Review 90*(3) (March), 54–61.

Poteat, V. P., Yoshikawa, H., Calzo, J. P., Gray, M. L., DiGiovanni, C. D., Lipkin, A., Mundy-Shephard, A., Perrotti, J., Scheer, J. R., and Shaw, M. P. (2014). Contextualizing gay-straight alliances: Student, advisor, and structural factors related to positive youth development among members. *Childhood Development, 86*(1), 176–193.

Puhl, R. M., Luedicke, J., and Heuer, C. (2011). Weight-based victimization toward overweight adolescents: Observations and reactions of peers. *Journal of School Health, 81*(11), 696–703.

Rakic, P., Bourgeois, J. P., and Goldman-Rakic, P. S. (1994). Synaptic development of the cerebral cortex: Implications for learning, memory, and mental illness. *Progress in Brain Research, 102*, 227–243.

Rasberry, C. N., Lee, S. M., Robin, L., Laris, B. A., Russell, L. A., Coyle, K. K., and Nihiser, A. J. (2011). The association between school-based physical activity, including physical education, and academic performance: A systematic review of the literature. *Preventive Medicine, 52*, S10–S20.

Ratelle, C. F., Guay, F., Larose, S., and Senécal, C. (2004). Family correlates of trajectories of academic motivation during a school transition: A semiparametric group-based approach. *Journal of Educational Psychology, 96*(4), 743–754.

Reardon, S. F. (2011). The Widening academic achievement gap between the rich and poor: New evidence and possible explanations. In G. J. Duncan and R. J. Murnane (Eds.), *Whither Opportunity? Rising Inequality, Schools, and Children's Life Changes*. Available: https://www.russellsage.org/publications/whither-opportunity.

Rivet, A. E., and Krajcik, J. S. (2004). Achieving standards in urban systemic reform: An example of a sixth grade project-based science curriculum. *Journal of Research in Science Teaching, 41*(7), 669-692.

Rogers, T., and Feller, A. (2018). Reducing student absences at scale by targeting parents' misbeliefs. *Nature Human Behaviour.* Publisher's Version.

Romeo, R. D. (2017). The impact of stress on the structure of the adolescent brain: Implications for adolescent mental health. *Brain Research, 1654*, 185–191.

Romeo, R. R., Segaran, J., Leonard, J. A., Robinson, S. T., West, M. R., Mackey, A. P., and Gabrieli, J. D. (2018). Language exposure relates to structural neural connectivity in childhood. *Journal of Neuroscience, 38*(36), 7870–7877.

Russell, S. T., Horn, S., Kosciw, J., and Saewyc, E. (2010). Safe schools policy for LBGTQ students and commentaries. *Social Policy Report, 24*(4), 1–25.

Russell, S. T., Ryan, C., Toomey, R. B., Diaz, R. M., and Sanchez, J. (2011). Lesbian, gay, bisexual, and transgender adolescent school victimization: Implications for young adult health and adjustment. *Journal of School Health, 81*(5), 223–230.

Santos, L., Elliott-Sale, K. J., and Sale, C. (2017). Exercise and bone health across the lifespan. *Biogerontology, 18*(6), 931–946.

Savitz-Romerj, M., and Bouffard, S. M. (2012). *Ready, Willing, and Able: A Developmental Approach to College Access and Success.* Cambridge, MA: Harvard Education Press.

Schwartz, M. B., Henderson, K. E., Read, M., Danna, N., and Ickovics, J. R. (2015). New school meal regulations increase fruit consumption and do not increase total plate waste. *Child Obesity, 11*(3), 242–247.

Schwartz, S. J., Côté, J. E., and Arnett, J. J. (2005). Identity and agency in emerging adulthood: Two developmental routes in the individualization process. *Youth & Society, 37*(2), 201–229.

Seiffge-Krenke, I., Kiuru, N., and Nurmi, J.E. (2010). Adolescents as "producers of their own development": Correlates and consequences of the importance and attainment of developmental tasks. *European Journal of Developmental Psychology, 7*(4), 479–510.

Sharkey, P. (2010). The acute effect of local homicides on children's cognitive performance. *Proceedings of the National Academy of Sciences of the United States of America, 107*(26), 11733–11738.

Shochat, T., Cohen-Zion, M., and Tzischinsky, O. (2014). Functional consequences of inadequate sleep in adolescents: A systematic review. *Sleep Medicine Reviews, 18*(1), 75–87.

Skiba, R. J., Chung, C-G., Trachok, M., Baker, T., Sheya, A., and Hughes, R. (2015). Where should we intervene? Contributions of behavior, student, and school characteristics to out-of-school suspension. In D. J. Losen (Ed.), *Closing the School Discipline Gap: Equitable Remedies for Excessive Exclusion* (pp. 132–146). New York, NY: Teachers College Press.

Smeding, A., Darnon, C., Souchal, C., Toczek-Capelle, M.-C., and Butera, F. (2013). Reducing the socio-economic status achievement gap at university by promoting mastery-oriented assessment. *PLoS ONE, 8*(8), e71678.

Snapp, S. D., Burdge, H., Licona, A. C., Moody, R. L., and Russell, S. T. (2015). Students' perspectives on LGBTQ-inclusive curriculum. *Equity & Excellence in Education, 48*(2), 249–265.

Steinberg, L. (2005). Cognitive and affective development in adolescence. *TRENDS in Cognitive Science, 9*(2), 69–74.

Steinberg, L. (2014). *Age of Opportunity: Lesson from the New Science of Adolescence.* Boston, MA: Houghton Mifflin Harcourt.

Steinberg, L., Cauffman, E., Woolard, J., Graham, S., and Banich, M. (2009). Are adolescents less mature than adults? Minors' access to abortion, the juvenile death penalty, and the alleged APA "flip-flop." *American Psychologist, 64*(7), 583–594.

Story, M., Holt, K., and Sofka, D. 2002. *Bright Futures in Practice: Nutrition.* 2nd ed. Arlington, VA: National Center for Education in Maternal and Child Health. [Online]. Available: http://www.brightfutures.org/nutrition/pdf/index.html.

Subcommittee of the President's Council on Fitness, Sports and Nutrition. (2012). *Physical Activity Guidelines for Americans—Midcourse Report: Strategies to Increase Physical Activity Among Youth.* Washington, DC: U.S. Department of Health and Human Services.

Tajfel, H., and Bruner, J. S. (1981). *Human Groups and Social Categories: Studies in Social Psychology.* New York: Cambridge University Press.

Tan, E., Healey, D., Gray, A. R., and Galland, B. C. (2012). Sleep hygiene intervention for youth aged 10 to 18 years with problematic sleep: A before-after pilot study. *BMC Pediatrics, 12,* 189.

Tenenbaum, H. R., and Ruck, M. D. (2007). Are teachers' expectations different for racial minority than for European American students? A meta-analysis. *Journal of Educational Psychology, 99*(2), 253–273.

Thompson, D. (2012). Where did all the workers go? 60 years of economic change in one graph. *The Atlantic.* January 26. Available: https://www.theatlantic.com/business/archive/2012/01/where-did-all-the-workers-go-60-years-of-economic-change-in-1-graph/252018/.

Tough, P. (2009). *Whatever It Takes: Geoffrey Canada's Quest to Change Harlem and America.* New York, NY: Houghton Mifflin Harcourt Publishing Company.

Umaña-Taylor, A. J., Quintana, S. M., Lee, R. M., Cross, W. E., Rivas-Drake, D., Schwartz, S. J., Syed, M., Yip, T., and Seaton, E. (2014). Ethnic and racial identity during adolescence and into young adulthood: An integrated conceptualization. *Child Development, 85*(1), 21–39.

Umaña-Taylor, A. J., Douglass, S., Updegraff, K. A., and Marsiglia, F. F. (2018). A small-scale randomized efficacy trial of the identity project: Promoting adolescents' ethnic-racial identity exploration and resolution. *Child Development, 89*(3), 862–870.

United States Census Bureau. (2017). *Highest Educational Levels Reached by Adults in the U.S. Since 1940*. Available: https://www.census.gov/newsroom/press-releases/2017/cb17-51.html.

United States Department of Agriculture, Food and Nutrition Service. (2017). *National School Lunch Program: Fact Sheet*. Available: https://fns-prod.azureedge.net/sites/default/files/cn/NSLPFactSheet.pdf.

Unterman, R. (2014). *Headed to College: The Effects of New York City's Small High Schools of Choice on Postsecondary Enrollment*. Policy brief. New York, NY: MDRC. Available: https://www.mdrc.org/sites/default/files/Headed_to_College_PB.pdf.

Vera-Estay, E., Dooley, J. J., and Beauchamp, M. H. (2015). Cognitive underpinnings of moral reasoning in adolescence: The contribution of executive functions. *Journal of Moral Education, 44*(1), 17–33.

Vitt, L. A., Anderson, C., Kent, J., Lyter, D. M., Siegenthaler, J. K., and Ward, J. (2000). *Personal Finance and the Rush to Competence: Financial Literacy Education in the U.S.* Middleburg, VA: Institute for Socio-Financial Studies. Available: https://www.isfs.org/documents-pdfs/rep-finliteracy.pdf.

Wahlstrom, K., Dretzke, B., Gordon, M., Peterson, K., Edwards, K., and Gdula, J. (2014). *Examining the Impact of Later High School Start Times on the Health and Academic Performance of High School Students: A Multi-Site Study*. Center for Applied Research and Educational Improvement. St. Paul, MN: University of Minnesota. Available: https://conservancy.umn.edu/handle/11299/162769.

Walker, H. M., and Shinn, M. R. (2002). Structuring school-based interventions to achieve integrated primary, secondary, and tertiary prevention goals for safe and effective schools. In M. R. Shinn, H. M. Walker, and G. Stoner (Eds.), *Interventions for Academic and Behavior Problems II: Preventive and Remedial Approaches* (pp. 1–25). Washington, DC: National Association of School Psychologists.

Walls, N. E., Kane, S. B., and Wisneski, H. (2009). Gay-straight alliances and school experiences of sexual minority youth. *Youth & Society, 41*(3), 307–332.

Warikoo, N., and Carter, P. (2009). Cultural explanations for racial and ethnic stratification in academic achievement: A call for a new and improved theory. *Review of Educational Research, 79*(1), 366–394.

Weaver C. M., and Heaney, R. P. 2006. Calcium. In M. E. Shils, M. Shike, A. C. Ross, B. Caballero, and R. J. Cousins (Eds.), *Modern Nutrition in Health and Disease*, 10th ed. Philadelphia, PA: Lippincott, Williams, and Wilkins.

West, M. (2014). Human capital and workforce development. In R. Phillips and R. H. Pittman (Eds.), *An Introduction to Community Development: Second edition* (pp. 241–255). New York, NY: Routledge.

Wright, Jr., K. P., Lowry, C. A., and LeBourgeois, M. K. (2012). Circadian and wakefulness-sleep modulation of cognition in humans. *Frontiers in Molecular Neuroscience, 5*, 50.

Wyse, A. E., Keesler, V., and Schneider, B. (2008). Assessing the effects of small school size on mathematics achievement: A propensity score-matching approach. *Teachers College Record, 110*(9), 1879–1900.

Yeager, D. S., and Dweck, C. S. (2012). Mindsets that promote resilience: When students believe that personal characteristics can be developed. *Educational Psychologist, 47*(4), 302–314.

Yeager, D. S., Purdie-Vaughns, V., Garcia, J., Apfel, N., Brzustoski, P., Master, A., Hessert, W. T., Williams, M. E., and Cohen, G. L. (2013). Breaking the cycle of mistrust: Wise interventions to provide critical feedback across the racial divide. *Journal of Experimental Psychology: General, 143*(2), 804–824.

Yeager, D. S., Romero, C., Paunesku, D., Hulleman, C. S., Schneider, B., Hinojosa, C., Lee, H. Y., O'Brien, J., Flint, K., and Roberts, A. (2016a). Using design thinking to improve psychological interventions: The case of the growth mindset during the transition to high school. *Journal of Educational Psychology, 108*(3), 374.

Yeager, D. S., Walton, G. M., Brady, S. T., Akcinar, E. N., Paunesku, D., Keane, L., Kamentz, D., Ritter, G., Duckworth, A. L., Urstein, R., Gomez, E. M., Markus, H. R., Cohen, G. L., and Dweck, C. S. (2016b). Teaching a lay theory before college narrows achievement gaps at scale. *Proceedings of the National Academy of Sciences of the United States of America, 113*(24), E3341.

Yeager, D. S., Dahl, R. E., and Dweck, C. S. (2018). Why interventions to influence adolescent behavior often fail but could succeed. *Perspectives on Psychological Science, 13*(1), 101–122.

Yip, T., Seaton, E. K., and Sellers, R. M. (2006). African American racial identity across the lifespan: Identity status, identity content, and depressive symptoms. *Child Development, 77*(5), 1504–1517.

Zenner, C., Herrnleben-Kurz, S., and Walach, H. (2014). Mindfulness-based interventions in schools—a systematic review and meta-analysis. *Frontiers in Psychology, 5*, 1–20.

CHAPTER 7

Abe-Kim, J., Takeuchi, D. T., Hong, S., Zane, N., Sue, S., Spencer, M. S., Appel, H., Nicdao, E., and Alegría, M. (2007). Use of mental health-related services among immigrant and US-born Asian Americans: Results from the National Latino and Asian American Study. *American Journal of Public Health, 97*(1), 91–98.

Adams, S. H., Park, M. J., Twietmeyer, L., Brindis, C. D., and Irwin, C. E., Jr. (2018). Association between adolescent preventive care and the role of the Affordable Care Act. *JAMA Pediatrics, 172*(1), 43–48.

Alegría, M., Vallas, M., and Pumariega, A. (2010). Racial and ethnic disparities in pediatric mental health. *Child and Adolescent Psychiatric Clinics of North America, 19*(4), 759–774.

Alegría, M., Carson, N. J., Goncalves, M., and Keefe, K. (2011). Disparities in treatment for substance use disorders and co-occurring disorders for ethnic/racial minority youth. *Journal of the American Academy of Child and Adolescent Psychiatry, 50*(1), 22–31.

Alegría, M., Green, J. G., McLaughlin, K. A., and Loder, S. (2015). Disparities in Child and Adolescent Mental Health Services in the U.S. William T. Grant Foundation Inequality Paper. New York, NY: William T. Grant Foundation. Available: https://wtgrantfoundation.org/library/uploads/2015/09/Disparities-in-Child-and-Adolescent-Mental-Health.pdf.

Alegría, M., Alvarez, K., Ishikawa, R. Z., DiMarzio, K., and McPeck, S. (2016). Removing obstacles to eliminating racial and ethnic disparities in behavioral health care. *Health Affairs, 35*(6), 991–999.

Alexander, S. C., Fortenberry, J. D., Pollak, K. I., Bravender, T., Davis, J. K., Ostbye, T., Tulsky, J. A., Dolor, R. J., and Shields, C. G. (2014). Sexuality talk during adolescent health maintenance visits. *JAMA Pediatrics, 168*(2), 163–169.

Alexandre, P., Martins, S., and Richard, P. (2009). Disparities in adequate mental health care for past-year major depressive episodes among Caucasian and Hispanic youths. *Psychiatric Services, 60*(10).

Allen, K. L., Byrne, S. M., Oddy, W. H., and Crosby, R. D. (2013). DSM–IV–TR and DSM-5 eating disorders in adolescents: Prevalence, stability, and psychosocial correlates in a population-based sample of male and female adolescents. *Journal of Abnormal Psychology, 122*(3), 720.

Allison, M. A., Crane, L. A., Beaty, B. L., Davidson, A. J., Melinkovich, P., and Kempe, A. (2007). School-based health centers: Improving access and quality of care for low-income adolescents. *Pediatrics, 120*(4), e887–e894.

Ambresin, A. E., Bennett, K., Patton, G. C., Sanci, L. A., and Sawyer, S. M. (2013). Assessment of youth-friendly health care: A systematic review of indicators drawn from young people's perspectives. *Journal of Adolescent Health, 52*(6), 670–681.

American Academy of Pediatrics, American Academy of Family Physicians, American College of Physicians, American Society of Internal Medicine. (2002). A consensus statement on health care transitions for young adults with special health care needs. *Pediatrics, 110*(Suppl. 3), 1304–1306.

Andreyeva, T., Puhl, R. M., and Brownell, K. D. (2008). Changes in perceived weight discrimination among Americans, 1995–1996 through 2004–2006. *Obesity, 16*(5), 1129–1134.

Austin, S. B., Nelson, L. A., Birkett, M. A., Calzo, J. P., and Everett, B. (2013). Eating disorder symptoms and obesity at the intersections of gender, ethnicity, and sexual orientation in U.S. high school students. *American Journal of Public Health, 103*(2), e16–e22.

Avila, R. M., and Bramlett, M. D. (2013). Language and immigrant status effects on disparities in Hispanic children's health status and access to health care. *Maternal and Child Health Journal, 17*(3), 415–423.

Baer J. S., Ginzler J. A., Peterson P. L. (2003). DSM-IV alcohol and substance abuse and dependence in homeless youth. *Journal of Studies on Alcohol, 64*(1), 5–14.

Beesdo, K., Knappe, S., and Pine, D. S. (2009). Anxiety and anxiety disorders in children and adolescents: Developmental issues and implications for DSM-V. *Psychiatric Clinics of North America, 32*(3), 483–524.

Belur, V., Dennis, M. L., Ives, M. L., Vincent, R., and Muck, R. (2014). Feasibility and impact of implementing motivational enhancement therapy–cognitive behavioral therapy as a substance use treatment intervention in school-based settings. *Advances in School Mental Health Promotion, 7*(2), 88–104.

Birmingham, C. L., Su, J., Hlynsky, J. A., Goldner, E. M., and Gao, M. (2005). The mortality rate from anorexia nervosa. *International Journal of Eating Disorders, 38*(2), 143–146.

Blum, R. W., Beuhring, T., Wunderlich, M., and Resnick, M.D. (1996). Don't ask, they won't tell: The quality of adolescent health screening in five practice settings. *American Journal of Public Health, 86*(12), 1767–1772.

Boyd, R. C., Butler, L., and Benton, T. D. (2018). Understanding adolescents' experiences with depression and behavioral health treatment. *Journal of Behavioral Health Services and Research, 45*(1), 105–111.

Brent, D. A., and Melhem, N. (2008). Familial transmission of suicidal behavior. *The Psychiatric Clinics of North America, 31*(2), 157–177.

Breslau, J., Gilman, S. E., Stein, B. D., Ruder, T., Gmelin, T., and Miller, E. (2017). Sex differences in recent first-onset depression in an epidemiological sample of adolescents. *Translational Psychiatry, 7*(5), e1139.

Brindis, C. D., and Moore, K. (2014). Improving adolescent health policy: Incorporating a framework for assessing state-level policies. *Annual Review of Public Health, 35*, 343–361.

Brindis, C. D., and Sanghvi, R. V. (1997). School-based health clinics: Remaining viable in a changing health care delivery system. *Annual Review of Public Health, 18*, 567–587.

Brindis, C., Park, M. J., Ozer, E. M., and Irwin, C. E., Jr. (2002). Adolescents' access to health services and clinical preventive health care: Crossing the great divide. *Pediatrics Annals, 31*(9), 575–581.

Brindis, C. D., Loo, V. S., Adler, N. E., Bolan, G. A., and Wasserheit, J. N. (2005). Service integration and teen friendliness in practice: A program assessment of sexual and reproductive health services for adolescents. *Journal of Adolescent Health, 37*(2), 155–162.

Britto, M. T., Tivorsak, T. L., and Slap, G. B. (2010). Adolescents' needs for health care privacy. *Pediatrics, 126*(6), e1469–e1476.

Britton, J. C., Grillon, C., Lissek, S., Norcross, M. A., Szuhany, K. L., Chen, G., and Pine, D. S. (2013). Response to learned threat: An fMRI study in adolescent and adult anxiety. *American Journal of Psychiatry, 170*(10), 1195–1204.

Brody, G. H., Lei, M.-K., Chae, D. H., Yu, T., Kogan, S. M., and Beach, S. R. H. (2014). Perceived discrimination among African American adolescents and allostatic load: A longitudinal analysis with buffering effects. *Child Development, 85*(3), 989–1002.

Brown, S. L., Teufel, J. A., and Birch, D. A. (2007). Early adolescents perceptions of health and health literacy. *Journal of School Health, 77*(1), 7–15.

Bucchianeri, M. M., Arikian, A. J., Hannan, P. J., Eisenberg, M. E., and Neumark-Sztainer, D. (2013). Body dissatisfaction from adolescence to young adulthood: Findings from a 10-year longitudinal study. *Body Image, 10*(1), 1–7.

Bulick, C. M., Blake, L., and Austin, J. (2019). Genetics of eating disorders: What the clinician needs to know. *Psychiatric Clinics, 42*(1), 59–73

Burgess, D. J., Fu, S. S., van Ryn, M. (2004). Why do providers contribute to disparities and what can be done about it? *Journal of General Internal Medicine, 19*(11), 1154–1159.

Busen, N. H., Hanks, R. G., Giardino, E. R., Cron, S. (2016). An assessment of the human papillomarvirus immunization knowledge, practices, and prevention among a cohort of urban college students. *Journal of Nursing & Interprofessional Leadership in Quality & Safety, 1*(1). Available: https://digitalcommons.library.tmc.edu/uthoustonjqualsafe/vol1/iss1/.

Calzo, J. P., Sonneville, K. R., Haines, J., Blood, E. A., Field, A. E., and Austin, S. B. (2012). The development of associations among body mass index, body dissatisfaction, and weight and shape concern in adolescent boys and girls. *The Journal of Adolescent Health: Official Publication of the Society for Adolescent Medicine, 51*(5), 517–523.

Campbell, K., and Peebles, R. (2014). Eating disorders in children and adolescents: State of the art review. *Pediatrics, 134*(3), 582–592.

Cancilliere, M. K., Yusufov, M., and Weyandt, L. (2018). Effects of co-occurring marijuana use and anxiety on brain structure and functioning: A systematic review of adolescent studies. *Journal of Adolescence, 65*, 177–188.

Carlisle, J., Shickle, D., Cork, M., and McDonagh, A. (2006). Concerns over confidentiality may deter adolescents from consulting their doctors: A qualitative exploration. *Journal of Medical Ethics, 32*(3), 133–137.

Carlo, G., Crockett, L. J., Wilkinson, J. L., and Beal, S. J. (2011). The longitudinal relationships between rural adolescents' prosocial behaviors and young adult substance use. *Journal of Youth and Adolescence, 40*(9), 1192–1202.

Carson, N., Le Cook, B., and Alegría, M. (2010). Social determinants of mental health treatment among Haitian, African American, and White youth in community health centers. *Journal of Health Care for the Poor and Underserved, 21*(2 Suppl.), 32–48.

Centers for Disease Control and Prevention. (2017). *Crude Prevalence Estimates for Currently Insured Among Adults Aged 18-64 Years, by State* and Sociodemographic Characteristics Behavioral Risk Factor Surveillance System, 2014* A.A.Y.B.R.F.S.S. Supplemental tables for: Surveillance for Health Care Access and Health Services Use, United States, 2014 (Ed.).

_____. (2018a). *HIV Among Youth*. Available: https://www.cdc.gov/hiv/group/age/youth/index.html.

_____. (2018b). *Trends in the Prevalence of Alcohol Use, National YRBS: 1991–2017*. Atlanta, GA: CDC.

_____. (2018c). *Trends in the Prevalence of Marijuana, Cocaine, and Other Illegal Drug Use, National YRBS: 1997–2017*. Atlanta, GA: CDC.

Chadi, N., Weisbaum, E., Malboeuf-Hurtubise, C., Ahola Kohut, S., Viner, C., Kaufman, M., Locke, J., and Vo, D. X. (2018). Can the Mindful Awareness and Resilience Skills for Adolescents (MARS-A) program be provided online? Voices from the youth. *Children* (Basel, Switzerland), 5(9), 115.

Charlton, B. M., Corliss, H. L., Missmer, S. A., Frazier, A. L., Rosario, M., Kahn, J. A., and Austin, S. B. (2011). Reproductive health screening disparities and sexual orientation in a cohort study of U.S. adolescent and young adult females. *Journal of Adolescent Health*, 49(5), 505–510.

Chernick, L. S., Schnall, R., Higgins, T., Stockwell, M. S., Castaño, P. M., Santelli, J, and Dayan, P. S. (2015). Barriers to and enablers of contraceptive use among adolescent females and their interest in an emergency department based intervention. *Contraception*, 91(3), 217–225.

Chithambo, T. P., Huey, S. J., Jr., and Cespedes-Knadle, Y. (2014). Perceived discrimination and Latino youth adjustment: Examining the role of relinquished control and sociocultural influences. *Journal of Latina/o Psychology*, 2(1), 54–66.

Christensen, H., Griffiths, K. M., and Korten, A. (2002). Web-based cognitive behavior therapy: Analysis of site usage and changes in depression and anxiety scores. *Journal of Medical Internet Research*, 4(1), 29–40.

Coates, T. J., Richter, L., and Caceres, C. (2008). Behavioural strategies to reduce HIV transmission: How to make them work better. *Lancet*, 372(9639), 669–684.

Coker, T. R., Sareen, H. G., Chung, P. J., Kennedy, D. P., Weidmer, B. A., and Schuster, M. A. (2010). Improving access to and utilization of adolescent preventive health care: The perspectives of adolescents and parents. *Journal of Adolescent Health*, 47(2), 133–142.

Copeland, W. E., Wolke, D., Shanahan, L., Costello, E. J. (2015). Adult functional outcomes of common childhood psychiatric problems: A prospective, longitudinal study. *JAMA Psychiatry*, 72(9), 892–899.

Copen, C. E., Dittus, P. J., Leichliter, J. S. (2016). *Confidentiality Concerns and Sexual and Reproductive Health Care Among Adolescents and Young Adults Aged 15-25*. NCHS Data Brief no. 266, 1-8. Available: https://www.cdc.gov/nchs/data/databriefs/db266.pdf.

Costello, E. J., He, J. P., Sampson, N. A., Kessler, R. C., and Merikangas, K. R. (2014). Services for adolescents with psychiatric disorders: 12-month data from the national comorbidity survey-adolescent. *Psychiatric Services*, 65(3), 359–366.

Craw, J. A., Gardner, L. I., Marks, G., Rapp, R. C., Bosshart, J., Duffus, W. A., Rossman, A., Coughlin, S. L., Gruber, D., Safford, L. A., Overton, J., Schmitt, K. (2008). Brief strengths-based case management promotes entry into HIV medical care: Results of the antiretroviral treatment access study-II. *Journal of Acquired Immune Deficiency Syndrome*, 47, 597–606.

Cummings, J. R., and Druss, B. G. (2011). Racial/ethnic differences in mental health service use among adolescents with major depression. *Journal of the American Academy of Child and Adolescent Psychiatry*, 50(2), 160–170.

Cummings, J. R., Case, B. G., Ji, X., Chae, D. H., and Druss, B. G. (2014). Racial/ethnic differences in perceived reasons for mental health treatment in U.S. adolescents with major depression. *Journal of the American Academy of Child and Adolescent Psychiatry*, 53(9), 980–990.

Curtin, S. C., Tejada-Vera, B., and Warner, M. (2017). *Drug Overdose Deaths among Adolescents Aged 15-19 in the United States: 1999-2015*. NCHS Data Brief no. 282. Hyattsville, MD: National Center for Health Statistics.

Daley, A. M., Polifroni, E. C., and Sadler, L. S. (2017). "Treat me like a normal person!" A meta-ethnography of adolescents' expectations of their health care providers. *Journal of Pediatric Nursing*, 36, 70–83.

Daniel, S. S., and Goldston, D. B. (2009). Interventions for suicidal youth: A review of the literature and developmental considerations. *Suicide and Life-threatening Behavior,* 39(3), 252–268.

Davies, B. R., and Allen, N. B. (2017). Trauma and homelessness in youth: Psychopathology and intervention. *Clinical Psychology Review, 54,* 17–28.

Davis, A. N., Carlo, G., Schwartz, S. J., Unger, J. B., Zamboanga, B. L., Lorenzo-Blanco, E. I., Cano, M. Á., Baezconde-Garbanati, L., Oshri, A., Streit, C., Martinez, M. M., Piña-Watson, B., Lizzi, K., and Soto, D. (2016). The longitudinal associations between discrimination, depressive symptoms, and prosocial behaviors in U.S. Latino/a recent immigrant adolescents. *Journal of Youth and Adolescence, 45*(3), 457–470.

Davis, S. A., Braykov, N. P., Lathrop, E., and Haddad, L. B. (2018). Familiarity with long-acting reversible contraceptives among obstetrics and gynecology, family medicine, and pediatrics residents: Results of a 2015 national survey and implications for contraceptive provision for adolescents. *Journal of Pediatric Adolescent Gynecology, 31*(1), 40–44.

Davison, K. K., and Birch, L. L. (2002). Processes linking weight status and self-concept among girls from ages 5 to 7 years. *Developmental Psychology, 38*(5), 735.

Deas, D., and Brown, E. S. (2006). Adolescent substance abuse and psychiatric comorbidities. *Journal of Clinical Psychiatry, 67,* 18.

DeCamp, L. R., and Bundy, D. G. (2012). Generational status, health insurance, and public benefit participation among low-income Latino children. *Maternal Child Health Journal, 16*(3), 735–743.

Diaz, A., and Peake, K. (2017). Administration of childhood physical and childhood sexual abuse screens in adolescents and young adults. *Annals of Global Health, 83,* 718–725.

_____. (In press). *Principles of Adolescent- and Young-Adult Friendly Care: Contributions to Reducing Health Disparities and Increasing Health Equity.* National Academy of Medicine, Leadership, Innovation, Impact for a Healthier Future.

Diaz, A., Edwards, S., Neal, W. P., Ludmer, P., Bitterman, J., and Nucci, A. T. (2004). CHIP: New opportunities in adolescent health care delivery. *Mt Sinai Journal of Medicine, 71*(3), 186–190.

DiLillo, D., DeGue, S., Kras, A., Di Loreto-Colgan, A. R., and Nash, C. (2006). Participant responses to retrospective surveys of child maltreatment: Does mode of assessment matter? *Violence and Victims, 21*(4), 410–424.

Divecha, Z., Divney, A., Ickovics, J., and Kershaw, T. (2012). Tweeting about testing: Do low-income, parenting adolescents and young adults use new media technologies to communicate about sexual health? *Perspectives on Sexual and Reproductive Health, 44*(3), 176–183.

Draucker, C. B. (2005). Processes of mental health service use by adolescents with depression. *Journal of Nursing Scholarship, 37*(2), 155–162.

Dunne, E .F., Unger, E. R., Sternberg, M., McQullan, G., Swan, D. C., Patel, S. S., and Markowitz, L. E. (2007). Prevalence of HPV infection among females in the United States. *JAMA, 297*(8), 813–819.

Edidin, J. P., Ganim, Z., Hunter, S.J., Karnik, N. S. (2012). The mental and physical health of homeless youth: A literature review. *Child Psychiatry and Human Development, 43*(3), 354–375.

Eiland, L., and Romeo, R. D. (2013). Stress and the developing brain. *Neuroscience, 26*(249), 162–171.

Eisinger, R. W., Dieffenbach, C. W., and Fauci, A. S. (2019). HIV viral load and transmissibility of HIV infection: Undetectable equals untransmittable. *JAMA, 321*(5), 451–452.

Eley, T. C., McAdams, T. A., Rijsdijk, F. V., Lichtenstein, P., Narusyte, J., Reiss, D., Spotts, E. L., Ganiban, J. M., and Neiderhiser, J. M. (2015). The intergenerational transmission of anxiety: A children-of-twins study. *American Journal of Psychiatry, 172*(7), 630–637.

English A., Bas, L., Boyle, A. D., and Eshragh, F. (2010). *State Minor Consent Laws: A Summary* (3rd ed.). Chapel Hill, NC: Center for Adolescent Health and Law.

English, A., Gold, R. B., Nash, E. and Levine, J. (2012). *Confidentiality for Individuals Insured as Dependents: A Review of State Laws and Policies.* Washington, DC: Guttmacher Institute. Available: https://www.guttmacher.org/report/confidentiality-individuals-insured-dependents-review-state-laws-and-policies.

English, A., Scott, J., and Park, M. J. (2014). *Implementing the Affordable Care Act: How Much Will It Help Vulnerable Adolescents and Young Adults?* San Francisco, CA: National Adolescent and Young Adult Health Information Center. Available: http://nahic.ucsf.edu/wp-content/uploads/2014/01/VulnerablePopulations_IB_Final.pdf.

ETR Associates. (2016). *Sex and the Teen Brain: Disrupting What We Think We Know.* Scotts Valley, CA: ETR Associates. Available: https://www.etr.org/kirby-summit/.

Feldstein Ewing, S. W., Houck, J. M., and Bryan, A. D. (2014). Neural activation during response inhibition is associated with adolescents' frequency of risky sex and substance use. *Addictive Behaviors, 44.*

Finer, L. B., and Zolna, M. R. (2014). Shifts in intended and unintended pregnancies in the United States, 2001–2008. *American Journal of Public Health, 104*(S1), S43–S48.

Fisak, B. J. Jr., Richard, D., and Mann, A. (2011). The prevention of child and adolescent anxiety: A meta-analytic review. *Prevention Science, 12*(3), 255–268.

Fitzgerald, K. D., Welsh, R. C., Stern, E. R., Angstadt, M., Hanna, G. L., Abelson, J. L. and Taylor, S. F. (2011). Developmental alterations of frontal-striatal-thalamic connectivity in obsessive-compulsive disorder. *Journal of the American Academy of Child and Adolescent Psychiatry, 50*(9), 938–948.

Food and Drug Administration. (2018). *2018 National Youth Tobacco Survey Finds Cause for Concern.* Washington, DC: Food and Drug Administration. Available: https://www.fda.gov/TobaccoProducts/PublicHealthEducation/ProtectingKidsfromTobacco/ucm405173.htm.

Ford, C. A. (1999). Foregone health care among adolescents. *JAMA, 282*(23), 2227.

Ford, C. A., Millstein, S. G., Halpern-Felsher, B. L., and Irwin, C. E., Jr. (1997). Influence of physician confidentiality assurances on adolescents' willingness to disclose information and seek future health care. A randomized controlled trial. *JAMA, 278*(12), 1029–1034.

Ford, J. A., Sacra, S. A., and Yohros, A. (2017). Neighborhood characteristics and prescription drug misuse among adolescents: The importance of social disorganization and social capital. *International Journal of Drug Policy, 46,* 4753.

Ford, J. L. (2011). Racial and ethnic disparities in human papillomavirus awareness and vaccination among young adult women. *Public Health Nursing, 28*(6), 485–493.

Ford, J., and Wright, L. (2017). Prescription drug misuse and arrest history. *Substance Use & Misuse, 52*(13), 1772–1777.

Forhan, S. E., Gottlieb, S. L., Sternberg, M. R., Xu, F., Datta, S. D., McQuillan, G. M., Berman, S. M., and Markowitz, L. E. (2009). Prevalence of sexually transmitted infections among female adolescents aged 14 to 19 in the United States. *Pediatrics, 124*(6), 1505–1512.

Fox, H. B., McManus, M. A., Klein, J. D., Diaz, A., Elster, A. B., Felice, M. E., Kaplan, D. W., Wibbelsman, C. J., and Wilson, J. E. (2010a). Adolescent medicine training in pediatric residency programs. *Pediatrics, 125*(1), 165–172.

Fox, H. B., Philliber, S. G., McManus, M. A., and Yurkiewicz, S. M. (2010b). *Adolescents' Experiences and Views on Health Care.* Washington, DC: National Alliance to Advance Adolescent Health. Available: https://www.thenationalalliance.org/publications/2017/7/14/adolescents-experiences-and-views-on-health-care.

Fox, H. B., McManus, M. A., and Arnold, K. N. (2010c). Significant multiple risk behaviors among U.S. high school students. *Fact Sheet No. 8*. Washington, DC: National Alliance to Advance Adolescent Health. Available: https://www.thenationalalliance.org/publications/2017/7/23significant-multiple-risk-behaviors-among-us-high-school-students.

Fox, H. B., McManus, M. A., Irwin Jr., C. E., Kelleher, K. J., and Peake, K. (2013). A research agenda for adolescent-centered primary care in the United States. *Journal of Adolescent Health, 53*(3), 307–310.

Frick, P. J., Lilienfeld, S. O., Ellis, M., Loney, B., and Silverthorn, P. (1999). The association between anxiety and psychopathy dimensions in children. *Journal of Abnormal Child Psychology, 27*(5), 383–392.

Fung, J., Kim, J. J., Jin, J., Chen, G., Bear, L., and Lau, A.S. (2018). A randomized trial evaluating school-based mindfulness intervention for ethnic minority youth: Exploring mediators and moderators of intervention effects. *Journal of Abnormal Child Psychology, 47*(1), 1–19.

Garland, J. E. (2001). Sleep disturbances in anxious children. In G. Stores and L. Wiggs (Eds.), *Sleep Disturbance in Children and Adolescents with Disorders of Development: Its Significance and Management* (pp. 155–160). London: Mac Keith Press.

Gilbert, A. L., McCord, A. L., Ouyang, F., Etter, D.J., Williams, R. L., Hall, J. A., Tu, W., Downs, S. M., and Aalsma, M. C. (2018). Characteristics associated with confidential consultation for adolescents in primary care. *Journal of Pediatrics, 199*, 79–84.

Gilmer, T. P., Ojeda, V. D., Fawley-King, K., Larson, B., and Garcia, P. (2012). Change in mental health service use after offering youth-specific versus adult programs to transition-age youths. *Psychiatric Services, 63*(6), 592–596.

Ginsburg, K. R., Forke, C. M., Cnaan, A., and Slap, G. B. (2002a). Important health provider characteristics: The perspective of urban ninth graders. *Journal of Developmental and Behavioral Pediatrics, 23*(4), 237–243.

Ginsburg, K. R., Winn, R. J., Rudy, B. J., Crawford, J., Zhao, H., and Schwarz, D. F. (2002b). How to reach sexual minority youth in the health care setting: The teens offer guidance. *Journal of Adolescent Health, 31*(5), 407–416.

Gleeson, C. R., Robinson, M. B., and Neal, R. D. (2002). A review of teenagers' perceived needs and access to primary health care: Implications for health services. *Primary Health Care Research and Development, 3*(3), 184–193.

Goldenberg, D., Telzer, E. H., Lieberman, M. D., Fuligni, A. J., and Galván, A. (2017). Greater response variability in adolescents is associated with increased white matter development. *Social Cognitive and Affective Neuroscience, 12*(3), 436–444.

Gray, N. J., Klein, J. D., Noyce, P. R., Sesselberg, T. S., and Cantrill, J. A. (2005). Health information-seeking behaviour in adolescence: The place of the internet. *Social Science and Medicine, 60*(7), 1467–1478.

Green, J. G., McLaughlin, K. A., Alegría, M., Costello, E. J., Gruber, M. J., Hoagwood, K., Leaf, P. J., Olin, S., Sampson, N. A., and Kessler, R. C. (2013). School mental health resources and adolescent mental health service use. *Journal of the American Academy of Child and Adolescent Psychiatry, 52*(5), 501–510.

Grilo, S. A., Catallozzi, M., Santelli, J. S., Yan, H., Song, X., Heitel, J., Kaseeska, K., Gorzkowski, J., Dereix, A. E., and Klein, J. D. (2019). Confidentiality discussions and private time with a health-care provider for youth, United States, 2016. *Journal of Adolescent Health, 64*(3), 311–318.

Gryczynski, J., Mitchell, S. G., Schwartz, R. P., Kelly, S. M., Dušek, K., Monico, L., and Hosler, C. (2019). Disclosure of adolescent substance use in primary care: Comparison of routine clinical screening and anonymous research interviews. *Journal of Adolescent Health, 64*(4), 541–543.

Guo, S., Kataoka, S. H., Bear, L., and Lau, A. S. (2013). Differences in school-based referrals for mental health care: Understanding racial/ethnic disparities between Asian American and Latino youth. *School Mental Health, 6*(1), 27–39.

Guse, K., Levine, D., Martins, S., Lira, A., Gaarde, J., Westmorland, W., and Gilliam, M. (2012). Interventions using new digital media to improve adolescent sexual health: A systematic review. *Journal of Adolescent Health, 51*(6), 535–543.

Gustafson, E. M. (2005). History and overview of school-based health centers in the U.S. *Nursing Clinics of North America, 40*(4), 595–606.

Guttmacher Institute. (2019a). *Minors' Access to STI Services.* Washington, DC: Guttmacher Institute.

_____. (2019b). *Minors' Access to Contraceptive Services.* Washington, DC: Guttmacher Institute.

Haber, S. N., Kim, K. S., Mailly, P., and Calzavara, R. (2006). Reward-related cortical inputs define a large striatal region in primates that interface with associative cortical connections, providing a substrate for incentive-based learning. *Journal of Neuroscience, 26*(32), 8368–8376.

Hafeez, H., Zeshan, M., Tahir, M.A., Jahan, N., and Naveed, S. (2017). Health care disparities among lesbian, gay, bisexual, and transgender youth: A literature review. *Cureus, 9*(4), e1184.

Hall, K. S., McDermott Sales, J., Komro, K. A., and Santelli J. (2016). The state of sex education in the United States, *AdHealth, 58,* 595.

Hamilton, B. E., Rossen, L. M., Branum, A. M. (2016). *Teen Birth Rates for Urban and Rural Areas in the United States, 2007–2015.* Washington, DC: Centers for Disease Control and Prevention. Available: https://www.cdc.gov/nchs/products/databriefs/db264.htm.

Han, B., Hedden, S. L., Lipari, R., Copello, E. A., and Kroutil, L. A. (2015). *Receipt of Services for Behavioral Health Problems: Results from the 2014 National Survey on Drug Use and Health.* Rockville, MD: Substance Abuse and Mental Health Services Administration.

Hansen, N. S., Thayer, R. E., Feldstein Ewing, S. W., Sabbineni, A., and Bryan, A. D. (2018). Neural correlates of risky sex and response inhibition in high-risk adolescents. *Journal of Research on Adolescence, 28*(1), 56–69.

Harris, B., Shaw, B., Lawson, H., and Sherman, B. (2016). Barriers to addressing adolescent substance use: perceptions of New York school-based health center providers. *Journal of School Health, 86*(2), 96–104.

Health Resources and Services Administration. (2015). *National Projections of Supply and Demand for Selected Behavioral Health Practitioners: 2013-2025.* Rockville, Maryland. Available: https://bhw.hrsa.gov/sites/default/files/bhw/health-workforce-analysis/research/projections/behavioral-health2013-2025.pdf.

Hettema J. M., Neale, M. C., and Kendler, K. S. (2001). A review and meta-analysis of the genetic epidemiology of anxiety disorders. *American Journal of Psychiatry, 158,* 1568–1578.

Hock-Long, L., Herceg-Baron, R., Cassidy, A. M., and Whittaker, P. G. (2003). Access to adolescent reproductive health services: Financial and structural barriers to care. *Perspectives on Sexual and Reproductive Health, 35*(3), 144–147.

Hudson, A. L., Nyamathi, A., Slagle, A., Greengold, B., Griffin, D. K., Khalilifard, F., Gedzoff, D., and Reid, C. (2009). The power of the drug, nature of support, and their impact on homeless youth. *Journal of Addictive Diseases, 28*(4), 356–365.

Hudson, A. L., Nyamathi, A., Greengold, B., Slagle, A., Koniak-Griffin, D., Khalilifard, F., and Getzoff, D. (2010). Health-seeking challenges among homeless youth. *Nursing Research, 59*(3), 212–218.

Hunt, J. B., Eisenberg, D., Lu, L., and Gathright, M. (2015). Racial/ethnic disparities in mental health care utilization among U.S. college students: Applying the institution of medicine definition of health care disparities. *Academic Psychiatry, 39*(5), 520–526.

Huppert, J. S., and Adams Hillard, P. J. (2003). Sexually transmitted disease screening in teens. *Current Women's Health Report, 3*(6), 451–458.

Insel, T. R. (2014). Mental disorders in childhood: Shifting the focus from behavioral symptoms to neurodevelopmental trajectories. *JAMA, 311*(17), 1727–1728.

Institute of Medicine (IOM) and National Research Council. (2004). *In the Nation's Compelling Interest: Ensuring Diversity in the Health-Care Workforce.* Washington, DC: The National Academies Press.

_____. (2014). *Capturing Social and Behavioral Domains and Measures in Electronic Health Records: Phase 2.* Washington, DC: The National Academies Press.

_____. (2015). *Investing in the Health and Well-being of Young Adults.* Washington, DC: The National Academies Press.

Irwin, C. E., Jr., Adams, S. H., Park, M. J., and Newacheck, P. W. (2009). Preventive care for adolescents: Few get visits and fewer get services. *Pediatrics, 123*(4), e565–e572.

Jarcho, J. M., Romer, A. L., Shechner, T., Galván, A., Guyer, A. E., Leibenluft, E., Pine, D. S., and Nelson, E. E. (2015). *Developmental Cognitive Neuroscience, 13,* 21–31.

Jin, H., Folsom, D. P., Lindamer, L., Bailey, A., Hawthorne, W., Garcia, P., and Jeste, D. V. (2003). Patterns of public mental health service use by age in patients with schizophrenia. *American Journal of Geriatric Psychiatry, 11*(5), 525–533.

Johnston L. D., O'Malley, P. M., Bachman, J. G., Schulenberg, J. E., and Miech, R. A. (2014). *Monitoring the Future National Survey Results on Drug Use, 1975–2013: Volume I, Secondary School Students.* Ann Arbor: Institute for Social Research, The University of Michigan.

Juszczak, L., Melinkovich, P., and Kaplan, D. (2003). Use of health and mental health services by adolescents across multiple delivery sites. *Journal of Adolescent Health, 32*(6), 108–118.

Kaiser Family Foundation. (2018). *Mental Health Care Health Professional Shortage Areas (HPSAs).* Available: https://www.kff.org/other/state-indicator/mental-health-care-health-professional-shortage-areas-hpsas/?currentTimeframe=0&sortModel=%7B%22colId%22:%22Location%22,%22sort%22:%22asc%22%7D.

_____. (2019). *Medicaid Enrollment by Age, FY2013.* Available: https://www.kff.org/medicaid/state-indicator/medicaid-enrollment-by-age/.

Kann, L., McManus, T., Harris, W. A., Shanklin, S. L., Flint, K. H., Hawkins, J., Queen, B., Lowry, R., O'Malley Olsen, E., Chyen, D., Whittle, L., Thornton, J., Lim, C., Yamakawa, Y. Brener, N., and Zaza, S. (2016). Youth Risk Behavior Surveillance – United States, 2015. *Surveillance Summaries, 65*(6), 1–174. Available: https://www.cdc.gov/mmwr/volumes/65/ss/ss6506a1.htm.

Kaye, W. H., Wierenga, C. E., Bailer, U. F., Simmons, A. N., and Bischoff-Grethe, A. (2013). Nothing tastes as good as skinny feels: The neurobiology of anorexia nervosa. *Trends in Neurosciences, 36*(2), 110–120.

Kendler, K., Myers, J., and Prescott, C. (2000). Parenting and adult mood, anxiety and substance use disorders in female twins: An epidemiological, multi-informant, retrospective study. *Psychological Medicine, 30*(2), 281–294.

Kennard, B. D., Goldstein, T., Foxwell, A. A., McMakin, D. L., Wolfe, K., Biernesser, C., Moorehead, A., Douaihy, A., Zullo, L., Wentroble, E., Owen, V., Zelazny, J., Iyengar, S., Porta, G., and Brent, D. (2018). As safe as possible (ASAP): A brief app-supported inpatient intervention to prevent postdischarge suicidal behavior in hospitalized, suicidal adolescents. *American Journal of Psychiatry, 175*(9), 864–872.

Kepley, H. O., and Streeter, R. A. (2018). Closing behavioral health workforce gaps: A HRSA program expanding direct mental health service access in underserved areas. *American Journal of Preventive Medicine, 54*(6), S190–S191.

Kershnar, R., Hooper, C., Gold, M., Norwitz, E.R., and Illuzzi, J. L. (2009). Adolescent medicine: Attitudes, training, and experience of pediatric, family medicine, and obstetric-gynecology residents. *Yale Journal of Biology and Medicine, 82*(4), 129–141.

Klapwijk, E. T., Goddings, A. L., Burnett Heyes, S., Bird, G., Viner, R. M., S. J. Blakemore. (2013). Increased functional connectivity with puberty in the mentalising network involved in social emotion processing. *Hormones and Behavior, 64*(2), 314–322.

Klein, J. D., and Wilson, K. M. (2002). Delivering quality care: Adolescents' discussion of health risks with their providers. *Journal of Adolescent Health, 30*(3), 190–195.

Knopf, D. K., Park, M. J., Brindis, C. D., Mulye, T. P., and Irwin, C. E., Jr. (2007). What gets measured gets done: Assessing data availability for adolescent populations. *Journal of Maternal and Child Health, 11*(4), 335–345.

Kogan, S. M., Berkel, C., Chen, Y. F., Brody, G. H., and Murry, V. M. (2006). Metro status and African-American adolescents' risk for substance use. *Journal of Adolescent Health, 38*(4), 454–457.

Ku, L., and Matani, S. (2001). Left out: Immigrants' access to health care and insurance. *Health Affairs, 20*(1), 247–256.

Kushel, M. B., Yen, I. H., Gee, L., and Courtney, M. E. (2007). Homelessness and health care access after emancipation. *Archives of Pediatrics and Adolescent Medicine, 161*(10), 986.

Lau, M., Lin, H., and Flores, G. (2012). Racial/ethnic disparities in health and health care among U.S. adolescents. *Health Services Research, 47*(5), 2031–2059.

Lau, J. S., Adams, S. H., Irwin, C. E., and Ozer, E. M. (2013). Receipt of preventive health services in young adults. *Journal of Adolescent Health, 52*, 42–49.

Lavender, J. M., Brown, T. A., and Murray, S. B. (2017). Men, muscles, and eating disorders: An overview of traditional and muscularity-oriented disordered eating. *Current Psychiatry Reports, 19*(6), 32.

Leder, M. R., Emans, S. J., Hafler, J. P., and Rappaport, L. A. (1999). Addressing sexual abuse in the primary care setting. *Pediatrics, 104*(2), 270–275.

Lee, K. H., Oppenheimer, C. W., Siegle, G. J., Ladouceur, C. D., Lee, G. E., Silk, J. S., and Dahl, R. E. (2018). Prefrontal cortical response to negative social words links social risk to depressive symptoms in adolescence. *Journal of Research on Adolescence, 28*(1), 87–102.

Lee, S., Juon, H. S., Martinez, G., Hsu, C. E., Robinson, E. S., Bawa, J., and Ma, G. X. (2009). Model minority at risk: Expressed needs of mental health by Asian American young adults. *Journal of Community Health, 34*(2), 144.

Lehrer, J. A., Pantell, R., Tebb, K., and Shafer, M. A. (2007). Forgone health care among U.S. adolescents: Associations between risk characteristics and confidentiality concern. *Journal of Adolescent Health, 40*(3), 218–226.

Lieb, R., Wittchen, H. U., Hofler, M., Fuetsch, M., Stein, M. B., and Merikangas, K. R. (2000). Parental psychopathology, parenting styles, and the risk of social phobia in offspring: A prospective-longitudinal community study. *Archives of General Psychiatry, 57*(9), 859–866.

Limbers, C. A., Cohen, L. A., and Gray, B. A. (2018). Eating disorders in adolescent and young adult males: Prevalence, diagnosis, and treatment strategies. *Adolescent Health, Medicine and Therapeutics, 9*, 111.

Lin, M. T., Burgess, J. F., Jr., and Carey, K. (2012). The association between serious psychological distress and emergency department utilization among young adults in the USA. *Social Psychiatry and Psychiatric Epidemiology, 47*(6), 939–947.

Lin, R. J., and Zhu, X. (2012). Leveraging social media for preventive care—a gamification system and insights. *Studies in Health Technology and Informatics, 180*, 838–842.

Lindberg, L., Santelli, J., and Desai, S. (2016). Understanding the decline in adolescent fertility in the United States, 2007-2012. *Journal of Adolescent Health, 59*(5), 577–583.

Lock, J. (2015). An update on evidence-based psychosocial treatments for eating disorders in children and adolescents. *Journal of Clinical Child & Adolescent Psychology, 44*(5), 707–721.

MacDonald, K., Fainman-Adelman, N., Anderson, K. K., and Iyer, S. N. (2018). Pathways to mental health services for young people: A systematic review. *Social Psychiatry and Psychiatric Epidemiology, 53*(10), 1005–1038.

Manganello, J. A. (2008). Health literacy and adolescents: A framework and agenda for future research. *Health Education Research, 23*(5), 840–847.

Manlove, J., Fish, H., and Moore, K.A. (2015). Programs to improve adolescent sexual and reproductive health in the U.S.: A review of the evidence. *Adolescent Health, Medicine, and Therapeutics, 6*, 47–79.

Markey, C. N. (2010). Invited commentary: Why body image is important to adolescent development. *Journal of Youth Adolescence, 39*(12):1387–1391.

Marshall, B. D., and Wood, E. (2010). Toward a comprehensive approach to HIV prevention for people who use drugs. *Journal of Acquired Immune Deficiency Syndrome, 55*(Suppl. 1), S23–S26.

Martin, J. A., Hamilton, B. E., Osterman, M. J., Driscoll, A. K., and Drake, P. (2018). *Births: Final Data for 2016.* Hyattsville, MD: National Center for Health Statistics.

Mashhoon, Y., Sava, S., Sneider, J. T., Nickerson, L. D., and Silveri, M. M. (2015). Cortical thinness and volume differences associated with marijuana abuse in emerging adults. *Drug and Alcohol Dependence, 155*, 275–283.

Mason-Jones, A. J., Crisp, C., Momberg, M., Koech, J., De Koker, P., and Mathews, C. (2012). A systematic review of the role of school-based healthcare in adolescent sexual, reproductive, and mental health. *Systematic Reviews, 1*(1), 49.

Masten, C. L., Eisenberger, N. I., Pfeifer, J. H., and Dapretto, M. (2013). Neural responses to witnessing peer rejection after being socially excluded: fMRI as a window into adolescents' emotional processing. *Developmental Science, 16*(5), 743–759.

Matthews-Ewald, M. R., Zullig, K. J., and Ward, R. M. (2014). Sexual orientation and disordered eating behaviors among self-identified male and female college students. *Eating Behaviors, 15*(3), 441–444.

Mazur, A., Brindis, C. D., and Decker, M. J. (2018). Assessing youth-friendly sexual and reproductive health services: A systematic review. *BMC Health Services Research, 18*(1), 216.

McEwen, B. S. (2005). Glucocorticoids, depression, and mood disorders: Structural remodeling in the brain. *Metabolism, 54*(5 Suppl. 1), 20–23.

McKee, M. D., Rubin, S. E., Campos, G., and O'Sullivan, L. F. (2011). Challenges of providing confidential care to adolescents in urban primary care: Clinician perspectives. *Annals of Family Medicine, 9*(1), 37–43.

Mechoulam, R., Peters, M., Murillo-Rodriguez, E., and Hanuš, L. O. (2007). Cannabidiol–recent advances. *Chemistry & Biodiversity, 4*(8), 1678–1692.

Merikangas, K. R., He, J. P., Burstein, M., Swanson, S. A., Avenevoli, S., Cui, L., Benjet, C., Georgiades, K., and Swendsen, J. (2010). Lifetime prevalence of mental disorders in U.S. adolescents: Results from the National Comorbidity Survey Replication—Adolescent Supplement (NCS-A). *Journal of the American Academy of Child and Adolescent Psychiatry, 49*(10), 980–989.

Merikangas, K. R., He, J. P., Burstein, M., Swendsen, J., Avenevoli, S., Case, B., Georgiades, K., Heaton, L., Swanson, S., and Olfson, M. (2011). Service utilization for lifetime mental disorders in U.S. Adolescents: Results of the national comorbidity survey-adolescent supplement. *Journal of the American Academy of Child and Adolescent Psychiatry, 50*(1), 32–45.

Mitchison, D., Hay, P., Slewa-Younan, S., and Mond, J. (2014). The changing demographic profile of eating disorder behaviors in the community. *BMC Public Health, 14*(1), 943.

Mojtabai, R., Olfson, M., and Han, B. (2016). National trends in the prevalence and treatment of depression in adolescents and young adults. *Pediatrics, 138*(6), e20161878–e20161878.

Molitor, F., Waltermeyer, J., Mendoza, M., Kuenneth, C., Aguirre, A., Brockmann, K., and Crump, C. (2006). Locating and linking to medical care HIV-positive persons without a history of care: Findings from the California Bridge Project. *AIDS Care, 18*, 456–459.

Mount Sinai Adolescent Health Center (MSAHC). (2017). *Blueprint for Adolescent and Young Adult Healthcare*. New York, NY: MSAHC. Available: https://teenhealthcare.org/wp-content/uploads/2018/05/MSAHC-Blueprint-Guide.pdf.

National Conference of State Legislatures . (2011). *The Affordable Care Act: Implications for Adolescents and Young Adults*. Washington, DC.

_____. (2017). *Immigrant Eligibility for Health Care Programs in the United States*. Washington, DC.

National Institute of Mental Health. (May 2018). *Health Information: Suicide Statistics*. Available: https://www.nimh.nih.gov/health/statistics/suicide.shtml#part_15496.

National Institute on Drug Abuse. (2018). *Opioids*. Available: https://www.drugabuse.gov/drugs-abuse/opioids.

National Research Council and Institute of Medicine (NRC and IOM). (2009). *Adolescent Health Services: Missing Opportunities*. Washington, DC: The National Academies Press.

National Rural Health Association. (2015). *The Future of Rural Behavioral Health*. Leawood, KS. Available: https://www.ruralhealthweb.org/NRHA/media/Emerge_NRHA/Advocacy/Policy%20documents/The-Future-of-Rural-Behavioral-Health_Feb-2015.pdf.

Nelson, E. E., Lau, J. Y., and Jarcho, J. M. (2014). Growing pains and pleasures: how emotional learning guides development. *Trends Cognitive Science, 18*(2), 99–108.

Neumark-Sztainer, D., Croll, J., Story, M., Hannan, P. J., French, S. A., and Perry, C. (2002). Ethnic/racial differences in weight-related concerns and behaviors among adolescent girls and boys. *Journal of Psychosomatic Research, 53*(5), 963–974.

Neumark-Sztainer, D., Paxton, S. J., Hannan, P. J., Haines, J., and Story, M. (2006). Does body satisfaction matter? Five-year longitudinal associations between body satisfaction and health behaviors in adolescent females and males. *Journal of Adolescent Health, 39*(2), 244–251.

New England Journal of Medicine Catalyst. (2018). *What Is Care Coordination?* Available: https://catalyst.nejm.org/what-is-care-coordination/.

Nishina, A., Juvonen, J., and Witkow, M. R. (2005). Sticks and stones may break my bones, but names will make me feel sick: The psychosocial, somatic, and scholastic consequences of peer harassment. *Journal of Clinical Child and Adolescent Psychology, 34*(1), 37–48.

Nock, M. K., Green, J. G., Hwang, I., McLaughlin, K. A., Sampson, N. A., Zaslavsky, A. M., and Kessler, R. C. (2013). Prevalence, correlates, and treatment of lifetime suicidal behavior among adolescents: Results from the National Comorbidity Survey Replication Adolescent Supplement. *JAMA Psychiatry, 70*(3), 300–310.

Norrholm, S. D., and Ressler, K. J. (2014). Genetics of anxiety and trauma-related disorders. *Neuroscience, 164*(1), 272–287.

Notah Begay III Foundation. (2018). *Active Living Story 2 – Engaging with the Zuni Pueblo Community to Promote Active Lifestyles: The Zuni Youth Enrichment Project*. Available: http://www.nb3foundation.org/9821-2/.

O'Doherty, J. P. (2004). Reward representations and reward-related learning in the human brain: Insights from neuroimaging. *Current Opinion in Neurobiology, 14*(6), 769–776.

Office of Adolescent Health. (2017). *United States Adolescent Mental Health Facts.* Available: https://www.hhs.gov/ash/oah/facts-and-stats/national-and-state-data-sheets/adolescent-mental-health-fact-sheets/united-states/index.html.

Ojeda, S. R., and Terasawa, E. (2002). Neuroendocrine regulation of puberty. In D. W. Pfaff et al., (Eds.), *Hormones, Brain and Behavior,* Vol. 4. (pp. 589–659). New York, NY: Elsevier.

Okoro, C. A., Zhao, G., Fox, J. B., Eke, P. I., Greenlund, K. J., and Town, M. (2017). Surveillance for health care access and health services use, adults aged 18-64 years— behavioral risk factor surveillance system, United States, 2014. *MMWR Surveillance Summaries, 66*(7), 1–42.

Olatosi, B. A., Probst, J. C., Stoskopf, C. H., Martin, A. B., and Duffus, W. A. (2009). Patterns of engagement in care by HIV-infected adults: South Carolina, 2004–2006. *AIDS, 23,* 725–730.

Olfson, M., Druss, B. G., and Marcus, S. C. (2015). Trends in mental health care among children and adolescents. *New England Journal of Medicine, 372*(21), 2029–2038.

Ostaszewski, K. (2015). Inadequate models of adolescent substance use prevention: Looking for options to promote pro-social change and engagement. *Substance Use and Misuse, 50*(8-9), 1097–1102.

Pace, J. E., Siberry, G. K., Hazra, R., and Kapogiannis, B. G. (2013). Preexposure prophylaxis for adolescents and young adults at risk for HIV infection: Is an ounce of prevention worth a pound of cure? *Clinical Infectious Disease, 561*(8), 1149–1155.

Pantin, H., Prado, G., Lopez, B., Huang, S., Tapia, M. I., Schwartz, S. J., Sabillon, E., Brown, C. H., and Branchini, J. (2009). A randomized controlled trial of Familias Unidas for Hispanic adolescents with behavior problems. *Psychosomatic Medicine, 71*(9), 987–995.

Park, I. J., Wang, L., Williams, D. R., and Alegría, M. (2017). Does anger regulation mediate the discrimination-mental health link among Mexican-origin adolescents? A longitudinal mediation analysis using multilevel modeling. *Developmental Psychology, 53*(2), 340–352.

Paschall, M. J., and Bersamin, M. (2018). School-based health centers, depression, and suicide risk among adolescents. *American Journal of Preventive Medicine, 54*(1), 44–50.

Patrick, M. E., Schulejnberg, J. E., O'Malley, P. M., Johnston, L. D., and Bachman, J. G. (2011). Adolescents' reported reasons for alcohol and marijuana use as predictors of substance use and problems in adulthood. *Journal of Studies on Alcohol and Drugs, 72*(1), 106–116.

Patton, G. C., Coffey, C., Romaniuk, H., Mackinnon, A., Carlin, J. B., Degenhardt, L., Olsson, C. A., and Moran, P. (2014). The prognosis of common mental disorders in adolescents: A 14-year prospective cohort study. *The Lancet, 383*(9926), 1404–1411.

Patton, G. C., Sawyer, S. M., Santelli, J. S., Ross, D. A., Afifi, R., Allen, N. B., Arora, M., Azzopardi, P., Baldwin, W., Bonell, C., Kakuma, R., Kennedy, E., Mahon, J., McGovern, T., Mokdad, A. H., Patel, V., Petroni, S., Reavley, N., Taiwo, K., Waldfogel, J., Wickremarathne, D., Barroso, C., Bhutta, Z., Fatusi, A. O., Mattoo, A., Diers, J., Fang, J., Ferguson, J., Ssewamala, F., and Viner, R. M. (2016). Our future: A Lancet commission on adolescent health and wellbeing. *The Lancet, 387*(10036), 2423–2478.

Pelkonen, M., Karlsson, L., and Marttunen, M. (2011). Adolescent suicide: Epidemiology, psychological theories, risk factors, and prevention. *Current Pediatric Reviews, 7*(1), 52–67.

Pennap, D., Burcu, M., Safer, D. J., and Zito, J. M. (2017). Hispanic residential isolation, ADHD diagnosis, and stimulant treatment among Medicaid-insured youth. *Ethnicity and Disease, 27*(2), 85–94.

Perez-Brumer, A., Day, J. K., Russell, S. T., and Hatzenbuehler, M. L. (2017). Prevalence and correlates of suicidal ideation among transgender youth in California: Findings from a representative, population-based sample of high school students. *Journal of the American Academy of Child & Adolescent Psychiatry, 56*(9), 739–746.

Perrino, T., Pantin, H., Prado, G., Huang, S., Brincks, A., Howe, G., Beardslee, W., Sandler, I., and Brown, C.H. (2014). Preventing internalizing symptoms among Hispanic adolescents: A synthesis across Familias Unidas trials. *Prevention Science, 15*(6), 917–928.

Peters, P., Pontones, P., Hoover, K. W., Patel, M. R., Galang, R. R., Shields, J., and Conrad, C. (2016). HIV infection linked to injection use of oxymorphone in Indiana, 2014–2015. *New England Journal of Medicine, 375,* 229–239.

Pfeifer, J. H., Kahn, L. E., Merchant, J. S., Peake, S. J., Veroude, K., Masten, C. L., and Dapretto, M. (2013). Longitudinal change in the neural bases of adolescent social self-evaluations: Effects of age and pubertal development. *Journal of Neuroscience, 33*(17), 7415–7419.

Philbin, M. M., Tanner, A. E., DuVal, A., Ellen, J. M., Xu, J., Kapogiannis, B., Bethel, J., Fortenberry, J. D., and Adolescent Trials Network for H.I.V.A.I. (2014). Factors affecting linkage to care and engagement in care for newly diagnosed HIV-positive adolescents within fifteen adolescent medicine clinics in the United States. *AIDS and Behavior, 18*(8), 1501–1510.

Pont, S. J., Puhl, R., Cook, S. R., and Slusser, W. (2017). Stigma experienced by children and adolescents with obesity. *Pediatrics, 140*(6), e20173034.

Prado, G., and Pantin, H. (2011). Reducing substance use and HIV health disparities among Hispanic youth in the USA: The Familias Unidas program of research. *Psychosocial Intervention, 20*(1), 63–73.

Prado, G., Huang, S., Cordova, D., Malcolm, S., Estrada, Y., Cano, N., Maldonado-Molina, M., Bacio, G., Rosen, A., Pantin, H., and Brown, C. H. (2013). Ecodevelopmental and intrapersonal moderators of a family based preventive intervention for Hispanic youth: A latent profile analysis. *Prevention Science, 14*(3), 290–299.

Prejean, J., Song, R., Hernandez, A., Ziebell, R., Green, T., Walker, F., Lin, L. S., An, Q., Mermin, J., Lansky, A., and Hall, H. I. (2011). Estimated HIV incidence in the United States, 2006–2009. *PLoS One, 6*(8), e17502.

Prinstein, M. J., and Aikins, J. W. (2004). Cognitive moderators of the longitudinal association between peer rejection and adolescent depressive symptoms. *Journal of Abnormal Child Psychology, 32*(2), 147–158.

Prinstein, M. J., Cheah, C. S., and Guyer, A. E. (2005). Peer victimization, cue interpretation, and internalizing symptoms: Preliminary concurrent and longitudinal findings for children and adolescents. *Journal of Clinical Child and Adolescent Psychology, 34*(1), 11–24.

Puhl, R. M., Luedicke, J., and Heuer, C. (2011). Weight-based victimization toward overweight adolescents: Observations and reactions of peers. *Journal of School Health, 81*(11), 696–703.

Quickfall, J., and Crockford, D. (2006). Brain neuroimaging in cannabis use: A review. *The Journal of Neuropsychiatry and Clinical Neurosciences, 18*(3), 318–332.

Reitsema, A. M., and Grietens, H. (2016). Is anybody listening? The literature on the dialogical process of child sexual abuse disclosure reviewed. *Trauma, Violence, and Abuse, 17*(3), 330–340.

Richardson, L. P., McCarty, C. A., Radovic, A., and Suleiman, A. B. (2017). Research in the integration of behavioral health for adolescents and young adults in primary care settings: A systematic review. *Journal of Adolescent Health, 60*(3), 261–269.

Rigby, K. (2003). Consequences of bullying in schools. *The Canadian Journal of Psychiatry, 48*(9), 583–590.

Riley, M., Patterson, V., Lane, J. C., Won, K. M., and Ranalli, L. (2018). The adolescent champion model: Primary care becomes adolescent-centered via targeted quality improvement. *Journal of Pediatrics, 193*, 229–236, e221.

Ringheim, K. (2007). Ethical and human rights perspectives on providers' obligation to ensure adolescents' rights to privacy. *Studies in Family Planning, 38*(4), 245–252.

Rivers, S., Reyna, V., and Mills, B. (2008). Risk taking under the influence: A fuzzy-trace theory of emotion in adolescence. *Developmental Review, 28*(1), 107–144.

Romero, L., Pazol, K., Warner, L., Cox, S., Kroelinger, C., Besera, G., Brittain, A., Fuller, T. R., Koumans, E., and Barfield, W. (2016). Reduced disparities in birth rates among teens aged 15-19 years – United States, 2006–2007 and 2013–2014. *MMWR Morbidity and Mortality Weekly Report 2016, 65*, 409–414.

Romero, L. M., Olaiya, O., Hallum-Montes, R., Varanasi, B., Mueller, T., House, D. L., Schlanger, K., and Middleton, D. (2017). Efforts to increase implementation of evidence-based clinical practices to improve adolescent-friendly reproductive health services. *Journal of Adolescent Health, 60*(3), S30–S37.

Roy, A. K., Fudge, J. L., Kelly, C., Perry, J. S. A., Daniele, T., Carlisi, C., Ernst. M. Intrinsic functional connectivity of amygdala-based networks in adolescent generalized anxiety disorder. *Journal of the American Academy of Child & Adolescent Psychiatry, 52*(3) (2013), 290–299.

Ruderfer, D. M., Walsh, C. G., Aguirre, M. W., Tanigawa, Y., Ribeiro, J. D., Franklin, J. C., and Rivas, M. A. (2019). Significant shared heritability underlies suicide attempt and clinically predicted probability of attempting suicide. *Molecular Psychiatry, 1*.

Russell, S. T., Sinclair, K. O., Poteat, V. P., and Koenig, B. W. (2012). Adolescent health and harassment based on discriminatory bias. *American Journal of Public Health, 102*(3), 493–495.

Sadler, L. S., and Daley, A. M. (2002). A model of teen-friendly care for young women with negative pregnancy test results. *The Nursing Clinics of North America, 37*(3), 523–535.

Santa Maria, D., Guilamo-Ramos, V., Jemmott, L. S., Derouin, A., and Villarruel, A. (2017). Nurses on the front lines: Improving adolescent sexual and reproductive health across health care settings. *American Journal of Nursing, 117*(1), 42–51.

Santelli, J. S. (2008). Medical accuracy in sexuality education: Ideology and the scientific process. *American Journal of Public Health, 98*(10), 1786–1792.

Santor, D. A., Poulin, C., Leblanc, J.C., and Kusumakar, V. (2007). Facilitating help seeking behavior and referrals for mental health difficulties in school aged boys and girls: A school-based intervention. *Journal of Youth Adolescence, 36*(6), 741–752.

Satterwhite, C. L., Torrone, E., and Meites, E. (2013). Sexually transmitted infections among U.S. women and men: Prevalence and incidence estimates, 2008. *Sexually Transmitted Disease Surveillance, 40*(3), 187–193.

Savell, S. (2005). Child sexual abuse: Are health care providers looking the other way? *Journal of Forensic Nursing, 1*(2), 78–82.

Schalet, A. T., Santelli, J. S., Russell, S. T., Halpern, C. T., Miller, S. A., Pickering, S. S., Goldberg, S. K., and Hoenig, J. M. (2014). Invited commentary: Broadening the evidence for adolescent sexual and reproductive health and education in the United States. *Journal of Youth Adolescence, 43*(10), 1595–1610.

Schoen, C., Abrams, M. K., and Davis, K. (1997). *The Commonwealth Fund Survey of the Health of Adolescent Girls*. New York, NY: The Commonwealth Fund.

School-Based Health Alliance. (2014). *2013-14 Digital Census Report*. Washington, DC: School-Based Health Alliance. Available: http://censusreport.sbh4all.org/.

Schuster, M. A. (1996). Communication between adolescents and physicians about sexual behavior and risk prevention. *Archives of Pediatrics & Adolescent Medicine, 150*(9), 906.

Scott, L. D., Jr., and Davis, L. E. (2006). Young, black, and male in foster care: Relationship of negative social contextual experiences to factors relevant to mental health service delivery. *Journal of Adolescence, 29*(5), 721–736.

Sedgh, G., Finer, L. B., Bankole, A., Eilers, M. A., and Singh, S. (2015). Adolescent pregnancy, birth, and abortion rates across countries: Levels and recent trends. *Journal of Adolescent Health, 56*(2), 223–230.

Sedlander, E., Brindis, C. D., Bausch, S. H., and Tebb, K. P. (2015). Options for assuring access to confidential care for adolescents and young adults in an explanation of benefits environment. *Journal of Adolescent Health, 56*(1), 7–9.

Shakibnia, E. B., Timmons, S. E., Gold, M. A., and Garbers, S. (2018). "It's pretty hard to tell your mom and dad that you're on a method": Exploring how an app could promote adolescents' communication with partners and parent(s) to increase self-efficacy in long-acting reversible contraception use. *Journal of Pediatric Adolescent Gynecology, 31*(2), 116–121.

Shaw, J. M., Mitchell, C. A., Welch, A. J., and Williamson, M. J. (2015). Social media used as a health intervention in adolescent health: A systematic review of the literature. *Digital Health, 1*, 205–207.

Sheftall, A. H., Mathias, C. W., Furr, R. M., and Dougherty, D. M. (2013). Adolescent attachment security, family functioning, and suicide attempts. *Attachment and Human Development, 15*(4), 368–383.

Siegel, R. S., and Dickstein, D. P. (2011). Anxiety in adolescents: Update on its diagnosis and treatment for primary care providers. *Adolescent Health, Medicine, and Therapeutics, 30*(3), 1–16.

Singh S. (2000). Adolescent pregnancy and childbearing: Levels and trends in developed countries. *Family Planning Perspectives 32*(1), 14–23.

Singh, S., Darroch, J., and Frost J. (2001). Socioeconomic disadvantage and adolescent women's sexual and reproductive behavior: The case of five developed countries. *Family Planning Perspectives, 33*(6), 251–289.

Society for Adolescent Health and Medicine (SAHM) and American Academy of Pediatrics. (2016). Confidentiality protections for adolescents and young adults in the health care billing and insurance claims process. *Journal of Adolescent Health, 58*(3), 374–377.

Sokolowski, M., Wasserman, J., and Wasserman, D. (2015). An overview of the neurobiology of suicidal behaviors as one meta-system. *Molecular Psychiatry, 20*(1), 56–71.

Soleimanpour, S., Brindis, C., Geierstanger, S., Kandawalla, S., and Kurlaender, T. (2008). Incorporating youth-led community participatory research into school health center programs and policies. *Public Health Reports, 123*(6), 709–716.

Soleimanpour, S., Geierstanger, S. P., Kaller, S., McCarter, V., and Brindis, C. D. (2010). The role of school health centers in health care access and client outcomes. *American Journal of Public Health, 100*(9), 1597–1603.

Spence, R., Owens-Solari, M., and Goodyer, I. (2016). Help-seeking in emerging adults with and without a history of mental health referral: A qualitative study. *BMC Research Notes, 9*(1), 415.

Steinberg, L. (2014). *Age of Opportunity: Lessons from the New Science of Adolescence.* New York, NY: First Mariner Books.

Stinson, F. S., Ruan, W. J., Pickering, R., and Grant, B. F. (2006). Cannabis use disorders in the USA: Prevalence, correlates and co-morbidity. *Psychological Medicine, 36*(10), 1447–1460.

Swanson, S. A., Crow, S. J., Le Grange, D., Swendsen, J., and Merikangas, K. R. (2011). Prevalence and correlates of eating disorders in adolescents: Results from the national comorbidity survey replication adolescent supplement. *Archives of General Psychiatry, 68*(7), 714–723.

Tang, S. S., Hudak, M. L., Cooley, D. M., Shenkin, B. N., and Racine, A. D. (2018). Increased Medicaid payment and participation by office-based primary care pediatricians. *Pediatrics, 141*(1).

Tebb, K. P., Sedlander, E., Pica, G., Diaz, A., Peake, K., and Brindis, C. (2014). *Protecting Adolescent Confidentiality Under Health Care Reform: The Special Case Regarding Explanation of Benefits (EOBs).* San Francisco, CA: Philip R. Lee Institute for Health Policy Studies.

Tebb, K. P., Sedlander, E., Bausch, S., and Brindis, C. D. (2015). Opportunities and challenges for adolescent health under the Affordable Care Act. *Maternal and Child Health Journal, 19*(10), 2089–2093.

Tebb, K. P., Pica, G., Twietmeyer, L., Diaz, A., and Brindis, C. D. (2018). Innovative approaches to address social determinants of health among adolescents and young adults. *Health Equity, 2*(1), 321–328.

Telzer, E. H., Fuligni, A. J., Lieberman, M. D., and Galván, A. (2014). Neural sensitivity to eudaimonic and hedonic rewards differentially predict adolescent depressive symptoms over time. *Proceedings of the National Academy of Sciences of the United States of America, 111*(18), 6600–6605.

Thomas, J. F., Temple, J. R., Perez, N., and Rupp, R. (2011). Ethnic and gender disparities in needed adolescent mental health care. *Journal of Health Care for the Poor and Underserved, 22*(1), 101–110.

Torian, L. V., Wiewel, E. W., Liu, K. L., Sackoff, J. E., and Frieden, T. R. (2008). Risk factors for delayed initiation of medical care after diagnosis of human immunodeficiency virus. *Archives of Internal Medicine, 168*, 1181–1187.

Trust for America's Health. (2018). *Braiding and Blending Funds to Support Community Health Improvement: A Compendium of Resources and Examples.* Washington, DC. Available: https://www.tfah.org/wp-content/uploads/2018/01/TFAH-Braiding-Blending-Compendium-FINAL.pdf.

Tylee, A., Haller, D. M., Graham, T., Churchill, R., and Sanci, L. A. (2007). Youth-friendly primary-care services: How are we doing and what more needs to be done? *The Lancet, 369*(9572), 1565–1573.

Umaña-Taylor, A. J. (2016). A post-racial society in which ethnic-racial discrimination still exists and has significant consequences for youths' adjustment. *Current Directions in Psychological Science, 25*(2), 111–118.

Valenzuela, J. M., and Smith, L. (2015). Topical review: Provider-patient interactions: An important consideration for racial/ethnic health disparities in youth. *Journal of Pediatric Pscyhology, 41*(4), 473–480.

Van Handle, M. M., Rose, C. E., Hallisey, E. J., Kolling, J. L., Zibbell, J. E., Lewis, B., Bohm, M. K., Jones, C. M., Flanagan, B. E., Siddiqi, A. E., Igbal, K., Dent, A. L., Mermin, J. H., McCray, E., Ward, J. W., and Brooks, J. T. (2016). County-level vulnerability assessment for rapid dissemination of HIV or HCV infections among persons who inject drugs, United States. *Journal of AIDS, 73*(3), 323–331.

Van Voorhees, B. W., Fogel, J., Pomper, B. E., Marko, M., Reid, N., Watson, N., Larson, J., Bradford, N., Fagan, B., Zuckerman, S., Wiedmann, P., and Domanico, R. (2009). Adolescent dose and ratings of an internet-based depression prevention program: A randomized trial of primary care physician brief advice versus a motivational interview. *Journal of Cognitive and Behavioral Psychotherapies, 9*(1), 1–19.

Vo, D. X., and Park, M. J. (2008). Racial/ethnic disparities and culturally competent health care among youth and young men. *American Journal of Men's Health, 2*(2), 192–205.

Voracek, M., and Loibl, L. M. (2007). Genetics of suicide: A systematic review of twin studies. *Wiener klinische Wochenschrift* [The Central European Journal of Medicine], *119*(15–16), 463–475.

Walker, T. Y., Elam-Evans, L. D., Singleton, J. A., Yankey, D., Markowitz, L. E., Fredua, M. S., Williams, C. L., Meyer, S. A., and Stokley, S. (2017). National, regional, state, and selected local area vaccination coverage among adolescents aged 13–17 years – United States, 2016. *Centers for Disease Control and Prevention, Morbidity and Mortality Weekly Report, 66*(33), 874–882.

Watson, R. J., Adjei, J., Saewyc, E., Homma, Y., and Goodenow, C. (2017). Trends and disparities in disordered eating among heterosexual and sexual minority adolescents. *International Journal of Eating Disorders, 50*(1), 22–31.

Weinreb, L., Nicholson, J., Williams, V., and Anthes, F. (2007). Integrating behavioral health services for homeless mothers and children in primary care. *American Journal of Orthopsychiatry, 77*(1), 142–152.

Wilson, J. D., Berk, J., Adger, H., and Feldman, L. (2018). Identifying missed clinical opportunities in delivery of overdose prevention and naloxone prescription to adolescents using opioids. *Journal of Adolescent Health, 63*(2), 245–248.

Wodtke, G. T. (2013). Duration and timing of exposure to neighborhood poverty and the risk of adolescent parenthood. *Demography, 50*(5), 1765–1788.

Wong, C. A., Merchant, R. M., and Moreno, M. A. (2014). Using social media to engage adolescents and young adults with their health. *Healthcare (Amsterdam), 2*(4), 220–224.

World Health Organization. (2003). *Adolescent Friendly Health Services: An Agenda for Change*: Geneva, Switzerland: World Health Organization.

_____. (2012*). Making Health Services Adolescent Friendly: Developing National Quality Standards for Adolescent Friendly Health Services.* Geneva, Switzerland: World Health Organization.

Yin, H. H., Mulcare, S. P., Hilario, M. R. F., Clouse, E., Holloway, T., Davis, M. I., and Costa, R. M. (2009). Dynamic reorganization of striatal circuits during the acquisition and consolidation of a skill. *National Neuroscience, 12*(3), 333–341.

Zanoni, B. C., and Mayer, K. H. (2014). The adolescent and young adult HIV cascade of care in the United States: Exaggerated health disparities. *AIDS Patient Care STDs, 28*(3), 128–135.

Zibell, J., Asher, A. K., Patel, R. C., Kupronis, B., Iqbal, K., Ward, J. W., and Holtzman, D. (2018). Increases in acute hepatitis C virus infection related to a growing opioid epidemic and associated injection drug use, United States, 2004 to 2014. *AJPH: Hepatitis C and Opioids, 108*(2), 175–181.

CHAPTER 8

Allen, E. C., Combs-Orme, T., McCarter Jr., R. J., and Grossman, L. S. (2000). Self-reported depressive symptoms in school-age children at the time of entry into foster care. *Ambulatory Child Health, 6*(1), 45–57.

Andersen, S. L., Tomada, A., Vincow, E. S., Valente, E., Polcari, A., and Teicher, M. H. (2008). Preliminary evidence for sensitive periods in the effect of childhood sexual abuse on regional brain development. *Journal Neuropsychiatry Clinical Neuroscience, 20*(3), 292–301.

Barth, R. P. (1990). On their own: The experiences of youth after foster care. *Child & Adolescent Social Work Journal, 7*(5), 419–440.

Burns, B. J., Phillips, S. D., Wagner, H. R., Barth, R. P., Kolko, D. J., Campbell, Y., and Landsverk, J. (2004). Mental health need and access to mental health services by youths involved with child welfare: A national survey. *Journal of the American Academy of Child & Adolescent Psychiatry, 43*(8), 960–970.

Chaffin, M., and Bard, D. (2006). Impact of intervention surveillance bias on analyses of child welfare report outcomes. *Child Maltreatment, 11*(4), 301–312.

Chamberlain, P. (2003). *Treating Chronic Juvenile Offenders: Advances Made Through the Oregon Multidimensional Treatment Foster Care Model*. Washington, DC: American Psychological Association.

Chamberlain, P., Price, J. M., Reid, J. B., Landsverk, J. A., Fisher, P. A., and Stoolmiller, M. (2006). Who disrupts from placement in foster and kinship care? *Child Abuse and Neglect, 30*, 409–424.

Chamberlain, P., Price, J., Reid, J., and Landsverk, J. (2008). Cascading implementation of a foster parent intervention: Partnerships, logistics, transportability, and sustainability. *Child Welfare, 87*, 27–48.

Child Trends. (2016). *Child Welfare Financing: A Survey of Federal, State, and Local Expenditures*. Bethesda, MD: Child Trends.

Children's Bureau. (2016). *Racial Disproportionality and Disparity in Child Welfare*. Washington, DC: U.S. Department of Health and Human Services, Administration for Children and Families.

Children's Bureau. (2017). *Child Maltreatment 2015*. Washington, DC: U.S. Department of Health & Human Services, Administration for Children and Families, Administration on Children, Youth and Families. Available: http://www.acf.hhs.gov/programs/cb/research-data-technology/statistics-research/child-maltreatment.

Courtney, M. E., and Piliavin, I. (1998). *Foster Youths Transitions to Adulthood: Outcomes 12 to 18 Months After Leaving Out-Of-Home Care*. Madison, WI: School of Social Work, University of Wisconsin-Madison.

Courtney, M. E., Okpych, N. J., Charles, P., Mikell, D., Stevenson, B., Park, K., Kindle, B., Harty, J. and Feng, H. (2016). *Findings from the California Youth Transitions to Adulthood Study (CalYOUTH): Conditions of Youth at Age 19*. Chicago, IL: Chapin Hall at the University of Chicago.

Cusick, G. R., Havlicek, J. R., and Courtney, M. E. (2012). Risk for arrest: The role of social bonds in protecting foster youth making the transition to adulthood. *American Journal of Orthopsychiatry, 82*(1), 19–31.

Dickes, A., Kemmis-Riggs, J., and McAloon, J. (2018). Methodological challenges to the evaluation of interventions for foster/kinship carers and children: A systematic review. *Clinical Child and Family Psychology Review, 21*(2), 109–145.

Dworsky, A., and DeCoursey, J. (2009). *Pregnant and Parenting Foster Youth: Their Needs, Their Experiences*. Chicago, IL: Chapin Hall Center for Children at the University of Chicago.

Fish, J. N., Baams, L., Wojciak, A. S., and Russell, S. T. (2019). Are sexual minority youth overrepresented in foster care, child welfare, and out-of-home placement? Findings from nationally representative data. *Child Abuse and Neglect, 89*, 203–211.

Fisher, P. A., Burraston, B. O., and Pears, K.C. (2005). The Early Intervention Foster Care Program: Permanent placement outcomes from a randomized trial. *Child Maltreatment, 10*, 61–71.

Fisher, P. A., Leve, L. D., Delker, B., Roos, L. E., and Cooper, B. (2016). A developmental psychopathology perspective on foster care research. *Developmental Psychopathology, 1*, 42.

Fisher, P. A., Stoolmiller, M., Gunnar, M. R., and Burraston, B. O. (2007). Effects of a therapeutic intervention for foster preschoolers on diurnal cortisol activity. *Psychoneuroendocrinology, 32*(8-10), 892–905.

Fowler, P. J., Marcal, K. E., Zhang, J., Day, O., and Landsverk, J. (2017). Homelessness and aging out of foster care: A national comparison of child welfare-involved adolescents. *Children and Youth Services Review, 77*, 27–33.

Geenen, S., Powers, L. E., Phillips, L. A., Nelson, M., McKenna, J., Winges-Yanez, N., Blanchette, L., Croskey, A., Dalton, L.D., Salazar, A., and Swank, P. (2015). Better futures: A randomized field test of a model for supporting young people in foster care with mental health challenges to participate in higher education. *Journal of Behavior Health Services and Research, 42*(2), 150–171.

Greeson, J. K., Thompson, A. E., Evans-Chase, M., and Ali, S. (2015). Child welfare professionals' attitudes and beliefs about child welfare-based natural mentoring for older youth in foster care. *Journal of Social Service Research, 41*(1), 93–112.

Hanson, J. L., Adluru, N., Chung, M. K., Alexander, A. L., Davidson, R. J., and Pollak, S. D. (2013). Early neglect is associated with alterations in white matter integrity and cognitive functioning. *Child Development, 84*(5), 1566–1578.

Institute of Medicine, and National Research Council (IOM and NRC). (2014). *New directions in child abuse and neglect research*. Washington, DC: The National Academies Press.

Juvenile Law Center and Juveniles for Justice. (2018). *Tools for Success: A Toolkit for Child Welfare Professionals to Achieve Permanency and Stability for Youth in Foster Care*. Philadelphia, PA: Juvenile Law Center and Juveniles for Justice. Available: https://jlc.org/sites/default/files/attachments/2019-02/2018-YFCPermanencyToolkit-FINAL-DIGITAL.pdf.

Juvenile Law Center. (2018a). *Failed Policies, Forfeited Futures: A Nationwide Scorecard on Juvenile Records*. Philadelphia, PA: Juvenile Law Center and Juveniles for Justice.

_____. (2018b). *National Extended Foster Care Review: 50-state Survey of Law and Policy*. Philadelphia, PA: Juvenile Law Center and Juveniles for Justice.

Keller, T. E., Cusick, G. R., and Courtney, M. E. (2007). Approaching the transition to adulthood: Distinctive profiles of adolescents aging out of the child welfare system. *Social Service Review, 81*(3), 453–484.

Kemmis-Riggs, J., Dickes, A., and McAloon, J. (2018). Program components of psychosocial interventions in foster and kinship care: A systematic review. *Clinical Child and Family Psychology Review, 21*(1), 13–40.

Kempe, C. H., Silverman, F. N., Steele, B. F., Droegemueller, W., and Silver, H. K. (1962). The battered-child syndrome. *JAMA, 181*, 17–24.

Kerr, D. C. R., Leve, L. D., and Chamberlain, P. (2009). Pregnancy rates among juvenile justice girls in two randomized controlled trials of multidimensional treatment foster care. *Journal of Consulting and Clinical Psychology, 77*(3), 588–593.

Kim, H. K., and Leve, L. D. (2011). Substance use and delinquency among middle school girls in foster care: A three-year follow-up of a randomized controlled trial. *Journal of Consulting and Clinical Psychology, 79*, 740–750.

Kupchik, A., Fagan, J., and Liberman, A. (2003). Punishment, proportionality, and jurisdictional transfer of adolescent offenders: Test of the leniency gap hypothesis. *Stanford Law Policy Review, 14*(1), 57–84.

Leve, L. D., and Chamberlain, P. (2007). A randomized evaluation of Multidimensional Treatment Foster Care: Effects on school attendance and homework completion in juvenile justice girls. *Research on Social Work Practice, 17*(6), 657–663.

Leve, L. D., Harold, G. T., Chamberlain, P., Landsverk, J. A., Fisher, P. A., and Vostanis, P. (2012). Practitioner review: Children in foster care–vulnerabilities and evidence-based interventions that promote resilience processes. *Journal of Child Psychology and Psychiatry, 53*(12), 1197–1211.

Leve, L. D., Kerr, D. C., and Harold, G. T. (2013). Young adult outcomes associated with teen pregnancy among high-risk girls in a randomized controlled trial of multidimensional treatment foster care. *Journal of Child & Adolescent Substance Abuse, 22*(5), 421–434.

McCoy, H., McMillen, J. C., and Spitznagel, E. L. (2008). Older youth leaving the foster care system: Who, what, when, where, and why? *Children and Youth Services Review, 30*(7), 735–745.

McCrory, E., De Brito, S. A., and Viding, E. (2012). The link between child abuse and psychopathology: A review of neurobiological and genetic research. *Journal of the Royal Society of Medicine, 105*(4), 151–156.

National Conference of State Legislatures. (2017). *Extending Foster Care Beyond 18.* Available: http://www.ncsl.org/research/human-services/extending-foster-care-to-18.aspx.

Okpych, N. J., Courtney, M., and Dennis, K. (2017). *Memo from CalYOUTH: Predictors of High School Completion and College Entry at Ages 19/20.* Chicago, IL: Chapin Hall at the University of Chicago.

Oosterman, M., Schuengel, C., Slot, N. W., Bullens, R. A. R., and Doreleijers, T. A. H. (2007). Disruptions in foster care: A review and meta-analysis. *Children and Youth Services Review, 29,* 53–76.

Orton, H. D., Riggs, P. D., and Libby, A.M. (2009). Prevalence and characteristics of depression and substance use in a U.S. child welfare sample. *Children and Youth Services Review, 31*(6), 649–653.

Pechtel, P., and Pizzagalli, D. A. (2011). Effects of early life stress on cognitive and affective function: An integrated review of human literature. *Psychopharmacology (Berlin), 214*(1), 55–70.

Pechtel, P., Lyons-Ruth, K., Anderson, C. M., and Teicher, M. H. (2014). Sensitive periods of amygdala development: The role of maltreatment in preadolescence. *Neuroimage, 97,* 236–244.

Pilowsky, D. J., and Wu, L. T. (2006). Psychiatric symptoms and substance use disorders in a nationally representative sample of American adolescents involved with foster care. *Journal of Adolescent Health, 38*(4), 351–358.

Price, J. M., Chamberlain, P., Landsverk, J., Reid, J. B., Leve, L. D., and Laurent, H. (2008). Effects of a foster parent training intervention on placement changes of children in foster care. *Child Maltreatment, 13,* 64–75.

RTI International. (2008). *Adolescents Involved with Child Welfare: A Transition to Adulthood.* Research Triangle Park, NC: RTI International.

Rubin, D. M., O'Reilly, A. L. R., Luan, X., and Localio, A. R. (2007). The impact of placement stability of behavioral well-being for children in foster care. *Pediatrics, 119,* 336–344.

Ryan, J. P., Herz, D., Hernandez, P. M., and Marshall, J. M. (2007). Maltreatment and delinquency: Investigating child welfare bias in juvenile justice processing. *Children and Youth Services Review, 29*(8), 1035–1050.

Shah, M. F., Liu, Q., Eddy, J. M., Barkan, S., Marshall, D., Mancuso, D., Lucenko, B., and Huber, A. (2016). Predicting homelessness among emerging adults aging out of foster care. *American Journal of Community Psychology, 60*(1-2), 33–43.

Southerland, D., Casanueva, C. E., and Ringeisen, H. (2009). Young adult outcomes and mental health problems among transition-age youth investigated for maltreatment during adolescence. *Children and Youth Services Review, 31*(9), 947–956.

Stotland, E., and Godsoe, C. (2006). The legal status of pregnant and parenting youth in foster care. *University of Florida Journal of Law and Public Policy, 17*(1).

Taussig, H. N., and Culhane, S. E. (2010). Impact of a mentoring and skills group program on mental health outcomes for maltreated children in foster care. *Archives of Pediatrics and Adolescent Medicine, 164,* 739–746.

The Annie E. Casey Foundation. (2011). *Disparities and Disproportionality in Child Welfare: Analysis of the Research – Papers from a Research Symposium Convened by the Center for the Study of Social Policy and the Annie E. Casey Foundation on Behalf of the Alliance for Racial Equity in Child Welfare.* Available: http://www.aecf.org/m/resourcedoc/AECF-DisparitiesAndDisproportionalityInChildWelfare-2011.pdf.

The Pew Charitable Trusts. (2018). *Juveniles in Custody for Noncriminal Acts.* Available: https://www.pewtrusts.org/en/research-and-analysis/data-visualizations/2018/juveniles-in-custody-for-noncriminal-acts?utm_campaign=2018-10-17+Rundown&utm_medium=email&utm_source=Pew.

Torres-García, A., Okpych, N. J., and Courtney, M. E. (2019). *Memo from CalYOUTH: Youths' and Child Welfare Workers' Perceptions of Youths' Educational Preparedness.* Chicago, IL: Chapin Hall at the University of Chicago.

Trickett, P. K., Noll, J. G., Susman, E. J., Shenk, C. E., and Putnam, F. W. (2010). Attenuation of cortisol across development for victims of sexual abuse. *Development and Psychopathology, 22*(1), 165–175.

Turney, K., and Wildeman, C. (2016). Mental and physical health of children in foster care. *Pediatrics, 138*(5).

U.S. Department of Health and Human Services. (2015). *The AFCARS Report.* Washington, DC: U.S. Department of Health and Human Services.

_____. (2018). *The AFCARS Report: Preliminary FY' 2017 Data.* Washington, DC.

Van der Put, C.E., Assink, M., Gubbels, J., and van Solinge, N.F.B. (2018). Identifying effective components of child maltreatment interventions: A meta-analysis. *Clinical Child and Family Psychology Review, 21*(2), 171–202.

Villagrana, M. (2017). Racial/ethnic disparities in mental health service use for older foster youth and foster care alumni. *Child and Adolescent Social Work Journal, 34*(5), 419–429.

Villegas, S., and Pecora, P.J. (2012). Mental health outcomes for adults in family foster care as children: An analysis by ethnicity. *Children and Youth Services Review, 34*(8), 1448–1458.

Westat, Inc. (1991). *A National Evaluation of Title IV-E Foster Care Independent Living Programs for Youth.* Washington, DC: U.S. Department of Health and Human Services.

Wulczyn, F., Hislop, K., and Chen, L. (2007). *Foster Care Dynamics 2000–2005: A Report from the Multistate Foster Care Date Archive.* Chicago, IL: Chapin Hall Center for Children at the University of Chicago.

Zlotnick, C., Tam, T., and Zerger, S. (2012). Common needs but divergent interventions for u.S. Homeless and foster care children: Results from a systematic review. *Health and Social Care in the Community, 20*(5), 449–476.

CHAPTER 9

Abram, K. M., Stokes, M. L., Welty, L. J., Aaby, D. A., and Teplin, L. A. (2017). Disparities in HIV/AIDS risk behaviors after youth leave detention: A 14-year longitudinal study. *Pediatrics, 139*(2).

Agan, A. Y. (2011). Sex offender registries: Fear without function? *The Journal of Law & Economics, 54*(1), 207–239.

Aizer, A., and Doyle, J. J. J. (2015). Juvenile incarceration, human capital, and future crime: Evidence from randomly assigned judges. *Quarterly Journal of Economics, 130*(2), 759–803.

Allen, J. P., Pianta, R. C., Gregory, A., Mikami, A.Y., and Lun, J. (2011). An interaction-based approach to enhancing secondary school instruction and student achievement. *Science, 333*(6045), 1034–1037.

American Academy of Pediatrics. (2011). Policy statement: Health care for youth in the juvenile justice system. *Pediatrics, 128*(6).

American Bar Association. (2018). *School-to-prison pipeline expands with innovative diversion efforts.* Washington, DC: American Bar Association.

American Civil Liberties Union. (2017). *Caged In: Solitary Confinement's Devastating Harm on Prisoners with Physical Disabilities.* New York, NY: American Civil Liberties Union.

Anderson, J. M., Buenaventura, M., and Heaton, P. S. (Forthcoming). The effects of holistic defense on criminal justice outcomes. *Harvard Law Review.*

Annie E. Casey Foundation. (2018). *Implementation of New York's Close to Home Initiative: A New Model for Youth Justice.* Baltimore, MD: The Annie E. Casey Foundation.

Arnett, J. J. (2000). Emerging adulthood: A theory of development from the late teens through the twenties. *American Psychologist, 55*(5), 469–480.

Arnold, D., Dobbie, W., and Yang, C. S. (2018). Racial bias in bail decisions. *Quarterly Journal of Economics, 133*(4), 1885–1932.

Arya, N. (2007). *Jailing Juveniles: The Dangers of Incarcerating Youth in Adult Jails in America.* Washington, DC: Campaign for Youth Justice.

Association of State Correctional Administrators and Yale Law School. (2016). *Aiming to Reduce Time-In-Cell: Reports From Correctional Systems on the Numbers of Prisoners in Restricted Housing and on the Potential of Policy Changes to Bring About Reforms.* Nampa, ID: Association of State Correctional Administrators.

Austin, J., Dedel, K., and Gregoriou, M. (2000). *Juveniles in Adult Prisons and Jails: A National Assessment.* Washington, DC: Bureau of Justice Assistance.

Barnert, E. S., Dudovitz, R., Nelson, B. B., Coker, T. R., Biely, C., Li, N., Chung, P. J. (2017). How does incarcerating young people affect their adult health outcomes? *Pediatrics, 139*(2), 1–9.

Bechtel, K., Lowenkamp, C. T., and Holsinger, A. (2011). Identifying the predictors of pretrial failure: A meta-analysis. *Federal Probation, 75*(2).

Bechtold, J., and Cauffman, E. (2014). Tried as an adult, housed as a juvenile: A tale of youth from two courts incarcerated together. *Law and Human Behavior, 38*(2), 126–138.

Beck, A. J., and Harrison, P. M. (2008). *Sexual Victimization in State and Federal Prisons Reported by Inmates, 2007.* Washington, DC: U.S. Department of Justice, Office of Justice Programs, Bureau of Justice Statistics. Available: https://www.bjs.gov/content/pub/pdf/svsfpri07.pdf.

Beery, A. K., and Kaufer, D. (2014). Stress, social behavior, and resilience: Insights from rodents. *Neurobiology of Stress, 1*, 116–127.

Bishop, D. M., and Frazier, C. (2000). Consequences of transfer. In J. Fagan and F. Zimmerman (Eds.), *The Changing Borders of Juvenile Justice.* Chicago, IL: University of Chicago Press.

Bishop, D. M, Frazier, C. E., Lanza-Kaduce, L., and Winner, L. (1996). The transfer of juveniles to criminal court: Does it make a difference? *Crime & Delinquency, 42*(2), 171–191.

Bureau of Justice Statistics. (2003). *Recidivism of Sex Offenders Released from Prison in 1994.* Washington, DC: U.S. Department of Justice, Office of Justice Programs.

Burke, J. D., Mulvey, E. P., Schubert, C. A., and Garbin, S. R. (2014). The challenge and opportunity of parental involvement in juvenile justice services. *Children and Youth Services Review, 39*, 39–47.

Burke, K. (2005). All grown up: Juveniles incarcerated in adult facilities. *Journal of Juvenile Law, 25*, 69–78.

Casey, B. J. (2015). Beyond simple models of self-control to circuit-based accounts of adolescent behavior. *Annual Review of Psychology, 66*, 295–319.

Cauffman, E., Lexcen, F. J., Goldweber, A., Shulman, E. P., and Grisso, T. (2007). Gender differences in mental health symptoms among delinquent and community youth. *Youth Violence and Juvenile Justice, 5,* 287–307.

Cauffman, E., Fine, A., Mahler, A., Simmons, C. (2018). How developmental science influences juvenile justice reform. *UC Irvine Law Review, 8*(10), 21–40.

Cavanagh, C., and Cauffman, E. (2017). What they don't know can hurt them: Mothers' legal knowledge of youth reoffending. *Psychology, Public Policy, & Law, 23,* 141–153.

Center for Substance Abuse Treatment. (2000) *Comprehensive Case Management for Substance Abuse Treatment. Treatment Improvement Protocol (TIP) Series, No. 27.* HHS Publication No. (SMA) 15-4215. Rockville, MD: Center for Substance Abuse Treatment.

Chaffin, M. (2008). Our minds are made up—don't confuse us with the facts: Commentary on policies concerning children with sexual behavior problems and juvenile sex offenders. *Child Maltreatment, 13*(2), 110–121.

Chein, J. M., Albert, D., O'Brien, L., Uckert, K., and Steinberg, L. (2011). Peers increase adolescent risk taking by enhancing activity in the brain's reward circuitry. *Developmental Science, 14*(2), F1–F10.

Child Trends. (2018). *Key Facts about Juvenile Incarceration.* Available: https://www.childtrends.org/indicators/juvenile-detention.

Circuit Court of Cook County Illinois. (2018). *Juvenile Temporary Detention Center Performance Measures and Population Statistics.* Available: http://www.cookcountycourt.org/ABOUTTHECOURT/OfficeoftheChiefJudge/JuvenileTemporaryDetentionCenter/PerformanceReports.aspx.

Coffey, O. D., and Gemignani, M. G. (1994). *Effective Practices in Juvenile Correctional Education: A Study of the Literature and Research, 1980-1992.* Washington, DC: U.S. Department of Justice, Office of Justice Programs, Office of Juvenile Justice and Delinquency Prevention.

Cook, P. J., and Laub, J. H. (1998). The unprecedented epidemic in youth violence. *Crime and Justice, 24,* 27–64.

Côté, J. E. (2014). The dangerous myth of emerging adulthood: An evidence-based critique of a flawed developmental theory. *Applied Developmental Science, 18*(4), 177–188.

Council of Juvenile Correctional Administrators. (2015). *Toolkit: Reducing the Use of Isolation.* Available: http://cjca.net/attachments/article/751/CJCA%20Toolkit%20Reducing%20the%20Use%20of%20Isolation.pdf.

Dank, M., Yu, L., Pelletier, J., Mora, M., and Conner, B. (2015). *Locked: Interactions with the Criminal Justice and Child Welfare Systems for LGBTQ Youth, YMSM, and YWSW Who Engage in Survival Sex.* Washington, DC: The Urban Institute.

Davies, H. J., and Davidson, H. A. (2001). *Parental Involvement Practices of Juvenile Courts.* Report to the Office of Juvenile Justice and Delinquency Prevention. Washington, DC: U.S. Department of Justice.

Davis, K. (2018). OJJDP Head Caren Harp wants to rebalance system from focus on "therapeutic intervention." *Juvenile Justice Information Exchange.* Available: https://jjie.org/2018/03/22/ojjdp-head-caren-harp-wants-to-rebalance-system-from-focus-on-therapeutic-intervention.

Dawes, R. M. (1971). A case study of graduate admissions: Application of three principles of human decision making. *American Psychologist, 26*(2), 180–188.

_____. (1979). The robust beauty of improper linear models in decision making. *American Psychologist, 34*(7), 571–582.

Dawes, R. M., Faust, D., and Meehl, P. E. (1989). Clinical versus actuarial judgement. *Science, 243,* 1668–1674.

DeLone, M. A., and DeLone, G. J. (2017). Racial disparities in juvenile justice processing. In C. J. Schreck (Ed.), *The Encyclopedia of Juvenile Delinquency and Justice*. Hoboken, NJ: Wiley & Sons, Inc.

DiClemente, R. J., and Wingood, G. M. (2017). Changing risk trajectories and health outcomes for vulnerable adolescents: Reclaiming the future. *Pediatrics, 139*(2).

Dmitrieva, J., Monahan, K. C., Cauffman, E., and Steinberg, L. (2012). Arrested development: The effects of incarceration on the development of psychosocial maturity. *Developmental Psychopathology, 24*(3), 1073–1090.

Durnan, J. Olsen, R., and Harvell, S. (2018). *State-led Juvenile Justice Systems Improvement: Implementation Progress and Early Outcomes*. Washington, DC: Urban Institute. Available: https://www.urban.org/sites/default/files/publication/98321/state-led_juvenile_justice_systems_improvement_3.pdf.

Durose, M. R., Cooper, A. D., and Snyder, H. N. (2014). *Recidivism of Prisoners Released in 30 States in 2005: Patterns from 2005 to 2010*. Washington, DC: U.S. Department of Justice, Office of Justice Programs, Bureau of Justice Statistics.

Engel, M., Jacob, B. A., and Curran, F. C. (2014). New evidence on teacher labor supply. *American Educational Research Journal, 51*(1), 36–72.

Fabelo, T., Thompson, M. D., Plotkin, M., Carmichael, D., Marchbanks, M. P., and Booth, E. A. (2011). *Breaking Schools' Rules: A Statewide Study of How School Discipline Relates to Students' Success and Juvenile Justice Involvement*. New York, NY: Council of State Governments Justice Center, Public Policy Research Institute. Available: https://knowledgecenter.csg.org/kc/system/files/Breaking_School_Rules.pdf.

Fader, J., Kurlychek, M. C., and Morgan, K. A. (2014). The color of juvenile justice: Racial disparities in dispositional decisions. *Social Science Research, 44*, 126–140.

Feierman, J., Keller, E.C., Glickman, M., and Stanton, R. (2011). *Navigating the Juvenile Justice System in Pennsylvania: A Guide for Parents and Guardians*. Philadelphia, PA: Juvenile Law Center.

Feierman, J., Goldstein, N., Haney-Caron, E., and Columbo, J. F. (2016) *Debtors' Prison for Kids? The High Cost of Fines and Fees in the Juvenile Justice System*. Philadelphia, PA: Juvenile Law Center.

Feierman, J., Lindell, K. U., and Eaddy, N. (2017). *Unlocking Youth: Legal Strategies to End Solitary Confinement in Juvenile Facilities*. Philadelphia, PA: Juvenile Law Center.

Feld, B. C. (1989). Right to counsel in juvenile court: An empirical study of when lawyers appear and the difference they make. *Journal of Criminal Law and Criminology, 79*.

Feld, B. C. (2003). Race, politics, and juvenile justice: The Warren court and the conservative "backlash." *Minnesota Law Review, 87*(5), 1447–1578.

Feld, B. C. (2006). Police interrogation of juveniles: An empirical study of policy and practice. *Journal of Criminal Law and Criminology, 97*.

Fine, A., and Cauffman, E. (2015). Race and justice system attitude formation during the transition to adulthood. *Journal of Development and Life-Course Criminology, 1*, 325.

Flores, A. W., Bechtel, K., and Lowenkamp, C. T. (2016). False positives, false negatives, and false analyses: A rejoinder to "machine bias: There's software used across the country to predict future criminals. And it's biased against Blacks." *Federal Probation, 80*(2).

Gaitan, D. D. (2004). *Involving Latino Families in Schools: Raising Student Achievement Through Home-School Partnerships*. Thousand Oaks, CA: Corwin Press.

Glowa-Kollisch, S., Kaba, F., Waters, A., Leung, Y. J., Ford, E., and Venters, H. (2016). From punishment to treatment: The "clinical alternative to punitive segregation" (CAPS) program in New York City jails. *International Journal of Environmental Research and Public Health, 13*(2), 182.

Goel, S., Shroff, R., Skeem, J. L., and Slobogin, C. (2019). The accuracy, equity, and juris- prudence of criminal risk assessment. *SSRN Electronic Journal.* Available: https://papers. ssrn.com/sol3/papers.cfm?abstract_id=3306723.

Goodwin-De Faria, C., and Marinos, V. (2012). Youth understanding and assertion of legal rights: Examining the roles of age and power. *International Journal of Children's Rights, 20,* 343–364.

Grassian, S. (2006). Psychiatric effects of solitary confinement. *Washington University Journal of Law and Policy, 22,* 325–383.

Grisso, T. (1980). Juveniles' capacities to waive Miranda rights: An empirical analysis. *California Law Review, 68*(6), 1134–1166.

_____. (1981). *Juveniles' Waiver of Rights: Legal and Psychological Competence.* New York, NY: Plenum Press.

_____. (2004). *Double Jeopardy: Adolescent Offenders with Mental Disorders.* Chicago, IL: University of Chicago Press.

Grisso, T., Steinberg, L., Woolard, J., Cauffman, E., Scott, E., Graham, S., Lexcen, F., Reppucci, N.D., and Schwartz, R. (2003). Juveniles' competence to stand trial: A comparison of adolescents' and adults' capacities as trial defendants. *Law and Human Behavior, 27*(4), 333–363.

Grove, W. M., Zald, D. H., Lebow, B. S., Snitz, B. E., and Nelson, C. (2000). Clinical versus mechanical prediction: A meta-analysis. *Psychological Assessment, 12*(1), 19–30.

Guassi Moreira, J. F., Tashjian, S. M., Galván, A., and Silvers, J. A. (2018). Parents versus peers: Assessing the impact of social agents on decision making in young adults. *Psychological Science, 29*(9), 1526–1539.

Gupta-Kagan, J. (Forthcoming). The intersection between young adult sentencing and mass incarceration. *Wisconsin Law Review, 2018*(4).

Hager, E. (2015). *Our Prisons in Black and White: The Race Gap for Adults Is Shrinking. Why Is It Widening for Juveniles?* Available: https://www.themarshallproject.org/2015/11/18/ our-prisons-in-black-and-white.

Hahn, R., McGowan, A., Liberman, A., Crosby, A., Fullilove, M., Johnson, R., Moscicki, E., Price, L., Snyder, S., Tuma, F., Lowy, J., Briss, P., Cory, S., and Stone, G. (2007). Effects on violence of laws and policies facilitating the transfer of youth from the juvenile to the adult justice system: A report on recommendations of the Task Force on Community Preventive Services. *MMWR: Recommendations and Reports, 56*(RR09), 1-11. Available: https://www.cdc.gov/mmwr/preview/mmwrhtml/rr5609a1.htm.

Haney, C. (2003). Mental health issues in long-term solitary and "supermax" confinement. *Crime & Delinquency, 49*(1), 124–156.

Hansen, B., and Waddell, G. (2014). *Walk Like a Man: Do Juvenile Offenders Respond to Being Tried as Adults.* Unpublished Manuscript, University of Oregon, Eugene.

Hanson, R. K., Harris, A. J. R., Helmus, L., Thornton, D. (2014). High-risk sex offenders may not be high risk forever. *Journal of Interpersonal Violence, 29*(15), 2792–2813.

Harcourt, B. E. (2015). Risk as a proxy for race. *The Dangers of Risk Assessment, 27*(4), 237–243.

Harding, N. N. (2006). Ethnic and social class similarities and differences in mothers' beliefs about kindergarten preparation. *Race, Ethnicity and Education, 9*(2), 223–237.

Harris, A. (2016). *A Pound of Flesh: Monetary Sanctions as Punishment for the Poor.* New York, NY: Russell Sage Foundation.

Hayek, C. (2016). *Environmental Scan of Developmentally Appropriate Criminal Justice Responses to Justice-Involved Young Adults.* Washington, DC: U.S. Department of Justice, Office of Justice Programs, National Institute of Justice.

Heller, S. B., Shah, A. K., Guryan, J., Ludwig, J., Mullainathan, S., and Pollack, H. A. (2017). Thinking, fast and slow? Some field experiments to reduce crime and dropout in Chicago. *Quarterly Journal of Economics, 132*(1), 1-54.

Higgins, L. (2010, February 11). Error was made during 2003 sex offense conviction of Matthew Freeman, attorney claims in motion. *The Ann Arbor News.* Available: http://www.annarbor.com/news/error-wasmade-during-2003-conviction-of-matthew-freeman-attorney-claims-inmotion.

Hockenberry, S., Wachter, A., and Sladky, A. (2016). *Juvenile Residential Facility Census, 2014: Selected Findings.* Washington, DC: U.S. Department of Justice, Office of Justice Programs, Office of Juvenile Justice and Delinquency Prevention.

Hoeve, M., Blokland, A., Dubas, J. S., Loeber, R., Gerris, J. R., and van der Laan, P. H. (2008). Trajectories of delinquency and parenting styles. *Journal of Abnormal Child Psychology, 36,* 223–235.

Hoeve, M., Dubas, J. S., Eischelsheim, V. I., van der Lann, P. H., Smeenk, W., and Gerris, J. R. (2009). The relationship between parenting and delinquency: A meta-analysis. *Journal of Abnormal Child Psychology, 37,* 749–775.

Holloway, S. D., Rambaud, M. F., Fuller, B., and Eggers-Piérola, C. (1995). What is "appropriate practice" at home and in child care? Low-income mothers' views on preparing their children for school. *Early Childhood Research Quarterly, 10,* 451–473.

Human Rights Watch. (2013). *Raised on the Registry: The Irreparable Harm of Placing Children on Sex Offender Registries in the US.* Washington, DC: Human Rights Watch.

Hunt, J., and Moodie-Mills, A. (2012). *The Unfair Criminalization of Gay and Transgender Youth: An Overview of the Experiences of LGBT Youth in the Juvenile Justice System.* Washington, DC: Center for American Progress.

Hurst, Y. G., Frank, J., and Browning, S. L. (2000). The attitudes of juveniles toward the police: A comparison of Black and White youth. *Policing: An International Journal, 23*(1), 37–53.

Hyer, M. M., and Glasper E. R. (2017) Separation increases passive stress-coping behaviors during forced swim and alters hippocampal dendritic morphology in California mice. *PLoS ONE 12*(4), e0175713.

Icenogle, G., Steinberg, L., Duell, N., Chein, J., Chang, L., Chaudhary, N., Di Giunta, L., Dodge, K. A., Fanti, K. A., Lansford, J. E., Oburu, P., Pastorelli, C., Skinner, A. T., Sorbing, E., Tapanya, S., Uribe Tirado, L. M., Alampaya, L. P., Al-Hassan, S. M., Takash, H. M. S., and Bacchini, D. (2019). Adolescents' cognitive capacity reaches adult levels prior to their psychosocial maturity: Evidence for a "maturity gap" in a multinational, cross-sectional sample. *Law and Human Behavior, 43*(1), 69–85.

Institute of Medicine and National Research Council. (2001). *Juvenile Crime, Juvenile Justice.* Washington, DC: National Academy Press.

_____. (2015). *Investing in the Health and Well-Being of Young Adults.* Washington, DC: The National Academies Press.

Irvine, A., and Canfield, A. (2016). The overrepresentation of lesbian, gay, bisexual, questioning, gender nonconforming and transgender youth within the child welfare to juvenile justice crossover population. *Journal of Gender, Social Policy, and the Law, 24*(2).

Jacob, B. A. (2007). The challenges of staffing urban schools with effective teachers. *Future of Children, 17*(1), 129–153.

Jennings, W. G., Piquero, A. R., and Hays, S. (2009). Investigating the continuity of sex offending: Evidence from the second philadelphia birth cohort. *Justice Quarterly, 26*(1), 58–76.

Jennings, W. G., Piquero, A. R., Zimring, F. E., and Reingle, J. M. (2015). Assessing the conti-
nuity of sex offending over the life course: Evidence from two large birth cohort studies.
In A. Blokland and P. Lussier (Eds.), *Sex Offenders: A Criminal Career Approach*.
Hoboken, NJ: John Wiley & Sons, Ltd.

Joint Criminal Justice Reform Committee. (2014). *Joint Criminal Justice Reform Committee
Final Report*. Springfield, IL: Illinois General Assembly.

Juvenile Law Center. (2014a). *Failed Policies, Forfeited Futures: A Nationwide Scorecard on
Juvenile Records*. Philadelphia, PA: Juvenile Law Center.

_____. (2014b). *Juvenile Records: A National Review of State Laws on Confidentiality, Seal-
ing, and Expungement*. Philadelphia, PA: Juvenile Law Center.

_____. (2016). *Future Interrupted: The Collateral Damage Caused by Proliferation of Juve-
nile Records*. Philadelphia, PA: Juvenile Law Center.

_____. (2018a). *Broken Bridges: How Juvenile Placements Cut Off Youth From Communities
And Successful Futures*. Philadelphia, PA: Juvenile Law Center.

_____. (2018b). *Failed Policies, Forfeited Futures: A Nationwide Scorecard on Juvenile Records*
Available: https://juvenilerecords.jlc.org/juvenilerecords/#!/map.

Kahneman, D. (2011). *Thinking, Fast and Slow*. New York, NY: Farrar, Straus and Giroux.

Kleinberg, J., Lakkaraju, H., Leskovec, J., Ludwig, J., and Mullainathan, S. (2018). Human
decisions and machine predictions. *Quarterly Journal of Economics, 133*(1), 237–293.

Kleinberg, J., Ludwig, J., Mullainathan, S., and Sunstein, C. R. (2019). *Discrimination in the Age
of Algorithms*. Available: https://papers.ssrn.com/sol3/papers.cfm?abstract_id=3329669.

Lehmann, P. S., Chiricos, T., and Bales, W. D. (2017). Sentencing transferred juveniles in the
adult criminal court: The direct and interactive effects of race and ethnicity. *Youth Violence and Juvenile Justice, 15*(2), 172–190.

Letourneau, E. J., Levenson, J. S., Bandyopadhyay, D., Sinha, D., and Armstrong, K. S. (2010).
Effects of South Carolina's sex offender registration and notification policy on adult
recidivism. *Criminal Justice Policy Review, 21*(4), 435–458.

Levenson, J. S., and Cotter, L. P. (2005). The effect of Megan's Law on sex offender reintegra-
tion. *Journal of Contemporary Criminal Justice, 21*(1), 49–66.

Listenbee, R. L., Torre, J., Boyle, G., Cooper, S. W., Deer, S., Durfee, D. T., James, T.,
Lieberman, A., Macy, R., Marans, S., McDonnell, J., Mendoza, G., and Taguba, A.
(2012). *Report of the Attorney General's National Task Force on Children Exposed to
Violence*. Washington, DC: U.S. Department of Justice, Office of Justice Programs, Office
of Juvenile Justice and Delinquency Prevention.

Lobel, J., and Akil, H. (2018). Law and neuroscience: The case of solitary confinement.
Daedalus, the Journal of the American Academy of Arts & Sciences, 147(4), 61–75.

Loeber, R., Farrington, D. P., and Petechuk, D. (2013). *Bulletin 1: From Juvenile Delinquency
to Young Adult Offending*. Washington, DC: U.S. Department of Justice.

Loeffler, C. E., and Chalfin, A. (2017). Estimating the crime effects of raising the age of majority. *Criminology & Public Policy, 16*(1), 45–71.

Loeffler, C. E., and Grunwald, B. (2015). Decriminalizing delinquency: The effect of raising
the age of majority on juvenile recidivism. *Journal of Legal Studies, 44*(2).

Lowenstein Center for the Public Interest. (2016). *Jurisdiction Survey of Juvenile Solitary
Confinement Rules in Juvenile Justice Systems*. Available: https://www.lowenstein.com/
pro-bono/pro-bono-briefs.

Luna, B., Padmanabhan, A., and O'Hearn, K. (2010). What has fMRI told us about the development of cognitive control through adolescence? *Brain and Cognition, 72*, 101–113.

MacArthur Foundation. (2015). *Juvenile Justice in a Developmental Framework: A 2015 Status
Report*. Chicago, IL: MacArthur Foundation. Available: http://www.modelsforchange.net/
publications/787.

Macomber, D., Skiba, T., Blackmon, J., Esposito, E., Hart, L., Mambrino, E., Richie, T., and Grigorenko, E. L. (2010). Education in juvenile detention facilities in the state of Connecticut: A glance at the system. *Journal of Correctional Education (Glen Mills)*, 61(3), 223–261.

Majd, K., Marksamer, J., and Reyes, C. (2009). *Hidden Injustice: Lesbian, Gay, Bisexual, And Transgender Youth In Juvenile Courts*. San Francisco, CA: National Juvenile Defender Center and National Center for Lesbian Rights.

Matthews, S., Schiraldi, V., and Chester, L. (2018). Youth justice in Europe: Experience of Germany, the Netherlands, and Croatia in providing developmentally appropriate responses to emerging adults in the criminal justice system. *Justice Evaluation Journal*, 1(1), 59–81.

McCormick, E. M., Qu, Y., and Telzer, E. H. (2016). Adolescent neurodevelopment of cognitive control and risk-taking in negative family contexts. *Neuroimage, 124*(Pt A), 989–996.

Mears, D. P., and Cochran, J. C. (2015). Mass incarceration and prisoner reentry: A problem that will not go away. *Academy of Criminal Justice Sciences Today 40*, 1, 4–10.

Mears, D. P., and Travis, J. (2004). *The Dimensions, Pathways, and Consequences of Youth Reentry*. Washington, DC: Urban Institute.

Medendorp, W. E., Petersen, E. D., Pal, A., Wagner, L. M., Myers, A. R., Hochgeschwender, U., and Jenrow, K. A. (2018). Altered behavior in mice socially isolated during adolescence corresponds with immature dendritic spine morphology and impaired plasticity in the prefrontal cortex. *Frontiers in Behavioral Neuroscience, 12*, 87.

Meehl, P. E. (1954). *Clinical Versus Statistical Prediction: A Theoretical Analysis and a Review of the Evidence*. Minneapolis, MN: University of Minnesota Press.

Mercado, C. C., Alvarez, S., and Levenson, J. (2008). The impact of specialized sex offender legislation on community reentry. *Sex Abuse, 20*(2), 188–205.

Miner-Romanoff, K. (2014). Juvenile offenders tried as adults: what they know and implications for practitioners. *Northern Kentucky Law Review, 41*, 205–224.

Moffitt, T. E. (1993). Adolescence-limited and life-course-persistent antisocial behavior: A developmental taxonomy. *Psychological Review, 100*(4), 674–701.

Monahan, K. C., Goldweber, A., and Cauffman, E. (2010). The effects of visitation on incarcerated juvenile offenders: How contact with the outside impacts adjustment on the inside. *Law and Human Behavior, 35*(2), 143–151.

Moran, M. (2014). AMA votes to oppose solitary confinement of juveniles. *Psychiatric News: Newspaper of the American Psychiatric Association, 49*(24).

Morgan, E., Salomon, N., Plotkin, M., and Cohen, R. (2014). *The School Discipline Consensus Report: Strategies from the Field to Keep Students Engaged in School and out of the Juvenile Justice System*. New York, NY: Council of State Governments Justice Center. Available: http://csgjusticecenter.org/wp-content/uploads/2014/06/The_School_Discipline_Consensus_Report.pdf.

Mulvey, E. P., and Schubert, C. (2011). Youth in prison and beyond. In B. C. Feld and D. M. Bishop (Eds.), *Oxford Handbook on Juvenile Crime and Juvenile Justice*. New York, NY: Oxford University Press.

_____. (2012). Some initial findings and policy implications of the pathways to desistance study. *Victims & Offenders, 7*(4), 407–427.

Mulvey, E. P., Schubert, C. A., and Piquero, A. (2014). *Pathways to Desistance: Summary Technical Report*. Washington, DC: U.S. Department of Justice.

Nagin, D. S., and Telep, C.W. (2017). Procedural justice and legal compliance. *Annual Review of Law and Social Science, 13*(1), 5–28.

Najdowski, C. J., Cleary, H. M. D, and Stevenson, M. C. (2016). Adolescent sex offender registration policy: Perspectives on general deterrence potential from criminology and developmental psychology. *Psychology, Public Policy, and Law, 22*(1), 114–125.

National Academies of Sciences, Engineering, and Medicine. (2018). *Proactive Policing: Effects on Crime and Communities.* Washington, DC: The National Academies Press. Available: https://www.nap.edu/catalog/24928/proactive-policing-effects-on-crime-and-communities.

National Center for Education Statistics. (2018). Spotlight 1: Prevalence, type, and responsibilities of security staff in k–12 public schools. *Indicators of School Crime and Safety.* Available: https://nces.ed.gov/programs/crimeindicators/ind_S01.asp.

National Center for Juvenile Justice. (2017). *Easy Access to the Census of Juveniles in Residential Placement: 1997-2015.* Available: https://www.ojjdp.gov/ojstatbb/ezacjrp/asp/selection.asp.

National Center for Mental Health and Juvenile Justice. (2007). *Trauma Among Youth in the Juvenile Justice System: Critical Issues and New Directions.* New York, NY: National Center for Mental Health and Juvenile Justice.

National Conference of State Legislatures. (2018). *Juvenile Justice 2017 Year-end Report.* Available: http://www.ncsl.org/research/civil-and-criminal-justice/juvenile-justice-2017-year-end-report.aspx.

_____. (2019a). Juvenile justice bills tracking database. Available: http://www.ncsl.org/research/civil-and-criminal-justice/ncsls-juvenile-justice-bill-tracking-database.aspx.

_____. (2019b, January 11). *Juvenile Age of Jurisdiction and Transfer to Adult Court Laws.* Available: http://www.ncsl.org/research/civil-and-criminal-justice/juvenile-age-of-jurisdiction-and-transfer-to-adult-court-laws.aspx.

National Council of Juvenile and Family Court Judges. (2016). *Resolution Regarding Reducing the Use of Solitary Confinement for Youth.* Reno, NV: National Council of Juvenile and Family Court Judges.

National Council on Crime and Delinquency. (2007). *And Justice for Some: Differential Treatment of Youth of Color in the Justice System.* Oakland, CA: National Council on Crime and Delinquency.

National Institute of Justice. (2016). *Restrictive Housing in the U.S.: Issues, Challenges, and Future Directions.* Washington, DC: U.S. Department of Justice, Office of Justice Programs.

National Juvenile Defender Center. (2016). *Defend Children: A Blueprint for Effective Juvenile Defender Services.* Washington, DC: National Juvenile Defender Center.

National Research Council. (2013). *Reforming Juvenile Justice: A Developmental Approach.* Washington, DC: The National Academies Press.

_____. (2014a). *The Growth of Incarceration in the United States: Exploring Causes and Consequences.* Washington, DC: The National Academies Press.

_____. (2014b). *Implementing Juvenile Justice Reform: The Federal Role.* Washington, DC: The National Academies Press.

Office of Juvenile Justice and Delinquency Prevention. (1997). *Juvenile Justice Reform Initiatives in the States: 1994-1996.* Available: https://www.ojjdp.gov/pubs/reform/preface.html.

_____. (2012). *Report of the Attorney General's National Task Force on Children Exposed to Violence.* Washington, DC: U.S. Department of Justice.

Pajer, K. A., Kelleher, K., Gupta, R. A., Rolls, J., and Gardner, W. (2007). Psychiatric and medical health care policies in juvenile detention facilities. *Journal of the American Academy of Child and Adolescent Psychiatry, 46*(12), 1660–1667.

Peck, J. H. (2015). Minority perceptions of the police: A state-of-the-art review. *Policing: An International Journal of Police Strategies and Management, 38*(1), 173–203.

Perker, S. S., and Chester, L. (2017). *Emerging Adults: A Distinct Population That Calls for an Age-Appropriate Approach by the Justice System*. Cambridge, MA: Program in Criminal Justice Policy and Management.

Piquero, A. R. (2008). Disproportionate minority contact. *Future of Children, 18*(2), 59–79.

Piquero, A. R., and Jennings, W. G. (2017). Research note: Justice system-imposed financial penalties increase the likelihood of recidivism in a sample of adolescent offenders. *Youth Violence and Juvenile Justice, 15*(3), 325–340.

Potter, C. C., and Jenson, J. M. (2003). Cluster profiles of multiple problem youth: Mental health problem symptoms, substance use, and delinquent conduct. *Criminal Justice and Behavior, 30*, 230–250.

Rademacher, E. M. (2016). The beginning of the end: Using Ohio's plan to eliminate juvenile solitary confinement as a model for statutory elimination of juvenile solitary confinement. *William & Mary Law Review, 57*(3).

Redding, R. E. (2008). Juvenile transfer laws: An effective deterrent to delinquency? *Juvenile Justice Bulletin*. Available: https://works.bepress.com/richard_redding/6/.

Redding, R. E., and Fuller, E. J. (2004). What do juvenile offenders know about being tried as adults? Implications for deterrence. *Juvenile and Family Court Journal, 55*, 35–44.

Ricks, A., and Esthappan, S. (2018). *States Are Looking Beyond the Juvenile Justice System to Address School Truancy*. Available: https://www.urban.org/urban-wire/states-are-looking-beyond-juvenile-justice-system-address-school-truancy.

Rocque, M., Serwick, A., and Plummer-Beale, J. (2017). Offender rehabilitation and reentry during emerging adulthood. In L. M. Padilla-Walker and L. J. Nelson (Eds.), *Flourishing in Emerging Adulthood: Positive Development During the Third Decade of Life*. Oxford, United Kingdom: Oxford University Press.

Rogers, T., and Feller, A. (2018). Reducing student absences at scale by targeting parents' misbeliefs. *Nature Human Behaviour, 2*(5), 335–342.

Rozzell, L. (2013). *The Role of Family Engagement in Creating Trauma-informed Juvenile Justice Systems*. Los Angeles, CA: National Center for Child Traumatic Stress.

Sample, L. L., and Bray, T. M. (2006). Are sex offenders different? An examination of rearrest patterns. *Criminal Justice Policy Review, 17*(1), 83–102.

Sampson, R. J., and Wilson, W. J. (1995). Toward a theory of race, crime, and urban inequality. In J. Hagan and R. D. Peterson (Eds.), *Crime and Inequality* (pp. 37–54). Stanford, CA: Stanford University Press.

Sampson, R. J., Wilson, W. J., and Katz, H. (2018). Reassessing "Toward a Theory of Race, Crime, and Urban Inequality": Enduring and new challenges in 21st century America. *DuBois Review: Social Science Research on Race, 15*(1), 13–34.

Sandler, J. C., Letourneau, E. J., Vandiver, D. M., Shields, R. T., and Chaffin, M. (2017). Juvenile sexual crime reporting rates are not influenced by juvenile sex offender registration policies. *Psychology, Public Policy, and Law, 23*(2), 131–140.

Schiraldi, V., Western, B., and Bradner, K. (2015). *Community-based Responses to Justice-Involved Young Adults*. Washington, DC: U.S. Department of Justice, National Insitute of Justice.

Scott, E. S., Bonnie, R. J., and Steinberg, L. (2016). Young adulthood as a transitional legal category: Science, social change, and justice policy. *Fordham Law Review, 85(641)*. Available: https://ir.lawnet.fordham.edu/flr/vol85/iss2/12.

Scott, E. S., and Grisso, T. (1997). The evolution of adolescence: A developmental perspective on juvenile justice reform. *The Journal of Criminal Law and Criminology, 88*(1).

Sedlak, A .J., and McPherson, K. S. (2010). *Conditions of Confinement: Findings from the Survey of Youth in Residential Placement*. Washington, DC: U.S. Department of Justice, Office of Justice Programs, Office of Juvenile Justice and Delinquency Prevention.

Sharkey, P. (2010). The acute effect of local homicides on children's cognitive performance. *Proceedings of the National Academy of Sciences of the United States of America, 107*(26), 11733–11738.

Sharkey, P., and Elwert, F. (2011). The legacy of disadvantage: Multigenerational neighborhood effects on cognitive ability. *American Journal of Sociology, 116*(6), 1934–1981.

Sharkey, P., and Faber, J. W. (2014). Where, when, why, and for whom do residential contexts matter? Moving away from the dichotomous understanding of neighborhood effects. *Annual Review of Sociology, 40*(1), 559–579.

Sharkey, P., Schwartz, A. E., Ellen, I. G., and Lacoe, J. (2014). High stakes in the classroom, high stakes on the street: The effects of community violence on students' standardized test performance. *Sociological Science, 1*, 199–220.

Sickmund, M., Sladky, A., and Kang, W. (2014). *Easy Access to Juvenile Court Statistics: 1985–2011.* Washington, D.C.: U.S. Department of Justice, Office of Juvenile Justice and Delinquency Prevention.

Steinberg, L. (2014). *Age of Opportunity: Lessons from the New Science of Adolescence.* New York: First Mariner Books.

_____. (2017). Adolescent brain science and juvenile justice policymaking. *American Psychological Association, 23*(4), 410–420.

Steinberg, L., and Monahan, K. C. (2007). Age differences in resistance to peer influence. *Developmental Psychology, 43*(6), 1531–1543.

Steinberg, L., Albert, D., Cauffman, E., Banich, M., Graham, S., and Woolard, J. (2008). Age differences in sensation seeking and impulsivity as indexed by behavior and self-report: Evidence for a dual systems model. *Developmental Psychology, 44*(6), 1764–1778.

Stevens, M. C., Kiehl, K. A., Pearlson, G. D., and Calhoun, V. D. (2007). Functional neural networks underlying response inhibition in adolescents and adults. *Behavioural Brain Research, 181*, 12–22.

Task Force on Community Preventive Services. (2007). Recommendation against policies facilitating the transfer of juveniles from juvenile to adult justice systems for the purpose of reducing violence. *American Journal of Preventive Medicine, 32*(4), 5–6.

Teplin, L. A., Abram, K. M., McClelland, G. M., Dulcan, M. K., and Mericle, A. A. (2002). Psychiatric disorders in youth in juvenile detention. *Archives of General Psychiatry, 59*(12), 1133–1143.

Tewksbury, R., and Lees, M. (2006). Perceptions of sex offender registration: Collateral consequences and community experiences. *Sociological Spectrum, 26*(3), 309–334.

The Pew Charitable Trusts. (2015). *Re-examining Juvenile Incarceration: High Cost, Poor Outcomes Spark Shift to Alternatives.* Baltimore, MD: The Pew Charitable Trusts.

The White House. (2016). *Fact Sheet: Department of Justice Review of Solitary Confinement.* Available: https://obamawhitehouse.archives.gov/the-press-office/2016/01/25/fact-sheet-department-justice-review-solitary-confinement.

Tottenham, N., and Galván, A. (2016). Stress and the adolescent brain: Amygdala-prefrontal cortex circuitry and ventral striatum as developmental targets. *Neuroscience and Biobehavioral Reviews, 70*, 217–227.

Travis III L. F., and Coon, J. K. (2005). *The Role of Law Enforcement in Public School Safety: A National Survey.* Center for Criminal Justice Research, University of Cincinnati.

Tyler, T. R. (1990). *Why People Obey the Law.* New Haven, CT: Yale University Press.

U.S. Commission on Civil Rights. (2017). *Targeted Fines and Fees Against Low-Income Communities of Color: Civil Rights and Constitutional Implications.* Washington, DC: The U.S. Commission on Civil Rights.

U.S. Department of Justice. (2018). *OJJDP Statistical Briefing Book.* Available: https://www.ojjdp.gov/ojstatbb/crime/JAR_Display.asp?ID=qa05200.

Urban Institute. (2014). *Juvenile Justice Pay for Success Initiative.* Available: https://pfs.urban. org/pfs-project-fact-sheets/content/juvenile-justice-pay-success-initiative.

Vermeiren, R., Jespers, I., and Moffitt, T. (2006). Mental health problems in juvenile justice populations. *Child and Adolescent Psychiatric Clinics of North America, 15*(2), 333–351, vii–viii.

Vidal, S., and Woolard, J. (2016). Parents' perception of juvenile probation: Relationship and interaction with juvenile probation officers, parent strategies, and youth's compliance on probation. *Children and Youth Services Review, 66,* 1–8.

Viljoen, J. L., Klaver, J., and Roesch, R. (2005). Legal decisions of preadolescent and adolescent defendants: Predictors of confessions, pleas, communication with attorneys, and appeals. *Law and Human Behavior, 29*(3), 253–277.

Welborn, B. L., Lieberman, M. D., Goldenberg, D., Fuligni, A. J., Galván, A., and Telzer, E. H. (2016). *Social Cognitive and Affective Neuroscience, 11*(1), 100–109.

Wilson, B. D. M., Jordan, S. P., Meyer, I. H., Flores, A. R., Stemple, L., and Herman, J. L. (2017). Disproportionality and disparities among sexual minority youth in custody. *Journal of Youth Adolescence, 46*(7), 1547–1561.

Winner, L, Lanza-Kaduce, L., Bishop, D. M., and Frazier, C. E. (1997). The transfer of juveniles to criminal court: Reexamining recidivism over the long term. *Crime and Delinquency, 43*(4), 548–563.

Woolard, J. L., Cleary, H. M. D., Harvell, S. A. S., and Chen, R. (2008). Examining adolescents' and their parents' conceptual and practical knowledge of police interrogation: A family dyad approach. *Journal of Youth and Adolescence, 37*(6), 685–698.

Youth.gov. (2018). *Juvenile Justice: Reentry.* Available: https://youth.gov/youth-topics/ juvenile-justice/reentry.

Zane, S. N., Welsh, B. C., and Mears, D. P. (2016). Juvenile transfer and the specific deterrence hypothesis. *Criminology & Public Policy, 15*(3), 901–925.

Zgoba, K. M., Miner, M., Levenson, J., Knight, R., Letourneau, E., and Thornton, D. (2016). The Adam Walsh Act: An examination of sex offender risk classification systems. *Sexual Abuse: Journal of Research and Treatment, 28*(8), 722–740.

Zimring, F. E. (2004). *An American Travesty: Legal Responses to Adolescent Sexual Offending.* Chicago, IL: The University of Chicago Press.

Zyvoloski, S. (2018). *Impacts of and Alternatives to Solitary Confinement in Adult Correctional Facilities.* Available: https://sophia.stkate.edu/msw_papers/841.

CHAPTER 10

Berg, M., Coman, E., and Schensul, J. J. (2009). Youth action research for prevention: A multilevel intervention designed to increase efficacy and empowerment among urban youth. *American Journal of Community Psychology, 43*(3-4), 345–359.

Brody, G. H., Yu, T., Chen E., and Miller, G. E. (2017.) Family-centered prevention ameliorates the association between adverse childhood experiences and prediabetes status in young black adults. *Preventive Medicine 100,* 117–122.

Cammarota, J., and Fine, M. (2008). *Revolutionizing Education: Youth Participatory Action Research in Motion.* New York: Routledge.

Dahl, R. E., Allen, N. B., Wilbrecht, L., and Suleiman, A. B. (2018). Importance of investing in adolescence from a developmental science perspective. *Nature, 554,* 441–450.

Fuligni, A. J., Dapretto, M., and Galván, A. (2018). Broadening the impact of developmental neuroscience on the study of adolescence. *Journal of Research on Adolescence, 28*(1), 150–153.

Galván, A. (2014). Insights about adolescent behavior, plasticity, and policy from neuroscience research. *Neuron, 83*, 262–265.

George, M. J., and Odgers, C. L. (2015). Seven fears and the science of how mobile technologies may be influencing adolescents in the digital age. *Perspectives on Psychological Science, 10*(6), 832–851.

Knopf, D. K., Jane Park, M., Brindis, C. D., Mulye, T. P., and Irwin, C. E. Jr. (2007). What gets measured gets done: Assessing data availability for adolescent populations. *Journal of Maternal and Child Health, 11*(4), 335–345.

Layard, R., Clark, A. E., Cornaglia, F., Powdthavee, N., and Vernoit, J. (2014). What predicts a successful life? A life-course model of well-being. *Journal of Economics (London), 124*(580), 720–738.

Orben, A., and Przybylski, A. K. (2019). The association between adolescent well-being and digital technology use. *Nature Human Behaviour, 3*, 173–182.

Ozer, E. J. (2016). Youth-led participatory action research. In L. A. Joason and D. S. Glenwick (Eds.), *Handbook of Methodological Approaches to Community-Based Research: Qualitative, Quantitative, and Mixed Methods* (pp. 263–272). New York: Oxford University Press.

Seabrook, E. M., Kern, M. L., and Rickard, N. S. (2016). Social networking sites, depression, and anxiety: A systematic review. *Journal of Mental Health, 3*(4), e50–e69.

Twenge, J. M. (2019). *The Sad State of Happiness in the United States and the Role of Digital Media. In World Happiness Report: 2019.* Available: https://s3.amazonaws.com/happiness-report/2019/WHR19_Ch5.pdf.

APPENDIX A

Angrist, J. D. (1990). Lifetime earnings and the Vietnam era draft lottery: Evidence from Social Security administrative records. *The American Economic Review, 80*(3), 313–336.

Angrist, J. D., and Pischke, J-S. (2009). *Mostly Harmless Econometrics: An Empiricist's Companion.* Princeton, NJ: Princeton University Press.

Connolly, P., Keenan, C., and Urbanska, K., (2018). The trials of evidence-based practice in education: A systematic review of randomized controlled trials in education research 1980–2016. *Educational Research, 60*(3), 276–291.

Fahle, E., and Reardon, S. F. (2018). How much do test scores vary among school districts? New estimates using population data, 2009–2015. *Educational Researcher, 47*(4).

Jackson, M., and Cox, D. R. (2013). The principles of experimental design and their application in sociology. *Annual Review of Sociology, 39*, 27–49.

Meyer, B. D. (1995). Natural and quasi-experiments in economics. *Journal of Business and Economic Statistics, 13*(2), 151–161.

APPENDIX B

Crone, E. A., and Dahl, R. E. (2012). Understanding adolescence as a period of social–affective engagement and goal flexibility. *Nature Reviews Neuroscience, 13*(9), 636.

DeJonckheere, M., Nichols, L. P., Moniz, M. H., Sonneville, K. R., Vydiswaran, V. V., Zhao, X., and Chang, T. (2017). MyVoice National Text Message Survey of Youth Aged 14 to 24 Years: Study Protocol. *JMIR Research Protocols, 6*(12).

Patton, G. C., Sawyer, S. M., Santelli, J. S., Ross, D. A., Afifi, R., Allen, N. B., and Kakuma, R. (2016). Our future: a Lancet commission on adolescent health and wellbeing. *The Lancet, 387*(10036), 2423–2478.

Region of Waterloo, Department of Social Services. (2012). *Lived Experience as Expertise: Considerations in the Development of Advisory Groups of People with Lived Experience of Homelessness and/or Poverty.* Available: https://www.homelesshub.ca/sites/default/files/PROMISING.PRACTICE.MANUAL.FINAL.pdf.

San Mateo County Health. (2017). *Lived Experience Is Expertise.* Available: https://www.smchealth.org/article/lived-experience-expertise.

UNICEF. 2003. *The State of the World's Children.* Available: https://www.unicef.org/sowc03/contents/pdf/SOWC03-eng.pdf.

United Nations. (2007). *World Youth Report.* New York, NY: United Nations. Available: https://www.un.org/esa/socdev/unyin/documents/wyr07_complete.pdf.

Appendix A

Assessing the Evidence

Members of the committee were drawn from different disciplines with different methodological and analytic approaches to developing and interpreting evidence. The committee relied on the range of experimental and observational approaches described in Table A-1.

One of the committee's central challenges was to summarize what is known about the causes of disparities in adolescent behavior, health, and well-being and the effects of those disparities on adult outcomes. Of course, these explanations depend on the synthesis of many studies, each of which has methodological strengths and limitations relating to the nature of the study design and the data collected. For example, researchers who have observed a positive association between student test scores and later adult economic outcomes are careful not to assume a causal relationship between educational performance and employment, due to the possibility of confounders—variables that are correlated with both test scores and economic outcomes—causing a spurious association between the two. By contrast, data generated by randomized controlled trials (RCTs) do not suffer from confounding, because the act of randomization severs any relationship between a confounder and the independent variable (e.g., education, in the example above). As such, data generated from an RCT can produce an estimate of the causal relationship between education and adult economic status without concern that confounders are biasing the estimate. RCTs are increasingly being used in social science research (Jackson and Cox, 2013). Nevertheless, RCTs are not appropriate in all settings, because they can be infeasible or expensive, and for some interventions

TABLE A-1 Description of General Uses of Experimental and Observational Approaches

Experimental Approaches	
Large-Scale Randomized Controlled Trials (RCTS)	RCTs are frequently used to assess the effects of a particular educational intervention, such as school infrastructure, teacher characteristics, or school organization, on student outcomes (see, e.g., Connolly et al., 2018). RCTs tend to be implemented only after observational research has provided evidence that a proposed intervention is likely to be effective. Reasonable assumptions can therefore be made about the likely risks and benefits of the research to participants.
Small-Scale Experiments	Small-scale experiments are often used as a precursor to an RCT and are used frequently in educational research in psychology and economics. They rely on small sample sizes and are frequently implemented without a strong observational evidence base. Because the effects of such experiments are more difficult to predict in advance, risks and benefits to participants are also more difficult to predict.

Observational Approaches	
Analysis of Administrative Data	Statistical analyses of administrative data are common in the educational context (see e.g., Fahle and Reardon, 2018). Data collected from administrative sources are "de-identified" and held in specialist data centers, so that risks to subjects are minimal.
Analysis of Survey Data	Statistical analyses of survey data are also common. They rely on data collected by individual researchers or survey agencies. Participation in surveys is voluntary, and risks to subjects are usually minimal.
Collection of Qualitative Data	In some disciplines, and especially in sociology, ethnographic and interview-based studies make up a substantial part of the evidence base on educational inequality. Due to the importance of thickly detailed description in such studies, anonymity is a special concern, so researchers go to considerable lengths to de-identify individuals and contexts when reporting research results.

randomization can be considered ethically objectionable if it denies an adolescent a service or treatment known to be beneficial.

Because of these concerns about RCTs, researchers have increasingly used "natural experiments" to estimate causal effects. Such studies harness changes in state and local policies that generate plausibly random or quasi-random variation in exposure to a given service or treatment to estimate its causal effect on outcomes of interest (see Meyer, 1995 and Angrist and Pishke, 2009 for an overview of these methods). One such example is the use of the draft lottery to estimate the impact on future earnings of service in the military among youth during the Vietnam War (Angrist, 1990).

Because one's draft number is randomly generated and draft numbers are very predictive (though not perfectly predictive) of military service, the draft generates variation in military service that is not confounded. A researcher using various statistical and econometric techniques can use this variation to generate a causal estimate.

Despite the limitations of estimation based on observational data, careful use of observational data has many advantages: First, it is very useful for identifying associations that can be more rigorously studied using other approaches; second, in some cases careful use of natural experiments or other research designs can minimize the bias from confounding; and finally, some questions are by their nature not amenable to randomized trials (such as the question of what the effects are of a new state law that changes the age of majority in the criminal justice system) and so can only be studied using observational data.[1]

---

[1] In addition to concerns over research design, there are significant ethical considerations related to research on adolescents. All research on vulnerable populations raises special ethical considerations, because members of these populations may be less capable of providing informed consent, of assessing the costs and benefits of participating in research, and of entering into research voluntarily. Adolescents are particularly likely to be vulnerable: their capacity for self-determination is understood to be related to maturity, they are particularly likely to be members of social and economic groups seen to require greater protection, and they may be members of institutionalized groups that are vulnerable by virtue of being institutionalized.

Appendix B

Youth Engagement

Youth cannot know how age thinks and feels, but old men are guilty if they forget what it is to be young.— J. K. Rowling

THE IMPORTANCE OF ENGAGING YOUTH

Meaningful participation of young people in all aspects of their personal and community development has been recognized by the United Nations as a fundamental right of youth (UNICEF, 2003). The United Nations defines youth engagement as "the active and meaningful involvement of young people in all aspects of their own development and that of their communities, including their empowerment to contribute to decisions about their personal, family, social, economic, and political development" (United Nations, 2007, p. 245). Such engagement requires recognition of young people's knowledge, perspectives, and experience as valuable contributions to decision making at all levels (United Nations, 2007), along with structures and systems put in place by adults to support them (Patton et al., 2016).

Adolescents exhibit agency in their development and have the power to shape the course of their own lives, as well as the well-being of their communities and society at large. Environment and experience critically sculpt the developmental process of adolescence, and youth themselves are shaping these experiences and environments. Moreover, adolescents are particularly primed for participation in civic life, and throughout history young people have used their energy, enthusiasm, and passion to inspire and lead social change (Patton et al., 2016).

Engaging adolescents is beneficial for both adolescents themselves and the community as a whole. Opportunities for social and emotional engagement are protective against mental disorders, many of which begin during adolescence (Crone and Dahl, 2012). In contrast, when such opportunities are absent, adolescents may be drawn into antisocial forms of engagement (such as violence, substance abuse, and extremism), which negatively impacts their health and the well-being of their communities (Patton et al., 2016).

In the process of its deliberation and the writing of this report, the committee recognized the value of learning from adolescents about how they perceive their communities, families, and themselves. There is a growing recognition that lived experience—the perceived understanding of day-to-day life—is evidence in its own right. For decades, qualitative researchers of adolescent health have used adolescents' lived experiences to understand the embodied experience of various health conditions (Patton et al., 2016). In addition, the public and nonprofit sectors have sought to engage individuals with lived experience in developing effective solutions to social problems, such as homelessness (Region of Waterloo Department of Social Services, 2012) and mental health services (San Mateo County Health, 2017).[1]

In this spirit, the committee sought the input of a diverse group of adolescents throughout its deliberative process to better understand how young people perceive and engage with the systems intended to serve them. Youth from across the country were engaged to share their knowledge, experiences, and insights with the committee. The methods and results of this youth engagement are described below.

METHODS

The committee engaged young people through a variety of methods, both in person and virtually. Adolescents from across the United States and from a variety of backgrounds contributed their insights and perceptions. In the course of all of these activities, the committee heard from youth about their priorities for the future and the greatest challenges they currently face.

First, the committee heard from a diverse group of youth panelists at two points during its deliberations. Six adolescents spoke to the committee at a public information-gathering session on June 6, 2018, in Washington, D.C.[2] Shyara Hill is a 24-year-old from Philadelphia, where she attends the Community College of Philadelphia and advocates for justice policy reform with the Juvenile Law Center. Marcus Jarvis is a 26-year-old from

---

[1] See https://www.smchealth.org/article/lived-experience-expertise.
[2] For videos of the session, see http://sites.nationalacademies.org/DBASSE/BCYF/DBASSE_187987.

Philadelphia and an alumnus of the Juvenile Law Center's Juveniles for Justice advocacy program. He entered the justice system at age 16 while in foster care and continues to advocate for change in the juvenile justice and child welfare systems. Nyla Mpofu is a 15-year-old from McLean, Virginia. She has participated in Girl Scouts for 10 years and volunteers extensively in her community. Jocelyn Nolasco is a senior at the University of Maryland, College Park. Since high school, she has worked as a student activist; her current focus is on supporting survivors of sexual assault and trauma. Ayanna Tucker is a master's degree student at the University of Maryland, College Park. A native of Charlotte, North Carolina, and a graduate of Howard University, she plans to pursue a career in public health communications. The young people on the panel responded to a series of questions about their experiences, such as:

- What are the biggest advantages and the biggest disadvantages of growing up in the 21st century?
- What are the biggest misconceptions about youth that adults hold?
- What role does your hometown/neighborhood play in shaping your life?
- How do you interact with your peers?
- How would you change the systems (education, health, justice system, child welfare system) that are supposed to be supporting you?
- What supports do you need to be prepared for the future?
- Who are the people most instrumental in helping you succeed? How could these people be better supported?
- What do you hope your future looks like?

The youth on the panel also shared their reflections on authentic youth engagement. They called for greater involvement of young people in deveoping and implementing programs targeted at them, because they have the firsthand experience to understand the issues. Each expressed a desire to reshape their environments for the benefit of future generations. They mentioned ending the school-to-prison pipeline, justice reform, reducing health disparities, and changing public perceptions of Black youth and youth involved in the justice and child welfare systems.

In addition, a second youth panel was conducted with the Maryland Youth Advisory Council (MYAC) to gather young people's input on the committee's recommendations. In December 2018, three committee members and project staff met with three adolescent members of MYAC in Annapolis, Maryland. Darius Craig is the former chair of the council. He is a student at the University of Maryland, College Park, where he studies political science and criminal justice, and a native of Baltimore

City. Caroline Larkin is the current chair of the council and a student at the University of Maryland, College Park. She participated in Air Force Reserve Officer Training Command and is interested in pursuing a career in law. Zachary Caplan served for 2 years on the council as a high school student. Today, he is a sophomore at the University of Maryland, College Park, where he studies government and politics; he is interested in pursuing a career in law. Their reflections informed the development of the committee's recommendations.

Second, the committee commissioned an analysis from the University of Michigan's MyVoice program to understand adolescents' own perceptions of the adolescence period and their understanding of and perspectives on inequality in their communities. MyVoice is a national mixed-methods text-message poll of youth ages 14 to 24. Each week, MyVoice sends a series of quantitative and qualitative survey questions via text message to a subset of the 1,400 young people who are enrolled in the poll. The poll allows youth to discuss in their ojwn words their opinions on topics such as health, health care policy, and related issues that affect their health and well-being (DeJonckheere et al., 2017). Participants are given modest incentives for each set of questions they answer.[3]

In October 2018, two polls with five questions each were administered to the MyVoice sample on behalf of the committee; these questions appear in Box B-1. Eight hundred and forty-six youth responded (a response rate of 75 percent). The responses were reviewed and coded by two investigators from the MyVoice team, who compiled summary statistics and identified major themes. The mean age of the respondents to both sets of questions was 18.5 years. Thirty-six percent identified as male, 57 percent as female, and 7 percent as other. Most (60%) respondents identified as non-Hispanic white, followed by other non-Hispanic races and ethnicities (20%), Hispanic (13%), and Black (8%). About one-third (32%) were enrolled in free and reduced price lunch at their school.

YOUTH PERSPECTIVES

Through these processes, the committee was able to better understand the lived experiences of adolescents from a range of backgrounds. Across the various modes of engagement with the committee, youth expressed both excitement and anxiety about growing up. In addition, they identified three priority areas where adults and systems could help:

1. provide support during the transition from adolescence to adulthood;
2. provide adequate resources for mental health; and

---

[3] Further details of MyVoice's research protocol are described in DeJonckheere et al. (2017).

BOX B-1
MyVoice Questions

In October 2018, the committee commissioned MyVoice to poll its sample using two sets of questions. The first set sought to understand the transition from childhood to adulthood from adolescents' perspectives:

1. Hi from MyVoice! Going from being a kid to an adult can be a big change. What has this transition been like for you? Why?
2. What has been hard about this transition?
3. What has been good about this time in your life?
4. What would have made this transition easier?
5. What advice would you give your younger self to help you through this transition?

The second poll asked questions regarding the community resources important to youth:

1. Hey {{name}}! Community resources are local places or services that help improve people's lives. What resources do you have in your community?
2. What are the most important community resources you feel like you need to live a safe and healthy life? Why?
3. What resources do you use most often? Why?
4. What gets in the way of you using the resources in your community?
5. What resources do you think are missing from your community? What makes you say that?

SOURCE: Information from MyVoice, 2019.

---

3. respectfully and authentically engage adolescents in decisions that affect them.

Mixed Emotions about Adulthood

I have been able to start thinking about what I'm really passionate about and start cultivating skills that benefit those passions. It's exciting to start finding myself and see what may be the future.
—17-year-old, non-Hispanic white female MyVoice participant

The gaining of responsibilities, more expectations, more opportunities for my life to fall off the rails.—MyVoice participant

The young people that the committee engaged with generally viewed their transition to adulthood with a mixture of excitement and trepidation. About a quarter of the youth in the MyVoice survey expressed excitement about their growing independence, while about 40 percent felt stressed or anxious about the changes. Another quarter expressed both positive and negative emotions. Similarly, youth panelists viewed growing up as both a challenge and an opportunity. As one participant said, "It is a very big change, but I think it allows you to grow a lot if you make the most of the opportunity."

Young people shared their excitement about shaping their own futures, leading independent lives, and igniting their passions. The young people in the MyVoice survey reported enjoying their growing freedoms, pursuing education and career paths that interested them, and fully exploring their sexual and/or gender identities. "It's been exciting learning about all the things I can do with myself and preparing my life [to be] fully independent," said one 21-year-old MyVoice participant. "I can start to see my future shaping up, which is cool."

Likewise, the youth panelists identified growth and identity formation as two of the markers of adolescence. "You learn about yourself. You become more comfortable with yourself. . . . You are building that identity again," said one panel participant. For others, developing an identity and future plans were challenging. "It's been pretty hard, trying to figure out what I believe, what standards I have, what kind of people I like and what kind of person I want to [be]," said one 15-year-old respondent.

The youth panelists also expressed some anxiety about the ongoing changes in their lives. Although some adolescents were excited by their growing autonomy from their families, many others reported struggling with their increased responsibilities and changes in their social and family lives. "I feel like we're kind of thrown into the real world, and we're trying to do well in school, maintain healthy relationships, and figure out who we are as a person," said one 15-year-old participant. "It's a lot to handle." A panel participant reiterated this concern, identifying the pressure placed on young people by adults as an additional challenge: "There is just such a pressure to be on top of it and like know who you are that we all kind of like can find a lot of stress within that." Others reported that the change was too sudden for their liking, and that they felt like they were thrown into adulthood without enough support. "There's a lot more responsibility you suddenly have, yet don't necessarily want," said one 22-year-old respondent.

The Need for Support

I wish there was a welcome to being an adult package.—18-year-old, other race, other gender MyVoice participant

I wish that people were more supportive and accepting that we are still teenagers who want to be young, while also shouldering responsibility.—17-year-old, non-Hispanic white, female MyVoice participant

I have the support of my family around me and that allows me to kind of ease into the transition and slowly build up to it.—21-year-old, non-Hispanic white, female MyVoice participant

Throughout the process, adolescents from various backgrounds reiterated the pressing need for support during their transition from adolescence to young adulthood. For many of the youth the committee spoke to, taking on adult responsibilities for the first time was a common source of stress, particularly when they felt they lacked the knowledge or experience to do things on their own. As one 15-year-old respondent said, "The hardest part has been people thinking I'm responsible and mature enough to do adult tasks that require more knowledge than I have."

Learning to pay bills, budget and save money, make doctor's appointments, and make decisions about their future were all identified as sources of stress by participants in the MyVoice poll. One 16-year-old participant said, "All of a sudden there are lots of expectations piled on you and in school you didn't learn enough about how taxes work or how you're going to support yourself." Likewise, the youth panelists recalled feeling stressed and confused when they had to do certain "adult tasks" on their own for the first time.

Many youth identified the lack of preparation for the "real world" as a cause of that stress. "There isn't a whole lot of preparation from being a kid to suddenly takin[g] care of yourself and other people and paying bills while going to school while getting good grades and figuring out what to do with your life," said a 22-year-old MyVoice respondent. For both the youth panelists and the MyVoice respondents, youth reported their desire for more structured classes in schools on how to perform necessary adult tasks such as taxes and finances. Participants asked for "clear, straightforward guidance" and a "primer on adult life" to help them take on their growing responsibilities. As one youth panelist said, "in school, they should be teaching you how to prepare for real-life situations. . . . I'm going to school to learn, I should be learning all that necessary stuff that I need for life too." In addition, youth called for more job training and shadowing opportunities so that they could explore different career paths and prepare for full-time work.

Similarly, the adolescents who participated identified mentorship as important for helping them navigate adolescence and the transition to adulthood. One panelist credited his success in college to mentors in his community: "I had community members that have helped shield me from everything—all of the noise in the background." Whether they wanted help exploring career paths or embodying their sexual and gender identities, adolescents expressed a need for trusted adults to take on a mentorship role in their lives.

Mental Health Supports

The young adults the committee engaged were very clear in their need for more and better mental health services. Adolescents in both the MyVoice survey and the youth panels identified a lack of mental health services in their communities, with one panelist describing the situation at her school as "dire." "Everyone feels stressed at some point," she noted, and "you should be able to have these resources" to cope with challenges available. Throughout the youth engagement process, young people called upon the systems that adolescents engage with and the adults who work within those systems to better serve their mental health needs.

In addition, youth noted the need to destigmatize mental illness. "Being young, having a mental disorder, it puts you at such vulnerability because you have to face the stigmas from everyone around you," one panelist noted. Although the participants expressed some optimism that the stigma around mental health was lessening, "it is still not even close to where it needs to be." They called upon adults to do more to change the culture around mental health, and noted that having positive relationships with the adults in their lives can help them navigate their mental health challenges.

Authentic Engagement

I think one of the most—a really harmful term is they're too young to know what they want. That has been used time and time again to insinuate that because we are young, because we are still developing, we don't know what we want. I think that is false.—panelist

A third theme that emerged from the committee's engagement with youth was the desire for authentic and respectful engagement of adolescents. The young people the committee engaged noted a lack of respect for youth. "People don't treat teenagers like kids, but they also don't treat us like adults yet," said one 17-year-old MyVoice participant. A youth panelist suggested that the perceived lack of urgency around policy issues that affect children and young people is due to their lesser power in the political sphere. "Because we are not a voting constituency, in my opinion, a lot of times, that is what makes the problem less important," he said. Although some adults are supportive of young people's engagement in policy issues, there is still a lack of respect for youth voices in decision making, he continued. "You can get a microphone. We can scream and make as much noise as we want. The thing is I would say very rarely is that actually like listened to. It is kind of held for the sake of, okay, we need to get some opinion as to what young people want, except then the thing is nothing is really done with that."

CONCLUSION

In recognition of the importance of engaging adolescents in research and policy, the committee used several mechanisms to hear directly from young people across the country. Through in-person meetings and virtual polls, adolescents from a range of backgrounds shared their insights and perspectives on the challenges and opportunities facing young people today. The adolescents that the committee engaged identified the need for supports for taking on adult responsibilities, better mental health resources, and authentic and respectful engagement from adults as their priorities. Society has a responsibility to listen to and engage with young people in decisions that affect them. By recognizing the importance of young people's knowledge and implementing structures and systems that enable youth to engage, society can ensure that youth voices are heard.

Appendix C

Biosketches of
Committee Members and Staff

RICHARD J. BONNIE (*Chair*) is Harrison Foundation professor of law and medicine, professor of public policy, professor of psychiatry and neurobehavioral sciences, and director of the Institute of Law, Psychiatry and Public Policy at the University of Virginia. He teaches and writes about health law and policy, bioethics, criminal law, and public policies relating to mental health, substance abuse, and public health, and has coauthored leading textbooks on criminal law and public health law. Bonnie has chaired numerous studies for the Academies on subjects ranging from elder mistreatment to juvenile justice reform to underage drinking, most recently a study on policies needed to end the opioid epidemic in the United States (2017). He received the Yarmolinsky Medal in 2002 for his contributions to the National Academies of Sciences, Engineering, and Medicine.

ANNA AIZER is a professor of economics at Brown University. A labor and health economist with interests in the area of child health and well-being. She is also codirector of the National Bureau of Economic Research's Program on Children. Her current work considers the mechanisms behind the intergenerational transmission of poverty. In particular, she focuses on the roles played by health insurance and access to medical care, domestic violence, exposure to environmental toxins, the role of stress, and poor children's greater interaction with the juvenile justice system in explaining why the children of poor mothers are more likely to grow up to be poor themselves. She completed a postdoctoral fellowship at Princeton University's Center for Research on Child Wellbeing in 2004. Aizer holds a Ph.D. in economics from the University of California, Los Angeles.

MARGARITA ALEGRÍA is chief of the Disparities Research Unit at Massachusetts General Hospital and professor in the Departments of Medicine and Psychiatry at Harvard Medical School. Alegría has published widely on the improvement of health care services delivery for diverse racial and ethnic populations, conceptual and methodological issues with multicultural populations, and ways to bring the community's perspective into the design and implementation of health services. She is currently the principal investigator (PI) of four National Institutes of Health–funded research studies that cover, among other subjects, the impact of Medicaid plans on access to and quality of substance use disorder treatment, community capacity building to prevent disability among minority elders, and causes of racial/ethnic disparities in mental disorders. She is also co-PI on a William T. Grant Foundation grant investigating strategies to reduce behavioral health inequality between adolescents of majority and minority racial/ethnic groups living in four different neighborhoods. Dr. Alegría obtained her Ph.D. in psychology from Temple University.

EMILY P. BACKES is a program officer for the Board on Children, Youth, and Families in the Division of Behavioral and Social Sciences and Education at the National Academies of Sciences, Engineering, and Medicine. She served as the study director for the Committee on the Neurobiological and Socio-behavioral Science of Adolescent Development and Its Applications. Previously, she served as study director for the report *Transforming the Financing of Early Care and Education*. In her time at the National Academies, she has provided analytical and editorial support to projects covering a range of topics, including juvenile justice, policing, illicit markets, education and literacy, science communication, and human rights. She holds an M.A. in history from the University of Missouri and a J.D. from the University of the District of Columbia's David A. Clarke School of Law.

CLAIRE D. BRINDIS is director of the Philip R. Lee Institute for Health Policy Studies and a professor in the Department of Pediatrics, Division of Adolescent Medicine and the Department of Obstetrics, Gynecology and Reproductive Health Sciences at the University of California, San Francisco (UCSF). She holds the Caldwell B. Esselstyn Chair in Health Policy. She is also codirector of the Adolescent and Young Adult Health National Resource Center and founding director of the Bixby Center for Global Reproductive Health at UCSF. A native of Argentina, Brindis conducts research addressing child, adolescent, and women's health policy, the implementation of health care reform and immigration health, and how disparities impact access to quality care, health outcomes, and health insurance coverage. Her work also focuses on program evaluation and the translation of research into policy at the local, state, and national levels. Other research interests include consumer engagement in health care system redesign, tracking the implementation of the Affordable Care Act on adolescents, young adults, and women, and research on the health and mental health needs of those who are part of the Deferred Action for Childhood Arrival Program (also known as Dreamers). Throughout these and other projects, Dr. Brindis is committed to closing the gap between evidence-based innovation and its application to policy and programs. She holds a doctoral degree in public health and behavioral sciences from the University of California, Berkeley.

ELIZABETH CAUFFMAN is a professor in the Department of Psychological Science at the University of California, Irvine (UCI), where she also holds courtesy appointments in the School of Education and the School of Law. At the broadest level, Cauffman's research addresses the intersection between adolescent development and juvenile justice. She has published widely on a range of topics in the study of contemporary adolescence, including adolescent brain development, risk taking and decision making, parent-adolescent relationships, and juvenile justice. Findings from Cauffman's research were incorporated into the American Psychological Association's amicus briefs submitted to the U.S. Supreme Court in *Roper v. Simmons*, which abolished the juvenile death penalty, and in both *Graham v. Florida* and *Miller v. Alabama*, which placed limits on the use of life without parole as a sentence for juveniles. As part of her larger efforts to help research inform practice and policy, she served as a member of the MacArthur Foundation's Research Network on Adolescent Development and Juvenile Justice and currently directs the Center for Psychology and Law at UCI as well as directs the Masters in Legal and Forensic Psychology Program at UCI. Cauffman holds a Ph.D. in developmental psychology from Temple University and completed a post-doctoral fellowship at the Center on Adolescence at Stanford University.

TAMMY CHANG is a health services researcher and practicing family physician with a passion for adolescent health, specifically for breaking the cycle of poverty and poor health among adolescent mothers and their children. Her National Institutes of Health–sponsored research is focused on improving access to reproductive health care and promoting healthy pregnancy weight gain among at-risk adolescents using text messaging, social media mining, and natural language processing (NLP). She is also the founding director of MyVoice, a national text-message poll of youth ages 14 to 24 that uses mixed methods and NLP with the goal of informing local and national policies in real time. Chang is a faculty member in the National Clinician Scholars Program, in which she trains junior faculty clinicians and teaches a master's level course in leadership and communication. She holds an M.D. and an M.P.H. in health policy and management from the University of Michigan. Chang completed residency training and served as co-chief resident in the Department of Family Medicine at the University of Michigan, and is an alumna of the University of Michigan Robert Wood Johnson Foundation Clinical Scholars Program.

MESMIN DESTIN is associate professor at Northwestern University in the School of Education and Social Policy and the Department of Psychology, as well as serving as a fellow of Northwestern's Institute for Policy Research. Destin directs a multidisciplinary lab group and investigates social psychological mechanisms underlying socioeconomic disparities in educational outcomes during adolescence and young adulthood. Using laboratory and field experiments, he studies factors that influence how young people perceive themselves and pursue their futures. At the university level, he examines how subtle social experiences and institutional messaging shape the motivation and educational trajectories of low-socioeconomic- status and first-generation college students. Destin holds a Ph.D. in social psychology from the University of Michigan.

ANGELA DIAZ is the Jean C. and James W. Crystal professor in the Department of Pediatrics and the Department of Environmental Medicine and Public Health at the Icahn School of Medicine at Mount Sinai. Diaz is also the director of the Mount Sinai Adolescent Health Center, which provides young people with comprehensive, interdisciplinary, integrated medical care, as well as sexual and reproductive health, mental health, and dental and optical services. Under her leadership, the center has grown significantly and is a major training site in the field of adolescent health and medicine. She has been a White House Fellow and a member of the Food and Drug Administration Pediatric Advisory Committee. She was formerly a member of the Board of Directors of the New York City Department of Health and Mental Hygiene. In 2003, she chaired the National Advisory Committee on Children and Terrorism for the Department of Health and Human Services. In 2009, she was appointed by Mayor Michael Bloomberg to the New York City Commission for Lesbian, Gay, Bisexual, Transgender and Questioning Runaway and Homeless Youth Taskforce. Diaz is active in public policy and advocacy in the United States and has conducted international health projects on several continents. She holds an M.D. from Columbia University College of Physicians and Surgeons, an M.P.H. from Harvard University, and a Ph.D. in epidemiology from Columbia University.

MARY GHITELMAN is a senior program assistant for the National Academies' Board on Children, Youth, and Families and the Committee on Population in the Division of Behavioral and Social Sciences and Education. She has been with the National Academies since April 2015, working on reports including *The Integration of Immigrants into American Society*; *Valuing Climate Damages: Updating Estimation of the Social Cost of Carbon Dioxide*; and *Transforming the Financing of Early Care and Education*. She received her B.A. in psychology from Beloit College and studied abroad in Copenhagen, Denmark, with a focus in cross-cultural psychology.

NANCY E. HILL is the Charles Bigelow professor of education in the Graduate School of Education at Harvard University. Her research focuses on parenting and adolescent development, especially examining issues across ethnicity, race, and socioeconomic status. She studies how parents and other adults can support youth as they engage in school, succeed academically, and hone their goals, aspirations, and sense of purpose. Her current research projects includes a longitudinal study following adolescents across high school, focusing on economically and ethnically diverse youth and their emerging sense of purpose and views of the economy as they influence postsecondary transitions to college and career. She received the William T. Grant Foundation's Distinguished Faculty Fellowship to support her engagement with the Massachusetts' Executive Office on Education and the Ernest R. Hilgard Lifetime Achievement Award from APA Division 1 for her contributions to psychology. She currently is the president-elect of the Society for Research in Child Development (SRCD) and has served on the Governing Council and as Secretary of SRCD. In addition, she has chaired the Board of Directors of ChildFund International, an international nongovernmental organization, which uses a developmental framework to better serve and empower disadvantaged children, youth, and families in 25 nations globally. Hill earned her Ph.D. in developmental psychology from Michigan State University.

MICHELLE JACKSON is assistant professor of sociology at Stanford University and an associate member of Nuffield College, Oxford. Her main research interests lie in social inequality, social mobility, and the sociology of education. Her research aims to understand how it is that social inequality is produced and reproduced by social institutions. Her work places institutional constraints and incentives at the center of an understanding of intergenerational inequality. Jackson is an editorial board member of *American Sociological Review*, *European Sociological Review*, *Research in Social Stratification and Mobility*, and *Social Forces*. She holds a Ph.D. in sociology from Nuffield College, Oxford.

ARLENE F. LEE is the former executive director of the Maryland Governor's Office for Children, where she chaired the Children's Cabinet and worked to support the governor's vision for the well-being of Maryland's children. Ms. Lee was also the director of policy at the Center for the Study of Social Policy, where she focused on helping federal and state elected officials develop research-informed policies and funding to improve results for children and families. In this last capacity, she oversaw PolicyforResults. org, a leading national resource for results-based policy. She has served as deputy director of the Georgetown University Center for Juvenile Justice Reform, director of the Federal Resource Center for Children of Prisoners, and youth strategies manager for the Governor's Office of Crime Control and Prevention. Ms. Lee is also the author of numerous articles. She holds a J.D. from Washington College of Law, American University. As a result of her work, Ms. Lee was named one of Maryland's Top 100 Women and has received three Governor's Citations.

LESLIE LEVE is associate director of the Prevention Science Institute, associate director of the Prevention Science graduate programs, and associate vice president for research in the Office of the Vice President for Research and Innovation at the University of Oregon. Her research and teaching interests are focused on child and adolescent development and preventive interventions. She leads federal research grants that focus on developmental pathways and intervention outcomes for children and families. This includes preventive intervention studies with youth in foster care and with adolescents in the juvenile justice system aimed at preventing risk behaviors and improving public health outcomes, and adoption studies that examine the interplay between biological (genetic, hormonal), psychological, and social influences on development. Her work also focuses on outcomes for girls and women. Leve holds a Ph.D. in developmental psychology from the University of Oregon.

JENS LUDWIG is the Edwin A. and Betty L. Bergman Distinguished Service Professor at the University of Chicago, director of the University of Chicago Crime Lab, and codirector of the University of Chicago Urban Education Lab. Ludwig also serves as a nonresident senior fellow in economic studies at the Brookings Institution, research associate of the National Bureau of Economic Research (NBER), and codirector of the NBER's working group on the economics of crime. His research focuses on social policy, particularly in the areas of urban poverty, crime, and education, and is recently focusing on ways of using new tools from the field of machine learning combined with the growing availability of large government administrative datasets ('big data') to try to make progress on these policy challenges. He is a member of the editorial board of the American Economic Review and is an elected member of the National Academy of Medicine. Ludwig holds both an M.A. and a Ph.D. in economics from Duke University.

SUSAN VIVIAN MANGOLD is chief executive officer of the Juvenile Law Center. She is professor emeritus at the University at Buffalo School of Law, where she taught for more than 20 years and served as vice dean for academics, with a scholarly focus on children and the law. Mangold also chaired a university-wide initiative on strategic strength in civic engagement and public policy. The author of numerous articles on the child welfare system, she was the primary investigator for a Robert Wood Johnson Foundation study of the impact of different types of funding on long-term outcomes for children in foster care. During her undergraduate years at Harvard University, she founded the Cambridge Youth Enrichment Program (now Summer Urban Program) to offer educational and recreational programs for youth in the summers, and later became program director for Girls Club (now Girls Inc.) in Massachusetts, which provided after-school services to inner-city girls, many of whom were involved in the child welfare and justice systems. This experience led her to Harvard Law School with the intent of becoming a children's attorney. During law school, she became executive director of Harvard Legal Aid and cofounded the Children's Rights Project. Upon graduation, she received a Harvard Law School Public Interest Fellowship to work at the Juvenile Law Center, where she worked as a staff attorney for 5 years. She writes and speaks frequently on current issues impacting older youth in the justice and child welfare systems. Mangold holds a J.D. from Harvard Law School.

BRUCE S. MCEWEN is the Alfred E. Mirsky Professor and head of the Harold and Margaret Milliken Hatch Laboratory of Neuroendocrinology at the Rockefeller University in New York. McEwen's laboratory has carried out groundbreaking research, discovering adrenal steroid receptors and, later, estrogen receptors in the hippocampus, a brain region that mediates memory and mood regulation. These discoveries, now expanded to other brain regions such as amygdala, prefrontal cortex, and nucleus accumbens, showed that circulating stress and sex hormones do more in the brain than just provide feedback to regulate neuroendocrine function, but rather influence cognitive and emotional processes throughout the life course, with major implications for anxiety and depressive disorders. This includes regulating ongoing adaptive remodeling of brain circuits and connections between neurons as well as regulating neurogenesis in the hippocampus of the adult brain. He is past president of the Society for Neuroscience and member of the National Academy of Sciences and the National Academy of Medicine. He has received many awards, including the Dale Medal of the British Endocrine Society, the Karl Spencer Lashley Award, American Philosophical Society, the Scolnick Prize in Neuroscience from MIT, the Ipsen Foundation Prize in Neuronal Plasticity, the Society for Biological Psychiatry Gold Medal, and the Thomas W. Salmon

Award from the New York Academy of Medicine. McEwen holds a B.A. in chemistry from Oberlin College and a Ph.D. in cell biology from The Rockefeller University.

STEPHANIE OH is an M.D./Ph.D. candidate in the Rutgers University/ Robert Wood Johnson Medical School/Princeton University Physician-Scientist Program, where she recently finished her Ph.D. in neuroscience and is in the process of completing her M.D. degree. Her thesis work focused on the neuroprotective role of novel-coding mRNA and non-coding microRNAs in Parkinson's disease. She is a director of the medical school's student-run free clinic, spearheading efforts to provide free, longitudinal, primary medical care to uninsured patients in the community and leading IRB-approved research projects for novel health care interventions and quality improvement. Prior to her doctoral studies, Oh received her B.Sc. in biological engineering at Massachusetts Institute of Technology, researched molecular mechanisms of neuronal plasticity at Johns Hopkins Medical Institute, and served as an AmeriCorps fellow at Mass Mentoring Partnership, a nonprofit dedicated to improving mentoring programs and youth development organizations.

STEPHEN T. RUSSELL is the Priscilla Pond Flawn Regents Professor in child development in the Department of Human Development and Family Sciences and a faculty member in the Population Research Center at the University of Texas at Austin. He studies adolescent development, with an emphasis on adolescent sexuality, LGBT youth, and parent-adolescent relationships. Beginning more than 15 years ago, Russell began a program of research on adolescent sexual orientation, minority stress, and the health and well-being of sexual minorities. He published a series of papers that were the first to document significant health risks among sexual-minority adolescents using the National Longitudinal Study of Adolescent to Adult Health (or Add Health Study). He continues to study health risk and resilience among this population, with an emphasis on gender and cultural differences. In addition, he is an expert in the role of school policies, programs, and practices in supporting adolescent adjustment, achievement, and health. He has been involved in community and professional organizations throughout his career, including as human relations commissioner in Durham, North Carolina; Davis, California; and Tucson, Arizona; and is currently on the Board of Directors of the Sexuality Information and Education Council of the United States. He has been an elected board member of the National Council on Family Relations and is past-president of the Society for Research on Adolescence. Russell holds a Ph.D. in sociology from Duke University.

DARA SHEFSKA is a research associate on the Board on Children, Youth, and Families. She joined the National Academies in 2015 as a research assistant on the Food and Nutrition Board, staffing the Roundtable on Obesity Solutions. In this role, she focused on publications, communications, and coordinating the Early Care and Education Innovation Collaborative. She was awarded the Health and Medicine Division's Fineberg Impact Award in 2016 for her efforts to increase the visibility of Roundtable workshops and publications. Prior to this, Ms. Shefska studied urban geography at McGill University in Montreal, Quebec, where she conducted research on how neighborhoods influence gestational diabetes.

ELIZABETH TOWNSEND is an associate program officer with the Board on Children, Youth, and Families (BCYF) at the National Academies, who in addition to supporting this study supported the Committee on Building an Agenda to Reduce the Number of Children in Poverty by Half in 10 Years. Prior to joining these studies, Townsend was a research associate for the Board on Behavioral, Cognitive, and Sensory Sciences' Decadal Survey on Social and Behavioral Sciences for Applications to National Security. Other BCYF studies she has worked on include Ethical Considerations for Research on Housing-Related Health Hazards Involving Children; Children's Health, the Nation's Wealth: Assessing and Improving Child Health; and Working Families and Growing Kids: Caring for Children and Adolescents. She holds a B.S. from Radford University and an M.P.H. from the University of Alabama at Birmingham, where she interned with the Comprehensive Cancer Center and volunteered with the Alabama Vaccine Research Clinic and 1917 Clinic.

JOANNA LEE WILLIAMS is an associate professor at the Curry School of Education and Human Development, University of Virginia, and is affiliated with Youth-Nex: The University of Virginia Center to Promote Effective Youth Development, and the Center for Race and Public Education in the South. Williams' research interests focus on race and ethnicity as social contexts for youth development. Specifically, her work examines issues of equity and diversity in the context of school-based peer social networks, and ethnic identity as an element of positive youth development. She also has applied interests in understanding diversity, peer relations, and positive outcomes in youth development programs and previously served as associate director of research for the Young Women Leaders Program, a mentoring program for middle school girls. Williams holds a Ph.D. in developmental psychology from Temple University.